Essentials of Physical Health in Psy

Essentials of Physical Health in Psychiatry

Edited by
Irene Cormac and David Gray

RCPsych Publications

RCPsych Publications is an imprint of the Royal College of Psychiatrists
17 Belgrave Square, London SW1X 8PG
www.rcpsych.ac.uk

British Library Cataloguing-in-Publication Data.
A catalogue record for this book is available from the British Library.

ISBN 978 1 908020 40 6

Distributed in North America by Publishers Storage and Shipping Company.

Printed in the UK by Bell & Bain Limited, Glasgow.

Contents

Foreword

This practical guide is a very welcome and, dare I say, overdue contribution towards giving the physical health needs of people with mental health problems a higher priority.

As a medical discipline with its own specialty areas, psychiatry inevitably focuses on the mental health needs of patients. But as our mission is to improve the lives of people with mental illness, 'improving lives' should include physical as well as mental health and well-being.

This marvellous book makes it clear that this is not just an issue for psychiatrists, but is also an area for general practitioners, nurses and other health professionals to consider.

Even a cursory examination of some of the statistics reveals the huge cost of poor physical illness to those with severe mental illness. For example, men with a diagnosis of psychosis live 20 years less than the general population, while women with the diagnosis live 15 years less, with evidence that this 'mortality gap' may be widening.

Of the 7500 people who develop a psychosis in England each year, many face a future compromised by poor physical health as well as psychological difficulties. Antipsychotic drugs often lead to rapid weight gain and increases in cholesterol, compromising broader health and well-being. We also know that, for a wide variety of reasons, smoking prevalence among those with a diagnosis of schizophrenia is much higher than it is in the general population.

But behind the human tragedy of premature mortality is the reality that mental and physical disorders frequently coexist, often intertwined with social exclusion, restricted opportunities and disadvantage. People with an enduring physical illness are also more likely to experience mental health problems.

With chapters covering a wide range of health issues and common problems that may affect psychiatric patients, I am sure this book will be a great help to mental health professionals and psychiatrists everywhere. I am proud that the Royal College of Psychiatrists has published it.

Sue Bailey

Consultant Child and Adolescent Forensic Psychiatrist,
Greater Manchester West Mental Health NHS Foundation Trust
President, Royal College of Psychiatrists, 2011–2014

Foreword

There is no doubt that physical and mental health should not be separated, as each affects the other. In medicine, however, mental health is often seen as the prerogative of psychiatrists and psychiatrists themselves are often ready to pass on the physical care of their patients to colleagues in other specialties. This creates further divisions between psychiatrists and physicians and surgeons.

Psychiatry is a medical specialty and psychiatrists spend a considerable period in their training learning the fundamentals of medicine. It is imperative that psychiatrists as part of their professional role and responsibility are aware of medical issues and are able to interpret basic medical investigations; equally, they must be aware of where they should seek help and, more importantly, when. Physical and mental health complement and influence each other and it is essential that all doctors are aware of these links. The mind–body dualism has had an unfortunate effect on medicine, and there appears to be an assumption that these two components of health do not communicate with each other. To understand the distress patients experience and how it affects their physical health and social functioning, a holistic approach is needed for assessment as well as management plans. Patients may use physical or psychological idioms to express their distress, depending on their socioeconomic, educational, cultural and social mores. That does not mean that one way of expressing distress is inferior to the other.

This volume brings together authors who are committed to reducing this dichotomy. The editors are to be congratulated for putting together such an expert team to collaborate on this vital topic. My fervent hope is that this book will encourage not only trainee psychiatrists but other mental health professionals as well as more senior colleagues to revisit their skills.

Dinesh Bhugra

Professor of Mental Health and Cultural Diversity, Institute of Psychiatry, King's College London

President, Royal College of Psychiatrists, 2008–2011

Preface

Physicians and psychiatrists have written this book, to cover the essential physical health topics that are most relevant to people with mental disorders and intellectual disabilities.

Of course, it is not possible to cover every eventuality, physical condition or disability in this book, but *Essentials of Physical Health in Psychiatry* will help you to increase your knowledge, and confidence, in managing at least some of the more common physical conditions that your patients may develop. In addition, we hope that *Essentials of Physical Health in Psychiatry* will stimulate you to read in more depth.

Finally, our authors, experts in their respective fields, have provided guidance on when to seek help from medical specialist colleagues; with their advice, this will enable psychiatrists and psychiatric nurses to care for the physical as well as mental health of their patients, whether in an institution or in the community.

I.C.
D. G.

Figures

Tables

Boxes

Contributors

Guruprasad P. Aithal MD PhD FRCP, NHS co-director, Nottingham Digestive Disease Centre: National Institute for Health Research Biomedical Research Unit, Queen's Medical Centre, Nottingham, UK.

David Anderson Consultant and Honorary Senior Lecturer in Old Age Psychiatry, Mossley Hill Hospital, Mersey Care NHS Trust, UK.

Charles N. Antonypillai MBBS MD MRCP, Department of Endocrinology, Oxford Centre for Diabetes, Endocrinology and Metabolism, Churchill Hospital, University of Oxford, UK

Theingi Aung MBBS, MRCP, Department of Endocrinology, Oxford Centre for Diabetes, Endocrinology and Metabolism, Churchill Hospital, University of Oxford, UK

Gordon Bates MBChB, MMedSc, FRCPsych, Consultant Child and Adolescent Psychiatrist, Huntercombe Hospital, Stafford

David Burton MBChB BMedSci, Porterbrook Clinic, Sheffield, and The University of Sheffield.

Iain C. Campbell DSc, Professor of Neurochemistry, Section of Eating Disorders, Institute of Psychiatry, King's College London.

Alan Cohen FRCGP, Director of Primary Care, West London Mental Health NHS Trust

Irene Cormac FRCPsych, Honorary Consultant Forensic Psychiatrist, Rampton Hospital, Nottinghamshire Healthcare NHS Trust.

Jonathan Corne MA PhD FRCP, Consultant Physician, Department of Respiratory Medicine, Nottingham University Hospitals, and Special Lecturer, University of Nottingham.

Ed Day MA BM BCh DM MRCPsych, Senior Lecturer in Addiction Psychiatry, University of Birmingham and Honorary Consultant in Addiction Psychiatry, Birmingham and Solihull Mental Health NHS Foundation Trust.

Tom Fox MB BS MCRP, Specialist Registrar, Endocrinology and Diabetes, Plymouth Hospitals NHS Trust, Derriford Hospital, Plymouth.

Evelyn Goodwin Exercise referral coordinator, GP referral instructor, Healthy Lifestyle Team, Nottinghamshire Healthcare NHS Trust, Rampton Hospital, Retford.

Stephen C. L. Gough PhD MD FRCP, Professor of Diabetes and Consultant Physician, Oxford Centre for Diabetes, Endocrinology and Metabolism Churchill Hospital, Headington, Oxford.

David Gray DM MPH BMedSci BM BS FRCP FRSPH MCSP, Reader in Medicine and Consultant Cardiologist, Nottingham University Hospitals.

Elspeth Guthrie MBChB MSc MD FRCPsych, Consultant in Psychological Medicine, Manchester Royal Infirmary.

Lisa Hart BSc Hons Health and Sports Studies, Healthy Lifestyle Team, Nottinghamshire Healthcare NHS Trust, Rampton Hospital, Retford.

Joanne Haswell Barrister, LLB (Hons) PGDip (Legal Practice)

Kate Hill BA (Hons) Solicitor, RadcliffesLeBrasseur

Will Irving MA MB BChir MRCP PhD FRCPath, Professor and Honorary Consultant in Virology, University of Nottingham and Nottingham University Hospitals NHS Trust.

Muhammad Ali Karamat MD MBBS MRCP, Consultant Physician and Honorary Senior Lecturer, Department of Diabetes, Heart of England NHS Foundation Trust, Bordesley Green East, Birmingham, and University of Birmingham.

Niki Karavitaki MSc PhD FRCP, Department of Endocrinology, Oxford Centre for Diabetes, Endocrinology and Metabolism, Churchill Hospital, University of Oxford, UK

Sanjay Khurmi BSc MBBS LLM MRCPsych, Consultant in Adult Psychiatry, Coventry Crisis Resolution and Home Treatment Team.

William Lee BSc MB ChB MSc MRCPsych, MRC Research Training Fellow, General Hospital Psychiatry, Psychological Medicine, Institute of Psychiatry, King's College London.

Christy Lowe BSc (Hons) MBBS FCEM, Maidstone and Tunbridge Wells NHS Trust, Tunbridge Wells Hospital, Tunbridge Wells.

Geoff Marston BM BS BMedSci FRCPsych, Consultant Psychiatrist for Adults with a Learning Disability, Caludon Centre, Clifford Bridge Road, Walsgrave, Coventry.

Lisa McNally MSc PhD CPsychol, Public Health Principal, NHS Surrey & Surrey County Council

Vidya Navaratnum BMedSci(Hons) BM BS MRCP(London), Clinical Lecturer in Respiratory Medicine, University of Nottingham.

Ayanangshu Nayak Consultant in Liaison Psychiatry, Porterbrook Clinic, Longley Centre, Sheffield Health and Social Care NHS Foundation Trust, Sheffield, UK.

David Osborn PhD MA MSc MRCPsych, Reader and Consultant Psychiatrist, University College London Mental Health Sciences Unit.

David Perry MB ChB MRCPsych FRSA, Consultant Psychiatrist for Adults with a Learning Disability, Caludon Centre, Clifford Bridge Road, Walsgrave, Coventry.

Michael Phelan BSc MBBS FRCPsych, Consultant Psychiatrist, West London Mental Health NHS Trust

Julie Phukan MB MRCPI PhD, Neurology Specialist Registrar, Royal Free Hospital, London.

Jonathan Pinkney MD FRCP, Professor of Medicine, Peninsula College of Medicine and Dentistry, University Department of Medicine, Plymouth Hospitals NHS Trust, Derriford Hospital, Plymouth.

Amy Pritty BSc Hons in Health and Physical Recreation, Healthy Lifestyle Team, Nottinghamshire Healthcare NHS Trust, Rampton Hospital, Retford.

Barbara Pryse (deceased) MA B Med Sci (Hons) RGN RMN Cert Ed (FE) ENB 199. Modern Matron Physical Healthcare and Infection Prevention and Control, Rampton Hospital, UK

James S. Rakshi MD FRCP, Consultant Neurologist, Royal Free and Barnet General Hospitals, Honorary Consultant Neurologist, National Hospital for Neurology and Neurosurgery, London, and Honorary Senior Lecturer, University College London.

Vidyasagar Ramappa MRCP, Specialist Registrar in Gastroenterology, Nottingham University Hospitals NHS Trust, Nottingham

Murad El-Salamani MB BCh FRCS FFAEM, Consultant in Emergency Medicine and Associate Clinical Director Emergency Medicine, Doncaster and Bassetlaw Hospitals.

Yusri Taha MBBS MRCP MD FRCPath, Consultant in Infectious Diseases and Clinical Virology, Nottingham University Hospitals NHS Trust.

Janet Treasure MRCP FRCPsych, Professor of Psychiatry, Institute of Psychiatry, King's College London.

Mark Tuthill BSc MB BS MRCP, Department of Oncology, Hammersmith Hospital, Imperial College NHS Trust, London.

Josephine Tuthill MBBS BSc (Hons) MRCP, University Hospital Lewisham, London.

John A. H. Wass MA MD FRCP, Department of Endocrinology, Oxford Centre for Diabetes, Endocrinology and Metabolism, Churchill Hospital, University of Oxford, UK

Jonathan Waxman BSc MD FRCP, Professor of Oncology, Department of Oncology, Hammersmith Hospital, Imperial College Healthcare NHS Trust, London.

Bronwen Williams MB ChB DGM DCH MRCGP, City and Hackney Teaching PCT, London

Adrian Wills MB BS BSc FRCP MMedSci MD, Nottingham University Hospitals NHS Trust.

Sabine Woerwag-Mehta MRCPCH MRCPsych, Consultant Child and Adolescent Psychiatrist, East Kent University Trust.

Kevan Wylie MD FRCP FRCPsych FRCOG, Porterbrook Clinic, Sheffield and The University of Sheffield.

Section I

Improving physical health

1

Meeting the physical health needs of people with mental disorders and disabilities

William Lee and Irene Cormac

All forms of mental disorder and intellectual disability carry increased risks of physical illness and premature mortality. This chapter provides information on common physical health risks, ways to improve physical health and the development of physical health services. An outline is given of the role of the psychiatrist as a doctor in psychiatric practice. The information in this chapter can be used as a guide. The authors have recommended sources of further information.

Health and well-being

In 1948, the World Health Organization (WHO) defined health in its constitution as 'A state of complete physical, mental and social well-being and not merely the absence of disease or infirmity'.[1] This definition has been criticised for being a better definition of happiness than of health. An alternative definition states 'Health is a condition of well-being free of disease or infirmity and is a basic and universal human right'.[2] This definition permits health to be measured, for example using mortality, morbidity and quality-of-life measures. Nevertheless, the WHO definition highlights the need to attend to mental and social aspects of health, which continue to affect so many people worldwide.

Ill health is a universal experience – everyone experiences acute or chronic physical or mental ill health during his or her lifetime. Ill health is caused by an array of often interacting intrinsic and extrinsic factors. In 2004, the two greatest causes of disability worldwide were estimated to be infections of the lower respiratory tract and diarrhoeal diseases.[3] These groups of conditions are caused by infective agents, which can be tackled by public health measures such as clean drinking water, sanitation, soap and anti-infective agents, for example disinfectants, and antiviral and antibiotic medications. However, the presence of infective agents alone is often not enough to cause ill health. Other factors unrelated to the eradication of pathogens can affect health, in particular nutrition, housing, education and climate, as well as law and order in society.

Ill health prevents people from contributing economically and socially to society, and thus perpetuates poverty and hinders economic development.[3] Increasingly in higher-income countries, governments have recognised the social and economic importance of health, especially the benefits from reducing modifiable health risk factors and chronic, non-communicable diseases. The WHO has global strategic plans to address four chronic diseases (cardiovascular diseases, cancer, chronic respiratory diseases and diabetes mellitus), which are responsible for causing 60% of all deaths worldwide; notably, 80% of these deaths occur in low- and middle-income countries.[4] These four diseases are mostly preventable – by eliminating tobacco use, unhealthy diet, physical inactivity and the harmful use of alcohol.[5]

Table 1.1 All causes of death in England and Wales in males and females aged 28 days and over, in 2008, by ICD-10 category

Cause of death	Total number of deaths	% of all deaths	ICD-10 code[6]
Circulatory system disorder	168 238	33	I00–I99
Neoplasm	141 143	28	C00–D48
Respiratory system disorder	71 751	14	J00–J99
Digestive system disorder	25 997	5	K00–K99
Mental and behavioural disorders	18 438	4	F00–F99
Disease of nervous system	17 521	3	G00–G99
Endocrine and metabolic disease	7 426	1	E00–E99

Source: Office for National Statistics, 2009.[5]

In England and Wales, causes of death in the general population are published by the Office for National Statistics. In 2008, the three commonest causes of death were cardiovascular diseases, neoplasms and respiratory diseases (Table 1.1).[5]

Public health guidance by the UK National Institute for Health and Clinical Excellence (NICE)[7] states that the risk of an adult dying prematurely is increased mainly by the following risk factors:

- a low income (or membership of a low-income family)
- being a recipient of state benefits
- being a member of some minority ethnic groups
- having mental health problems
- having intellectual disabilities
- living in public or social housing
- living in an institution (including convicted prisoners)
- being homeless.

This guidance recommends reducing premature deaths from cardiovascular diseases and other smoking-related diseases by finding those who are most at risk and delivering strategies known to improve health according to other NICE guidelines, for example on the use of statins[8] and on smoking cessation[9] (see also Chapter 6).

Primary care trusts and local authorities can identify areas of social deprivation in England using the Index of Multiple Deprivation 2007 system, which combines economic, social and housing factors to provide a single deprivation score.[10] Similar systems are specific to other parts of the UK.

Table 1.2 Standardised mortality ratios (SMRs) for selected mental disorders derived from a meta-analysis

Mental disorder	SMR: all deaths	SMR: unnatural deaths	Notes
All forms of mental disorder	150	–	
Schizophrenia	157	434	
Bipolar disorder	202	918	
Depression	133–135	551/720 (M/F)	
Panic disorder	206	429	
Eating disorders	538	1269	Self-starvation caused 65% of deaths
Alcohol misuse/dependence	197	442	
Substance misuse	453	1503	69% of deaths unnatural
Personality disorders	184	371	52% of deaths unnatural
Organic mental disorders	326	324	4% of deaths unnatural
Mental retardation	633	103	Deaths from natural causes: SMR = 783

Source: Harris & Barraclough, 1998.[12]

Physical health of people with mental disorders and disabilities

Premature death and ill health

People suffering from mental health problems have an increased risk of poor physical health and of dying earlier than people in the general population (Table 1.2).[11–13] Standardised mortality ratios (SMRs) vary according to the type of mental disorder. Eating disorders and addictions carry the highest risks. Deaths from unnatural causes (essentially accidents, suicide and homicide) were found to be high for schizophrenia and major depression and deaths from natural causes were increased for people with organic mental disorders.

People with intellectual disabilities are 58 times more likely to die before the age of 50 than the rest of the population (see Chapter 26) and to have more unmet health needs than people in the general population.[14] Even after adjustments are made for social deprivation, death rates remain higher in people with mental health problems than in the general population.[14]

Poor health in people with mental problems is due to a combination of factors, including increased rates of tobacco smoking,[15] increased use of alcohol and illicit drugs,[16] decreased levels of physical activity and increased rates of obesity.[11] Specific processes by which mental ill health could affect the body include reduced heart-rate variability and changes in platelet aggregation.[17] These processes would predict excess mortality only from certain causes, as found by some researchers,[18] but not all,[19] so this question remains open.

In people with schizophrenia, there are more deaths from injuries, accidents, suicides and homicides than in the general population (Table 1.3).[20,21] The risk of death from homicide is increased 6 times, for suicide 12–13 times, and from accidents the risk of death is increased 3–5 times. In a Scottish study, 70% of men and 86% of women with schizophrenia were found to be overweight or obese.[22] About 70% of people with schizophrenia smoke tobacco.[23] Men and women with schizophrenia have a 90% increased risk of developing bowel cancer and women with schizophrenia have a 42% increased risk of developing breast cancer.[13] Rates of coronary heart disease, diabetes, stroke and respiratory disease are higher than in the general population and death rates in a 5-year period are higher.[13]

Addiction to alcohol and substance misuse increase the risk of acquiring infections with blood-borne viruses (e.g. human immunodeficiency viruses) due to increased rates of unprotected sex and intravenous drug misuse.[24] People with mental disorders are also less likely to take medication for communicable diseases, for example for the treatment of tuberculosis. Other associations of poor health and schizophrenia are listed in Box 1.1.

Healthcare

Healthcare professionals have been found to search less thoroughly for physical problems in people with mental disorders, and symptoms may be wrongly attributed to the mental disorder or are ignored, so-called 'diagnostic overshadowing', further increasing the health divide.[25]

Psychotropic medications, especially newer antipsychotic medications, have physical side-effects including weight gain, obesity and abnormalities in lipid metabolism, and some medications are associated with increased rates of type 2 diabetes, hypertension and cardiovascular events.[26] The risk of sudden death increases with each additional antipsychotic medication

Table 1.3 Rates of disease and earlier death in people with schizophrenia, with age-adjusted rates

Physical health diagnosis	Rates in people with schizophrenia	Rates in general population
Coronary heart disease	31% (22%)	18% (8%)
Diabetes	41% (19%)	30% (9%)
Cerebrovascular accident	21% (28%)	11% (12%)
Respiratory disease/COPD	23% (28%)	17% (15%)

Figures in parentheses are age-adjusted death rates within 5 years of the physical health diagnosis.
COPD: chronic obstructive pulmonary disease.

Source: Hippisley-Cox et al, 2006.[13]

Box 1.1 Examples of health risks in people with mental disorders and disabilities

- Risk behaviours, such as sexual behaviour, addiction
- Less likely to be registered with a general practitioner and dentist
- Low attendance rates for health screening
- Late presentation or non-presentation with significant symptoms
- Difficulty keeping appointments with healthcare providers
- Diagnostic overshadowing (mental disorder given priority over physical health)
- Side-effects of psychotropic medications
- Direct effects of specific mental illnesses on the body

taken: the relative risk of taking more than one antipsychotic medication is 2.50 (95% CI 1.46 to 4.30) per increment of one psychotropic medication.[27]

Prescribers should monitor the psychiatric and physical effects of psychotropic medication, avoid potential drug interactions and check for pre-existing conditions such as pregnancy and diabetes, as well as whether the patient is taking other medications. Further information for prescribers about psychotropic medication, including doses, side-effects and drug interactions, is available in the *Maudsley Prescribing Guidelines*.[28]

Health improvement

Government, regulation and commissioning

In the UK, government health policies focus mainly on health promotion, disease prevention and delivery of effective healthcare, which should meet certain standards and achieve consistent quality. In England and Wales, the 2004 White Paper *Choosing Health* outlined ways to reduce health inequalities between sociodemographic groups by motivating, supporting and providing opportunities for people to lead healthier lives by improving their diet, physical activity and mental health, and by reducing other modifiable health risks.[29] The Chief Medical Officer has recommended that people of all ages should increase their physical activity, and also noted the beneficial effects of exercise on mental health.[29] Change4Life is a movement supported by the UK Department of Health designed to improve the health of families by promoting changes to diet and exercise.[30]

Health policies for the general population should apply to people with mental disorders and intellectual disabilities. In 2011 a cross-governmental strategy was introduced, 'No health without mental health', which applies to people of all ages; key aims include improving the mental health of more people, improving the physical health of people with mental health problems, reducing their risk of premature mortality, reducing avoidable harm, stigma and discrimination, as well as improving the mental health of people with physical health problems.[31]

In England, the Care Quality Commission (CQC)[32] regulates health services and adult social care, in both the National Health Service (NHS) and the private sector, as well as in ambulance and blood transfusion services. The CQC sets standards for care, registers health facilities and regulates health providers. Health providers must meet essential quality standards to maintain their registration.[32] The CQC has legal powers to remove registration and implement financial penalties or fines if CQC standards are unmet, and of note, these powers apply to mental health settings.

In 2006, a commissioning framework integrated various initiatives into a single plan for primary care trusts (PCTs) to improve the physical health of people with mental health problems by identifying physical health needs and then developing and commissioning health services such as annual health checks for people with mental health problems (backed up by a case register), specifically targeted smoking cessation services[33] and organised exercise programmes.

Guidance on health conditions

In Scotland, the Scottish Intercollegiate Guidelines Network (SIGN; www.sign.ac.uk) publishes guidance on the treatment of several physical health conditions. In England and Wales, the National Institute for Health and Clinical Excellence (NICE) produces independent, national guidance on promoting good health, and on preventing and treating ill health, which is based on best available research evidence and value for money (Box 1.2). Guidance from NICE is available for a range of clinical conditions and public health topics. In addition, NICE technology appraisals make recommendations on

Box 1.2 The nature of guidelines from the National Institute for Health and Clinical Excellence and the Scottish Intercollegiate Guidelines Network

Both sets of guidelines:

- provide expert opinion, algorithms and protocols for healthcare
- set standards for physical healthcare, based on research evidence
- improve adherence to evidence-based standards of healthcare.

the use of new and existing medicines and treatments, within the NHS in England and Wales. In 2009, NICE issued its first guidance on the treatment of depression in people with chronic physical health problems.[34]

In other branches of medicine, checklists, algorithms and guidelines are widely used to ensure patients receive evidence-based care or care based on standards agreed by a consensus of experts. Nevertheless, clinical judgement must also be used to ensure the needs of individual patients are met, otherwise the clinician's role may become limited to the transcription of data or to following instructions.

Numerical approaches have produced superior outcomes to judgement in many differing spheres of human activity,[35] so it is timely to focus on using research evidence to inform clinical decisions and view this as the formalised and disciplined use of the best evidence, rather than as a debate between formulaic and judgement-based care.

As medical practice continually changes, psychiatrists should undertake continuous professional development (CPD) on relevant physical health topics to meet the needs of their patients.

Patient care: standards

Standards of physical healthcare

In 2009, the Royal College of Psychiatrists published physical health standards for psychiatric services for adults, children and young people, for those with intellectual disabilities, and for forensic psychiatric settings. These standards can be used for policies, service development and audit of physical health services.[14]

Guidelines from both the National Institute for Health and Clinical Excellence (NICE) and the Scottish Intercollegiate Guidelines Network (SIGN) are applicable to people with mental disorders and intellectual disabilities.

Everyone with a mental disorder or intellectual disability should have access to the same standard of physical healthcare as others in the general population. Patients should be empowered to manage their own health and to register with a general practitioner (GP) (Chapter 3). Patients should be offered an annual health review (Chapter 9). They may benefit from the initiatives arising in primary care through the Quality Outcome Framework[36] (QOF) incentive and reward scheme (Chapter 3), which has indicators for clinical and organisational practice and nationally agreed standards for the delivery of healthcare. Steps should be taken to reduce the barriers to access to secondary care services through facilitating appointments, improving communication and reducing the stigma associated with mental health problems.

Quality of services

High-quality services should deliver care consistently to high standards and without significant variation or waste. In 2008, the Darzi report, *High Quality Care For All*, stated the areas where quality improvements should be undertaken in the NHS, and priorities for commissioning services, to meet needs of patients; the report mainly focused on aims and standards.[37]

Another approach to improving quality is the adoption of cross-organisational management techniques such as the Lean and Six Sigma system, which reduces variation and waste in processes, to achieve consistent delivery such that there are only a few 'failures' per million opportunities (to fail), thus improving reliability and efficiency. Topics or processes for improvement are chosen, then are defined, measured and analysed, before changes are implemented, together with monitoring and control systems. In the Lean and Six Sigma system, staff of varying levels of expertise can use a range of management tools to improve quality. The Lean and Six Sigma was devised at the US electronics firm Motorola in the 1980s but has found wide application elsewhere, including within healthcare systems and the NHS.

Box 1.3 Tips that can help patients access physical healthcare

- Offer support/information about registering with a GP and dentist
- Request longer or shorter appointments, if needed, with GP
- Suggest using telephone consultations with GP, when appropriate
- Plan regular physical health checks
- For hospital appointments, arrange for 'reminder' text messages to be sent
- Suggest patients keep a list of useful contact telephone numbers

Governance

Clinicians should contribute to the management of clinical services. In the NHS, management and control systems are often based on central and local standards or targets, for example key performance indicators (KPIs) and targets for payment by results (PBR). Systems that are widely used to monitor and improve services include clinical audit, committees, complaints systems, policies and procedures, and internal reviews – such as apply after sudden untoward incidents (SUIs) – and shared learning from incidents which nearly, or actually, led to serious harm.

Systems are required to track progress and to measure achievements. An example of a monitoring system is the 'balanced scorecard', on which a topic is recorded. Then, alongside this topic, the percentage rates of performance or achievement of targets or standards are recorded in colour to mark compliance. Within a red, amber, green (RAG) system of flagging, red means non-compliance, amber shows partial compliance and green indicates full compliance.

If certain actions are agreed, action plans can be used to monitor and facilitate progress. Columns are used to list the desired action, next to a list of those responsible for the action, and the stage of compliance is marked in RAG colours in the final column, enabling everyone to see at a glance the progress of the plan.

Responsibilities of mental health professionals

Mental health professionals and psychiatrists should offer assistance to patients to maintain and improve their physical health (Box 1.3). It is crucial to address factors that may directly or indirectly affect a patient's physical health such as their income (including state benefits), employment, social contact and living conditions (heating, hot water, electricity, food, personal hygiene and clothing). Some useful resources for patients are listed in Box 1.4.

Roles and responsibilities of psychiatrists

As doctors, psychiatrists must follow guidance from the General Medical Council (GMC) contained in *Good Medical Practice*[38] and other GMC guidance on topics such as confidentiality[39] and patient consent, both for clinical activity and for research.[40]

The Royal College of Psychiatrists has set specific standards for psychiatrists on their role in physical healthcare:[41]

- Psychiatrists must be competent to undertake a physical examination and to arrange investigations.
- Psychiatrists must ensure that they understand the therapeutic and adverse effects of prescribed

Table 1.4 Useful websites for physical health information for psychiatric patients

NHS Choices	www.nhs.uk
NHS Direct	www.nhsdirect.nhs.uk
MIND	www.mind.org.uk
Patient.co.uk	www.patient.co.uk
Rethink	www.rethink.org
The Princess Royal Trust for Carers	www.carers.org

medication, and that they report suspected adverse drug reactions.

- Psychiatrists should communicate with general practitioners (with patient consent) and must ensure they include relevant information about physical health in their referrals.

Legal issues relating to psychiatric practice are addressed in Chapter 11.

The NHS and the voluntary sector provide a wealth of information on physical health topics for patients and carers. Mental health professionals should inform patients where to access health information. Some examples are given in Table 1.4.

Box 1.4 Information for mental health professionals

Oxford Handbook Series (Oxford University Press):

- Longmore M, Wilkinson I, Davidson E, *et al. Oxford Handbook of Clinical Medicine*, 8th edition, 2010
- Simon C, Everitt H, Kendrick T. *Oxford Handbook of General Practice*, 3rd edition, 2010
- Wyatt JP, Illingworth RN, Graham CA, Hogg K. *Oxford Handbook of Accident and Emergency Medicine*, 4th edition, 2012

Kumar P, Clark ML (eds) *Clinical Medicine*, 8th edition. Saunders, 2012

Houghton AR, Gray D. *Chamberlain's Symptoms and Signs in Clinical Medicine: An Introduction to Medical Diagnosis*. Hodder Arnold, 2010

Joint Formulary Committee. *British National Formulary*. British Medical Association and Royal Pharmaceutical Society (http://bnf.org/bnf/index.htm)

GP notebook (www.gpnotebook.co.uk/homepage.cfm)

Norfolk and Suffolk NHS Foundation Trust: Choice and Medication website provides information leaflets on psychotropic medications (www.choiceandmedication.org/nsft/pages/printableleaflets/)

Improving Physical and Mental Health, resources for health professionals (www.rcpsych.ac.uk/mentalhealthinfo/improvingphysicalandmh.aspx)

Psychiatrists and mental health professionals must take care of their own health, should register with a GP and avoid treating themselves, their family or friends.

Developing physical health services

The health needs of patients vary with demographic and social characteristics and disease prevalence. Needs assessments should therefore be undertaken before a physical health service is developed (Box 1.5).

Box 1.5 Checklist for development of services

Preliminary information

- Population size and demographics
- Socioeconomic status
- Physical comorbidities (e.g. rates of diabetes, asthma, epilepsy, obesity)
- Mental conditions (e.g. diagnostic categories, comorbidities with addictions)
- Length of stay in in-patient or institutional setting
- Current physical health services and efficacy
- Views of patients and carers, and other stakeholders
- Evidence-base for new service
- Policies and procedures which exist or which are needed

Key steps

- Develop the service concept, its importance/relevance
- Obtain support from key decision-makers
- Obtain support from colleagues, senior and local management
- Undertake an options appraisal of benefits, disadvantages and alternatives
- Address barriers to change
- Estimate costs and funding options
- Recruitment or secondment of staff
- Evaluation of the service

Service development

New projects, especially larger ones, require leadership, management and often funding. Support from management is essential, whether in the community or in in-patient settings. The recruitment process is often the most time-consuming part of organising a new service, so it is best to obtain guidance from experienced colleagues, and from staff in finance and human resources departments. For significant changes, it is advisable to use a comprehensive communications strategy.[42]

From day one, clinical services need effective clinical and managerial supervision. Staff will need adequate working facilities, resources and supervision. Staff who are poorly trained or poorly supervised tend to be less productive and to have higher sickness rates.

Box 1.6 Checklist for a comprehensive in-patient physical healthcare service

Employees

- General practitioner, nurse, administrator, infection control staff, and staff trained to deliver screening or monitoring such as ECG (electrocardiography)

Service-level agreements

- Dietetics, physiotherapy, podiatry, haematology, biochemistry, radiology, anaesthesiology, audiology, optometry and dentistry

Management

- Contracts, monitoring/audit, service development, links with other hospitals, clinical governance

Secondary care

- Referral pathways, contracts for services (e.g. neurology, cardiology, eating disorders services, old age, drugs and alcohol services)

Standards

- Care pathways and delivery of care should be based on acceptable standards (e.g. guidance from the National Institute for Health and Clinical Excellence). Services should be monitored/audited to ensure agreed standards are met

Communication

- Safe and effective systems of communication are needed between clinical teams and primary care services

Primary care services for in-patient settings

In many in-patient psychiatric services, psychiatrists provide physical healthcare. They should ensure that every patient has a physical health check on admission. Weekly GP sessions can be helpful to provide physical healthcare and to support psychiatrists with physical healthcare provision, but this is not always possible. During brief hospital admissions, patients may continue to visit their GP for physical healthcare. However, long-stay patients require comprehensive physical health services delivered in the psychiatric setting (Box 1.6).[43]

Making changes in health

When confronted by an event or a transition, individuals and organisations can reach a 'tipping point' and make sudden changes. Normally, changes are more gradual or step-wise, passing through different stages of change: pre-contemplation, contemplation, preparation, maintenance and relapse.[44] By assessing the stage of change, clinicians can gauge how likely it will be that a person or group will engage with an intervention. For individuals to change, they have to believe it is possible to change, to want the change or outcome proposed, and to believe the change is achievable by them. The criteria in this 'expectancy theory' are entirely based on beliefs (Box 1.7).[45]

Box 1.7 Key components of the expectancy theory

- *Expectancy*: strength of a person's belief that their efforts will lead to success (i.e. the task can be done within available resources)
- *Valence*: level of satisfaction expected from the outcome (i.e. the extent to which the person values the anticipated outcome)
- *Instrumentality*: the belief that the level of performance can be directly linked to the amount of effort (i.e. hard work brings more chance of success)

Source: Vroom, 1990.[45]

Motivational factors are different for each person. Financial rewards are not always the most effective motivators. Internal motivators may include the desire to achieve personal goals, to be recognised as successful, to overcome fear and gain control over unwanted feelings or behaviour. Examples of external motivators that are used in mental health settings for patients are the opportunity to gain more freedom and to win praise, certificates and prizes for achievements.

Motivational interviewing can be used to help patients to make changes. Role models are also useful to promote changes in behaviour, for example to encourage patients to take exercise. Attitudes and expectations of staff and patients can be changed by training and education. Staff who are regarded as capable and competent are more likely to be trusted by patients. If staff have a positive attitude towards maintaining health and well-being, this can help to provide the necessary leadership to achieve improvements in healthcare services.

Public health guidance from NICE provides information on the most appropriate generic and specific interventions to support changes in attitude and behaviour change at population and community levels.[46]

Research

Research is essential for creating an evidence base for relating to the improvement of the physical health of psychiatric patients. Clinicians and academics should work together to prioritise research topics and where feasible to conduct randomised controlled trials and service evaluations.

Research projects do not have to be large to make a difference. However, it is important to design them properly, to complete the data analysis and to avoid the temptation to allow findings from a study to gather dust in a drawer, or to rest forgotten in a computer file. Audit and other types of service evaluation should not be ignored.

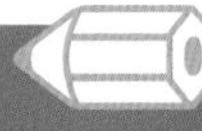

Learning points

- According to the WHO, the four main diseases that are preventable are cardiovascular disease, stroke, cancer and type 2 diabetes mellitus.
- In the UK, the major causes of death are diseases of the circulatory system, neoplasms and diseases of the respiratory system.
- Eating disorders and alcohol misuse carry the highest risks of premature mortality.
- People with schizophrenia have a higher risk of developing bowel cancer and women with schizophrenia have a higher risk of developing breast cancer.
- Addiction to alcohol and substances increases the likelihood of acquiring infection with blood-borne viruses.
- Addiction to alcohol and substances reduces compliance with treatment for tuberculosis.
- Health professionals search less thoroughly for physical health conditions in people with mental disorders and intellectual disabilities (so-called 'diagnostic overshadowing').
- Risk of sudden death increases incrementally with each additional antipsychotic medication prescribed.
- Guidelines from NICE and SIGN should apply to people with mental disorders and intellectual disabilities as much as the rest of the community.
- Standards for physical health services are available from the Royal College of Psychiatrists.
- Management systems should be used to monitor and improve physical health services, such as the Lean Six Sigma system, balanced score cards and action plans.

Summary

There is much to be done to improve the physical health of patients with mental health problems and intellectual disabilities, to reduce the inequalities of health and to improve inclusion of patients in mainstream health services. The following chapters are designed to inform clinicians about physical health topics and the physical health conditions relating to the psychiatric specialties.

References

1 World Health Organization. *Constitution of the World Health Organization.* WHO, 2006 (http://www.who.int/governance/eb/who_constitution_en.pdf).

2 Saracci R. The World Health Organisation needs to reconsider its definition of health. *BMJ* 1997; **314**: 1409–10.

3 World Health Organization. *The Global Burden of Disease, 2004 Update.* WHO, 2004 (http://www.who.int/healthinfo/global_burden_disease/2004_report_update/en/index.html).

4 World Health Organization. *2008–2013 Action Plan for the Global Strategy for the Prevention and Control of Noncommunicable Diseases.* A53/14. WHO, 2008 (http://whqlibdoc.who.int/publications/2009/9789241597418_eng.pdf).

5 Office for National Statistics. *Mortality Statistics: Deaths Registered in 2008.* ONS, 2009.

6 World Health Organization. *The ICD-10 Classification of Mental and Behavioural Disorders: Clinical Descriptions and Diagnostic Guidelines.* WHO, 1992.

7 National Institute for Health and Clinical Excellence. *Reducing the Rate of Premature Deaths from Cardiovascular Disease and Other Smoking-Related Diseases: Finding and Supporting Those Most at Risk and Improving Access to Services (Public Health Guidance PH15).* NICE, 2008.

8 National Institute for Health and Clinical Excellence. *Statins for the Prevention of Cardiovascular Events in Patients at Increased Risk of Developing Cardiovascular Disease or Those with Established Cardiovascular Disease (Technology Appraisal TA94).* NICE, 2006.

9 National Institute for Health and Clinical Excellence. *Smoking Cessation Services in Primary Care, Pharmacies, Local Authorities and Workplaces, Particularly for Manual Working Groups, Pregnant Women and Hard to Reach Communities (Public Health Guidance PH10).* NICE, 2008.

10 Department for Communities and Local Government. *Indices of Deprivation.* DCLG, 2011 (http://www.communities.gov.uk/communities/research/indicesdeprivation/deprivation10/).

11 Brown S, Birtwistle J, Roe L, *et al.* The unhealthy lifestyle of people with schizophrenia. *Psychol Med* 1999; **29**: 697–701.

12 Harris EC, Barraclough B. Excess mortality of mental disorder. *Br J Psychiatry* 1998; **173**: 11–53.

13 Hippisley-Cox J, Coupland C, Langford G, *et al. A Comparison of Survival Rates for People with Mental Health Problems and the Remaining Population with Specific Conditions.* Disability Rights Commission, 2006.

14 O'Brien G, Bullock R, Black S, *et al. Physical Health in Mental Health (Occasional Paper OP67).* Royal College of Psychiatrists, 2009.

15 Hughes JR, Hatsukami DK, Mitchell JE, *et al.* Prevalence of smoking among psychiatric outpatients. *Am J Psychiatry* 1986; **143**: 993–7.

16 Grant BF, Stinson FS, Dawson DA, *et al.* Prevalence and co-occurrence of substance use disorders and independent mood and anxiety disorders: results from the National Epidemiologic Survey on Alcohol and Related Conditions. *Arch Gen Psychiatry* 2004; **61**: 807–16.

17 Carney RM, Freedland KE, Miller GE, *et al.* Depression as a risk factor for cardiac mortality and morbidity: a review of potential mechanisms. *J Psychosom Res* 2002; **53**: 897–902.

18 Osborn DP, Levy G, Nazareth I, Petersen I, Islam A, King MB. Relative risk of cardiovascular and cancer mortality in people with severe mental illness from the United Kingdom's General Practice Research Database. *Arch Gen Psychiatry* 2007; **64**: 242–9.

19 Mykletun A, Bjerkeset O, Dewey M, Prince M, Overland S, Stewart R. Anxiety, depression, and cause-specific mortality: the HUNT study. *Psychosom Med* 2007; **69**: 323–31.

20 Brown S, Inskip H, Barraclough B. Causes of the excess mortality of schizophrenia. *Br J Psychiatry* 2000; **177**: 212–7.

21 Hiroeh U, Appleby L, Mortensen PB, *et al.* Death by homicide, suicide, and other unnatural causes in people with mental illness: a population-based study. *Lancet* 2001; **358**: 2110–2.

22 McCreadie RG. Diet, smoking and cardiovascular risk in people with schizophrenia: descriptive study. *Br J Psychiatry* 2003; **183**: 534–9.

23 Meltzer H. *Economic Activity and Social Functioning of Residents with Psychiatric Disorders.* TSO (The Stationery Office), 1996.

24 Prince M, Patel V, Saxena S, *et al.* No health without mental health. *Lancet* 2007; **370**: 859–77.

25 Roberts L, Roalfe A, Wilson S, *et al.* Physical health care of patients with schizophrenia in primary care: a comparative study. *Fam Pract* 2007; **24**: 34–40.

26 De Hert M, Dekker JM, Wood D, *et al.* Cardiovascular disease and diabetes in people with severe mental illness: Position statement from the European Psychiatric Association (EPA), supported by the European Association for the Study of Diabetes (EASD) and the European Society of Cardiology (ESC). *Eur Psychiatry* 2009; **24**: 412–24.

27 Joukamaa M, Heliovaara M, Knekt P, *et al.* Schizophrenia, neuroleptic medication and mortality. *Br J Psychiatry* 2006; **188**: 122–7.

28 Taylor D, Paton C, Kapur S. *Maudsley Prescribing Guidelines (10th edn).* Taylor and Francis, 2010.

29 Department of Health. *Choosing Health: Making Healthy Choices Easier.* Department of Health, 2004.

30 Department of Health. *Change4Life.* Department of Health, 2010.

31 HM Government. *No Health Without Mental Health: A Cross-Government Mental Health Strategy for People of All Ages.* Department of Health, 2011.

32 Care Quality Commission. *Essential Standards of Quality and Safety.* CQC, 2010.

33 Department of Health. *Choosing Health: Supporting the Physical Needs of People with Severe Mental Illness – Commissioning Framework.* Department of Health, 2006.

34 National Institute for Health and Clinical Excellence. *The Treatment and Management of Depression in Adults with Chronic Physical Health Problems (Clinical Guidelines CG91).* NICE, 2009.

35 Ayres I. *Super Crunchers: Why Thinking-by-Numbers Is the New Way To Be Smart.* John Murray, 2007, p. 272.

36 National Institute for Health and Clinical Excellence. *About the Quality and Outcomes Framework.* NICE, 2012 (www.nice.org.uk/aboutnice/qof/qof.jsp).

37 Darzi AW. *High Quality Care for All: NHS Next Stage Review Final Report.* TSO (The Stationery Office), 2008.

38 General Medical Council. *Good Medical Practice.* GMC, 2012.

39 General Medical Council. *Confidentiality: Protecting and Providing Information.* GMC, 2009.

40 General Medical Council. *Consent Guidance: Patients and Doctors Making Decisions Together.* GMC, 2008.

41 Royal College of Psychiatrists. *Good Psychiatric Practice (College Report CR154).* Royal College of Psychiatrists, 2009.

42 Cormac I, McNally L. How to implement a smoke-free policy. *Adv Psychiatr Treat* 2008; **14**: 198–207.

43 Cormac I, Martin D, Ferriter M. Improving the physical health of long-stay psychiatric in-patients. *Adv Psychiatr Treat* 2004; **10**: 107–15.

44 Prochaska JO, DiClemente CC. Stages and processes of self-change of smoking: toward an integrative model of change. *J Consult Clin Psychol* 1983; **51**: 390–5.

45 Vroom VH. *Manage People, Not Personnel: Motivation and Performance Appraisal.* Harvard Business Press, 1990.

46 National Institute for Health and Clinical Excellence. *Behaviour Change at Population, Community and Individual Levels (Public Health Guidance PH6).* NICE, 2007.

2

Lifestyle and risks to physical health

David Gray

Premature mortality and morbidity attributable to acute infectious disease have been replaced by chronic degenerative disease, largely as the consequence of lifestyle changes. This chapter outlines the prevention, investigation and treatment of obesity, coronary heart disease, metabolic syndrome and diabetes mellitus with special reference to psychiatric patients. People with mental health conditions are at greater risks of an 'unhealthy' lifestyle through poor dietary choices, inactivity and smoking. They are also likely to be prescribed medication which encourages weight gain and not to have access to general practitioner services that we take for granted.

Introduction

In Western societies, infectious diseases such as diphtheria, whooping cough, scarlet fever, measles and tuberculosis were once common causes of morbidity and premature mortality, accounting for one-third of all deaths. Long before vaccination, immunisation and antibiotics were widely available, the proportion of deaths caused by infection was in decline. Industrialisation accompanied by economic development and urbanisation led to a reduction in poverty, more secure sources of nutrition and improved housing; these contributed greatly to human survival and quality of life, particularly in the past hundred years or so.

In Western society today, the 'control' achieved over infectious disease has changed the nature of mortality and morbidity, although HIV/AIDS, MRSA and sporadic bacterial and viral epidemics are never far away. An increasing proportion of the population can now expect to survive to old age. The average male baby born today in Western society can look forward to almost 80 years of life, and a female baby even longer. Many low- and middle-income countries are also undergoing this transition away from prevalent acute infectious disease, and falling neonatal and infant mortality rates are interpreted as an important marker of economic progress.[1]

Economic development has brought significant changes to daily life and lifestyle, leading to shorter working hours (for most), improved working conditions, greater disposable income and increased leisure time. The daily struggle to make a living is no longer a reality in our relatively affluent society, especially where social services in the state sector (at least in the UK) provide a safety net. But there is a 'downside' to this affluence. Despite increased leisure time, our society has become more sedentary, with television almost a national pastime in some countries; computer games have displaced activity-based play; home-cooked meals using seasonal, local produce are easily replaced with commercially processed, relatively low-cost convenience food (usually with high fat and carbohydrate content); and governments are fighting a rearguard action in the face of rising alcohol consumption and cigarette smoking.

With increasing affluence, the character of morbidity and mortality has changed. Infectious disease has been replaced by chronic, non-communicable, degenerative diseases, notably type 2 diabetes, coronary heart disease, cerebrovascular disease, peripheral vascular disease, obesity and the metabolic syndrome, and even some cancers have been labelled 'lifestyle diseases'.[2]

Chronic degenerative diseases will inevitably present difficulties for health services as the result of epidemiological and demographic change. With population growth comes an increasing number who may become liable to and are affected by chronic disease. With an ageing population, prolonged exposure to environmental factors through a lengthened life span increases the likelihood of accruing more chronic diseases. Even high-income countries are struggling to afford modern healthcare systems, partly due to these changes, made worse by increasing reliance on medical technology and compounded by rising expectations. Most European countries spend 7–11% of their gross domestic product on healthcare; the USA spends the most, in 2010 estimated at 18% and this is predicted unlikely to fall despite reform.[3]

Greater spending, however, does not guarantee better health.[4] Spending on health services does not buy added years. Tables of average life expectancy rank the USA 27th, with many countries spending considerably less on healthcare enjoying greater length of life. Nor does it mean that public health objectives will be met; whereas 15% of the objectives of the US Department of Health and Human Services' initiative 'Healthy People 2000' have been met, and good progress has been made towards another 44% of the objectives, obesity, physical activity and adolescent cigarette use (comprising 20% of the objectives) have got worse.[5]

As the population ages and longevity increases, more individuals are subject to a range of chronic degenerative diseases; before industrialisation, few worried about chronic diseases because life expectancy was too short for these diseases to emerge. The result of our affluence and current lifestyle is to expose the individual to these diseases at an earlier age.

Type 2 diabetes

The prevalence of diabetes has more or less doubled in the past 20 years or so. For the UK, this means nearly 2 million people, or about 4% of the population, are affected,[6] and this is expected to rise to 4.7% by 2025, driven largely by an increase in type 2 diabetes.[7] Worldwide, about 150 million people are affected, with diabetes responsible for about 5 million deaths per year.[8] But this is only part of the story, as not everyone with diabetes is diagnosed – in the UK, about 3% of men and 1.5% of women have diabetes but are unaware of this.[9]

The symptoms of diabetes are easy to control yet it is a far from benign disease process. Although its more severe consequences may not be seen for many years, nevertheless affected individuals get off to a bad start. The diagnosis reduces life expectancy by as much as 10 years.[10] This is just the start because diabetes is a major risk factor for vascular disease in the long term, and those with the condition face the prospect of eye, cardiovascular, cerebrovascular, renovascular and peripheral vascular disease.

Several factors may contribute to the development of diabetes, such as Cushing's syndrome, myotonic dystrophy, Friedrich's ataxia and (more commonly) steroid use. There is a strong genetic predisposition to type 1 diabetes and an even stronger one to type 2. However, environmental factors, age, physical inactivity, a high-fat diet and weight gain leading to central and chronic obesity also predispose to type 2 diabetes. By any measure, diabetes is a health crisis in the making (see chapter 16, on diabetes and its treatment).

Diagnosing and preventing diabetes

Type 1 diabetes, due to a lack of insulin secretion, is an autoimmune condition so is not *directly* preventable.

Type 2 diabetes, which is more common than type 1, occurs when there is resistance to the effects of insulin. Its diagnosis is outlined in Box 2.1. The risk of developing diabetes seems to be *lowest* in those who

Box 2.1 Diagnosing diabetes mellitus

Suspect diabetes if a patient presents with 'classic' symptoms such as thirst, polyuria and unexplained weight loss. The diagnosis of diabetes is usually straightforward:

- venous plasma glucose level (from a randomly obtained sample) is 11.1 mmol/l or more, *or*
- the fasting plasma glucose level is ≥ 7.0 mmol/l (whole blood ≥ 6.1 mmol/l), *or*
- the plasma glucose level is ≥ 11.1 mmol/l at 2 h after administration of 75 g anhydrous glucose (oral glucose tolerance test).

have high activity levels, eat a healthy diet (comprising high fibre, high polyunsaturated/saturated fat ratio), do not smoke, consume only moderate amounts of alcohol and are of normal weight. It does not suddenly develop but is preceded by *pre-diabetes*, characterised by a higher than normal blood glucose level, but below that at which diabetes is diagnosed. Early and aggressive treatment through lifestyle change can slow down or halt the development of type 2 diabetes.[11]

As activity levels decline, weight tends to increase and with it insulin resistance may emerge, so that normal levels of insulin have less effect on muscle and adipose cells and glucose levels stay higher for longer; this stimulates the pancreas to secrete more insulin. The effect on fat cells is to cause a rise in fatty acids in plasma; on muscle cells, glucose uptake is reduced; and on liver cells, glucose production is increased. Each makes a contribution to high circulating blood glucose levels. High plasma levels of insulin and glucose are believed to lead to type 2 diabetes, with all its consequences.

Weight loss and increased physical activity can reduce the risk of developing diabetes by about 50%.[12] In those with pre-diabetes, the risk can be reduced by 30% using metformin (see chapter 16).[13]

Obesity and metabolic syndrome

Prevalence

There is evidence that obesity is becoming more prevalent, in both adults[14] and, more worryingly, in young children.[15] From 1993 to 2001, the prevalence of obesity – defined as a body mass index (BMI) of over 30 kg/m^2 – rose from 13.2% to 21.0% in men and from 16.4% to 23.5% in women.[9]

Why are we getting fatter?

The main reasons for the increase in obesity appear to be increased reliance on and consumption of convenience and 'fast' foods and decreased activity, especially at a young age[16] (including a decrease in school sports activities and increased gaming on computers rather than 'real' play). The extent of the advertising and availability of 'junk' food such as crisps, chips and chocolate bars attests to the demand and size of the market.[17] Things are changing for the worse. For instance, the size of a McDonald's burger has increased, from 333 g in 1990 to 590 g today.[18]

> The metabolic syndrome is 'A cluster of risk factors for diabetes and cardiovascular disease occurring more frequently than would be the case by chance alone'.[19]

Obesity – why it matters

Obesity has adverse effects on physical and psychological health, at least by association if not causation. These effects include osteoarthritis, obstructive sleep apnoea, diabetes mellitus, some forms of cancer, cardiovascular disease, hypertension, renal failure, stroke and heart failure, non-insulin-dependent diabetes mellitus (NIDDM), atherosclerosis, non-alcoholic fatty liver disease and a pro-inflammatory and pro-thrombotic state. Obesity almost doubles the risk of premature death from all causes, relative to individuals with a healthy weight.

Obesity, especially morbid obesity (BMI >35 kg/m^2), is frequently associated with a high-fat diet, raised blood pressure and lack of exercise. For each kilogram weight gain the increase in risk is about 4.5–9%.[19]

Lifestyle, obesity and the metabolic syndrome

The metabolic syndrome is a 'cluster of risk factors for diabetes and cardiovascular disease occurring more frequently than would be the case by chance alone'.[20] The existence of the syndrome has been questioned,[21] but whether it exists or not is immaterial – it is a clinically useful indicator that excess risk needs to be addressed. There is no universally agreed definition; several definitions exist, each based on expert opinion from world, American, European and international panels, but most include central obesity and the presence of varying levels of blood pressure, cholesterol or triglyceride or blood glucose. Waist circumference is pivotal in the definition provided by the International Diabetes Foundation (IDF) because it correlates very closely with excess visceral fat and abdominal obesity predicts metabolic syndrome.[22]

Putting waist circumference at the centre of diagnosis makes identification of risk straightforward and it has

Table 2.1 The International Diabetes Foundation definition of metabolic syndrome: waist circumference by ethnicity

Ethnic group	Men	Women
European	≥94 cm (37.0 in)	≥80 cm (31.5 in)
South Asian	≥90 cm (35.4 in)	≥80 cm (31.5 in)
Chinese	≥90 cm (35.4 in)	≥80 cm (31.5 in)
Japanese	≥85 cm (33.5 in)	≥90 cm (35.4 in)

been suggested that 'waist circumference measurement should become a routine part of global assessment of metabolic and cardiovascular risk and should be integrated into standard clinical practice'.[23]

The IDF definition also takes into account the different body habitus due to ethnicity, as shown in Table 2.1.

Body mass index or waist circumference as a risk marker?

Body mass index (BMI), calculated by dividing weight (in kilograms) by height (in metres) squared, was initially adopted as a risk marker by life assurance companies, as it predicts life expectancy. There is plenty of evidence that BMI is associated with ill health (Table 2.2): cardiovascular disease, type 2 diabetes, sleep apnoea, some cancers and osteoarthritis. It is assumed to be a measure of how thin or fat an individual is. For example, most catwalk models are 'thin', with a BMI below 20 kg/m^2, while about 20% of the UK population is obese.[24] However, it is not a true measure of body fat; for example, most of the England rugby team are 'mesomorphs' and would meet a definition of obese, with a BMI typically in excess of 30 kg/m^2.

Unlike BMI, waist circumference explains obesity-related health risk.[25] Consequently, armed with a tape measure and completely lacking mathematical ability, any clinician can readily identify an individual who is at increased health risk (unlike BMI), albeit crudely. In some cases, even the tape measure may be unnecessary and a simple 'eyeball test' will suffice.

Table 2.2 Body mass index (BMI) and risk of premature death

BMI kg/m^2	Relative risk of death
25–26.9	1.3
27–28.9	1.6
29–31	2.1

The World Health Organization has accepted BMI as the standard for recording obesity statistics. Nonetheless, BMI makes gross assumptions about body composition, and may overestimate adiposity in athletes (who have a lean body mass) while underestimating adiposity on the elderly, who generally have a less lean body mass.

In Fig. 2.1 the dashed lines represent subdivisions within a major class (e.g. 'Underweight' may be divided into 'severe', 'moderate' and 'mild' subclasses).

Management of the metabolic syndrome

The aim is to reduce risk through a broad range of strategies including:

- appropriate and aggressive therapy of all vascular risk factors
- lifestyle measures
  - modified diet, which may be supplemented with drug therapy (at present, the only licensed medication for obesity is the lipase inhibitor orlistat)
  - smoking cessation
  - increased exercise
- reduction of hypertension
- management of dyslipidaemia
- medication, for any or all of the above.

Management of obesity

Drugs should be used only as part of a general treatment plan for obesity. The only drug licensed for its role in obesity management is orlistat (marketed as Xenical by Roche and available over the counter), a lipase inhibitor that reduces fat absorption by about 30%. If the fat content of the diet is not reduced before the patient starts taking the drug, as evidenced by weight loss, the patient will complain (predictably) of loose stools and even soiling or oily discharge. Appropriate advice on diet and exercise is essential, as is behaviour management and appropriate support.

What constitutes success?

It is best to be realistic and not set or agree to extreme goals. It is better to achieve a goal and start again than to consider inability to achieve an impossible goal a

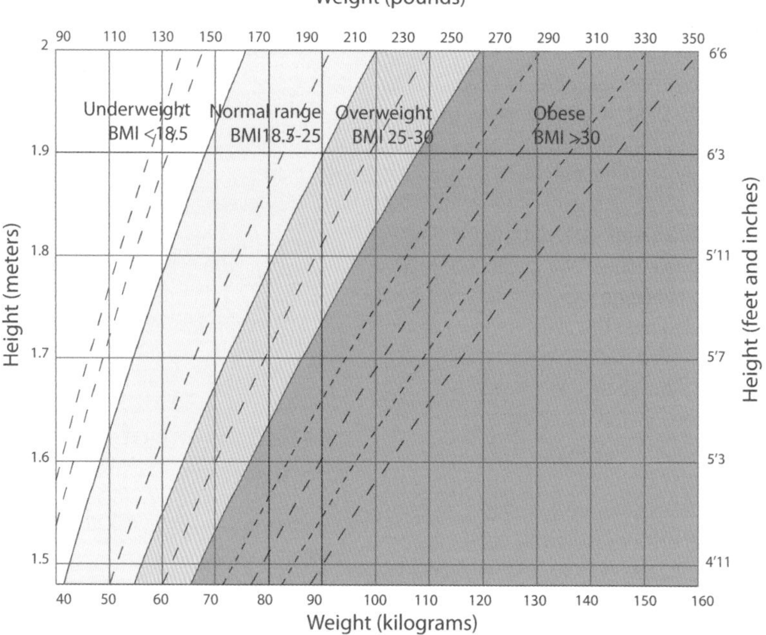

Fig. 2.1 Body mass index chart.

failure. Any weight loss is better than none. Suggested targets are:

- weight loss – 5–10% of pre-diet weight
- waist circumference – 5–10 cm reduction
- improved nutrition
- improved physical activity levels
- improved comorbid disease control and reduced medication
- improved risk markers
  - blood pressure
  - cholesterol and triglyceride levels
  - glucose, and $HbA1_c$ levels
- improved Quality and Outcomes Framework targets
- improved well-being
- increased self-esteem.

The patient may have other goals, often along the lines of dresses fit, rings not too tight, increased belt 'comfort', improved quality of life (such as knees not hurting).

The benefits of weight loss

Weight loss of 10% brings specific benefits to those who are morbidly obese:

- reduction in mortality
  - 20% fall in total mortality
  - > 30% fall in diabetes-related deaths
  - > 40% fall in obesity-related deaths
- reduction in blood pressure
  - fall of 10 mmHg systolic pressure
  - fall of 20 mmHg diastolic pressure
- improved control of diabetes
  - > 50% decreased risk of developing diabetes
  - 30–50% fall in fasting glucose
  - 15% decrease in $HbA1_c$
- reduced hyperlipidaemia
  - 10% decrease in total cholesterol
  - 15% decrease in low-density lipoprotein cholesterol
  - 30% decrease in triglycerides
  - 8% increase in high-density lipoprotein cholesterol.

Relevance of body weight to psychiatric patients

Patients with a psychiatric illness are prone to weight gain for many reasons, but the chief ones are that, generally, they take less exercise than the general population and many medications encourage weight gain and changes in body composition (Box 2.2). Weight gain has been recognised as a side-effect of the first psychotropic drugs to be used. Drug treatment of a psychiatric disorder is often accompanied by increased appetite or food craving and subsequent weight gain, most commonly in those on second-generation antipsychotic drugs, mood stabilisers and some (but not all) tricyclic antidepressants; 'conventional' antipsychotics tend to cause only slight to moderate weight gain.[27] This is fully discussed in other chapters. The tendency to weight loss in the early weeks after starting a serotonin reuptake inhibitor may be followed by weight gain with long-term treatment; obesity and its associated morbidity may lead to discontinued treatment.

Strategies to contain weight gain are essential to minimise the health risks due to concomitant hypertension, coronary heart disease, ischaemic stroke, impaired glucose tolerance, diabetes mellitus, dyslipidaemia, respiratory problems, osteoarthritis and cancer.

In addition, weight gain has psychosocial consequences, such as a sense of demoralisation, physical discomfort and substantial social stigma, which may be so intolerable that a patient may discontinue therapy even if it is effective.

If a patient was overweight prior to treatment, it is important to establish why. There may be fondness for sweet and fatty foods, 'food craving' or comfort eating. These may become even more apparent on treatment.

Box 2.2 Drugs associated with weight gain and changes in body composition

- Insulin
- Sulfonylureas
- Thiazolidinediones
- Steroids
- Some anticonvulsants (phenytoin and valproate)
- Pizotifen
- Some forms of hormonal contraception
- Psychiatric drugs
- Some antipsychotics
- Some antidepressant medications

Source: Haslam & James, 2005.[26]

Options for combating weight gain in psychiatric patients

Only trial and error will establish what method of weight loss (or at least maintenance) is best for each patient.

Diet and exercise and lifestyle modification are the usual initial interventions.[28] Depression, anxiety, bipolar disorder or schizophrenic disorder can diminish cooperation and compliance with medication but it is still important to warn each patient before they start treatment that weight gain is a likely side-effect and to offer counselling, combined with regular monitoring of weight, BMI, blood pressure, biological parameters (baseline and then 3-monthly evaluations of fasting glucose level, fasting cholesterol and triglyceride levels, and glycosylated haemoglobin).

Review any concomitant medications such as steroids that may facilitate weight gain or increase appetite.

If the clinical response to a psychiatric drug has been less than ideal, consider switching to another drug of the same or another class, as the tendency to encourage weight gain is less with some than others.

Review the patient's diet. This will require expert input as the source of calories may not be obvious. In some institutions, 'good' behaviour may be rewarded by providing access to the 'tuck' shop; if so, consider changing the shop's stock content gradually until there are only 'healthy' options. Avoid foods with a high-fat content and replace with low-fat options.[29]

Increasing physical activities may be feasible in some institutions. Even where this presents practical difficulties, a small amount of daily exercise can be beneficial. There is excellent advice on the web on simple daily recreational activities and the energy expenditure required to achieve these (see for example www.brianmac.co.uk/energyexp.htm).

A good start is a target of 10 000 steps a day. This can be assessed using simple belt-worn pedometers, which are accurate enough for most purposes.

If the patient is already overweight or obese, another option is treatment with orlistat (see above and Chapter 7). Reduction in dietary intake of fat is essential when taking orlistat, as it may cause oily rectal leakage, flatulence and faecal urgency.

Bulk-forming agents such as methyl cellulose give a feeling of satiety but there is little evidence of efficacy in weight control (see chapter 7, on obesity and weight management.

Vascular diseases

There is evidence that many cases of chronic vascular disease could be avoided by: adopting a Mediterranean-type diet,[30] increasing physical activity and stopping smoking. Even in countries in transition, cardiovascular risk appears early in life; in urban Tunisia, for example, schoolchildren are exposed to excess risk, with high rates of obesity, blood pressure, hypercholesterolaemia and smoking.[31]

In those countries where cardiovascular disease is in decline, such as Finland and the USA, the prevalence of risk factors is also greatly reduced.[32,33]

Cardiovascular disease

The Framingham Study (see Chapter 12) identified various factors that are associated with increased cardiovascular risk. Half of premature mortality is related to risky behaviour like cigarette smoking, alcohol misuse, lack of exercise, poor diet and substance misuse. These, in turn, are closely related to factors such as socioeconomic status, education and the availability of social supports in the community.

Summary

A 'modern' lifestyle has its undoubted advantages but these come at a price: reduced physical activity, increased calorie and fat intake and weight gain, and, with these, diabetes, the metabolic syndrome and vascular disease. Patients with psychiatric disorders are at even greater risk. All those involved in their care need to be proactive in reducing these risks as much as possible, especially as many patients do not have access to the medical services and facilities which those without psychiatric problems take for granted. Members of mental health teams must be prepared to act as surrogates, especially in in-patient units patients detained under mental health legislation.

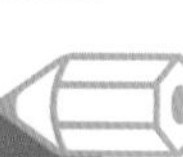

Learning points

- Modern lifestyle has changed both the nature of the diseases we acquire during life and the modality of death.
- With increasing affluence, chronic, non-communicable, degenerative diseases, notably type 2 diabetes, coronary heart disease, cerebrovascular disease, peripheral vascular disease, obesity and the metabolic syndrome and some cancers, have become increasingly common.
- Half of premature mortality is related to risky behaviour, often related to socioeconomic factors, education level and social support.
- The metabolic syndrome is a cluster of risk factors for diabetes and cardiovascular disease that occurs more frequently than by chance alone.
- Obesity is becoming more prevalent; it has adverse effects on physical and psychological health.
- Psychiatric patients are at increased risk because screening (taken for granted by those without psychiatric illness) is often not available.
- Members of mental health teams must be prepared to provide surrogate general practitioner services.
- Weight gain in psychiatric patients is problematic, and a range of strategies need to be considered to contain an increased BMI secondary to psychotropic medication.

References

1 World Health Organization. WHO Mortality Database: Tables. WHO, 2005 (http://www.who.int/healthinfo/morttables/en/index.html).

2 Bandolier. Effect of lifestyle on death and disease (http://www.medicine.ox.ac.uk/bandolier/booth/hliving/Lifedeath.html).

3 Himmelstein DU, Woolhandler S. Obama's reform: no cure for what ails us. *BMJ* 2010; **340**: 742.

4 UC Atlas of Global Inequality. Health care spending (http://ucatlas.ucsc.edu/spend.php).

5 US National Center for Health Statistics. Priority Area Progress Figures. In *Healthy People 2000 Final Review*. Public Health Service, 2001 (http://www.cdc.gov/nchs/data/hp2000/hp2k01.pdf).

6 Diabetes UK. *Diabetes in the UK in 2010: Key Statistics on Diabetes.* Diabetes UK, 2010.

7 International Diabetes Federation. *Diabetes Atlas* (5th edn). *IDF,* 2011 (http://www.idf.org/diabetesatlas).

8 World Health Organization. *WHO Chronic Disease Information Sheets: Diabetes.* WHO, 2006.

9 Department of Health. *Health Survey for England 2003. DH,* 2004.

10 Franco OH, Steyerberg EW, Hu FB, *et al.* Associations of diabetes mellitus with total life expectancy and life expectancy with and without cardiovascular disease. *Arch Intern Med* 2007; **167**: 1145–51.

11 Crandall JP, Knowler WC, Kahn SE, *et al.* The prevention of type 2 diabetes. *Nat Clin Pract Endocrin Metab* 2008; **4**: 382–93.

12 Toumielehto T, Lindström J, Erikkson JG, *et al.* Finnish Diabetes Prevention Study. *Prevention of type 2* diabetes mellitus by changes in lifestyle among subjects with impaired glucose tolerance. *N Engl J Med* 2001; **344**: 1343–50.

13 Knowler WC, Barrett-Connor E, Fowler SE, *et al.* Reduction in the incidence of type 2 diabetes with lifestyle intervention or metformin. *N Engl J Med* 2002; **346**: 393–403.

14 National Obesity Observatory. *Trends in Obesity Prevalence.* NOO, 2010 (http://www.noo.org.uk/NOO_about_obesity/trends).

15 Sahota P, Barth JH, Rudolf MCJ, *et al.* Obesity in childhood frequently leads to obesity in adulthood. *BMJ* 2001; **322**: 1094–5.

16 Pereira MA, Kartashov AI, Ebbeling CB, *et al.* Fast-food habits, weight gain, and insulin resistance (the CARDIA study): 15-year prospective analysis. *Lancet* 2005; **365**: 36–42.

17 Select Committee on Health. *Health – Third Report.* Health Committee Publications, 2004.

18 Young LR, Nestle M. Portion sizes and obesity: responses of fast-food companies. *J Publ Health Policy* 2007; **28**: 238–48.

19 Eckel RH for the Nutrition Committee. Obesity and Heart Disease: A Statement for Healthcare Professionals from the Nutrition Committee, American Heart Association. *Circulation* 1997; **96**: 3248–50.

20 International Diabetes Federation. *The IDF Consensus Worldwide Definition of the Metabolic Syndrome.* IDF, 2006.

21 Kahn R, Buse J, Ferranninni E, *et al.* The metabolic syndrome: time for a critical appraisal: joint statement from the American Diabetes Association and the European Association for the Study of Diabetes. *Diabetes Care* 2005; **28**: 2289–304.

22 Han TS, Williams K, Sattar N, *et al.* Analysis of obesity and hyperinsulinaemia in the development of the metabolic syndrome (San Antonio Heart Study). *Obes Res* 2002; **10**: 923–31.

23 Pouliot MC, Despres JP, Lemieux S, *et al.* Waist circumference and abdominal sagittal diameter: best simple anthropometric indexes of abdominal visceral adipose tissue accumulation and related cardiovascular risk in men and women. *Am J Cardiol* 1994; **73**: 460–8.

24 The NHS Information Centre. *Statistics on Obesity, Physical Activity and Diet: England, 2006.* The Information Centre, 2006.

25 Janssen I, Katzmarzyk PT, Ross R. Waist circumference and not body mass index explains obesity-related health risk. *Am J Clin Nutr* 2004; **79**: 379–84.

26 Haslam DW, James WP. Obesity. *Lancet* 2005; **366**: 1197–209.

27 Ruetsch O, Viala A, Bardou H, *et al.* Psychotropic drugs induced weight gain: a review of the literature concerning epidemiological data, mechanisms and management. *Encephale* 2005; **31**: 507–16.

28 Scottish Intercollegiate Guidelines Network. *Management of Obesity: Quick Reference Guide.* SIGN, 2010.

29 Weststrate JA. Fat and obesity. *Int J Obes Relat Metab Disord* 1995; **19** (suppl): S38–43.

30 Sofi F, Cesari F, Abbate R, *et al.* Adherence to Mediterranean diet and health status: meta-analysis. *BMJ* 2008; **337**: a1344

31 Ghannem H, Darioli R, Limam K, *et al.* Epidemiology of cardiovascular risk factors among schoolchildren in Sousse, Tunisia. *J Cardiovasc Risk* 2001; **8**: 87–91.

32 Vartiainen E, Laatikainen T, Peltonen M, *et al.* Thirty-five-year trends in cardiovascular risk factors in Finland. *Int J Epidemiol* 2010; **39**: 504–18.

33 Arnett DK, McGovern PG, Jacobs DR Jr, *et al.* Fifteen-year trends in cardiovascular risk factors (1980–1982 through 1995–1997): the Minnesota Heart Survey. *Am J Epidemiology* 2002; **156**: 929–935.

3
General practice in the UK

Alan Cohen

This chapter describes the role of the general practitioner as a point of first contact in providing healthcare and preventive care; coordinating care as part of the multidisciplinary team; and interacting with the mental health team. It also suggests how patients may be helped to get the best out of the general practitioner service.

Introduction

Describing primary care, and hence its role in caring for people with mental health problems, is not entirely straightforward. Primary care can be described in terms of:

- those who provide care
- where that care is provided
- the type of care available/provided, or
- for whom that care is provided.

In practice, to understand primary care and its role, all these aspects need to be understood.

Primary care provides the patient's first point of contact with the National Health Service (NHS), apart from accidents and emergencies. In addition, the primary care role includes acting as a gatekeeper to other services to ensure that those who need to be seen by secondary care are referred (and that those who do not need referral are managed appropriately) and offering continuity of care for a wide range of chronic diseases.

The range of services available in primary care is great. The sector serves people with acute, self-limiting conditions as well as those with long-term conditions such as asthma or diabetes. It also provides care across the life-span, from prenatal and antenatal care, through monitoring child development (Fig. 3.1) to end-of-life care.

Primary care additionally incorporates advice on health promotion and illness prevention, such as childhood vaccinations; it also provides rehabilitation services, care coordination, care commissioning and in some cases service development and research. Primary care offers healthcare for people with social, psychological

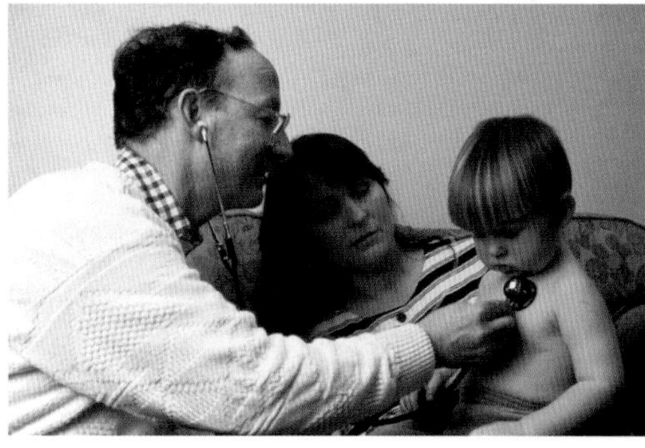

Fig. 3.1 Home visit, chest examination.

or physical health needs. Services are provided to individuals within a fixed or defined population.

Primary care services are community-based, being part of the community, with staff who are often community residents who reflect local community characteristics and contribute to their community. The staff are professionals operating in a multidisciplinary team that is frequently led by the general practitioner (GP), trained to deliver healthcare that starts with the 'undifferentiated' or 'unorganised' presentation of symptoms, and to organise those symptoms into an assessment and classification that acknowledges the social, psychological and biological needs of the individual. This chapter focuses on GPs and others who work in primary care.

It is important to distinguish the difference between primary care services and the services provided by general practice surgeries:

- General practitioners are self-employed doctors, who work from premises that they either own or rent; they usually employ their own staff, including nurses and other health professionals, and the doctor sets the characteristics of how that group of individuals will work together.
- Primary care services are more loosely defined but include those provided by district nurses, health visitors, midwives, social workers, 'end of life' teams, primary care mental health teams, and other healthcare providers who work predominantly in the community rather than in the hospital environment. Sometimes members of primary care services such as district nurses, health visitors and social workers may also be part of the GP team, while not being directly employed by the GP. This is a pragmatic approach to what is organisationally rather confusing and has a particular name – the primary healthcare team (PHCT). The PHCT is an extremely effective multidisciplinary team that addresses the biopsychosocial needs of individuals within a fixed population.

General practitioners

One of the most frequently quoted descriptions of a GP is the 1974 definition from Leeuwenhorst (the 'Leeuwenhorst Declaration'):

> The general practitioner is a licensed medical graduate who gives personal, primary and continuing care to individuals, families and a practice population irrespective of age, sex and illness. It is the synthesis of these functions which is unique.[1]

General practice has been described as organising the chaos of the first presentation.

While there continues to be a debate about the exact definition,[2] the most widely accepted version comes from the Royal College of General Practitioners:[3]

> General practitioners/family doctors are specialist physicians trained in the principles of the discipline. They are personal doctors, primarily responsible for the provision of comprehensive and continuing care to every individual seeking medical care irrespective of age, sex and illness.
>
> They care for individuals in the context of their family, their community and their culture, always respecting the autonomy of their patients.
>
> They recognise they will also have a professional responsibility to their community.
>
> In negotiating management plans with their patients they integrate physical, psychological, social, cultural and existential factors, utilising the knowledge and trust engendered by repeated contacts.
>
> General practitioners/family physicians exercise their professional role by promoting health, preventing disease and providing cure, care or palliation. This is done either directly or through the services of others according to health needs and the resources available within the community they serve, assisting patients where necessary in accessing these services.
>
> They must take the responsibility for developing and maintaining their skills, personal balance and values as a basis for effective and safe patient care.

Some key facts about GPs

Here are some key facts about general practitioners.[3]

- GPs refer 14% of the population to hospital specialties, meaning that 86% of all health needs are managed within primary care.
- Over 250 million consultations take place annually in general practice, with 15% of the population seeing a GP in any 2-week period.
- Around 42 000 GPs work in 10 500 surgeries in the UK. There are more GPs than all consultants in all specialties combined.
- The average patient will visit their GP about four times a year, with 78% of people consulting their GP at least once during each year.
- Each GP looks after 2000 patients on average and conducts about 7000 consultations per year.
- About 40% of the GP workforce in England is female, compared with 25% a decade ago.

- About a quarter of all practices in the UK are single-handed (i.e. operating with only one GP).

Characteristics of a GP

These criteria are based on the Royal College of General Practitioners information leaflet.[4]

First point of contact

Normally, GPs are the point of first medical contact within the healthcare system. They provide healthcare 'free at the point of access' for all people registered with the practice, irrespective of age or sex. Practices provide care for a specific (geographically defined) population – they have a registered list of people for whom they are responsible.

Everybody has the right to be registered with a GP. If the patient is unable to find a GP, the local primary care trust (PCT) can allocate that patient to a GP, who, under the terms of contract, is obliged to accept the patient. Except in emergencies, GPs are not entitled to provide care for people who are not part of their registered list. The absolute need to treat only patients on the registered list is frequently important when considering people with a severe mental illness whose carer is not registered with the patient's practice. The GP cannot intervene directly with the carer of their patient in a medical sense, and so where the health of the carer is an issue, the usual route is to speak to the carer's GP directly.

Coordinate care

General practitioners work as part of a multidisciplinary team – the PHCT. GPs are also responsible for referring patients to clinical specialists for care, when it is appropriate – this is their gatekeeping role.

There are some similarities between the community mental health team and the PHCT. Both act as the first point of contact, and both have the opportunity to refer patients to a more specialist service if appropriate. In primary care, there seem to be fewer issues relating to how teams work, such as who is the team leader. This may be because of the dual role of the GP as both a colleague to, and in some cases as employer of, other members of the team. While this can clearly have some complicated and perhaps difficult consequences, it does make the leadership very clear, which brings benefits in terms of decision-making.

Only 14% of all patients are referred to specialists, but less than 10% of patients with mental health problems are referred to specialist mental health teams.[5]

> No medical specialty, other than mental health, returns patients to general practice because they are not ill enough. For those with the most common diagnosis seen in primary care, depression and anxiety, being told they are not ill enough, added to their own feelings of negativity, makes engagement with healthcare services difficult.

This means that over 90% of people with mental health problems are managed entirely in primary care. The process of referral to a specialist is complicated so far as the therapeutic relationship with the patient is concerned; it can be interpreted by the patient as though the GP no longer wishes to care for the patient, or is unable to provide the care that they believe is needed.

For that referral to be made and then rejected by the specialist mental health trust because the patient does not have a severe and enduring mental illness – the National Service Framework (NSF) recommends that specialist mental health trusts prioritise those with a severe and enduring mental illness – sends a very confusing message to both patient and GP. There is no other medical specialty where patients are returned to general practice because they are not ill enough. For the GP, this suggests a distant and uninterested organisation behaving unlike any other medical specialty. For patients, the message is even more confusing; they do not merit a specialist opinion. For people who are referred for depression and anxiety – the most common diagnoses seen in primary care – to be told that they are not ill enough, on top of their own feelings of negativity, makes further support and engagement with healthcare services difficult.

As attention is increasingly focused on the physical health of people with mental health problems, the role of the GP as a coordinator of care becomes more important. People with schizophrenia are more likely to suffer from diabetes and metabolic syndrome. Later chapters in this book describe the detailed management of these conditions. However, few psychiatrists, and fewer mental health teams, have the experience and knowledge to manage these conditions, which, like schizophrenia, are complex, long-term disorders. In the same way that it is inappropriate – in most cases – for a GP to manage a patient with schizophrenia, it is equally inappropriate – in most cases – for a mental health team to believe that they can manage a person with diabetes or metabolic syndrome.

It is clearly the role of GPs to coordinate the care of an individual who has both schizophrenia and some other long-term condition. GPs may manage the long-term condition themselves, or, if they feel it appropriate, refer the patient to a specialist team for advice. Caring for people with schizophrenia and diabetes is more complicated than caring for people with diabetes alone, and requires a greater knowledge and specialist support than would otherwise be the case.

Long-term physical conditions in individuals with other forms of severe and enduring mental illness are more common but also more complicated to manage, making the role of the GP in coordinating care essential. It has often been suggested that these vulnerable patients may not wish to register with a GP, or have difficulty finding a practice that will accept them. Every patient has the right to be registered with a practice, and a patient can be allocated to a practice. It should be the responsibility of every mental health team to ensure that each of the patients for whom they provide care is registered with a general practice.

The person-centred approach

General practitioners identify people and their problems in the context of their life circumstances, developing a person-centred approach orientated towards the individual, the family and their community. In addition to dealing with the disease process, a good GP understands how the patient copes with and views the illness. This approach is one that is shared with mental health professionals. It describes the biopsychosocial approach to healthcare, and begins to address the individual patient's understanding of what symptoms, and diagnoses might mean.

The unique consultation process

General practitioners have a unique consultation process, which, through effective communication between doctor and patient, over time establishes a relationship. Each contact between the patient and family doctor contributes to an evolving story and each individual consultation can draw on this prior shared experience. The value of this relationship is determined by the communication skills of the family doctor and the relationship can be therapeutic in itself.

Extensive research has shown that, on average, GPs identify only about 50% of people with a mental health problem. The research has all been carried out in a similar fashion: patients in the waiting room are given a questionnaire – originally the General Health Questionnaire (GHQ) – and then after the consultation the finding from that questionnaire is compared with the clinical view of the GP. The finding is validated against a 'gold standard' – an interview, usually lasting at least an hour, by a research psychiatrist. The research is therefore rather imbalanced, in that it compares a 10-minute unorganised consultation with an hour-long interview with a psychiatrist. Consider a GP with six 10-minute consultations with the patient; the GP identifies half of the patients with a mental health problem in the first consultation, and then half the remainder at the second and subsequent consultations; by the end of the sixth consultation, both GP and research psychiatrist would have achieved the same identification rate. This demonstrates the importance of the evolving story, the importance of time, the importance of the therapeutic relationship between patient and GP that research fails to acknowledge.

General practitioners are skilled communicators and this helps them sort out and organise the presenting problem. GPs must distinguish between potential diagnoses, for example abdominal pain caused either by an ulcer or by the stress of unemployment. More likely, the GP may find that both an ulcer and unemployment are significant features in the presentation, and manage both problems.

Continuity of care

General practitioners provide 'longitudinal' continuity of care, meaning that care is provided by as few professionals as possible, and is consistent with the patient's other needs. The general practice patient record provides a narrative of the health and care of patients throughout the whole of their life. It is the task of family doctors to be responsible for providing direct care to their patients during core hours, or commissioning and coordinating care when they are unable to provide it personally.

Almost unique in the world, the medical record for an individual receiving care from an NHS GP follows the patient to another GP surgery if the patient moves house. Thus the GP record provides a narrative that describes the health and social care needs of that individual. As the electronic practice record becomes more common, there is a need to ensure that the narrative aspect of the clinical record is not lost. A more complete understanding of the mental health needs of

A more complete understanding of the mental health needs of an individual can often be provided by a careful review of the clinical records held by the GP.

an individual can often be provided by a careful review of the clinical records held by the GP.

Multiple illnesses

General practitioners simultaneously manage both acute and chronic health problems of individual patients. The patient often consults for several complaints at the same time, the number increasing with age. The doctor has to manage multiple and complex problems by setting and negotiating priorities with the patient.

People with schizophrenia also get common illnesses such as an upper respiratory tract infection. Similarly, people with diabetes may also get depressed. GPs need to be able to manage and distinguish between the various disorders and the symptoms that relate to those diagnoses. In some groups of people, it is more likely that they will have more than one disorder, and this includes those with a severe mental illness – which provides in part the rationale for this book.

Diagnostic uncertainty

General practitioners manage 'undifferentiated' or imprecise symptoms, often at early stages in the development of an illness. This means that important decisions for patients have to be taken on the basis of limited information, with early signs of disease often non-specific to a particular condition. Having excluded an immediately serious outcome, the decision may well be to await further developments and review later. Frequently, the job of the family doctor is to reassure those with understandable anxieties about illness – having first determined that such illness is not present.

Understanding whether a person who complains of abdominal pain has a duodenal ulcer or is stressed by being made unemployed is the art of general practice. At the first consultation a patient may not be identified as suffering from a mental health condition – perhaps because they present with a physical symptom, and it is necessary to address that as well as any underlying emotional problem. Disentangling whether abdominal pain is due to an ulcer or emotional stress takes time; to expect a single 10-minute consultation to cover

One of the skills of the GP is the ability to tolerate the uncertainty of not knowing precisely what is happening, but to continue to provide support while symptoms progress or resolve. One example of this is 'watchful waiting' for people with depression.

the presentation of the symptoms, diagnosis, any investigations and the agreement of a treatment plan is unrealistic.

Frequently, even after several consultations it may not be clear exactly what is happening. One of the skills or characteristics of the GP is the ability to tolerate the uncertainty of not knowing precisely what is happening, but to arrange the consultation process to continue to provide support while symptoms progress or resolve. One example of this is 'watchful waiting' for people with depression. It is recommended[6] that primary care professionals keep a watching brief and regularly review people with mild depression, especially those in the early stages, as the condition may resolve spontaneously, or it may become clearer over time that the underlying condition is some other problem, such as post-traumatic stress disorder (PTSD).

There is a period of diagnostic uncertainty, which needs to be managed in a supportive fashion, with the GP offering advice to the patient, while not being in a position to make a definitive diagnosis, or making clear recommendations about treatment. This is a major part of the art of general practice.

The GP contract and the Quality and Outcomes Framework

General practitioners, unlike consultants or other medical staff employed by specialist mental health trusts, are self-employed. In 2004, a new contract was introduced for them, which introduced several new concepts.[7] For the first time it defined what was considered essential care:

To expect a single 10-minute consultation to cover the patient's history, diagnosis, investigations and treatment plan is unrealistic.

- management of patients who are ill, or who believe themselves to be so, with conditions from which recovery is generally expected, for the duration of that condition, including relevant health promotion advice and referral as appropriate, reflecting patient choice wherever practicable
- general management of terminally ill patients
- management of chronic disease in the manner determined by the practice, in discussion with the patient.

Defining essential services allows the principle that any care above and beyond this level of care should be separately remunerated, and is classed as an 'enhanced service'. The issue of how to ensure high-quality evidenced-based essential care was managed through the development of the Quality and Outcomes Framework (QOF). In outline, this is a system by which practices can score points for achieving certain targets or goals in specific different clinical and management areas. Each point has a monetary value, which (in theory) increases year on year. In total there are some 1050 points available to practices, of which 550 relate to clinical areas of care.

The clinical areas cover a number of different domains, such as diabetes and asthma. For each domain, there are a number of separate indicators; for the depression domain, for example, there are three indicators (discussed in more detail below).

Every 2 years, the clinical evidence supporting the various clinical indicators is reviewed by a group of experts who make recommendations for change to the negotiators of the contract. Sometimes these recommendations are accepted and sometimes they need to be altered to convert the sense of the recommendation into something that will work effectively as an indicator.

In 2010 the process was changed so that the review was undertaken by the National Institute for Health and Clinical Excellence (NICE). The intention was that there would be an explicit link between published guidelines and the development of QOF indicators. NICE's first amendments to the QOF were published in April 2011.

Mental health and the Quality and Outcomes Framework

There are two clinical domains that relate to mental healthcare: 'mental health' and 'depression'.

Mental health domain

The mental health domain has changed from its introduction in 2004 (see Table 3.1). Other changes over time indicate how the QOF is an evolving process; the first indicator in this domain (MH1) was changed in 2006 to be more specific about the sort of people to be included. Other changes include the omission of MH3 – which incentivises an aspect of the care of people taking lithium,

Table 3.1 The mental health domain in the QOF for 2004 and 2006

Domain	Indicator	Points
MH8	The practice can produce a register of patients with schizophrenia, bipolar disorder and other psychoses	4
MH9	The percentage of patients with schizophrenia, bipolar affective disorder and other psychoses with a review recorded in the preceding 15 months. In the review there should be evidence that the patient has been offered routine health promotion and prevention advice appropriate to their age, gender and health status	23
MH4	The percentage of patients on lithium therapy with a record of serum creatinine and thyroid stimulating hormone in the preceding 15 months	1
MH5	The percentage of patients on lithium therapy with a record of lithium levels in the therapeutic range within the previous 6 months	2
MH6	The percentage of patients on the register who have a comprehensive care plan documented in the records agreed between individuals, their family doctor and/or carers, as appropriate	6
MH7	The percentage of patients on the register who do not attend the practice for their annual review who are identified and followed up by the practice team within 14 days of non-attendance	3

QOF, Quality and Outcomes Framework

Table 3.2 The mental health domain in the QOF for 2012

Domain	Indicator	Points
MH8	The practice can produce a register of people with schizophrenia, bipolar disorder and other psychoses	4
MH11	The percentage of patients with schizophrenia, bipolar affective disorder and other psychoses who have a record of alcohol consumption in the preceding 15 months	4
MH12	The percentage of patients with schizophrenia, bipolar affective disorder and other psychoses who have a record of BMI in the preceding 15 months	4
MH13	The percentage of patients with schizophrenia, bipolar affective disorder and other psychoses who have a record of blood pressure in the preceding 15 months	4
MH14	The percentage of patients aged 40 years and over with schizophrenia, bipolar affective disorder and other psychoses who have a record of total cholesterol:HDL ratio in the preceding 15 months	5
MH15	The percentage of patients aged 40 years and over with schizophrenia, bipolar affective disorder and other psychoses who have a record of blood glucose in the preceding15 months	5
MH16	The percentage of patients (aged 25–64 in England and Northern Ireland, 20–60 in Scotland and 20–64 in Wales) with schizophrenia, bipolar affective disorder and other psychoses who had a cervical screening test in the preceding 5 years	5
MH17	The percentage of patients on lithium therapy with a record of serum creatinine and TSH in the preceding 9 months	1
MH18	The percentage of patients on lithium therapy with a record of lithium levels in the therapeutic range in the preceding 4 months	2
MH10	The percentage of patients on the register who have a comprehensive care plan documented in the records agreed between individuals, their family and/or carers as appropriate	6

BMI, body mass index; HDL, high-density lipoprotein; QOF, Quality and Outcomes Framework; TSH, thyroid-stimulating hormone.

Table 3.3 The depression domain in the QOF 2012

Domain	Indicator	Points
DEP1	The percentage of patients on the diabetes register and/or the coronary heart disease (CHD) register for whom case finding for depression has been undertaken on one occasion during the previous 15 months using two standard screening questions	8
DEP2	In those patients with a new diagnosis of depression, recorded between the preceding 1 April and 31 March, the percentage of patients who have had an assessment of severity at the outset of treatment using an assessment tool validated for use in primary care	25
DEP3	In those patients with a new diagnosis of depression and assessment of severity recorded between the preceding 1 April and 31 March, the percentage of patients who have had a further assessment of severity 5–12 weeks (inclusive) after the initial recording of the assessment of severity. Both assessments should be completed using an assessment tool validated for use in primary care	20

QOF, Quality and Outcomes Framework

Ensure that the practice receives the documentation for the care programme approach (CPA) , as this allows the practice to complete MH6 – the practice does *not* need to duplicate the CPA process, but can use the trust papers. It also allows the practice to concentrate on patients who are not in contact with the mental health trust.

and the inclusion of two new indicators, MH6 and MH7, which incentivise the recording of the presence of a care plan and incentivises the active, assertive follow-up of patients who do not attend a planned appointment. There were no changes to this part of the QOF in 2008.

In April 2011, the mental health domain was further reviewed, and the rather nebulous and poorly described MH9 was omitted to be replaced with six new indicators specifying new evidence-based measures (Table 3.2).

The total number of points available for these six new indicators is the same as for the indicator that they replaced.

Depression domain

In 2006 a new clinical domain was introduced for the care of people with depression. It had two indicators; in 2008 a third indicator was added (Table 3.3).

Although only two indicators were originally agreed, the intention was to implement some of the recommendations that were made in the NICE guidelines for depression.[6] People with some long-term conditions are more likely to suffer from depression, and therefore case-finding, as recommended in the NICE guidelines, is considered excellent practice. The indicator (DEP2) introduced the principle of assessing the severity of depression so that the intervention offered could be linked to the stepped-care approach recommended by NICE. In 2008, a further indicator (DEP3) was introduced, which incentivised follow-up at 3 months of patients with depression, by the use of the same severity questionnaire.

Other members of the primary healthcare team

Other members of the PHCT include nursing and administrative staff.

The practice nursing staff has three broad levels of seniority: nurse practitioners (the most senior), then practice nurses and then healthcare assistants. Not all practices will have nurses of all levels of seniority, and there are considerable levels of overlap between the first two levels. A nurse practitioner is a nurse competent to practise independently and in some cases to prescribe independently of the GP. Nurse practitioners can take responsibility for managing long-term conditions such as diabetes and ischaemic heart disease, and as part of that management will consult with their GP only when the management is complex or not straightforward. Nurse practitioners may be responsible for triaging patients who attend and request an emergency appointment. Practice nurses have a similar role, but less independence to manage these conditions, so their contact with GPs and degree of supervision will be greater. Both nurses and nurse practitioners undertake the more standard nursing procedures in a practice, such as dressings and vaccinations. Healthcare assistants are a relatively new addition to the practice team and undertake less complex tasks such as venesection and recording blood pressure and temperatures.

Administrative staff may include a practice manager, receptionists and computer technicians (though not necessarily all of these). The practice manager runs the practice, ensuring that all the administrative functions such as appointments, employment law, accounts, and information technology (IT) systems are in place and working effectively. Receptionists are the first point of contact with patients, and although they may have a reputation as a 'dragon', this is frequently not the case. Receptionists are trained to manage people's anger and frustration, and understand that these emotions are related to patients' concerns about their health. A practice depends on its computer system, as in most practices all clinical records are kept only on the IT system. Computer records are regularly scrutinised remotely to calculate the payments that practices receive from the QOF. Thus IT systems are essential for both clinical care and payments. Most practices employ a specialist to ensure that the practice system is up to date and working efficiently.

Practice-attached mental health staff, who have mental health training, make up about 3% of nurses working in primary care; only about 50% of PCTs employ counsellors or psychologists. It is unclear how many individual practices employ their own counsellor or a psychologist.

The advent of the Improving Access to Psychological Therapies (IAPT) programme is changing this picture considerably. This programme ensures a consistent approach, with a consistent set of outcome data to assess progress, for those people who are not appropriate to be managed in secondary care but who cannot be managed with confidence in primary care. While the IAPT programme is welcomed by GPs, there is still an underlying anxiety that failure to directly employ the staff providing the psychological therapies means that there is less control over the patients who are seen. In part this has been overcome, by ensuring that the IAPT staff work from GP surgeries and maintain a personal relationship with the practice staff, which generates trust and more appropriate referrals.

Proactive *v.* reactive care

Primary care provides preventive care. Primary prevention is the provision of care to prevent illness. This is best exemplified by the administration of childhood vaccinations – preventing the development of infections such as tetanus, polio and measles. The vaccination programme is delivered by the practice nurse and requires an up-to-date list of all patients of a particular age, so that the children can be offered appropriate vaccinations according to a schedule set out by the Department of Health. Screening programmes could be seen as very early secondary prevention; these include cervical cancer screening and breast mammography. A programme has recently been introduced for the detection of cancer of the bowel, and another is planned for people with cardiovascular disease. The development of the former is of particular interest to people with schizophrenia, as they appear to have an increased risk of carcinoma of the bowel, from the evidence provided to the Disability Rights Commission.[8] The move towards more preventive care is a major priority for the current government.

Secondary prevention is the care of those patients who have or have had symptoms that suggest an underlying disease, such as coronary heart or cerebrovascular disease.

Tertiary prevention is generally understood to be the rehabilitation of those with a chronic condition such as stroke. However, a better definition is the care provided to people with chronic disorders. Chronic or long-term conditions account for the major part of hospital admissions, and NHS costs. Long-term conditions include:

- diabetes
- ischaemic heart disease
- chronic neurological conditions
- chronic renal disease
- chronic obstructive pulmonary disease (COPD).

Without the ability to search computer databases, it is not possible to identify people who are at risk, be it of diabetes or depression, and to offer proactive care. If computer systems are used in psychiatric settings for physical health, they should have the same capability as GPs' systems.

The management of these conditions is undertaken by the nurse practitioner or practice nurse. There is a system for 'call and recall' of patients with long-term conditions to special clinics held at the surgery, to provide the standardised care set out in 'best practice' guidelines. The 'call and recall' system requires an up-to-date and effective IT system that can identify the correct patients and follow up of those who fail to attend.

Information technology

Primary care introduced IT systems over 20 years ago to support high-quality clinical care (Fig. 3.2).

Data are entered as codes, rather than free text, to facilitate searches. The codes are based on a system initially developed many years ago by a GP, Dr Read. The Read code system is hierarchical and originally did not relate to the World Health Organization's *International Classification of Disease* (ICD), or, in the area of mental health, the American Psychiatric Association's *Diagnostic and Statistical Manual of Mental Disorder* (DSM). The Read code system differs from the ICD or DSM by including processes other than diagnoses, such as codes for history and examination findings, operations and family history.

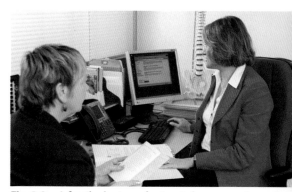

Fig. 3.2 A family doctor referring to her computer and printed literature in order to help a patient.

Over the years, the Read code system has changed and evolved to become closer to the codes used in the ICD and DSM. So, in mental health, the Read 'E' codes relate to the ICD-10 'F' codes. However, as old codes are not deleted, there may be a number of codes for a particular condition; for those codes that relate specifically to ICD, the 'E' prefix is followed by a 'u', indicating that it is the same code in the ICD and DSM systems. Hence the code for generalised anxiety disorder in the Read code system is Eu411, and the code for this disorder in ICD is F41.1. Over the past few years, attempts have been made to bring these codes together, in a system called SNOMED-CT.

The IT system used by practices on which clinical records are stored also allows the database to be interrogated to allow payments made under the QOF. For example, practices are incentivised to provide high-quality care to people with diabetes, and a measure of excellent control of diabetes is a glycosylated haemoglobin ($HbA1_c$) level under 6%. Practices are financially rewarded if 90% of diabetic patients meet this criterion. Practice computer systems are interrogated to assess how closely a practice comes to this target. Computer systems will also identify patients who are not achieving this level of care so that they can be recalled to review their care. Screening and proactive care are greatly facilitated by a modern IT system.

Registering with a general practice

Everybody is entitled to be registered with a GP. In the general population, 97% of people are registered with a general practice. However, there is some anecdotal evidence that some groups of people find it difficult to register with a particular practice. The 2004 General Medical Services (GMS) contract attempted to deal with this problem by requiring practices to describe their list as being 'open' or 'closed':

- an 'open list' requires GPs to accept any patient living within an area previously agreed with the PCT
- a 'closed list' does not have to accept any new patients, usually because the number registered was already greater than could be reasonably managed by the practice. Since a practice with a 'closed list' was busy, it faced financial sanctions, as the practice was unable to bid for extra services that could generate extra income.

The intention of the GMS contract was clear – to provide a financial incentive to encourage open lists. However, there was a rider inserted into the contract that acknowledged that, in some cases, an 'open' practice might be unable to accept new patients because, for example, a nurse or doctor might be ill. Such a list was described as 'open but full' and in theory allowed practices to be more selective about which patients they accepted.

The Department of Health has attempted to deal with this problem by incentivising the development of new practices in areas that are relatively under-doctored, and by allowing the development of new practices in areas where there is a particular population with specific needs. Thus, in areas where there may be a large number of refugees and asylum seekers, who on their own would not be sufficient to sustain a general practice, alternative funding streams are available to ensure that these vulnerable groups receive primary care services. These are known as personal medical services (PMS) practices.

Psychiatric patients

Community mental health teams (CMHTs) will often be aware which local practices are willing to take patients with particular problems. Continued effective care is more likely to be achieved by close personal working relationships (Box 3.1) and appropriate support to a practice than is the apparent 'dumping' of a difficult patient by the PCT. A 'give and take' approach is essential for the effective management of difficult patients.

As a last resort, a patient who has difficulty registering with a practice may be allocated by the PCT to a practice without the agreement of the GP, who must provide care

Box 3.1 Effective collaboration between mental health and primary care

Community mental health teams (CMHTs) and primary healthcare teams need to resolve different pressures and this may be facilitated by regular face-to-face meetings. The South-West London Mental Health Trust pioneered such meetings, which staff found very helpful. The CMHT ran through all the patients for which it cared, who were registered with that practice, to discuss their progress and ongoing care. General practice staff could air concerns about patients who might otherwise be referred, and could learn from specialists about the management of difficult patients. This resulted in improved care for patients and a better understanding of how the other team worked.

for 3 months before removing the patient from the list. This occurs infrequently but sadly includes some with a mental health problem and particularly those who are violent or potentially violent. For a restricted number of such patients each PCT has identified one practice that is set up to deal with violent and abusive patients. The surgery premises are designed to manage violent patients and the staff are specially trained.

In the same way that a patient may choose to leave a practice, so a practice may choose to remove a patient from the registered list. Anecdotally this occurs more frequently with patients with a severe mental illness, but there is little hard evidence to support this. Whatever the reason for a patient being removed from a GP's list, the advice from the General Practitioner Committee of the British Medical Association is clear; the patient should be informed of the reason, preferably face to face but at least in writing. The PCT should be informed and patients should not be removed during an active course of treatment. Ideally, patients should be given some warning that their behaviour is threatening their registration at the practice. Despite all this advice, there are still instances when patients arrive at the surgery only to be told that they have been removed from the practice list for no apparent (in the patient's view) reason.

For patients who have been removed from a practice list, the PCT will help them find another practice and, as described above, can if necessary allocate the patient to a practice.

Patients sometimes ask if they can 'appeal' against the decision of the practice. There is no specific process for appeal as such, unless the decision was taken because of a mistaken belief that the patient had moved out of the practice catchment area. Trying to repair a relationship between doctor and patient that has been so badly damaged that the practice has removed the patient from their list may not be realistic. It may be possible, however, for the CMHT to intercede early on behalf of a patient, especially if they are aware that the behaviour is deteriorating due to a mental illness.

Communication with a general practice

Communication with the practice is an area fraught with difficulty. The PHCT and the CMHT work in different ways and this often means that communication is sometimes difficult. CMHTs tend to provide care to a number of practices and it would be very convenient if all those practices communicated in a similar way. However, practices are all different and have different communication preferences. Some practices like a pro forma; others hate them. Some practices prefer to speak over the telephone about a patient; others will prefer a letter. Some would like a consultant psychiatrist to see a patient; others will not mind if another specialist assesses the patient. CMHTs have their own and their trust's requirements about receiving referrals, and how CMHTs work also varies considerably. All of these variables make effective and consistent communication difficult.

> Suggest a patient makes a list of questions beforehand to ask the GP. For example, a useful question is 'Do I need to come back if the symptoms don't resolve?' This allows the GP to put a timescale on resolution of symptoms, and prompts a follow-up appointment to be made. Suggest that a member of the community mental health team or carer/friend also attend the consultation, to act as an advocate if necessary.

The response from the CMHT can also vary. Some CMHTs use the initial assessment of the patient both as a response to the referring GP and as a clinical record of the assessment. This means that the practice may receive a four- or five-page letter, from which it is hard for GPs to ascertain the diagnosis and determine what responsibility they may have in the future. In some areas CMHTs have followed the line taken by neurosurgeons who either separate out the letter for the GP from the clinical assessment or have a summary in bold at the beginning of the letter.

Getting the best from a consultation in primary care

Visiting a GP can be stressful. It is well known that people remember only a third of what they are told, whether in a general practice or a specialist psychiatric consultation. For those with a mental health problem, the feeling of stress and anxiety may be even greater, making it harder for them to remember and benefit from the consultation. Another problem is 'diagnostic overshadowing', where a presenting symptom is explained by the doctor as a consequence of the patient's mental illness.

> Find out from the carer where he/she is registered and discuss care with that GP. Do not *assume* that a patient is registered at the same practice as the carer.

Carers

For mental health staff, understanding and responding to carers is an important part of the care. The difficulty in primary care is that there is an absolute responsibility not to care for people who are registered with another practice. This means that if the patient is registered with practice A, but the carers, perhaps the parents of a person with schizophrenia, are registered with practice B, then the GP who cares for the person with schizophrenia cannot become involved with the care of the parents, who remain the responsibility of the GP at practice B.

For any GP, taking the biopsychosocial approach means that understanding that a patient may be a carer is as relevant as knowing whether or not the patient has diabetes, or if their accommodation is damp. It is one other aspect of the life that needs to be considered when developing and providing care for an individual. The carer is not 'just' a carer, but has their own needs that need to be met by their GP, and the caring put in the perspective of the patient's health.

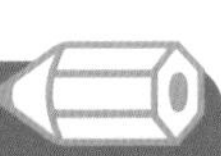

Learning points

- General practice works in a team, much in the same way that CMHTs work together.
- As CMHTs cover larger areas than a general practice, each CMHT should:
  - know the number of practices in its area
  - know how best to contact each practice
  - know the best format in which to send clinical information to each practice
  - be able to provide a list to each practice identifying which of its patients the CMHT is treating.
- CMHTs should also know how to contact the PCT, so that if necessary a patient can be allocated to a GP list, if that patient is currently unregistered.
- Mental health staff should have agreed protocols/guidelines for the identification and management of patients who may have a long-term condition.
- Mental health staff should know how best to work with general practice so that the physical care provided is not the sole responsibility of mental health staff.

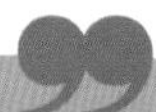

Summary

There are over 250 million consultations with GPs each year, of which at least a third have a mental health component. GPs address the healthcare needs of these patients by using the biopsychosocial model, using information that is generated through continuity of care, and the delivery of longitudinal family-centred care.

An important characteristic of care is the ability to manage the 'chaos of the first presentation' and to tolerate the uncertainty that this approach entails. In addition, GPs are well versed in managing patients with multiple comorbidities; this is particularly helpful as individuals with schizophrenia are more likely to suffer from diabetes and metabolic syndrome.

Over 90% of people with mental health problems are managed entirely in primary care. Referral can be frustrating for both patient and GP because the NSF recommendation that specialist mental health trusts prioritise those with a severe and enduring mental illness leads to rejection of the referral. This practice, of returning patients to general practice because they are not ill enough, seems unique among the medical specialties. As attention is more and more focused on the physical health of people with mental health problems, the role of the GP as a coordinator of care becomes more important.

References

1 Heyrman J, Spreeuwenbergh C (eds). *Vocational Training in General Practice.* Katholieke Universiteit Leuven, 1987.

2 Olesen F, Dickinson J, Hjortdahl P. General practice: time for a new definition. *BMJ* 2000; **320**: 354–7.

3 Hill AP, Freeman GK. *Promoting Continuity of Care in General Practice.* RCGP, 2011.

4 Royal College of General Practitioners. *The Future Direction of General Practice – A Roadmap.* RCGP, 2007.

5 Department of Health. *National Service Framework for Mental Health.* Department of Health, 1999.

6 National Institute for Health and Clinical Excellence. *Depression: Management of Depression in Primary and Secondary Care (Clinical Guidelines CG23).* NICE, 2004.

7 British Medical Association. *Investing in General Practice – The New General Medical Services Contract.* BMA and NHS Confederation, 2004.

4

The role of nurses

Barbara Pryse

This chapter describes the key roles nurses have in clinical care, including the routine monitoring of physical health parameters. It covers how to assess vital and neurological signs, monitoring oxygen therapy, weight management and nutrition assessments, tissue viability, falls prevention, infection control, and health promotion.

Introduction

Within mental health nursing, the physical well-being of the patient is not always recognised as a priority in care planning. The Department of Health's *Chief Nursing Officer Review of Mental Health Nursing*[1] recommends that mental health nurses (MHNs) should have sufficient skills and opportunities to improve the physical well-being of people's mental health problems.

Within intellectual disability services (also known as learning disability services), registered nurses have promoted the physical health of patients by using 'health action plans', as recommended by the Department of Health.[2] Health action plans had to be in place by 2005 and are especially useful for those with communication difficulties. This chapter sets out to identify the key areas that MHNs should take into consideration when delivering care within in-patient settings and, to some extent, in the community, in line with national standards for physical healthcare.

It is essential that nurses equip themselves with the basic skills and knowledge to manage the physical health of patients under their care. In-patients should have access to medical care, and initial care planning for physical health must take place with the multidisciplinary team. All newly admitted patients must have a physical examination, which should take into consideration their mental health state and level of risk. It may not, though, be possible to complete a full physical health assessment in a single session.

Physical examination

Within a high secure forensic setting, the target for undertaking a physical examination is within 24 hours following admission; this is a key performance indicator, reported quarterly to the strategic health authority for monitoring across the UK's three high secure services. While performance targets may not be set for all in-patient facilities, standards should be set and practice monitored.

Medical staff should use an agreed assessment tool for recording the physical examination and any areas of concern can be set out in an action plan, which should be given review dates and to which all members of the

Box 4.1 Information recommended for admission assessment and from baseline observations

- Medical history
- Family history
- Immunisation history
- Full physical examination
- Electrocardiography (ECG)
- Blood tests, including full blood count, urea and electrolytes
- Weight and height
- MUST (Malnutrition Universal Screening Tool) score
- Screening for blood-borne viruses

Source: Royal College of Psychiatrists, *Physical Health in Mental Health* (2009).[3]

multidisciplinary team should refer. The information that should be recorded is set out in Box 4.1.

It is important to involve physical healthcare teams in the care of in-patients at an early stage. If the psychiatric facility is on the same site as an acute general hospital, it will be easier for a ward manager or staff nurse to seek advice from various professions; for example, lead specialist nurses are able to advise on wound management or to provide education and training on the management of self-harm. Their involvement may need to be formalised through a service-level agreement (SLA) with the acute trust (Box 4.2), as the benefits to patients are likely to outweigh the cost of access to appropriate expertise.

Box 4.2 Service-level agreements (SLAs)

An SLA is a formal contract of services provided by one National Health Service (NHS) trust for another and includes the cost incurred. For example, dietetic services could be provided for an acute mental health trust by either an acute trust or a primary care trust; and the dietitian could work for one day a week seeing psychiatric patients with weight-management issues. The terms of the SLA would be clearly stated and reviewed by both parties on a regular basis, with costs agreed and reviewed annually. A major advantage of an SLA is access to experts who can deliver evidenced-based practice in their field of expertise when a full-time post is not required.

Many resources are available for MHNs. *The Royal Marsden Manual of Clinical Nursing Procedures*[4] is an excellent resource for all physical healthcare issues. It is available for purchase as a book and as a CD-ROM; it can be made available for hospitals via their internet services, with a yearly fee for multiple use.

Vital signs monitoring

When a patient is admitted to a mental health in-patient facility, baseline observation should be recorded by nursing staff as soon as is practicable, taking into account the patient's mental health status. Observations should include:

- temperature
- pulse
- blood pressure
- respiration
- oxygen saturation
- body mass index (BMI).

Data should be recorded and documented on relevant observation charts and within the patient's healthcare record. It is important to record observations using the correct documentation, which should be both easy to review and readily accessible to staff. Original forms, approved by trust boards, must be used; using blank photocopied documentation is not acceptable.

Education of qualified nursing staff and support workers is essential so they can recognise which clinical observations are within normal parameters and know what actions to take if any are outside the normal range. The frequency of observations must be agreed with medical teams and review dates must be set. Early Warning Scores (EWS)[5] or Patient at Risk (PAR) scores are 'track and trigger' systems used to identify the 'deteriorating' patient and to alert clinicians. Each set of physiological parameters is given a score, depending on whether it is within or outside the normal range. The total score, or an individual score, can be used to trigger the appropriate level of response from other clinicians (see Chapter 31, Table 31.1 on p. 424).

The EWS is well established within acute hospital settings and can be adapted for use in mental health settings. It provides clear guidance for nursing staff on actions to take if observations indicate a deterioration in the patient's physical condition. This is particularly important when 24-hour medical cover is not provided by a resident or non-resident doctor.

The AVPU score is widely used as an immediate assessment of conscious level. For long-term neurological observation, the Glasgow Coma Scale should be used.

Scoring tools are also available for monitoring, particularly after rapid tranquillisation and patient sedation. The AVPU score (Box 4.3) is widely used by first-aiders, ambulance crew and healthcare professionals as an immediate assessment of conscious level. It is not appropriate for long-term neurological observation,[6] for which the Glasgow Coma Scale (GCS)[7] is more appropriate (Box 4.4). The National Institute for Health and Clinical Excellence (NICE) recommends the use of the GCS (or other more complex tools) in the care of patients who self-injure by head-banging or of those who have undergone rapid tranquillisation.[8]

Box 4.3 The AVPU score

In the AVPU system, the patient is assessed working from the best (A) to the worst (U), with the best outcome being recorded. If a patient remains alert, this should be documented clearly in the nursing records.

A. Is the patient **A**lert?
Patient is fully awake but not necessarily fully oriented
Eyes will spontaneously open
Patient will respond to voice
Motor functions present

V. Does the patient respond **V**erbally?
Patient makes some response, however small, when prompted (may be with eyes, voice or motor response)

P. Does the patient respond to **P**ain?
Makes a response

U. Is the patient **U**nresponsive?
No response

Starting at 'A', record the best response. If the AVPU score is below 'A', the patient should be assessed using the Glasgow Coma Scale (Box 4.4). In-patient areas must have a reporting system to alert medical staff if a patient's AVPU score is 'V' or below. For areas without on-site full-time medical staff cover, systems must be identified to alert nursing staff of the actions to be taken (e.g. requesting an ambulance). Trust policy must reflect this.

Source: NursingTimes.net.[6]

The ABCDE (airway, breathing, circulation, disability and exposure) principles of resuscitation must be followed (see Chapter 31).[9] Training of staff in basic, intermediate or advanced levels of life support should be mandatory. Advanced level hospital life support can be developed in house to suit the needs of the service and all qualified staff should undertake a higher level of training. For health support workers a basic level of life support training is a minimum.

Box 4.4 The Glasgow Coma Scale

Eye-opening	**E**
Spontaneous	4
To noise/verbal	3
To pain	2
No response	1

Best verbal response	**V**
Oriented and converses	5
Confused	4
Inappropriate words	3
Incomprehensible sounds/grunts	2
No response	1

Best motor response	**M**
Normal spontaneous movements	6
To painful stimulus	
Localises pain	5
Withdraws in response to pain	4
Abnormal flexion to pain	3
Extension to pain	2
No response	1

Scores are added: E + V + M (3 – 15)
8 is the critical score

Scores ≤ 8	90% are in a coma
Scores ≤ 8 at 6 hours	mortality is 50%
Scores ≥ 9	not in coma
Scores 9–11	moderate severity
Scores ≥ 12	minor injury

Coma is defined as:
not opening eyes
not obeying commands
not uttering understandable words

Monitoring oxygen saturation: pulse oximetry

Pulse oximetry is a non-invasive measurement of arterial oxygen saturation that uses a finger probe.[10] The equipment costs between £100 and £800 and is easy to maintain. Training and education are usually provided by representatives from the company from which the equipment was purchased. Technique is important, as, for example, nail varnish or nicotine staining can interfere with readings. All medical devices must be checked on purchase and thereafter yearly by a medical engineering maintenance department; these are usually within the acute trust services.

For in-patients, it is important to record baseline oxygen saturations on admission and to discuss the results with a medical colleague who will advise on the action to take if predetermined parameters are exceeded. Measurement of oxygen saturation can also be included in an early warning system.

A decrease in oxygen saturation can be a key indicator of a patient, especially if the patient is suffering from a cardiac or respiratory disorder, is becoming unwell, or the findings are in association with, for example, raised or lowered temperature, pulse rate, blood pressure or respiration rate.

Patients in the community

Patients who are admitted for a brief stay may not need any changes to the management of their chronic disease; even so, MHNs must be aware of current treatment pathways and patient compliance. While they are staying in hospital, patients may miss key interventions such as foot checks for diabetes, so liaison is important, through discharge planning, with the practice nurse or the community psychiatric nurse. Also, liaison between MHN in the community and primary care services is essential. In general practice, the practice nurse often has a pivotal role in managing chronic diseases as well as performing telephone triage for acute illnesses.

While the management of chronic diseases is the responsibility of primary care teams, care plans should involve the MHN, who has a key role in recognising when a patient's physical health is deteriorating and when to seek help.

Given appropriate portable equipment, the community MHN has a role in recording physical health observations. Often the MHN may be able to engage with the patient to address physical health needs and issues, especially if the patient is reluctant to visit the general practitioner. Collaboration with practice nurses can help to ensure that access to health services is satisfactory.

> It is good practice for mental health nurses working with patients in the community to advise patients on diet and also to assist patients with blood sugar monitoring, advising on the risks of a high or low blood sugar level and alerting the practice nurse if blood sugar recordings are out of the normal range.

Weight management

On admission, it is important to record a patient's weight, height and BMI, as well as MUST (Malnutrition Universal Screening Tool) score.[11] This screening tool, available at www.bapen.org.uk/must_tool.html, can be applied to all adults and is appropriate for use in acute general hospital care and mental health settings. Often, obese patients are malnourished. The MUST can assist in recognising this and in helping to formulate management plans (Box 4.5).

An unwanted side-effect of most antipsychotic medications is weight gain, so weight should be monitored and recorded at a frequency determined by the multidisciplinary team and discussed on the ward round. Liaison with pharmacy may trigger a weight management programme for the patient. Referral of patients starting antipsychotic medication to a dietitian may help patients to manage their dietary intake and to keep their weight stable. The dietitian is also a valuable educational resource for MHNs when introducing MUST and in teaching how to record BMI correctly.

Tissue viability management (skin care)

In-patients are usually self-caring and staff may not feel it is relevant to check the condition of the patient's skin. Skin care procedures may feel intrusive for the nurse and patient, so retaining a patient's privacy and dignity is imperative.

Box 4.5 MUST (Malnutrition Universal Screening Tool)

There are five 'MUST' steps.

Step 1

Measure height and weight to obtain the patient's body mass index (BMI). If unable to obtain height and weight, use alternative procedures shown on the website

Step 2

Note percentage of unplanned weight loss and score using tables provided (view the scoring on the web page).

Step 3

Establish acute disease effect and score.

Step 4

Add scores from steps 1, 2 and 3 to obtain overall risk of malnutrition.

Step 5

Use management guidelines and/or local policy to develop care plan.

Source: This summary of MUST (Malnutrition Universal Screening Tool) is reproduced with the kind permission of BAPEN (British Association for Parenteral and Enteral Nutrition). The full MUST is not represented here but can be accessed at www.bapen.org.uk/must_tool.html (the site includes BMI charts and other materials).

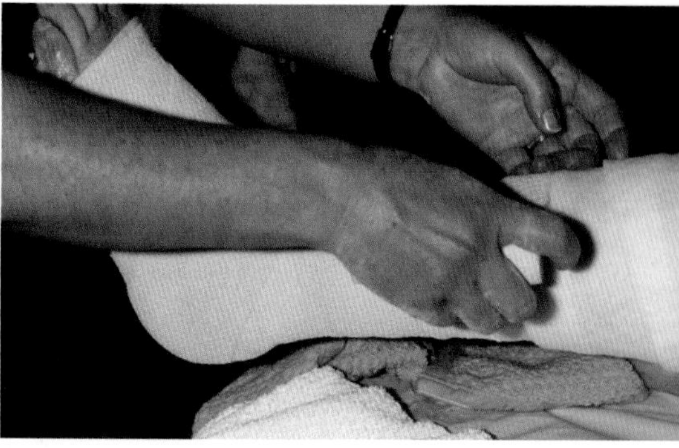

Fig. 4.1 Leg ulcer clinic: dressings procedure. Crepe bandage is applied over top of lint binding.

Assessment on admission is essential for the older patient, especially one admitted for respite or from an acute hospital, to identify any pressure ulcers that may have developed before admission. Any breaks in the skin or pressure ulcers should be measured and documented fully in the patient's healthcare record. Guidance from NICE is available for the management of pressure ulcers.[12] Patients with diabetes are at particular risk of leg or foot ulcers; if an ulcer is found, review by nurses specialising in wound management is essential and it is necessary to devise a care plan for management. Acute trusts and primary care trusts have tissue viability lead nurses who can assist in the management if a pressure ulcer or sore develops and in developing prevention strategies for the vulnerable patient.

For the initial assessment of a patient, as well as for the prevention of pressure sores, the Waterlow Tool can be used to identify risk factors (Box 4.6). After assessment, discussion of patient management with individuals leading tissue viability services is essential.

For a patient with reduced mobility, position changes every 4 hours may be necessary to ensure relief of pressure on threatened tissue. If a patient is at high risk due to prolonged periods of bed rest, tissue-relieving aids, such as cushions for chairs and air mattresses for management of the patient in bed, are available. Air mattresses will provide a support surface with two functions: they redistribute pressure, helping to prevent the formation of pressure ulcers; and they provide a comfortable surface for the patient.[13] An air mattress does not replace the need for position changes and skin

Box 4.6 The Waterlow Tool

The tool is used for the assessment and prevention of pressure sores. It incorporates:

- build/weight for height, skin type and visual areas of risk
- gender and age, continence, mobility
- special risks such as neurological deficit, diabetes, multiple sclerosis, stroke
- tissue malnutrition (arising from, for example, single-organ failure, anaemia, smoking).

Depending on the score obtained, the recommendations for review and management may include position changes every 2 hours, the monitoring of bony prominences (sacral area, elbow, shoulders and heels), and the use of pressure-relieving aids.

Full details and purchase options are available from www.judy-waterlow.co.uk

An air mattress does not replace the need for position changes and skin checks.

checks, however. Specialist tissue viability nurses can advise on products and many articles are available.

Falls prevention strategy

National guidance recommends that trusts have a falls prevention strategy.[14] Within mental health trusts, the strategy is usually developed for services for older people but it will be relevant for any patient who has reduced mobility. An integrated falls service will help to reduce the number of falls that result in serious injury and ensure effective treatment and rehabilitation for those who have fallen.[14]

'Falls assessment' documents can be developed in conjunction with back-care managers and physiotherapists. In many cases, documentation may need to be completed only on patient admission and reviewed if the service user experiences difficulty. Frequency of falls, time of day and circumstance must be recorded and monitored using relevant reporting documentation for the trust.[14] This will help in developing falls prevention strategies.

Before cot sides are fitted to a patient's bed a risk assessment must be undertaken.[15] Guidance on the type of cot side and the correct gap between the rails is also available to ensure the risk of entrapment is minimised. The National Patient Safety Agency (NPSA) has produced robust documentation and assessment tools (Fig. 4.2) that can be adapted.[15]

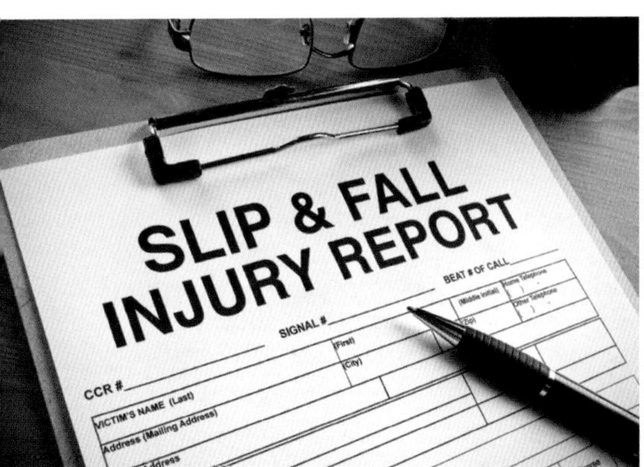

Fig. 4.2 A slip and fall injury report.

An e-learning programme that will develop staff competency in the safe use of bed rails is available on the Health and Safety Executive website (www.hse.gov.uk/foi/internalops/sectors/public/070706.htm).

Health promotion

Prevention strategies (health promotion) are important in both in-patient and out-patient settings. Mental health nurses can access many freely available resources for health promotion. For instance, the website of the British Heart Foundation (www.bhf.org.uk) has several booklets suitable for use by patients, for example, *Cholesterol and what you can do about it*, and *Angina*. These leaflets may be ordered from the British Heart Foundation. The Diabetes UK website (www.diabetes.org.uk) is an excellent resource for professionals and patients to gain further information regarding their condition. Health promotion notice boards and leaflet racks are a useful means of sharing health information.

Adaptations will be necessary for patients with intellectual disability; speech and language therapists can advise on the use of Makaton (which utilises signs and symbols to enhance communication, language and literacy skills) with those with communication and intellectual difficulties (see www.makaton.org).

Essence of Care (EOC) benchmarks include topics such as privacy and dignity, nutrition, communication and health promotion, and were introduced by the Chief Nurse in 2001. The benchmarking provides a tool to assist health practitioners to take a patient-focused and structured approach to sharing and comparing practice.[16]

Guidance on obesity from NICE raises many public health issues that should be reviewed by organisations and action should be taken where necessary.[17]

Infection prevention and control

Infection prevention and control (IPC) are as important in a mental health setting as in acute care facilities. Training materials are available on the Department of Health website (www.dh.gov.uk). These cover, among other topics, the use of personal protective equipment and advice on hand-washing.

Guidance from NICE (Clinical Guideline 139) outlines the basic principles of infection control in hospitals and in the community, including access to materials for the decontamination of hands, sharps containers and personal protective equipment.[18] The Care Quality Commission (CQC) will assess all National Health Service (NHS) trusts on their compliance with the regulations under section 20(5) of the Health and Social Care Act 2008.[19] The CQC provides guidance for providers on what is required to meet the registration requirements relating to healthcare-associated infections. Mental health trusts are not exempt from the Code of Practice.

Training in hand hygiene is essential and the NHS 'Clean Your Hands' campaign is relevant to mental health settings (Fig. 4.3). Within such settings, the use of alcohol hand gel may not be appropriate in all areas, as there has been at least one patient death following ingestion of alcohol hand gel.[20] It is best to discuss the use of alcohol hand gel and the location of dispensers with the infection prevention and control team.

An NHS trust may employ an infection prevention and control practitioner or have an SLA in place from a local acute provider to ensure that annual audits are conducted of the environment, and that action plans are available to deal with infection control issues, monitor outbreaks of infection and advise clinical teams on how to manage patients with infections such as meticillin-resistant *Staphylococcus aureus* (MRSA) (Fig. 4.4).

Screening for MRSA is infrequently performed in mental health settings. If a patient is found to be MRSA positive on swabbing/screening, nursing staff must have the confidence to manage the patient effectively and have robust care plans in place. After an outbreak of infection on a ward, such as diarrhoea and vomiting, the infection prevention and control team will advise on ward access, ward closures, obtaining samples and general hygiene within the ward. When the ward is reopened, a 'deep clean' of the environment, including curtain replacement, and close liaison with housekeeping staff are essential. If a 'cluster outbreak' occurs (i.e. more than two wards are affected), the infection prevention and control team should undertake a root cause analysis to detect common themes or causes.

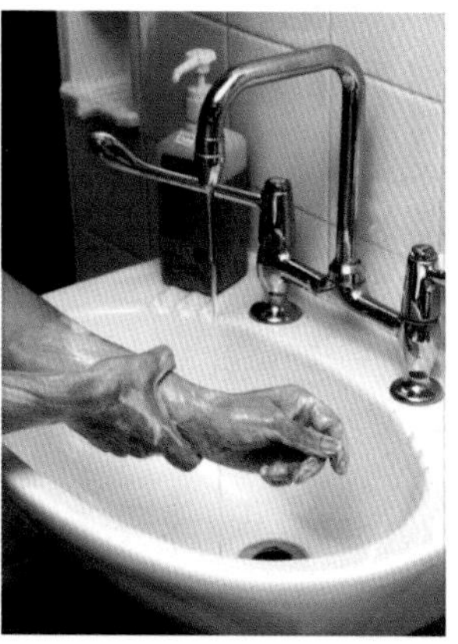
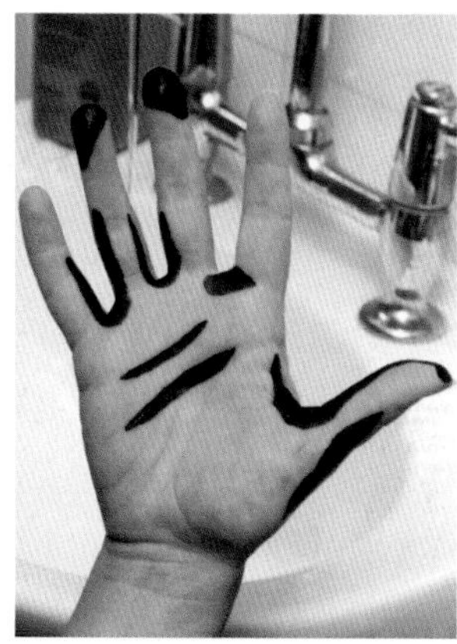

Fig. 4.3 Effective hand-washing. Technique and areas commonly missed.

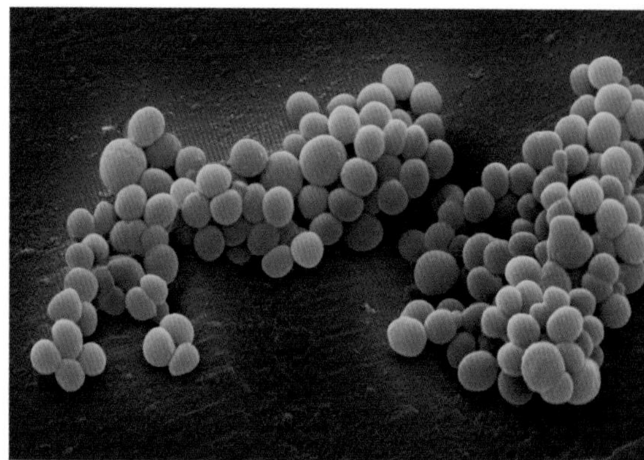

Fig. 4.4 A culture of meticillin-resistant *Staphylococcus aureus* (MRSA).

When transferring any patient with a known healthcare-associated infection, robust information must be shared before transfer and in some cases the transfer may have to be delayed.

Immunisation programmes

For long-term patients in mental health settings, immunisation programmes will be required after individual patient assessments. With the patient's permission, immunisation can be given for hepatitis B, for example. Medical staff will follow guidance as set out in the Department of Health's *Green Book: Immunisation Against Infectious Diseases*.[21]

Learning and development

The skills to manage physical healthcare can be imparted to mental health nurses using various techniques. Face-to-face teaching is effective when the recording of physical health observations is to be demonstrated, for example. Skill stations can give staff the opportunity

Table 4.1 Three sources of online education for mental health nurses

Body	Website	Provision
Resuscitation Council	www.resus.org.uk	Various publications, courses and posters which can be downloaded for staff training
NHS Choices	www.nhs.uk	Excellent resource for management of physical health conditions. The site can be searched by using key words, by entering signs and symptoms and by searching for disease management
NHS Direct	www.nhsdirect.nhs.uk	Can be used to check symptoms of service users

to practise with equipment in a safe environment with appropriately qualified staff.

E-learning modules (Table 4.1) or workbooks are suitable alternatives when it is difficult to release staff for training. Resources can be purchased 'off the shelf' or developed in-house in conjunction with the local education department. An excellent website with detailed instruction on how to set up e-learning can be found at www.nottingham.ac.uk/is/services/e-learning.

The NHS and Social Care e-learning resource database (www.connectingforhealth.nhs.uk/systemsandservices/icd/informspec/etd/elearning) has a health education section that gives examples of packages available, some of which are available for purchase.

If training in resuscitation is not provided in-house, it may be obtained from a local acute NHS trust that is recognised as a training site. Many providers also have intermediate and advanced life-support courses that can be accessed by medical and nursing staff.

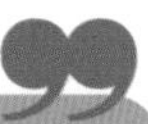

Summary

Mental health nurses may have limited or no experience of several aspects of managing physical healthcare. Nevertheless, nurses should equip themselves with the basic skills and knowledge to manage the physical health conditions of patients under their care. Nurses should be encouraged to obtain education and development to enhance key skills and their knowledge base, to ensure robust standards of physical healthcare are met.

Medical staff should use an agreed physical assessment tool (see Chapter 9). As a minimum, this should include a full physical examination, selected (baseline) blood tests, weight, height and body mass index, score on MUST (Malnutrition Universal Screening Tool), an electocardiogram (ECG) and immunisation history. Within a high secure forensic setting, a key performance indicator is full physical examination within 24 hours of admission.

All members of the multidisciplinary team, especially within in-patient settings, should work together to coordinate required actions and follow-up to improve and maintain the physical health of all their patients.

Learning points

- Ensure newly admitted patients have a full examination as soon as practicable.
- Record weight, BMI and MUST score and review regularly.
- Multidisciplinary team review of patients must include physical healthcare and an action plan for any issues identified.
- Educate staff in recognition of a deteriorating patient.
- Educate staff in life support and the use of the AVPU system.
- Ensure effective communication with all care providers internally and externally.
- Identify 'at risk' patients for skin integrity.
- Create robust care plans with review dates.
- Involve external experts where possible.

References

1 Department of Health. *The Chief Nursing Officer Review of Mental Health Nursing.* Department of Health, 2006.

2 Department of Health. *Action for Health: Health Action Plans and Health Facilitation.* Department of Health, 2002.

3 Royal College of Psychiatrists. *Physical Health in Mental Health: Final Report of a Scoping Group (Occasional Paper OP67).* Royal College of Psychiatrists, 2009.

4 Dougherty L (ed). *The Royal Marsden Hospital Manual of Clinical Nursing Procedures (7th edn).* Wiley-Blackwell, 2008.

5 Mann S, Bowler M. Using an early warning score tool in community nursing. *Nursing Times* 2008; **104**: 30–1.

6 Jevan P. Neurological assessment 1: assessing level of consciousness. Nursing Times.net 2008; 8 July (http://www.nursingtimes.net/nursing-practice/clinical-specialisms/neurology/neurological-assessment-1-assessing-level-of-consciousness/1703021.article).

7 Teesdale G, Jennett B. Assessment of coma and impaired consciousness: a practical scale. *Lancet* 1974; **ii**: 81–4.

8 National Institute for Health and Clinical Excellence. *Head Injury: Triage, Assessment, Investigation and Early Management of Head Injury in Infants, Children and Adults (Clinical Guidelines CG56).* NICE, 2007.

9 Resuscitation Council (UK). *Resuscitation Guidelines 2005.* Resustication Council (UK) .

10 Higgins D. Pulsoximetry. *Nurs Times* 2006; **101**: 34.

11 British Association for Parenteral and Enteral Nutrition. *Malnutrition Universal Screening Tool.* BAPEN, 2004 (http://www.bapen.org.uk/pdfs/must/must-full.pdf).

12 National Institute for Health and Clinical Excellence. *Pressure Ulcer Management (Clinical Guidelines CG29).* NICE, 2005.

13 Rithalia S, Kenney L. Mattress and beds – reducing and relieving pressure. *Nurs Times* 2000; **96**: 9.

14 Department of Health. *National Service Framework for Older People.* Department of Health, 2001.

15 National Patient Safety Agency. *Bedrails Safer Practice Notice.* NPSA, 2007 (http://www.nrls.npsa.nhs.uk/resources/?EntryId45=59815).

16 Department of Health. *Essence of Care: Patient-Focused Benchmarking for Healthcare Practitioners.* Department of Health, 2001.

17 National Institute for Health and Clinical Excellence. *Obesity (Clinical Guidelines CG43).* NICE, 2007.

18 National Institute for Health and Clinical Excellence. *Infection – Prevention and Control of Healthcare-Associated Infections in Primary and Community Care (Clinical Guidelines CG139).* NICE, 2012.

19 Department of Health. *Health and Social Care Act 2008 Code of Practice (Revised).* Department of Health, 2009.

20 National Patient Safety Agency. *Clean Hands Save Lives: Data for Incidents Related to Alcohol Hand Rub.* NPSA, 2008.

21 Department of Health. *Immunisation Against Infectious Diseases – 'The Green Book'* (2006 updated edn). Department of Health, 2007.

5

The role of health professionals allied to medicine

Irene Cormac

A wide range of health professionals provide healthcare and their roles are described in this chapter. They include audiologists, dentists, dietitians, occupational therapists, optometrists, pharmacists, physiotherapists, podiatrists, and speech and language therapists. The chapter describes simple tests that health practitioners should do before a patient is referred. It also gives advice on when to refer, to enable clinicians to get the best for patients with mental disorders.

Introduction

In the UK, everyone who is eligible to receive healthcare from the National Health Service (NHS) may register with a general practitioner (GP) and with a general dental practitioner (dentist). GPs and dentists may refer their patients to health professionals allied to medicine for assessment, advice and treatment.

Health professionals allied to medicine may work in the NHS, private practice or within commercial organisations, such as pharmacies and opticians. They include audiologists, podiatrists/chiropodists, dentists, dietitians, optometrists, speech and language therapists, occupational therapists, physiotherapists and pharmacists. Their expertise is essential for the physical care of people with mental disorders and disabilities. In this chapter, their roles are described; recommendations for further reading are made at the end of each section, as there is much more to learn about each specialty than is possible to include in this chapter. In addition, the NHS website www.nhscareers.nhs.uk gives a useful overview of each profession.

Audiology

Audiologists obtain a university degree and undertake clinical placements before qualifying to register with the Registration Council for Clinical Physiologists. The role of an audiologist is to test, diagnose, treat and prevent hearing and balance disorders. Audiologists mainly work within multiprofessional teams.

Patients referred to a specialist otolaryngology service (e.g. a hospital ear, nose and throat/ENT department) may receive an audiology assessment. Some criteria for referral to ENT services are listed in Box 5.1.

Hearing tests

In the UK, babies and children should have hearing tests.[1,2] In adults, it is important to enquire about hearing difficulties and loss.[3,4] Patients may experience some or most of the problems described in Box 5.2.

Hearing tests are normally conducted in a soundproof room or booth. Patients wear headphones, through which sounds of varying frequency and volume

Box 5.1 Criteria for referral for ENT assessment

Assessment may include audiology testing. Criteria include:

- history of deafness (especially if unilateral and of rapid onset)
- complaint of difficulty hearing
- pain or discomfort in the ear
- foreign body in the ear
- persistent discharge from the ear
- communication difficulties (e.g. poor language skills)
- medical history of conditions which may cause deafness (e.g. meningitis, rubella infection, syphilis, Ménière's disease and Paget's disease)
- congenital disorders associated with deafness (e.g. Usher syndrome)
- intellectual disabilities, especially those with Down syndrome
- neurological disorders (e.g. neurofibromatosis)
- medication side-effects (e.g. gentamicin toxicity)
- trauma (blow to the side of the head)
- job-related deafness (noise from machinery).

Adapted from du Feu & Fergusson;[5] Steiger.[6] ENT, ear, nose, throat.

are transmitted to each ear by an audiometer. Patients indicate whether they hear a sound and the audiologist plots the frequencies and volumes of sounds heard by each ear on a chart. This shows the pattern of hearing at different frequencies and can reveal hearing deficits.

To test for conduction deafness, a vibrating tuning fork should be placed on a mastoid process and when the sound disappears the tuning fork should then be held in front of the ear. The sound will continue to be heard unless there is conduction deafness.

To test for sensorineural deafness, a vibrating tuning fork should be placed on the centre of the patient's forehead. The sound of the vibrating tuning fork should be heard just as well in both ears unless there is sensorineural deafness, when the sound will be quieter in the affected ear.

Deafness may be congenital or acquired. Causes of acquired deafness (hearing loss) may include persistent otitis media with an effusion, cerumen (ear wax), loud noise, trauma and foreign bodies. Cerumen can be softened by various proprietary preparations before removal. Cotton buds are not recommended for removing cerumen as they can compact it, and the compacted cerumen can block the auditory canal.

Box 5.2 Common problems experienced by adults with hearing loss or deafness

Difficulty hearing when:

- another conversation is taking place nearby
- there is background noise
- talking on the telephone
- women and children are speaking.

Patients may notice that:

- other people seem to be talking too quietly
- they have to concentrate hard to hear speech
- they ask others to repeat what has been said
- it is difficult to hear the other person on the telephone
- the direction of sounds is hard to identify
- they did not hear the door bell or telephone ringing.

Other people may:

- complain that the television, radio or music is too loud
- become irritated when the person responds incorrectly
- suggest that the person may have hearing problems.

This list is based on questionnaires for hearing loss: Hearing Loss Questionnaire from the University of Wisconsin–Madison (www.uwhealth.org/audiology-hearing/hearing-loss-questionnaire/11423); NHS Choices: questions for patients on common symptoms of hearing impairment, with information about normal hearing and types of hearing loss (www.nhs.uk/Conditions/Hearing-impairment/Pages/Diagnosis.aspx); and Action on Hearing Loss, online self-assessment questionnaire (www.actiononhearingloss.org.uk/your-hearing/look-after-your-hearing/am-i-losing-my-hearing/am-i-losing-my-hearing.aspx).

The care of profoundly deaf people with mental disorders and intellectual disabilities requires specialist psychiatric services. These are available in both the NHS and the private sector. In addition to conduction and sensorineural deafness, people with intellectual disabilities may also have problems with cortical auditory processing in the brain.[7]

Various aids are available for deaf people (Box 5.3).

It is advisable to screen everyone with intellectual disabilities for sensory impairments. Remember that there may be problems in more than one sensory modality.

Box 5.3 Aids for people who are deaf or have hearing impairment

- Alert systems – lights, visual display, vibration and 'hearing' dogs
- Amplification systems – hearing aids, loop systems
- Visual – lip reading, subtitles, British sign language (BSL), text messages, signs and electronic displays.

Adapted from du Feu & Fergusson[5]

Communication difficulties from sensory impairment.

Speech and language therapists may assist with assessment and the development of communication strategies, and provide help to educate others (e.g. carers). A strategy should be developed for effective communication.

Useful websites

- Deafness in adults: http://www.patient.co.uk/doctor/Deafness-in-Adults.htm
- British Sign Language and facilities for deaf people: http://www.royaldeaf.org.uk/
- Down Syndrome: http://www.dsmig.org.uk/library/articles/guideline-hear-8.pdf

Recommended reading

Kiani R, Miller H. Sensory impairment and intellectual disability. *Adv Psychiatr Treat* 2010; **16**: 228–35.

Yueh B, Shapiro N, MacLean CH, *et al.* Screening and management of adult hearing loss in primary care. *JAMA* 2003; **289**: 1976–85.

Podiatry

Podiatrists are also called chiropodists. They specialise in the prevention, assessment and treatment of disorders and problems of the lower limbs, and advise on foot care and gait (Fig. 5.1). A GP or practice nurse may make referrals for NHS treatment, although private foot care can be obtained by individuals. In the UK, podiatrists and chiropodists should be registered with the Health Professions Council (www.hpcheck.org).

The role of the podiatrist is:

- to advise on general foot health and care
- to diagnose and treat foot pain and skin lesions (e.g. verrucas, corns and calluses)
- to provide screening and foot care for diabetic patients, for those with bony change or deformity, and those with poor circulation or neuropathy
- to assess and treat deformities of the feet (e.g. bunions and arthritis)
- to assess gait, both walking and running
- to alter balance of movement of the feet with orthotic soles, shoes and other devices to improve gait or balance
- to advise those at risk of foot injury (e.g. from sport)
- to provide nail surgery under local anaesthetic (e.g. for in-growing toenails)
- to provide information and training to carers or nurses, when appropriate.

The referral information needed by a podiatrist includes the following:

- reason for referral
- medical history
- current medication
- allergies
- health risk factors (e.g. clotting disorders, neutropenia, infection with blood-borne viruses).

Foot care for people with type 2 diabetes

Guidance on this from the National Institute for Health and Clinical Excellence should be followed.[8] This includes examination of the patient's feet, with tests of foot sensation with a 10 g monofilament (or testing for

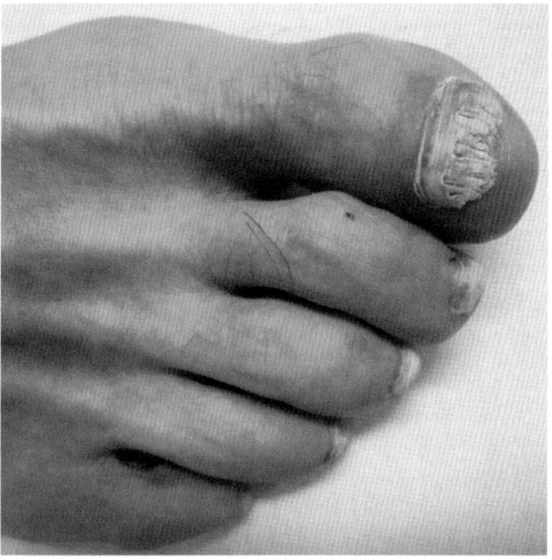

Fig. 5.1 Foot with fungal infection of toenails.
© James Heilman, MD.

vibration sense), palpation of foot pulses, and inspection of foot deformity and footwear. The frequency and type of interventions will depend on the degree of foot risk or presence of ulceration.

Care of toenails

Nails should be cut following the shape of the toe. They can be softened first by soaking the foot in a bath of warm water. Cutting toenails too short can predispose to in-growing toenails. Toenails can also be shaped with an emery board.

Recommended reading

The Society of Chiropodists and Podiatrists. *A Guide to the Benefits of Podiatry to Patient Care* (leaflet). Available at www.feetforlife.org

Dentistry and oral health

Dental professionals

Dentists are general dental practitioners who provide dentistry, in the NHS and/or in private practice (www.bda.org/dentists/representation/gdps). Dentists work in the community, hospitals, occupational health services, prisons and psychiatric settings. In the UK, dentists, dental hygienists, dental therapists, clinical dental technicians, orthodontic therapists and dental nurses must register with the General Dental Council (www.gdc-uk.org).

Dental nurses assist dentists by preparing dental instruments and materials for dental work, such as fillings. They may make clinical records, sterilise instruments and take X-rays.

Dental hygienists and dental therapists should work under the prescription of a dentist, who must examine the patient first. Dental hygienists use instruments and ultrasound to remove stains and deposits from the teeth and gums, and polish the teeth. They educate patients about oral health, tooth brushing and dental flossing. In addition, dental therapists may undertake a range of treatments, including fillings and extractions.

Dental technicians make dentures, crowns, bridges and dental braces, to the specification of a dentist, using a variety of materials such as gold, porcelain and plastic.

Specialist maxillofacial technicians make prostheses for patients with damaged or diseased faces.

Dental services

Dental services may be provided by NHS dentists, private dentists and community dentists or by dentists working in psychiatric settings. Dental surgeries must have up-to-date equipment and follow appropriate procedures for infection control, sterilisation, waste disposal (e.g. mercury amalgam) and dental X-rays.

Oral health

Dental caries (tooth decay) is caused by bacteria in dental plaque which destroy hard layers of the teeth. Sugary foods increase growth of these bacteria, leading to further damage to enamel. Acidic foods such as citrus fruits and carbonated drinks can erode tooth enamel. To reduce the risk of caries and erosion of enamel, it is essential to restrict consumption of acidic, carbohydrate and sugary foods.

Periodontal disease (gum disease or gingivitis) is an infection of the gums (Fig. 5.2), which may damage the periodontal ligaments of teeth, leading to loosening and loss of teeth. Gingivitis is mostly preventable and often presents with bleeding gums associated with tooth brushing. The temptation is to brush teeth less but gum health is improved by tooth brushing, because it removes bacteria and food debris, which contribute to the infection and inflammation of gums.

Oral cancer accounts for 1% of all cancers in the UK. It is more common in older people (those over 40) and in those who chew or smoke tobacco and in people who drink alcohol. In young non-smokers, oral cancer is associated with infection with the human papilloma virus (HPV). Oral cancer is often painless in the early stages and consequently is usually recognised late, giving a poor prognosis.

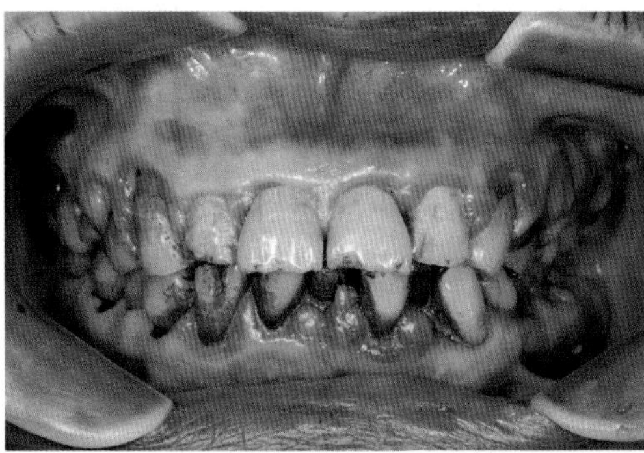

Fig. 5.2 Poorly maintained mouth with staining, gum disease and chronic infection.

Teeth can become sensitive to cold temperatures due to gums receding and consequent exposure of dentine. Patients can be reassured that the use of specially formulated toothpaste for sensitive gums can reduce pain on eating, without the need to seek dental advice.

Role of the dentist

History and examination

Dentists must be informed about their patient's physical and mental health, medical history, medication, allergies, and whether there is any possibility of pregnancy. The dentist must be aware of the current psychotropic medication, including side-effects such as dry mouth (xerostomia). Other information the dentist needs *before* treatment begins includes:[9]

- bleeding disorders – haemophilia, other coagulation defects and their severity
- use of anticoagulants – there is increased risk of bleeding if the international normalised ratio (INR) is >3
- heart valve disease – if there is risk of infective endocarditis, advice about prophylaxis with antibiotics should be sought[10]
- ischaemic heart disease – after myocardial infarction, defer elective dental treatment for 3 months
- immunocompromise – patients who are taking steroids or who are HIV positive are more likely to have oral candidiasis, herpetic infection and mouth ulcers; those with HIV are more likely to have certain cancers (e.g. Kaposi's sarcoma)
- allergies – latex allergy, allergy to antibiotics, reactions to local anaesthetics
- risk of cross-infection – hepatitis B, hepatitis C, HIV (e.g. associated with drug or alcohol misuse)
- mental state – risk of biting and poor cooperation.

The dentist will inspect the oral cavity using a mirror to identify caries, periodontal disease, malocclusion, wear of the teeth, and abnormalities of hard or soft tissues, including oral cancer. If necessary, X-rays will be taken to identify dental disease not visible to the naked eye, such as a root abscess or caries beneath the gingiva (gums). A chart is usually used to note decayed, missing or filled teeth (DMFT) and a DMFT score may be recorded. The dentist may examine the temporomandibular joint (TMJ), including jaw movement and lymph nodes, for signs of disease or infection.

Box 5.4 Taking dental history

Dental history may include (see also Table 5.1):

- difficulties with chewing or biting
- broken, missing or stained teeth
- bleeding from the gums
- infections
- toothache
- soreness or lesions in the mouth.

A dental history may include some of the items in Box 5.4.

Treatment

Dentists remove caries using a high-speed drill, mainly under local anaesthetic, and restore teeth through the fitting of fillings, veneers or crowns. Severely carious teeth may be extracted under local or general anaesthetic. If the tooth nerve has died, dentists may operate to remove the nerve and fill the root canal. Dental treatment may also involve making dental bridges, tooth implants and dentures (Box 5.5). Dentists take oral impressions and dental technicians can make dentures or false teeth to replace all or some missing teeth.

Patients with severe challenging behaviour may be offered diagnostic dental examinations and treatment under sedation or general anaesthesia.

Dentists who specialise in orthodontics treat malocclusion.

In the NHS most dental prescriptions are for antibacterial medications, drugs acting on the oropharynx, minerals, analgesia, hypnotics and anxiolytics.[11]

Box 5.5 Dentures

Dentures can be partial, replacing some missing teeth, or full, replacing an entire arch (upper or lower) or both arches. Dentures should fit gums without rubbing or pinching. They can be fixed in place with dental fixative and should be removed at least once daily for cleaning. Dentures should be cleaned with a denture brush and proprietary cleaning solutions or fluids/foaming tablets, to remove hard deposits. They should be stored overnight in clean water and rinsed before use. It is best to massage the gums gently with a soft toothbrush when dentures are left out.

Table 5.1 Dental problems and possible causes

Pain	Causes
Pain with hot and cold liquids	Caries, crack in tooth, loose filling, periodontal disease
Pain on biting or on tapping tooth	Caries, cracked tooth, loose filling
Constant throbbing pain	Tooth abscess
Constant dull ache	Sinus infection, ear infection
Intermittent dull pain	Referred pain from angina, lesions in head and neck, lung cancer
Pain and soreness in mouth	Oral candidiasis, dietary deficiencies (e.g. vitamin B, iron)
Ulcers	Aphthous ulcers, ill-fitting dentures, herpes simplex infection
Burning pain in mouth	Local lesions, psychogenic pain, dietary deficiency (e.g. vitamin B, folate, iron), medication (e.g. captopril)
Pain in cheek and gum	Trigeminal neuralgia, referred pain, blocked salivary duct (calculus)
Pain in temporomandibular joint	Bruxism (tooth grinding)

Source: Scully & Shotts, 2000.[12]

Oral health problems in psychiatric patients

Psychiatric patients are more likely than other people to have some of the factors that lead to poor oral health, including dental caries:[13]

- poor oral hygiene
- less access to dental care
- high dietary intake of carbohydrates
- smoking (increases risk of oral cancer)
- high alcohol intake (increases risk of oral cancer).

Saliva has an important role in maintaining oral health and a dry mouth (xerostomia) increases the risk of caries. Psychotropic medications that cause xerostomia include:

- lithium carbonate
- antidepressants
- sedatives (e.g. benzodiazepines)
- anticholinergics.

Hypersalivation is a common problem with clozapine. Vomiting in bulimia nervosa may lead to acid erosion of the lingual (tongue) side of the teeth. Delusions about dental caries/pain may lead an unwary dentist into treating a patient with healthy teeth for caries.

People with mental disorders and intellectual disabilities may take longer to settle in the dental chair and so require longer dental appointments. They may not be able to provide their medical history; information from others will be needed.

> Consent (normally verbal consent) must be obtained before dental procedures are undertaken. Patients without mental capacity to consent to treatment may receive treatment under relevant mental capacity legislation (e.g. the Mental Capacity Act 2005 in England and Wales). It may be necessary to obtain legal advice about consent issues.

> After vomiting, using fluoridated mouth washes instead of tooth brushing is advised, to reduce acid erosion of teeth.

Prevention of dental problems

Diet and lifestyle

Foodstuffs should be avoided that:

- adhere to teeth and stick to tooth crevices
- ferment to promote growth of the bacteria which form plaque
- cause acid erosion of enamel
- cause wear of tooth surfaces.

Such foodstuffs include carbonated and syrup drinks, confectionery, sugary foods and acidic fruit juices. Alcohol, smoking or chewing tobacco and infection with human papilloma virus can predispose to oral cancer. Prolonged smoking of tobacco in a hookah can lead to gum recession.

Systemic diseases, drugs and radiotherapy can cause oral ulcers, dental pain, halitosis (bad breath) and difficulty eating. Oral cancers can be painless and can present as ulcers, which are slow to heal.

Box 5.6 Emergency dental care

In an emergency outside normal working hours, patients should call their dental surgery to obtain the telephone number of the local emergency dental service. Patients not registered with a dentist may call NHS Direct (tel. 0845 4647) for advice, or telephone the number of the emergency dental service, provided by the primary care trust (England) or the local health board (Wales). Patients with urgent dental needs will normally be seen within 24 hours. Hospital accident and emergency departments deal with serious oral or facial injuries such as jaw fractures.

Oral hygiene

Teeth should be brushed twice daily using fluoride-containing toothpaste and a medium or soft toothbrush which has a small head and rounded bristles. Tooth brushing should be done with small circular movements, on every side of the teeth, for at least two minutes. Interdental cleaning (between the teeth) with dental floss and interdental toothbrushes removes food debris and reduces plaque. Waxed floss or dental tape can be easier to use if gaps between teeth are narrow. Good oral hygiene alone is insufficient to prevent dental caries but helps to prevent gum disease. Dentists advise against vigorous tooth brushing, especially with hard toothbrushes, as it can damage teeth and gums.

If it is difficult to use a normal toothbrush, a modified toothbrush or an electric toothbrush can be used. Toothbrushes and heads of electric toothbrushes should be replaced after 3–4 months, or sooner if the bristles are worn.

Fluoride hardens tooth enamel and is added to many brands of toothpaste. It occurs naturally in certain areas of the UK, or is added to tap water as a public health intervention. Excess fluoride consumed while teeth are developing can lead to spots of white flecking or discoloration of the teeth (dental fluorosis). This can be treated in the majority of cases if aesthetics are of concern.

Dental check-ups

Many people attend the dentist only if they have problems with their mouth or teeth. NICE guidance[14] states that routine dental check-ups can vary in frequency according to risk of dental problems, from every 3 months to yearly for patients under 18 years and from every 3 months to every 2 years for those over 18 years old. Dental risk assessments are based on the patient's medical and social history, dietary habits, use of fluoride, oral hygiene and salivary flow rates.

Between check-ups, dental treatment of a routine or emergency nature may be necessary (Box 5.6).

Sharing toothbrushes will increase the risk of exchange of bodily fluids and of transmission of blood-borne viruses, such as hepatitis C. Patients infected with blood-borne viruses should ensure that they do not share toothbrushes. They should inform their dentist and oral hygienist of their infection before treatment commences.

Recommended reading

Crispin S. *ABC of Oral Health*. BMJ Books, 2009.

Dietetics and nutrition

Dietitians have qualifications in nutrition and dietetics. They apply the science of nutrition to the feeding and education of people, in health and disease. There is a European Federation of the Associations of Dietitians (www.efad.org), to which the British Dietetic Association belongs (www.bda.uk.com). In the UK, dietitians must register with the Health Professions Council (www.hpc-uk.org).

Roles of a dietitian

- *Administrative*. Dietitians work with catering services to ensure that food is of adequate quality and has sufficient macro- and micronutrients to meet normal requirements for health, as well as meeting specialist requirements for health, culture and religion.

- *Individual case management.* Dietitians assess the nutritional status and needs of their patients, prepare and implement individual dietary prescriptions (eating plans), educate patients, staff and carers, and monitor progress.
- *Lifestyle and therapeutic interventions.* Dietitians design dietary interventions for patients who need advice and supervision to become healthy, for example for people who are overweight or obese.
- *Education and health promotion.* Dietitians promote health in the general population. They educate patients and health professionals about food, nutrition and a healthy diet. Dietitians may give advice about oral nutritional supplements, for example for people unable to fulfil their total nutritional requirements with a normal diet as well as for those who cannot eat or who refuse to eat.
- *Implementation of government policy.* Dietitians play a key role in the implementation of NICE guidance, for example for obesity and diabetes.[15,16]
- *Research and development.* Dietitians play an active role in research and development.

Institutional catering

Institutions must provide food that is sufficient in macro- and micronutrients. The menu should be rotated regularly to avoid menu fatigue (a minimum of every 4 weeks). Dietitians can assist with menu planning and modification of standard recipes so that dishes meet government guidelines.[17] Recipes can be analysed using computer software to aid compliance with recommended daily nutritional intake. Food that is deemed to be a 'healthy option' can be marked on the menu. The website of the Hospital Caterers Association has a section devoted to 'better hospital food' (www.hospitalcaterers.org/better-hospital-food).

Factors to consider about catering in in-patient psychiatric settings are indicated in Box 5.7.

Box 5.7 Factors to consider about catering in mental health in-patient settings

- Meals may be served within a 9-hour period or less (8 a.m. – 5 p.m.)
- Many patients want to have large portions and second helpings
- Many patients miss meals, especially breakfast
- Patients may restrict their menu choices
- Menu fatigue may occur
- Fresh fruit and vegetables are often perceived as unappetising
- Food is prepared early and stored for long periods in heated trolleys
- Convenience foods are often served, with high calorie, fat, salt and sugar content
- Chips and other 'high-fat' foods may be provided frequently (e.g. at least once per day)
- Meals are interrupted by clinical activities
- Patients may overeat through boredom and lack of other interests
- Appetite can be increased as a side-effect of psychotropic medication

Lifestyle and disease prevention

Dietitians advise on healthy eating and weight management, which should comply with current recommendations of the Food Standards Agency for the consumption of least five portions of fruit or vegetables daily and at least one portion of oily fish per week (two portions of fish per week) (see www.nhs.uk/Livewell/healthy-eating/Pages/Healthyeating.aspx). A Mediterranean type of diet is associated with longevity. A diet with a high intake of red meats and cured meats is associated with a greater risk of cancer. In the community, patients should be encouraged to buy fresh food and to cook nutritious meals.

Chapter 7, on obesity, describes the principles for weight management. When patients are prescribed psychotropic medication with known a side-effect of weight gain, it is essential to inform the patient and to monitor their weight at least monthly.

Individual dietary interventions

For nutritional screening, information is needed on body mass index, appetite, dietary intake, any unexplained weight loss or gain, and physical and mental conditions. Referrals should be made to dietitians if there are concerns about under- or over-nutrition (Table 5.2), nutritional deficiencies and health problems requiring dietary intervention (Box 5.8).

Table 5.2 Causes of under- or over-nutrition in mental health settings

Problem	Examples of causes
Under-nutrition	
Low body weight (body mass index < 18.5 kg/m^2)	Anorexia nervosa, starvation
Poor appetite	Dementia, severe depressive disorder
Inability to eat/swallow	Poor dentition, dysphagia
Refusal to eat	Emotional difficulties, anorexia nervosa
Unexplained weight loss	Physical disorder not yet diagnosed
Restricted diet	Paranoia about food being poisoned
Dietary deficiencies (e.g. lack of calcium, vitamin D)	Poor diet
Self-neglect	Addictions, severe mental illness
Dysphagia	Side-effects of psychotropic medication
Difficulty eating	Intellectual disabilities, challenging behaviour, dementia
Self-induced vomiting (which may lead to electrolyte imbalance, e.g. hypokalaemia)	Bulimia nervosa
Over-nutrition	
Overweight, with comorbidities	Hypothyroidism, diabetes mellitus, coronary heart disease
Obesity	Side-effects of psychotropic medication, consumption of too much confectionery, ready meals and 'take-away' foods
Binge eating	Bulimia nervosa
Excess eating	Prader–Willi syndrome, frontotemporal dementia, Pick's disease, Klüver–Bucy syndrome
Inactivity	Restricted access to exercise

Box 5.8 Examples of health problems requiring dietary management

- Diabetes mellitus
- Food intolerance (e.g. gluten in wheat)
- Bowel disorders (e.g. Crohn's disease)
- Cancer (e.g. oral cancer, cancer of oropharynx or larynx, cachexia, complications of chemotherapy)
- Post-operative recovery following surgery (especially abdominal surgery)
- Percutaneous endoscopic gastrostomy (PEG) feeding tube *in situ*
- Nasogastric feeding tube *in situ*

Dietetic and nutrition services

These services are normally provided in the community, general hospitals, and in psychiatric in- and out-patient settings, in the NHS and the private sector. Referral information should include:

- name, date of birth, NHS number and patient contact details
- name of referring clinician and contact details
- reason for referral
- diagnosis and clinical information
- past medical history
- medication including allergies
- body measurements, e.g. height, weight, waist size
- results of nutritional screening and assessment, if available

Dietary assessment

The dietitian will make a clinical, dietary and lifestyle assessment that incorporates the following elements:

- dietary history (foods normally eaten, frequency of consumption, portion sizes)
- current problem/presenting complaint
- eating patterns, including periods of starvation, binge eating, eating at abnormal times, restricted diet
- current physical health
- weight history (e.g. pregnancy-induced weight gain not lost after delivery, unintentional weight loss)
- previous interventions (e.g. restrictive or fad diets, previous re-feeding)
- motivation to change (stage of change, i.e. pre-contemplation, contemplation, preparation, action, maintenance, termination)
- body image
- body measurements (height, weight, waist size, body fat percentage)
- biochemical profiles.

Dietary interventions

These may include:

- motivational interviewing to initiate change
- goal setting and advice on how to reach goals
- specialist advice on management of eating disorders
- nutritional support and provision of artificial nutritional support (e.g. enteral feeding)
- prescriptive diets (e.g. healthy eating, weight-reducing diet, low-fat diet, diabetic diet)
- prescribed oral nutritional supplements (approved by the Advisory Committee on Borderline Substances), such as milk-style drinks and semi-solid desserts
- texture-modified diets or finger foods
- advice on eating environment (e.g. dining areas, posture at meals, cutlery and utensils).

Educational materials are available from local NHS trusts and from the Nutrition and Diet Resources website (www.ndr-uk.org).

Algorithms and protocols are available for weight management from NICE.[15]

Recommended reading

Webster-Gandy J, Madden A, Holdsworth M. *Oxford Handbook of Nutrition and Dietetics* (2nd edn). Oxford University Press, 2011.

Optometry

An optometrist (ophthalmic optician) is trained to examine eyes, test vision, and prescribe and fit spectacles and contact lenses. Systemic diseases may affect the eye and routine retinal screening is available for people with diabetes. Optometrists may refer a patient to a doctor (with the patient's consent) when they detect or suspect that an eye disease or systemic disease is present. Some optometrists are independent prescribers and can treat conditions of the eye and surrounding tissues.

Annual sight tests are advised for people aged under 16 years and over 70 years, for people with diabetes and for those with potentially progressive eye disease such as glaucoma, age-related macular degeneration, cataract, corneal dystrophy or ocular hypertension.

Sight tests include inspection of the eye, surrounding structures and the ocular fundus. Visual acuity is tested using a Snellen chart (Fig. 5.3). Normal vision is called '6/6 vision' because the person can see the letter on the chart at 6 metres (or 20 feet, as indicated in Fig. 5.3) that is expected to be accurately perceived by a normal eye at a distance of 6 metres. If vision is poor, the denominator

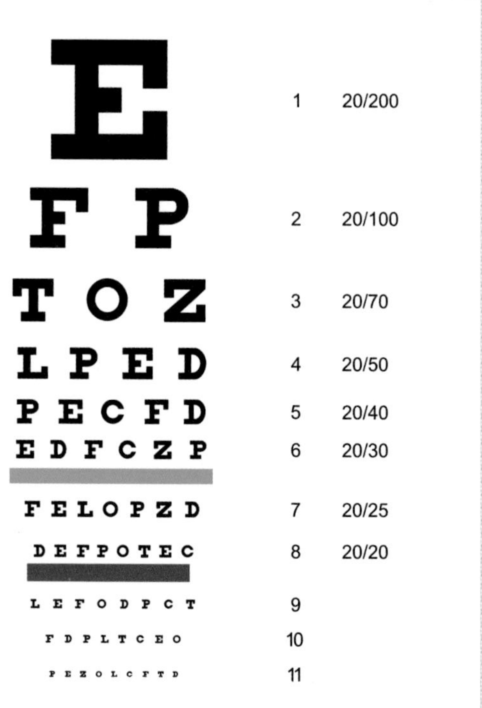

Fig. 5.3 Snellen chart.

will increase (e.g. 6/60) and it will decrease if vision is good (e.g. 6/4).

The optometrist will also measure the refractive error of the eyes and assess binocular vision to determine whether spectacles are required. Visual fields, ocular movements and intraocular pressure should also be checked. A slit-lamp can be used to examine the anterior chamber of the eye.

In England, the National Screening Programme for Diabetic Retinopathy (www.retinalscreening.nhs.uk) aims to reduce loss of sight in people with diabetes. Digital photographs of the retina (Fig. 5.4) are taken and are graded to identify stages of retinopathy and whether treatment is necessary.

In-patients in psychiatric facilities are *not* recalled automatically for screening and so this must be specifically arranged.

Referrals of patients with eye conditions are not always to an optometrist. In some instances referral to a hospital accident and emergency service is appropriate (Table 5.3) and in others referral may be made to an ophthalmic surgeon. The latter would require the following information:

- eye history – pain, photophobia, loss of visual acuity, loss of areas in visual fields, change in pupil size or reactivity to light
- history of eye disease (e.g. shingles affecting the eye)
- medical history (e.g. head injury, rheumatoid arthritis, temporal arteritis, diabetes mellitus, multiple sclerosis, infection)
- change in prescription of medication (e.g. anti-cholinergic side-effects may precipitate glaucoma)
- family history of eye disease or blindness (e.g. glaucoma)
- findings on examination (e.g. distribution of redness, eye movements, corneal abrasion, cataract, pupil size, regularity and reaction to light, fundoscopy)
- findings of the optometrist from an examination during routine eye test or retinal screening.

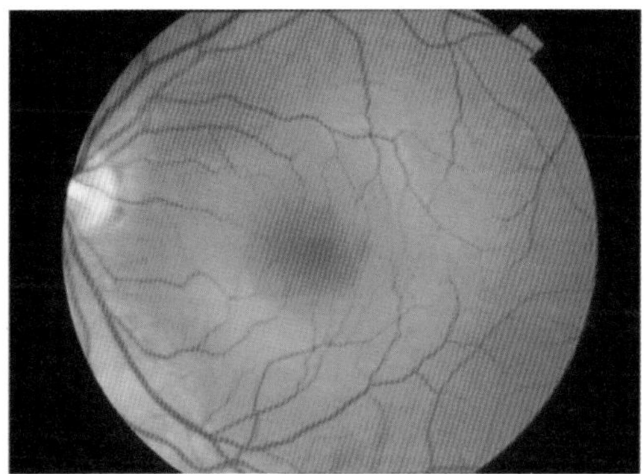

Fig. 5.4 A normal retina.

Recommended reading

Khaw PT, Shah P, Elkington AR. *ABC of Eyes*. BMJ Publishing, 2004.

Table 5.3 Reasons for assessment of eyes by accident and emergency services and recommended first aid

Condition	Recommended treatment
Eye injury: cuts, scratches, trauma, cuts to eyelid or eyebrow, chemical burns (acid or alkalis)	Avoid rubbing or wiping the eye. In case of chemical injury, irrigate the eye immediately with sterile saline or water. For injuries, seek an urgent ophthalmic opinion
Foreign body in the eye: e.g. grit, sand, glass, wood or metal splinters	Do not try to remove an object that penetrates the eye. Seek an urgent ophthalmic opinion
Infection: e.g. cellulitis of the tissues surrounding the eye, infection with shingles involving the cornea	Seek an urgent ophthalmic opinion
Sudden loss of vision in one or both eyes	Seek emergency assessment from ophthalmology services
Suspected acute onset of glaucoma, with painful, red eye, loss of vision	Seek an urgent ophthalmic opinion

Speech and language therapy

Speech and language therapists (SLTs) assess and treat people with speech, language and communication problems, and problems with eating and swallowing. In the UK, SLTs must obtain a degree in speech and language therapy and be registered with the Health Professions Council (www.hpc-uk.org).

Speech, language, communication

Communication skills are affected by many factors, including the strength and coordination of orofacial musculature, hearing, and the ability and motivation to listen and to maintain attention and concentration, as well as intellectual function, mental illness and institutionalisation. Communication difficulties can range from absent speech to significant impairment in the use of language in social situations (pragmatics).

Communication problems may exist independently or be caused by congenital disorders (e.g. Down syndrome, cleft lip), developmental disorders (e.g. autism) and acquired disorders (e.g. mental illness, multiple sclerosis, stroke). Patients may have different levels of ability in the various components of language and communication.

Disorders of communication

Speech

Disorders of speech may affect the ability to initiate talking and may also affect the clarity, sound and flow of the voice. Problems with speech production can be caused by a range of factors, including weakness and poor coordination of orofacial and respiratory muscles.

Language

Expressive language disorders are those that impair the ability to formulate and produce verbal and written communication.

Receptive language disorders are those that affect the ability to process and understand verbal and written communications. Problems may occur with use of language in social situations (pragmatics).

Linguistics

Linguistic disorders are those that affect comprehension of the meaning of language and of non-verbal communications, such as signs, diagrams or symbols. Other linguistic problems affect the construction of sentences and syntax.

Cognition

Problems with cognition can affect verbal memory, as well as logical and inferential thinking, which in turn can impair communication.

Referral

The referral criteria for SLT assessment include:

- absence, delay or abnormality of speech
- problems with understanding or making self understood
- difficulties with interpersonal relationships.

Assessment

The assessment by an SLT will cover the following principal areas:

- history – developmental delays, medical history, difficulties with understanding, speech, reading and writing in different contexts
- examination of pragmatic skills, voice production, breath control, attention, concentration, memory and problem-solving skills
- tests of vocabulary, grammar, hearing, intellectual abilities, comprehension and memory
- hearing and visual impairments may be detected by an SLT, who may recommend further assessment.

Treatment

A range of treatment strategies can be used to improve speech, language and communication:

- exercises to improve speech production, articulation and intelligibility
- interventions to increase self-awareness and awareness of others
- education to increase understanding of communication in social contexts
- strategies to improve hearing (arranging for hearing tests, referral for an ENT opinion or treatment)
- individual communication strategies, developed with the SLT
- alternative communication strategies or aids such as Makaton symbols (see www.makaton.org) or pictorial systems (e.g. cards to display needs or emotions).

Communication skills may be taught and enhanced using a comprehensive system of teaching, discussion and experiential learning. Treatment will be individualised to meet the patient's specific needs. Improved communication skills can increase confidence and self-esteem, improve interpersonal relationships and facilitate access and success with other treatment programmes.

British Sign Language (BSL; see www.british-sign.co.uk) is a system of communication for the deaf comprising standardised sign language, with finger spelling, hand signs and pictorial signs (Fig. 5.5). BSL interpreters can be employed to convey the communication of deaf signing patients to hearing staff and visa versa. However, it is beyond the scope of this book to describe BSL in detail.

- Check for understanding: ask patients to say what they understand has been said. Give written and pictorial material to aid understanding and retention of information.
- When appropriate, communication and other care plans should be shared with the patient, family, carers, health professionals and educators.
- New staff/carers should be made aware of communication strategies.
- Seek advice from an SLT if communication needs cannot easily be addressed.
- If communication deteriorates, check the patient's mental state, hearing and vision or consult an SLT.

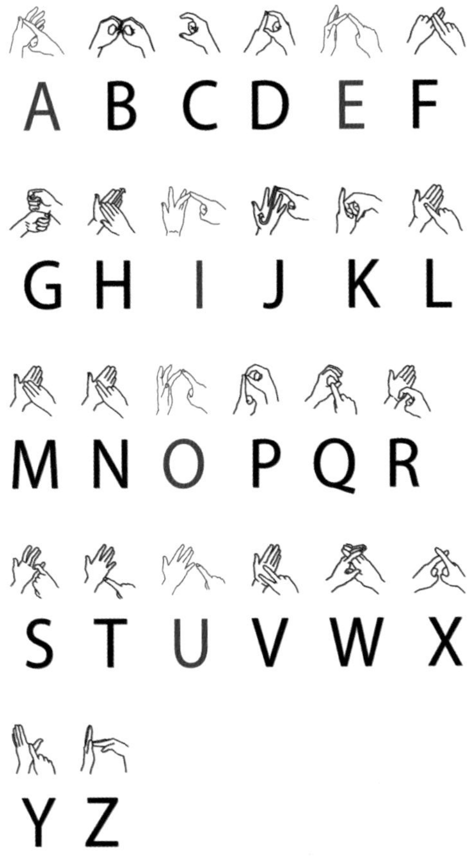

A B C D E F

G H I J K L

M N O P Q R

S T U V W X

Y Z

Fig. 5.5 The BSL finger-spelling alphabet. (Courtesy of www.british-sign.co.uk).

Dysphagia

Dysphagia is difficulty eating foods and drinking liquids. Difficulties can arise at any stage of the swallowing process, from chewing, formation of a bolus to the transfer of a bolus into the pharynx (i.e. the oral preparatory phase, oral phase and pharyngeal phase of swallowing). Causes of dysphagia include trauma, obstruction and neuromuscular disorders (e.g. stroke, multiple sclerosis, Parkinson's disease) and medication side-effects (e.g. extrapyramidal side-effects of psychotropic drugs) (Box 5.9). Dysphagia may also be caused by carcinoma of the oesophagus and oropharynx, which are associated with heavy drinking and smoking. Information on dysphagia after stroke is available from the Scottish Intercollegiate Guidelines Network.[18] Poisoning with corrosive liquids is a rare cause of dysphagia.

Dysphagia is common among those with intellectual disabilities.

Assessment

The patient history will cover the following areas:

- slow pace of eating or drinking
- food lodging in cheek sulcus
- dribbling or drooling
- sensation of food sticking in the throat
- coughing during eating or drinking, or after a meal
- choking or laryngeal spasm
- 'wet voice', caused by secretions collecting in the laryngeal vestibule
- recurrent respiratory infections

Box 5.9 Medications with side-effects that may affect swallowing

- Antipsychotic medications with extrapyramidal side-effects
- Any sedatives or medications that impair the level of consciousness
- Bisphosphonates (used for treatment of osteoporosis)
- Potassium supplements

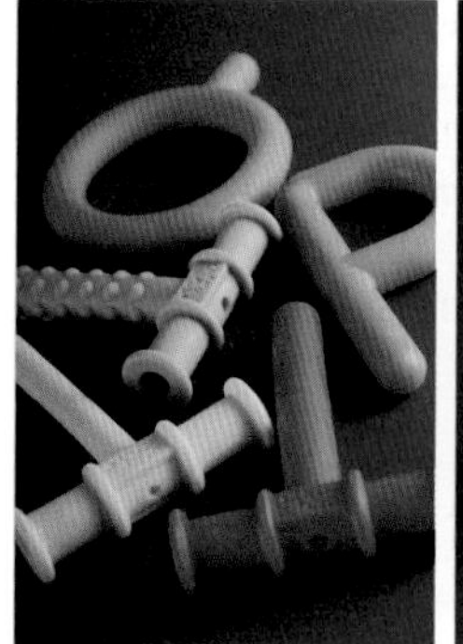
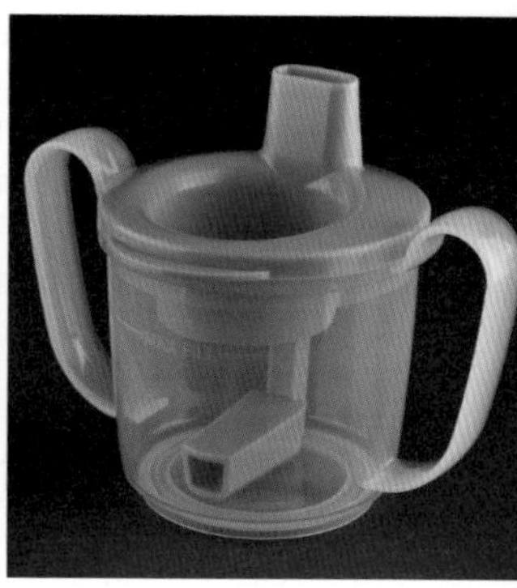

Fig. 5.6 Chewy Tubes™ (left) are used to develop chewing and biting skills and Drink Rite™ cup (right) for drinking liquids safely, without head tilting. By kind permission of Kapitex Healthcare.

- medication with extrapyramidal side-effects
- medical history of stroke, Parkinson's disease or other neurological disorders.

A speech and Language therapist (SLT) will observe the patient's posture, saliva management and oral hygiene, and check whether food debris collects in the buccal sulcus.

The patient will be observed drinking teaspoons of water (water swallow test). If it is safe to proceed, the SLT will observe the patient swallowing liquids and food with different textures. The SLT will also palpate the throat while the patient swallows.

Further examination may incorporate:

- video-fluoroscopy with food of various consistencies mixed with barium
- fibre-optic endoscopic evaluation of the pharyngeal and laryngeal stages of swallowing, using a flexible nasoendoscope inserted through the nares.

Treatment

Treatment will aim to rectify the underlying cause of dysphagia. The SLT may:

- recommend oral and facial exercises to improve muscle strength
- recommend changing the psychotropic medication or adding an anti-muscarinic drug
- make dietary modifications (e.g. avoid certain foods, puree meals, thicken drinks and offer carbonated or iced drinks)
- teach the patient postural manoeuvres to use when eating or drinking
- offer advice about taking small mouthfuls, reduced distraction during meals, allowing more time to eat and drink
- modify the environment for eating (e.g. seating and posture when eating)
- recommend special implements (Fig. 5.6).

The therapist will recommend the patient is referred to a physician, neurologist or ENT specialist if a serious underlying cause is suspected or if a nasogastric or gastronomy feeding is necessary.

No one should attempt to insert a nasogastric tube unless they have been trained to do so. A patient may die if a feed or medication is accidentally administered into the lungs via a nasogastric tube. The National Patient Safety Agency has issued guidance for the safe insertion of nasogastric feeding tubes.[19]

Recommended reading

France J, Kramer S. *Communication and Mental Illness: Theoretical and Practical Approaches.* Jessica Kingsley, 2005.

Hargie O (ed.) *The Handbook of Communication Skills.* Routledge, 2006.

Occupational therapy services

Occupational therapists assess and treat people with physical and mental conditions with purposeful activity to prevent disability, and to promote recovery and independence in daily life. They assist people with maintaining, enhancing and developing their occupation, leisure, work, self-care and daily living skills, individually or in group settings. The procedures typically undertaken are set out in Box 5.10.

Occupational therapists require a university degree or a postgraduate diploma in Occupational Therapy and registration with the Health Professions Council.

Assessment

Occupational therapists assess the physical, cognitive, psychological and environmental needs of people with various mental and physical disorders (e.g. dementia) and conditions, for example following injury, stroke and surgery. Therapists typically assess their patients' functional abilities, skills, knowledge, interests, routines, values and risks.

Clinical assessment

A clinical assessment will be undertaken to evaluate the patient's functional abilities, for example concentration, hand–eye coordination, dexterity, mobility, ability to sequence activities, risk of falling, as well as sight, hearing and environment. An example of a standardised assessment is the Assessment of Motor and Process Skills (AMPS, details of which are available at www.ampsintl.com), which has standards for the assessment of over 100 activities of daily living (Fig. 5.7).

Cognitive assessment

Occupational therapists may assess cognitive function and devise strategies to help patients to cope with memory deficits, improve coordination, sequencing of tasks, decision-making and time management.

Activity analysis

Occupational therapists may undertake an activity analysis with regard to the patient's choice of valued activities, and identify where rehabilitation, adaptations or aids can meet the specific needs of individual patients. For example, the process of making a hot drink involves several abilities:

- to judge how much water to put in the kettle
- to lift and tip a kettle
- to manipulate a cup, spoon and containers
- to sequence the adding of ingredients to a cup.

Patients with weakness of their dominant hand may be able to make a hot drink independently if they use

Box 5.10 Occupational therapy assessment and treatment procedures

- Informal assessment by observation of the patient in various settings
- Formal assessment of specific activities or tasks
- Standardised assessments
- Discussions with patients and carers
- Formulation of problems or difficulties
- Analysis of component parts of activities
- Negotiation of priorities with patients
- Collaborative working between the patient and therapist
- Remedy of deficits: changing physical, social or institutional environment
- Action plans, using activity as a therapeutic tool
- Enabling patients to achieve set goals
- Monitoring progress and achievements
- Reporting of progress
- Return to initial stages of the process

Source: Adapted from Creek, 2003.[20]

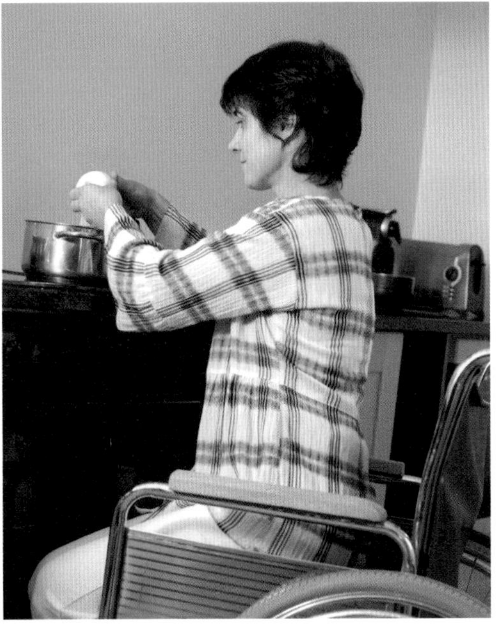

Fig. 5.7 A woman in a wheelchair cooking dinner, one of the standard activities of daily living.

a jug to fill the kettle with small amounts of water, and if they cannot tip the kettle then a kettle tipper device could be used instead.

Physical modifications and aids

Occupational therapists may recommend physical modifications of the environment, such as grab rails in toilet and bathing areas, access via a ramp and emergency call systems. A wide range of aids can be used to overcome the impact of disabilities, ranging from aids to put on socks, special cutlery and drinking cups, to mobility aids such as walking frames and wheelchairs.

Rehabilitation

Occupational therapists work with patients, carers and multidisciplinary teams to facilitate rehabilitation, the aim of which will be, for example, to enable patients to improve their confidence and skills with shopping, cooking, money management (e.g. paying bills), travelling on public transport and with making telephone calls.

Roles in life

Roles in life are important because they underpin a person's sense of self-worth and place in society. Occupational therapists can assist patients to recognise their roles in life, whether as family members, members of a social or religious group, or members of the workforce.

Recommended reading

Creek J. *Core Concepts of Occupational Therapy: A Dynamic Framework for Practice.* Jessica Kingsley, 2010.

Curtin M, Molineux M, Supyk J. *Occupational Therapy and Physical Dysfunction: Principles, Skills and Practice.* Elsevier, 2010.

Physiotherapy

Physiotherapists complete a 3- or 4-year university course and register to practise with the Health Professions Council. Their professional body is the Chartered Society of Physiotherapy (www.csp.org.uk).

The role of the physiotherapist is to improve or recover patients' movements, function and independence by using manual therapies and techniques such as ultrasound, as well as active and passive mobilisation.

Physiotherapists undertake diagnostic assessments and use instruments to measure range of movement, strength and physical characteristics of an area of the body. They design programmes of exercise, with active and passive movements, and teach patients how to complete their programme.

Physiotherapists are trained to assess the movements of joints and muscles by palpation, to identify damaged tissues and areas where joint surfaces are not gliding properly over one another. Manipulation, stretching and exercises are used to overcome restrictions on movement.

The role of the physiotherapist is also to assess and advise on safe mobilisation using aids such as latex bands, walking sticks and crutches, walking frames and wheelchairs. Physiotherapists play a key role in mobilisation of patients who have had surgery or a recent fall, and of those with balance or coordination problems.

Ultrasound may be used to improve the healing of soft tissues, improve blood flow and reduce tension in muscles. Similarly, ice packs are used to reduce swelling from recent injury and heat treatment is used to treat painful, tense areas.

In mental health settings, patients have various mental and physical health needs, so exercise programmes should be tailored to individual patients. Patients tend to prefer precise instructions for their exercises, rather than less structured instructions such as 'little and often'. For some patients, it is advisable to explain the exercises to staff and carers too.

Prevention is a key area of work for physiotherapists. Where patients are at risk of weight gain, the physiotherapist may encourage more cardiovascular exercise. They may lead 'healthy living' groups, promote exercise and motivate patients to lead a healthy lifestyle.

Recommended reading

Chartered Society of Physiotherapy and Chartered Physiotherapists in Mental Health. *A Framework for the Role of Physiotherapy in Mental Health and Wellness.* 2008.

Pope C. Recovering mind and body: a framework for the role of physiotherapy in mental health and well-being. *J Publ Ment Health* 2009; **8**: 36–9.

Pharmacy services

Pharmacists

Pharmacists complete a 4-year university course, followed by a pre-registration year and final examinations. In the UK, the General Pharmaceutical Council was established in 2010 to regulate the profession. The Royal Pharmaceutical Society has retained its role as the professional body for pharmacists. Pharmacists may work in community settings, general hospitals or psychiatric facilities, normally where there is a dispensary. Some pharmacists undertake additional training to enable them to register and practise as non-medical prescribers. Pharmacy technicians, assistants and administrators work closely with pharmacists.

Functions of pharmacy services

Medication

The role of the pharmacy service is to purchase, prepare, supply and distribute medicines safely within existing legislative frameworks, quality standards and guidelines (Fig. 5.8). Additional legal obligations apply to certain drugs such as controlled drugs.

Clinical pharmacy

Pharmaceutical knowledge, skill and judgement are applied to patient care to ensure that the benefits of pharmacological treatments outweigh any potential problems such as side-effects and interactions with other treatments. Pharmacy clinical practice encompasses prescription monitoring, medication reviews, close liaison with other health professionals, provision of medicines, information services, drug education, clinical audit and practice research.

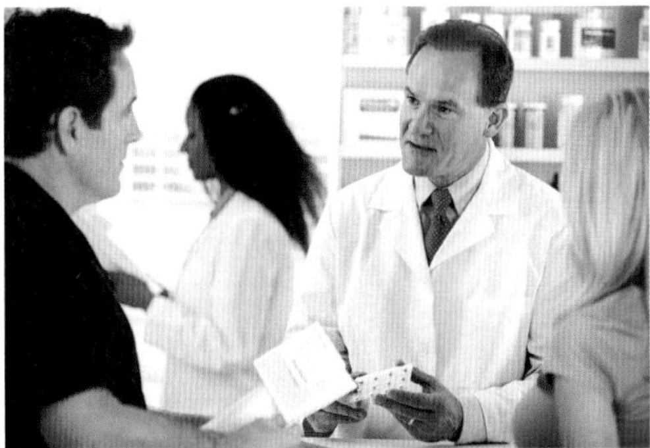

Fig. 5.8 Clinical pharmacist. A key role of clinical pharmacists is to advise and inform prescribers, as well as to check that the correct medication is dispensed and administered.

Safety and regulatory agencies

Safe and effective use of medicines is promoted nationally by bodies such as the National Patient Safety Agency (NPSA; www.npsa.nhs.uk), the Medicines and Healthcare products Regulatory Agency (MHRA; www.mhra.gov.uk/index.htm) and the National Institute for Health and Clinical Excellence (NICE; www.nice.org.uk). These agencies are responsible for issuing guidance and recommendations that pharmacists must incorporate into their working practice. The NPSA reports[21] that the most common type of incidents involving medication are:

- wrong dose, strength or frequency of medicine
- omitted medicine
- wrong medicine.

National Reporting and Learning System

In 2003, the NPSA set up the Reporting and Learning System (RLS; www.nrls.npsa.nhs.uk/report-a-patient-safety-incident) so that patients, carers and healthcare professionals can report 'unintended or unexpected incidents which could have, or did lead to harm' in a patient receiving NHS care. The RLS does not investigate reports but the information received is used to improve patient safety. The RLS publishes guidance to prevent harm to patients.

Role of pharmacists in mental health settings

Medication

Pharmacists will:

- check prescriptions, and dispense, check and record the dispensed medication
- use labelled containers, for named individuals
- provide written information and advice on the safe administration of medication
- advise clinicians of any incorrect prescriptions and medication interactions
- record allergies/contraindications, and alert clinicians to inappropriate prescriptions
- note past and current medical history (e.g. pregnancy, concomitant physical illness).

Monitoring

Pharmacists will monitor:

- drug interactions and side-effects
- tests required, as well as their frequency and results (e.g. electrocardiology, blood tests, drug serum levels)
- compliance with relevant Mental Health Act legislation for administration of treatment
- records of medication history (medication, length of treatment, efficacy, problems, etc.)
- storage and administration of medication in in-patient settings.

Liaison with others

Pharmacists will liaise with:

- clinical teams and ward staff
- monitoring services (e.g. for clozapine)
- healthcare services (e.g. local general hospital, general practitioner, community teams)
- wholesalers selling medication.

They will discuss treatment plans with the second-opinion appointed doctor (SOAD) for patients who are detained under the Mental Health Act 1983 in England and Wales.

Education and information

Pharmacists will:

- provide access to written or electronic guidelines on a range of medications
- advise clinicians, patients and carers
- provide advice on medication for physical disorders.

Clinics

Pharmacists may hold clinics for specific patient groups:

- patients at high risk of weight gain due to certain medications (e.g. clozapine, olanzapine)
- patients taking depot medication
- patients taking lithium.

Clinical governance and medicines management

Pharmacists will:

- monitor medication errors, omissions and near misses
- be members of drugs and therapeutics committee
- develop a formulary of medication
- notify relevant authorities if a serious incident has occurred
- conduct research and audit.

Community pharmacists

In addition to providing a prescription dispensing service, community pharmacists may sell certain medications over the counter for minor ailments and provide small quantities of medications to patients without a prescription in the event that an emergency supply is necessary. Pharmacists who have undertaken additional training can be registered as non-medical prescribers, allowing them to write prescriptions for prescription-only medicines within their area of expertise. Increasingly, community pharmacists are taking on other clinical roles, such as the management of asthma and diabetes, and blood pressure measurement, as well as providing lifestyle information on topics such as healthy eating and smoking cessation.

Adverse reactions to medication

Pharmacists have a key role in ensuring that adverse reactions are reported to relevant authorities. In the UK, the Medicines and Healthcare products Regulatory Agency (MHRA) is responsible for ensuring that medicines and medical devices both work and are safe. It does this by collecting information on suspected adverse drug reactions and takes action to protect the public if there is a problem. Patients and health professionals should use the Yellow Card Scheme (Fig. 5.9) to report suspected adverse reactions (www.mhra.gov.uk/Safetyinformation/Howwemonitorthesafetyofproducts/Medicines/TheYellowCardScheme/index.htm).

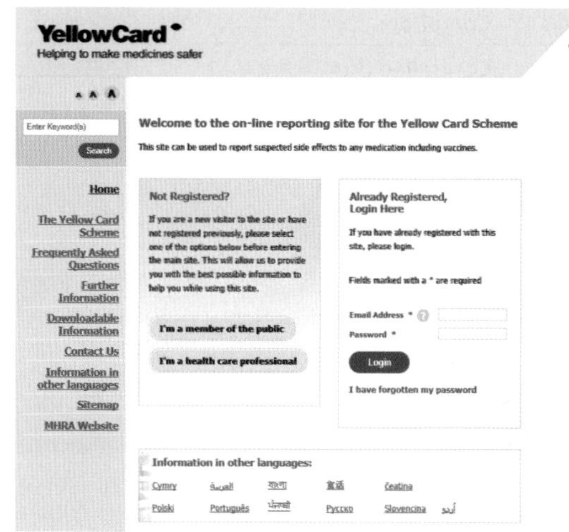

Fig. 5.9 Yellow Card Scheme for reporting suspected adverse drug reactions. Courtesy of MHRA.

The MHRA also collects reports of defects in medicinal devices and serious side-effects involving blood and blood components.

Controlled drugs

The Misuse of Drugs Act 1971 controls the export, import, production, supply and possession of 'dangerous or otherwise harmful drugs' which are designated 'controlled drugs'. The Act imposes a total prohibition on the possession, supply, manufacture, import or export of controlled drugs except as allowed by the Secretary of State. The legitimate use of controlled drugs is permitted under the Act by the Misuse of Drugs Regulations 2001, as amended, which classify controlled drugs into five schedules, in descending order of control. A summary of the schedules of the Act is presented in Table 5.4.

Pharmacists have a general authority to possess, supply and dispense all controlled drugs except drugs in schedule 1. Other classes of people who are required to possess and supply controlled drugs in the course of their business (e.g. wholesalers) must be granted a licence by the Home Office.

Pharmacists have responsibilities for the recording, monitoring and inspection of controlled drugs, maintaining running balances, making arrangements for the destruction of unusable stock, and for dealing with legal and ethical issues. Changes to legislation in the wake of the Shipman inquiry resulted in the Controlled Drugs (Supervision of Management and Use) Regulations 2006, which require every healthcare organisation prescribed as a designated body to appoint a 'controlled drugs accountable officer' to take organisational responsibility for controlled drugs. This individual is often (but not always) the chief pharmacist within the organisation.

The National Prescribing Centre (www.npc.nhs.uk) has resources and information on good practice and the management of controlled drugs in various settings, mainly for pharmacists and prescribers.

- Seek advice from a pharmacist before prescribing controlled drugs (CDs).
- Do not prescribe controlled drugs for anyone unless you are licensed to do so.
- Learn the correct way to write prescriptions for controlled drugs.
- Learn the correct process for giving prescriptions to others.
- Never prescribe controlled drugs for friends, relatives or yourself.

Table 5.4 A summary of the schedules of the Misuse of Drugs Act 1971

Schedule	Conditions applied	Comments	Examples of drugs classified
1	Controlled drug licence	It is illegal to possess these drugs without a licence	Cannabis, coca leaf, lysergic acid diethylamide (LSD)
2	Controlled drugs, with a register	These drugs have to be stored, prescribed and administered according to specific conditions	Morphine, pethidine, secobarbital, amphetamine, cocaine
3	Controlled drugs, without a register	Includes stimulant drugs and drugs with less potential for misuse	Barbiturates (except secobarbital), buprenorphine, midazolam, pentazocine and temazepam
4	Special requirements for the import, export and manufacture of drugs		Benzodiazepines (except temazepam and midazolam) and fencamfamine and most androgenic steroids and growth hormone
5	Requirement to retain invoices for purchase for 2 years		Low-strength preparations of codeine, pholcodeine and morphine

Adapted from www.patient.co.uk/doctor/Controlled-Drugs.htm

Recommended reading

Appelbe GE, Wingfield J. *Dale and Appelbe's Pharmacy Law and Ethics (9th Edn)*. Pharmaceutical Press, 2009.

Bazire S. *Psychotropic Drug Directory*. Lloyd-Reinhold Communications, 2012.

Ciraulo D, Greenblat D, Shader R, *et al*. *Drug Interactions in Psychiatry (3rd Edn)*. Lippincott Williams & Wilkins, 2005.

Summary

Providing comprehensive health care requires a team of health professionals. Health professionals allied to medicine play a key role in the detection, assessment and treatment of various aspects of physical health.

Mental health professionals should facilitate access to these health services so patients can benefit from the knowledge and expertise of these health professionals, in the community and during admission to psychiatric in-patient settings

Acknowledgements

With grateful thanks to the following health professionals for their assistance and guidance with this chapter.

Dentistry: Richard McCallum, Head of Oral Health, NHS Nottinghamshire County

Dietetics: Vera Todorovic, Consultant Dietitian in Clinical Nutrition, Doncaster and Bassetlaw Hospitals NHS Foundation Trust

Occupational therapy: Elizabeth Rowbottam, Occupational Therapist, Nottinghamshire Healthcare NHS Trust

Optometry: John Duffy, Optometrist, Nottinghamshire Healthcare NHS Trust

Physiotherapy: John Isaacs, Chartered Physiotherapist, Nottinghamshire Healthcare NHS Trust

Pharmacy: John White, Chief Pharmacist (Forensic Services), Nottinghamshire Healthcare NHS Trust.

Podiatry: Steve Winfield, Podiatrist, Rampton Hospital, Nottinghamshire Healthcare NHS Trust

Speech and language therapy: Kim Turner, Speech, Language and Communication Therapist, Central and North West London NHS Foundation Trust, and Lesley Tierney, Speech and Language Therapist with a special interest in dysphagia, Nottinghamshire Healthcare NHS Trust

References

1 NHS Screening Programmes. NHS Newborn Hearing Screening Programme, 2012 (http://hearing.screening.nhs.uk).

2 Deafness Research UK. *Hearing Tests for Babies and Young Children*. Deafness Research UK, 2010 (www.deafnessresearch.org.uk/factsheets/hearing-tests-for-babies.pdf).

3 Davis A, Smith P, Ferguson M, *et al*. Acceptability, benefit and costs of early screening for hearing disability: a study of potential screening tests and models. *Health Technol Assess* 2007; **11** (http://www.hta.ac.uk/fullmono/mon1142.pdf).

4 Department of Health. *Transforming Adult Hearing Services for Patients with Hearing Difficulty – A Good Practice Guide*. Department of Health, 2007.

5 Du Feu M, Fergusson K. Sensory impairment in mental health. *Adv Psychiatr Treat* 2003; **9**: 95–103.

6 Steiger JR. Audiologic referral criteria: sample clinic guidelines. *Hearing J* 2005; **58**: 38–42.

7 Kiani R, Miller H. Sensory impairment and intellectual disability. *Adv Psychiatr Treat* 2010; **16**: 228–35.

8 National Institute for Health and Clinical Excellence. *Type 2 Diabetes: Prevention and Management of Foot Problems (Clinical Guidelines CG10)*. NICE, 2004.

9 Davies R, Bedi R, Scully C. Oral health care for patients with special needs. *BMJ* 2000; **321:** 495–8.

10 National Institute for Health and Clinical Excellence. *Prophylaxis Against Infective Endocarditis: Antimicrobial Prophylaxis Against Infective Endocarditis in Adults and Children Undergoing Interventional Procedures (Clinical Guidelines CG64)*. NICE, 2008.

11 NHS Information Centre for Health and Social Care. *Prescribing by Dentists, 2008: England*. NHS, 2009.

12 Scully C, Shotts R. Mouth ulcers and other causes of orofacial soreness and pain. *BMJ* 2000; **321**: 162–5.

13 Matevosyan NR. Oral health of adults with serious mental illnesses: a review. *Comm Ment Health J* 2010; **46**: 553–62.

14 National Institute for Health and Clinical Excellence. *Dental Recall: Recall Intervals Between Dental Examinations (Clinical Guidelines CG19)*. NICE, 2004.

15 National Institute for Health and Clinical Excellence. *Obesity (Clinical Guidelines CG43)*. NICE, 2010.

16 National Institute for Health and Clinical Excellence. *Type 2 Diabetes: The Management of Type 2 Diabetes (Update; Clinical Guidelines CG66)*. NICE, 2008.

17 Department of Health. *Better Hospital Food Programme*. Department of Health, 2010.

18 Scottish Intercollegiate Guidelines Network. *Management of Patients with Stroke: Identification and Management of Dysphagia (National Clinical Guideline 78)*. SIGN, 2004.

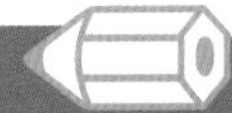

Learning points

- In the UK, babies and children should have hearing tests.
- Everyone with intellectual difficulties should be screened for sensory impairments.
- People with type 2 diabetes should receive foot care according to standards in NICE guidelines CG10.
- Gum health is improved by tooth brushing, which removes the bacteria and food debris that contribute to infection and inflammation of gums.
- Oral cancer accounts for 1% of cancers in the UK and is more common in people aged over 40 years, in those who use tobacco and in people who drink alcohol.
- Oral cancers can be painless and may present as ulcers, which are slow to heal.
- Guidance from NICE is available on prophylaxis against infective endocarditis.[8]
- Systemic diseases, drugs and radiotherapy can cause oral ulcers, dental pain, halitosis (bad breath) and difficulty eating.
- Dietetics referrals should be made when there are concerns about under- or over-nutrition, nutritional deficiencies and health problems requiring dietary intervention.
- Annual sight tests are available on the NHS for people under 16 years old, those over 70 years old, people with diabetes and for all those who have a potentially progressive eye disease such as glaucoma, age-related macular degeneration, cataract, corneal dystrophy or ocular hypertension.
- First aid for chemical burns of the eyes should be lengthy irrigation with sterile saline or water, which may save a person's sight.
- Improved communication skills can increase patients' confidence and self-esteem, and facilitate success with other treatment programmes.
- Never attempt to insert a nasogastric tube unless you have been trained to do so.
- A patient may die if a feed is accidentally administered into the lungs via a nasogastric tube.
- Occupational therapists can use standardised tools to assess activities of daily living.
- In physiotherapy in mental health settings, patients tend to prefer precise instructions for their exercises, rather than less structured instructions such as 'little and often'.
- For adverse drug reactions, patients and health professionals can use the Yellow Card System to report suspected adverse reactions.
- There is a correct process for giving prescriptions of controlled drugs to others and prescribers should never prescribe controlled drugs for friends, relatives or themselves.

19 National Patient Safety Agency. *Reducing the Harm Caused by Misplaced Nasogastric Feeding Tubes in Adults, Children and Infants.* NPSA, 2011.

20 Creek J. *Occupational Therapy Defined as a Complex Intervention.* Royal College of Occupational Therapists, 2003.

21 National Patient Safety Agency. *Safety in Doses: Medication Safety Incidents in the NHS (The Fourth Report from the Patient Safety Observatory).* NPSA, 2007.

6

Tobacco smoking

Lisa McNally

Smoking is an important risk factor for many diseases that cause premature morbidity and mortality. Smoking is particularly prevalent in psychiatric settings. This chapter discusses the factors that influence smoking and those that encourage patients to stop smoking. It also describes the treatments and devices that may be of help.

Introduction

Smoking is the single most preventable cause of death and disability in the world today.[1] Tobacco is an addictive substance that affects smokers' physical, mental, social and economic well-being. However, its use still thrives within the culture of mental healthcare.

This chapter provides an overview of the effects of smoking, with a particular focus on the users of mental healthcare services; it gives guidance on the important assessments, interventions and strategies related to smoking. Both in-patient and community healthcare settings are considered, along with the role of healthcare partners such as the Stop Smoking Services provided by the National Health Service (NHS).

The prevalence of smoking in psychiatric settings

In the UK estimates suggest that around 10 million adults are regular smokers according to a 2007 survey, representing some 21% of the adult population.[2] Among people with mental health problems, smoking rates are much higher. People with depressive episodes, phobias or obsessive–compulsive disorders are twice as likely to smoke as the general population,[3] while those with schizophrenia are nearly six times more likely to be smokers.[4]

Factors influencing smoking in psychiatric settings

There are three 'hypotheses' relating to why smoking is so prevalent among people with mental health problems (Box 6.1). All three factors cited may be present and may interact to influence smoking.[5]

First, the 'self-medication' hypothesis suggests that smoking is motivated primarily by negative reinforcement and its potential to offset some adverse features of mental health conditions. Nicotine stimulates the subcortical reward system and the prefrontal cortex, which both appear to be hypofunctional in schizophrenia.[6] There is contradictory evidence that smoking provides little benefit.[7] Indeed, as discussed

Box 6.1 Factors that can promote smoking in psychiatric settings

- *Self-medication.* Patients try to use smoking to alleviate adverse symptoms
- *The culture of mental healthcare.* Staff and other service users facilitate smoking
- *Filling a void.* Patients use cigarettes to alleviate boredom or as a daily coping strategy

Box 6.2 The impact of smoking

- Poor physical health
- Premature mortality
- Increased depression and anxiety
- Drained economic resources
- Aged physical appearance
- Difficulty in no-smoking settings

below, smoking has been implicated in the onset and worsening of mental health problems.

Second, the 'cultural' hypothesis suggests that the prevalence of smoking is raised and maintained by its central place in the 'culture' of mental healthcare. A large proportion of staff are also smokers[8] and they often use cigarettes to appease or engage patients.[9] It is therefore unsurprising that smoking-related interventions and policy have been found to be significantly less popular among mental health staff than among other healthcare professionals.[10]

Finally, the 'void hypothesis' is based on the idea that smoking, for mental health patients, is 'all they have in life' and stopping smoking will leave a significant void in their lives. However, it is worth noting that this theory may operate, at least in part, as a 'self-fulfilling prophecy'. A more positive approach to a perceived 'void' in a patient's life, rather than simply using it to justify smoking, may be actually addressing the void via smoking cessation programmes. Smoking cessation treatment, because of its person-centred and facilitative approach, can be used to empower a service user to find new activities and new ways of coping with stress.

Physical conditions

Smoking is a major cause of mortality. It is estimated that between 1950 and 2000 around 60 million people died from tobacco-related diseases in the 40 countries studied.[11] In England, around 18% of deaths (among those aged 35 years or more) were attributable to smoking in 2007.[12] Non-fatal illness and disability are also a consequence of smoking, notably asthma, peripheral vascular disease, infertility and dental problems. This places a large burden on healthcare services; one estimate suggested that in 2005–6 the direct cost of smoking to the NHS was £5.2 billion (Box 6.2).[13]

Stopping smoking is associated with numerous physical health gains, even when chronic illness has already developed due to smoking. Smoking cessation improves respiratory symptoms and bronchial hyper-responsiveness, and prevents accelerated decline in lung function, in all smokers, with or without chronic obstructive pulmonary disease (see Chapter 13).[14]

Impact of smoking on mental health

Taken as a whole, the research evidence suggests that any psychological 'gains' from smoking are, at best, transient and unsustainable. In fact, there is substantial evidence to suggest that smoking is actually detrimental to mental health, including depression[15,16] and anxiety.[17,18] Notably, stopping smoking seems to lead to a significant decrease in anxiety from the first week of abstinence.[19]

There are a number of possible mechanisms for the adverse effects of smoking on mental health. Explanations have made reference to the relationship between nicotine and serotonin[20] and the psychological effects of impaired respiration.[18]

Investigations and monitoring

Before a programme of smoking cessation is begun, it is essential to conduct an assessment, covering the four elements discussed below. This takes only about 5 minutes and should ideally take place within the context of a brief intervention (see later in the chapter). Such an assessment should be carried out routinely with all smokers, not just with those expressing the desire to quit.

1. Carbon monoxide breath test

An assessment related to smoking should always begin with a carbon monoxide test. As well as giving some indication of the extent to which smoking is affecting the patient, it can serve to highlight this to the patient, possibly thereby boosting their motivation to quit. A carbon monoxide breath monitor (Fig. 6.1) allows a quick, simple and non-invasive procedure. For purposes of interpretation, the normal carbon monoxide level for a non-smoker is usually less than 10 parts per million. The level for a smoker is usually much higher, and will vary according to the number of tobacco products smoked, how the smoke is inhaled and the time between smoking a cigarette and the assessment.

2. Motivation to quit

It is helpful to gauge the extent to which the patient wants to stop smoking. Patients can be asked to rate how important quitting smoking currently is to them, on a numerical scale such as 1 to 10, or 0 to 100%. A patient who rates the importance of quitting as very low should not be referred for support to stop smoking. Patients expressing a moderate or high desire to quit should always be referred for treatment, after the additional assessments discussed below.

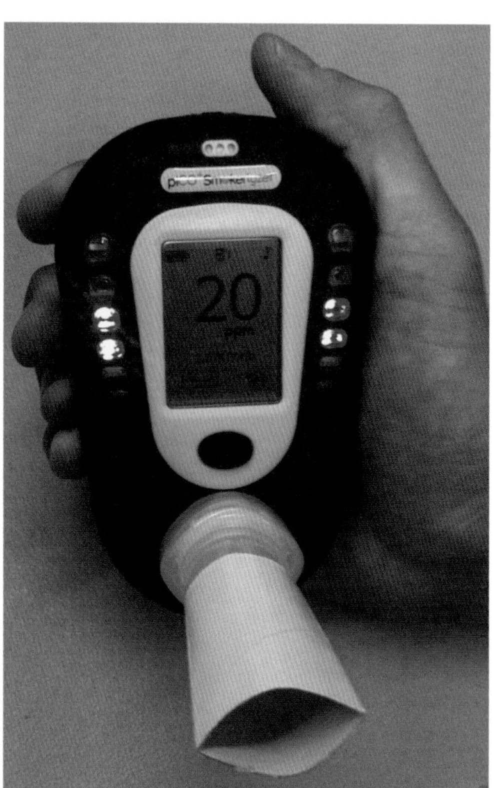

Fig. 6.1 Carbon monoxide breath testing device.

3. Self-efficacy

Self-efficacy can be defined as an individual's belief that he or she can succeed in the face of challenges. Research has found low self-efficacy to be a major predictor of relapse in smoking cessation.[21] Poor self-efficacy is likely to lead to the perception that stopping smoking will be difficult and, in turn, discourage attempts to quit. Tools aimed at assessing self-efficacy or perceived difficulties specifically in relation to smoking, along with methods to enhance self-efficacy, have been developed. One such tool is the Smoking Cessation Assessment of Need (SCAN).[22] Low self-efficacy should not be seen as a contraindication for a referral to stop smoking support, although low ratings should be briefly discussed and communicated to the team delivering this support.

4. Medication

Hydrocarbon by-products of smoking induce production of cytochrome P450 enzymes 1A2 (CYP1A2).[23] These are involved in the metabolism of some forms of psychotropic medication and, as a result, smokers often require higher doses. It follows that if a service user stops smoking, then a fall in CYP1A2 enzymes may occur over the course of a few days. An increase in plasma levels of some medications can therefore result if the same dosage is maintained, presenting a risk of adverse effects.

A number of different medications may be affected (Box 6.3). A notable example is the atypical anti-psychotic clozapine (Clozaril®), often prescribed for treatment-resistant schizophrenia. There can be a 1.5-fold rise in clozapine plasma concentrations in the 2–4 weeks following smoking cessation[24] and in some instances a 50–70% increase within 2–4 days. If baseline plasma concentrations are high – particularly over 1 mg/l – the plasma concentration may rise dramatically, owing to non-linear pharmacokinetics. If patients who are smoking more than 7–12 cigarettes per day while taking clozapine decide to quit, the dose may need to be reduced by 50%.[25,26] Baseline plasma levels of clozapine should be obtained before a patient

Box 6.3 Some medications affected by smoking

The levels of the following drugs (among others) are likely to increase in the days after a patient stops smoking:

clozapine	haloperidol
olanzapine	ziprasidone
chlorpromazine	mesoridazine
thiothixene	amitriptyline
fluphenazine	fluvoxamine
trifluoperazine	clomipramine
imipramine	desipramine
mirtazapine	nortriptyline
doxepin	duloxetine
trazodone	lorazepam
diazepam	warfarin
insulin	

stops smoking. Subsequently, monitoring should take place (by both staff and the patient themselves) for signs of toxicity, such as drowsiness or myoclonic spasms. If these signs emerge then the dose should be reduced and plasma levels monitored more frequently.[27]

It should be noted that, because the effects of smoking on medication metabolism described above are not a direct result of nicotine consumption, the strategy of attempting to counteract the increase in plasma clozapine (or other medications) is unlikely to be effective. The only valid course of action is an appropriate reduction in the prescribed dose of the medication. Similarly, if a patient is non-smoking and recommences smoking, the dose of clozapine should be increased.

Smoking induces production of cytochrome P450 enzymes that may be involved in the metabolism of some psychotropic medications. As a result, the risk of adverse effects may increase because smokers often require higher doses of medication; a fall in CYP1A2 enzymes may occur within days of quitting smoking; and the plasma levels of some medications may then increase without a change in drug dosage.

The only valid course of action to counteract an increase in plasma concentration is an appropriate reduction in the prescribed dose of medication. If a non-smoking patient commences smoking, the dose of clozapine should be increased.

Pharmaceutical treatment to assist smoking cessation

The aim of pharmacological support (Box 6.4) is to ease the experience of withdrawal, making a successful attempt to quit more likely. While these aids to smoking cessation have great potential, they cannot completely eliminate cravings, and should normally be used as part of a full programme of stop smoking support. The only exception to this is when nicotine replacement products are used to alleviate withdrawal within the context of a smoke-free policy.

Nicotine replacement therapy

Nicotine replacement therapy (NRT) is designed to replace some of the nicotine previously gained from cigarettes and thereby to reduce withdrawal symptoms. It is available in several forms, including: skin patches (Fig. 6.2), chewing gum, lozenges, sublingual tablets, inhalators and a nasal spray.

Adding NRT to stop smoking support increases the rate of quitting by 50–70%.[28] While NRT is considered a relatively non-invasive medication, side-effects can include skin irritation (when taken using patches), stomach problems (when taken using gums or lozenges) or irritation to the eyes and nose (when taken as a nasal spray). Particular care should be taken when prescribing NRT to pregnant or breastfeeding women, as well as those with unstable cardiovascular problems.

Box 6.4 Pharmacotherapy aids for smoking cessation

- Nicotine patches
- Nicotine gum, lozenges or tabs
- Nicotine inhaler
- Nicotine nasal spray and mouth spray
- Bupropion (Zyban®) (with caution)
- Varenicline (Champix®) (with caution)

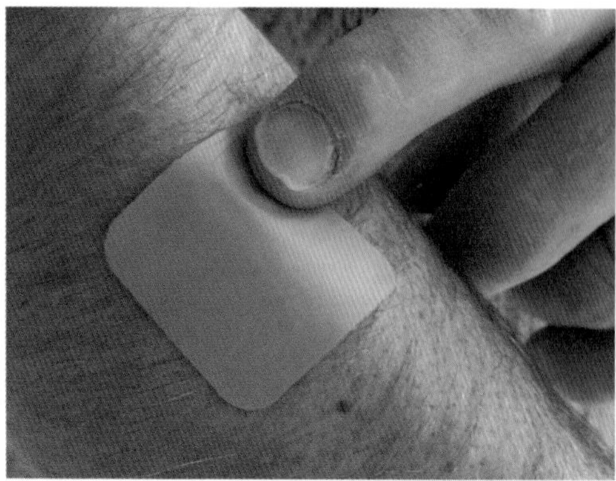
Fig. 6.2 Nicotine replacement patch.

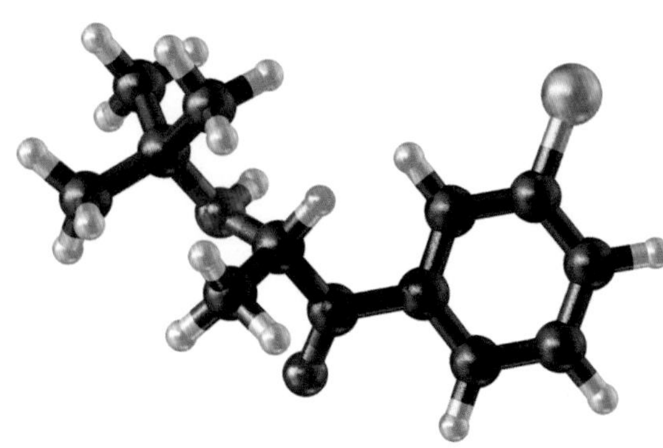
Fig. 6.3 Chemical structure of bupropion.

Bupropion

Bupropion (Zyban®) is an atypical antidepressant that acts as a noradrenaline and dopamine reuptake inhibitor. Studies suggest that it is an effective aid to smoking cessation.[29] However, it should be used in mental health settings with caution. One reason is that it has the potential to lower the seizure threshold and therefore may be dangerous when used in conjunction with other drugs known to have this effect, which include some antipsychotics and antidepressants.

Varenicline

The third and newest option available in relation to pharmacotherapy for smoking cessation is varenicline (Champix®). Varenicline is an alpha$_4$beta$_2$ nicotinic acetylcholine receptor partial agonist, which both relieves withdrawal and interferes with any rewarding effects of a lapse back to smoking. Treatment with varenicline begins before the quit date, with the dose being increased on cessation of smoking.

There is evidence to suggest that varenicline represents an effective smoking cessation pharmacotherapy.[30] The potential of varenicline is further boosted by its apparent lack of interactions with other medicines and its few side-effects (the most common effect in trials was mild to moderate nausea).

Some concern about varenicline has arisen due to the relatively high number of adverse event reports relating to suicidal thoughts or behaviour associated with its use. Although little evidence of an effect of varenicline on depression or suicidal behaviour has emerged in systematic research, prescribing guidance does highlight that care should be taken when prescribing varenicline to patients with a history of psychiatric illness. Mental well-being should be monitored through the quit attempt, and patients who develop suicidal thoughts or behaviour should stop their treatment and contact their doctor immediately.[31]

Referring to other services

All mental healthcare settings, including in-patient settings, should have clear referral pathways in place to the local NHS Stop Smoking Service. These services are usually delivered or commissioned by the local primary care trust, and offer treatment (usually over 6–8 weeks) within regular group-based or one-to-one sessions. The services also offer advice and training to other health professionals. Advice on when to refer is laid out in Box 6.5.

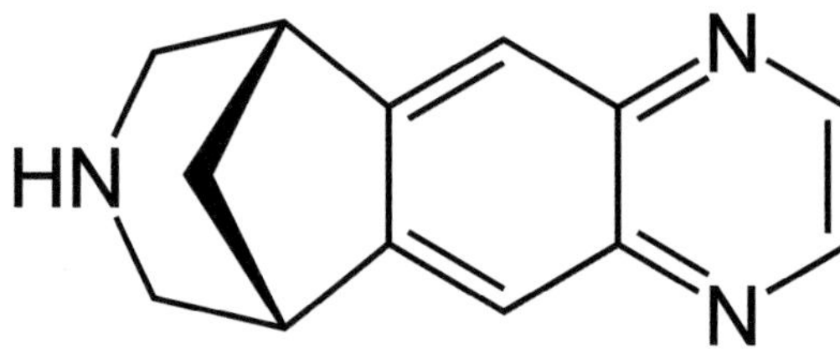

Fig. 6.4 Structure of varenicline.

Brief interventions

Brief interventions related to smoking should be delivered routinely to all smokers, not just those expressing a desire to quit. A brief intervention takes no more than 5 minutes and can follow a simple four 'A's procedure (Box 6.6). The four 'A's are:

- ask
- advise
- assist
- arrange.

The 'ask' stage begins with an assessment of the level of smoking by the patient (e.g. how many cigarettes per day) and supplements this with a carbon monoxide breath test (see above), the results of which should be recorded in the notes and fed back to the patient. At this stage, assessments of the patient's readiness to quit should also be carried out (see sections on motivation and self-efficacy above).

Whatever the patient's level of motivation to quit, the intervention should continue with the 'advise' stage. Some clear information about smoking and its impact should be given. Ideally, before the practitioner gives advice, patients should be encouraged to 'advise' themselves by being invited to say what they believe the drawbacks of smoking to be. These drawbacks may go beyond health issues and include the financial, cosmetic or social disadvantages of being a smoker.

Next, the 'assist' stage aims to raise self-efficacy by telling the patient about the treatments and support available. Reference should be made to the patient's earlier rating of self-efficacy. For example, a practitioner may ask why a moderate self-efficacy rating was given rather than a low rating and elicit positive statements such as 'Well, I have quit before for a while' or 'After all, I usually stick at things once I start them'.

The brief intervention ends with the 'arrange' stage, which, given an appropriate level of motivation, should include a referral for treatment. It is important at this stage to carry out the assessments related to medication interactions and pharmacotherapy. The patient's care coordinator should always be informed if a referral is made, as the NHS Stop Smoking Service will need to liaise throughout the quit attempt.

Box 6.5 When to refer to specialist smoking cessation services

- Conduct brief interventions with all patients who smoke
- If keen to stop, refer to any appropriate NHS agency providing advice and support on how to stop smoking
- Offer pharmacotherapy pending attendance

Box 6.6 The four 'A's of a brief intervention for smoking cessation

- *Ask.* Gauge the extent and impact of smoking. Assess readiness to quit.
- *Advise.* What does the patient see as the costs of smoking? Give clear advice.
- *Assist.* Give an overview of the treatments and support available.
- *Arrange.* Referral? Arrange pharmacotherapy and medication checks.

What to take into account in an in-patient setting

Smoking rates are high within residential and in-patient units[32] and such settings therefore present many opportunities for addressing smoking. In mental health settings, the 'smoking room' often acted as a social hub for patients. Attempts to address smoking should take these 'cultural' issues into account and deliver interventions within an environment that promotes quitting rather than smoking. Simple measures such as the display of pro-quitting posters and regular sessions on healthy living can contribute to this.

By far the most effective way of ensuring that a ward environment does not facilitate smoking is the introduction of a smoke-free policy. While the primary aim of banning smoking in ward settings is the protection of non-smoking patients and staff, moving smoking out of indoor areas, or even out of hospital grounds altogether, carries a clear message that smoking is no longer part of the ward culture. What is more, the fears of many staff that smoke-free policies will bring about ward disruption seem not to be borne out. In a systematic review of studies on ward-based smoking bans, the frequency of aggression, the use of seclusion, discharge against medical advice and the use of 'as needed' medication were found not to increase following policy implementation.[33]

Strategies for the introduction of a smoke-free policy in mental health settings are discussed in detail by Cormac & McNally.[27] Smoking indoors or within enclosed places became illegal in the UK in 2007, and was extended to mental health settings in 2008. While there is no longer a legal option to allow smoking on wards, there are still fundamental decisions that must be made. These include whether or not to provide outdoor smoking areas within hospital grounds, whether to allow designated 'smoking breaks' and the extent to which a policy is backed up with elements of smoking cessation support.

Smoking cessation support in the context of a smoke-free policy can have several benefits. The provision of nicotine replacement and advice on dealing with cravings will make patients more comfortable after their admission. By supporting patients with temporary abstinence from smoking induced by the smoke-free policy, it is possible to encourage more voluntary attempts to quit permanently, by enabling patients to assert control over their smoking.

Not all in-patient settings will be consistently appropriate for a full programme of stop smoking support (Box 6.7). In acute admissions wards, it may often be the case that, by the time a patient is well enough to engage in a programme of behavioural support, he or she may be close to being discharged. Acute-care in-patient settings can still fully engage in withdrawal support followed up by a brief intervention, and referral to stop smoking support in the community (see above for how to deliver a brief intervention).

However, in-patient settings providing for a longer admission, such as forensic services, are more able to accommodate a full, internal programme of stop smoking support.[34] These programmes should be developed and run in conjunction with local NHS Stop Smoking Services, which can provide expert advice, promotional resources, staff training and the co-facilitation of group-based sessions.

Box 6.7 Elements of NHS stop smoking support services for psychiatric patients

- Brief intervention and referral
- Checks on psychotropic medication
- Pharmacotherapy
- Setting of a 'quit date'
- Weekly support sessions
- Follow-up and relapse prevention

NHS, National Health Service.

What should happen in the community?

Community-based mental healthcare provides an excellent opportunity for the delivery of stop smoking support. The local NHS Stop Smoking Service can provide this in most cases, with mental health patients accessing the same range of services as other local people. A patient's care coordinator should always be central to the stop smoking support and be informed and consulted at every stage of treatment.

The care coordinator's role is important for a number of reasons, including the fact that he or she will need to ensure that the stop smoking treatment enhances rather than hinders other aspects of the patient's care. An obvious example of this is making sure that the potential effects of smoking cessation on psychotropic medication levels are addressed (see above). A care coordinator may also support the quit attempt directly, by offering encouragement and advice on quitting within their usual sessions with a patient.

The role of community care coordinators should not be restricted to supporting stop smoking programmes. They can also play a role in initiating quit attempts with a view to enhancing their patient's physical, mental and economic well-being. Community-based patients should therefore be offered routine brief interventions as part of their regular care. Care coordinators may be particularly well placed to offer these interventions due to their on-going relationship with the patient and their understanding of the factors that may be influencing the patient's smoking.

Interface between community and in-patient settings

The most important consideration in relation to the interface between community and in-patient settings is the establishment of efficient referral pathways to stop smoking support. There will usually be an opportunity for a brief intervention and referral towards the end of a patient's admission. If a referral is accepted then this should be communicated to both the local NHS Stop Smoking Service and the patient's care coordinator.

In establishing these referral pathways, effort should be made to ensure that stop smoking treatment is offered swiftly, in order to utilise the motivational 'momentum'. Arrangements for pharmacotherapy and medication checks should be made immediately (ideally before discharge) so that, on engaging with stop smoking support in the community, the patient does not experience any delays that may threaten a quit attempt.

Another important factor in the interface between community and in-patient settings relates to medication. The potential for smoking (and smoking cessation) to influence medication metabolism was discussed above. It follows from this that if a patient taking a medication that is affected by smoking restarts smoking, the dose may have to be increased to maintain an appropriate therapeutic level. This may be relevant when patients move from a non-smoking environment (e.g. a hospital ward) to a community setting in which smoking is allowed.

Summary

Addressing smoking is the responsibility of everyone in the healthcare system, including mental health settings. Ward staff and community-based professionals alike are well placed to encourage and facilitate patients' attempts to stop smoking, and by doing so make a real contribution to their overall physical, mental and economic well-being.

There are challenges, however, with none more important than the place of smoking within the culture of mental healthcare. The motivation of individual professionals to address smoking needs to be harnessed within an overall strategic approach that allows patients to find stop smoking support wherever they may be in the system. This, in turn, will require widespread training, effective partnership working and focused commissioning plans, all aimed at bringing about sustainable changes to how smoking is seen and addressed.

References

1 World Health Organization. *WHO Report on the Global Tobacco Epidemic, 2008: The MPOWER Package.* WHO, 2008 (http://www.who.int/tobacco/mpower/en/index.html).

2 Office for National Statistics. *General Household Survey: Smoking and Drinking Among Adults.* ONS, 2007.

3 Coultard M, Farrell M, Singleton N, *et al. Tobacco, Alcohol and Drug Use and Mental Health. TSO (The Stationery Office),* 2000.

4 de Leon J, Diaz FJ. A meta-analysis of worldwide studies demonstrates an association between schizophrenia and tobacco smoking behaviors. *Schizophr Res* 2005; **15**: 35–57.

5 McNally L. Smoking and mental health: influences on smoking. In *Quitting in Mind: A Guide to Influencing Stop Smoking Support in Mental Health Settings.* London Development Centre, 2009 (http://www.quittinginmind.net).

6 Chambers RA, Krystal JH, Self DW. A neurobiological basis for substance abuse comorbidity in schizophrenia. *Biol Psychiatry* 2001; **50**: 71–83.

7 Barnes M, Lawford BR, Burton SC, *et al.* Smoking and schizophrenia: is symptom profile related to smoking and which antipsychotic medication is of benefit in reducing cigarette use? *Aust N Z J Psychiatry* 2006; **40**: 575–80.

8 Trinkoff AM, Storr CL. Substance use among nurses: differences between specialties. *Am J Public Health* 1998; **88**: 581–5.

9 Mester R, Toren P, Ben-Moshe Y, *et al.* Survey of smoking habits and attitudes of patients and staff in psychiatric hospitals. *Psychopathology* 1993; **26**: 69–75.

10 McNally L, Oyefeso A, Annan J, *et al.* A survey of staff attitudes to smoking-related policy and intervention in psychiatric and general health care settings. *J Public Health* 2006; **28**: 192–6.

11 Peto R. *Mortality from Smoking in Developed Countries, 1950–2000.* Oxford Medical Publications, 1994.

12 The NHS Information Centre. *Statistics on Smoking: England, 2008.* The Information Centre, 2008 (http://www.ic.nhs.uk/pubs/smoking08).

13 Allender S, Balakrishnan R, Scarborough P, *et al.* The burden of smoking related ill health in the UK. Tobacco Control (online) 2009 (http://tobaccocontrol.bmj.com/cgi/content/abstract/tc.2008.026294v1).

14 Willemse BWM, Postma DS, Timens W, *et al.* The impact of smoking cessation on respiratory symptoms, lung function, airway hyperresponsiveness and inflammation. *Eur Respir J* 2004; **23**: 464–76.

15 Pasco JA, Williams LJ, Jacka FN, *et al.* Tobacco smoking as a risk factor for major depressive disorder: population-based study. *Br J Psychiatry* 2008; **193**: 322–6.

Learning points

- Smoking rates are much higher among people with mental health problems than among the general population.
- The highest smoking rates are found among patients with schizophrenia.
- The reasons why people with mental health problems are more likely to smoke include the potential for self-medication that comes with smoking, as well as cultural influences and a lack of alternative coping strategies.
- Regular smoking is detrimental to mental well-being as well as physical health.
- Routine assessments of smokers should include carbon monoxide breath tests, as well as brief measures of motivation and self-efficacy.
- Smoking affects enzymes involved in the metabolism of some forms of psychotropic medication and, as a result, smokers often require higher doses. An increase in the plasma levels of some medications can therefore result following cessation of smoking.
- Pharmacotherapy found to be effective for smoking cessation includes nicotine replacement therapy, bupropion and varenicline.
- Both nicotine replacement therapy and varenicline may be used by people with mental health conditions, although the latter should be used with caution. Bupropion is not generally recommended for smoking cessation in mental health settings.
- Brief interventions related to smoking should be delivered routinely with all smokers. This should result in a referral to specialist support if appropriate.
- Effective referral pathways for smoking cessation treatment should be developed between in-patient and community settings. Treatment should always involve the local NHS Stop Smoking Service.
- Smoke-free policies should be implemented and enforced within all mental health settings. In England and Northern Ireland, legislation prohibiting smoking in enclosed spaces now covers mental health settings.

16 Pedersen W, von Soest T. Smoking, nicotine dependence and mental health among young adults: a 13-year population based longitudinal study. *Addiction* 2009; **104**: 129–37.

17 Breslau N, Novak SP, Kessler RC. Daily smoking and the subsequent onset of psychiatric disorders. *Psychol Med* 2004; **34**: 323–33.

18 Johnson J, Cohen P, Pine D. Association between cigarette smoking and anxiety disorders during adolescence and early adulthood. *JAMA* 2000; **284**: 2348–51.

19 West R, Hajek P. What happens to anxiety levels on giving up smoking? *Am J Psychiatry* 1997; **154**: 1589–92.

20 Malone K, Waternaux C, Haas G. Cigarette smoking, suicidal behavior, and serotonin functioning in major psychiatric disorders. *Am J Psychiatry* 2003; **160**: 773–9.

21 Ockene JK, Emmons KM, Mermelstein RJ, *et al.* Relapse and maintenance issues for smoking cessation. *Health Psychol* 2000; **19** (1 suppl): 17–31.

22 McNally L. Psychological treatment dimensions: working with self-efficacy. In *Quitting in Mind: A Guide to Influencing Stop Smoking Support in Mental Health Settings*. London Development Centre, 2009.

23 Bazire S. *Psychotropic Drug Directory.* Fivepin, 2005.

24 de Leon J. Atypical antipsychotic dosing: the effect of smoking and caffeine. *Psychiatr Serv* 2004; **55**: 491–3.

25 Haslemo T, Eikeseth PH, Tanum L, *et al.* The effect of variable cigarette consumption on the interaction with clozapine and olanzapine. *Eur J Clin Pharmacol* 2006; **62**: 1049–53.

26 Ashir M. Smoking bans and cloazapine levels. *Adv Psychiatr Treat* 2008; **14**: 398–400.

27 Cormac I, McNally L. How to implement a smoke-free policy. *Adv Psychiatr Treat* 2008; **14**: 198–207.

28 Stead LF, Perera R, Bullen C, *et al.* Nicotine replacement therapy for smoking cessation. *Cochrane Database Syst Rev* 2008; **issue 1**: CD000146.

29 Hughes J, Stead L, Lancaster T. Antidepressants for smoking cessation. *Cochrane Database Syst Rev* 2007; **issue 1**: CD000031.

30 Cahill K, Stead LF, Lancaster T. Nicotine receptor partial agonists for smoking cessation. *Cochrane Database Syst Rev* 2008; **issue 3**: CD006103.

31 Medicines and Healthcare Products Regulatory Agency. *Drug Safety Update: Latest Advice for Medicines Users.* Volume 2, Issue 4, November 2008 (www.mhra.gov.uk/home/groups/pl-p/documents/publication/con030924.pdf).

32 Meltzer H, Gill B, Petticrew M, *et al. Economic Activity and Social Functioning of Residents with Psychiatric Disorders: OPCS Surveys of Psychiatric Morbidity in Great Britain, Report 6.* TSO (The Stationery Office), 1996.

33 Lawn SJ, Pols RG. Smoking bans in psychiatric inpatient settings? A review of the research. *Aust N Z J Psychiatry* 2005; **39**: 874–93.

34 Topping CA. *Smoking Cessation within the Forensic Mental Health Service with Conditions of Special Security.* NHS Scotland, 2008 (http://www.ashscotland.org.uk/ash/files/The%20State%20Hospital%20Exec%20Summary%20200808.pdf).

7

Obesity and weight management

Tom Fox and Jonathan Pinkney

People with mental disorders are particularly prone to weight gain and obesity. This chapter contains information on how to take a comprehensive dietary history, the routine investigations required for assessing an obese person; and the role of diet, medication, exercise and surgery in weight management. It also describes how psychiatric patients can be treated for their obesity in the community.

Introduction

Nature has blessed humans with a remarkable ability to survive famine. Intricate neuroendocrine pathways wed appetite and satiation to hedonism and emotion. It is scarcely surprising, therefore, that in an environment where food is so plentiful, many people with psychiatric illnesses experience considerable weight gain and obesity.[1] For example, in a survey of patients with bipolar disorder, 58% were classified as overweight, 21% as obese and 5% as extremely obese.[2] Until recently, however, the origins and consequences of this weight gain received scant attention and caused little concern. In the era of modern psychiatry, it has been recognised increasingly that psychiatric illness itself and psychotropic medications both contribute significantly to weight gain and metabolic problems such as diabetes mellitus.[3,4] There are always specific reasons why any individual becomes obese, but weight gain will be explained by a sustained period of positive energy balance, during which energy from excessive calorie ingestion exceeds energy losses (mainly from voluntary physical activity).

Obesity is commonly defined on the basis of body mass index – weight in kilograms divided by height in metres squared (kg/m^2) (Table 7.1). Obesity can be one of the most serious physical consequences of psychiatric disorders, sowing the seeds for a host of physical health problems (Box 7.1). Weight gain is one important reason why diabetes mellitus is increasingly recognised in patients treated with psychotropic medications, although drugs such as clozapine and olanzapine may also increase the risks of diabetes independently of weight gain.[4,5] Weight gain is undesirable, not least since obesity reduces life expectancy, mainly as a result of increased deaths from heart disease and cancer, and the risk of such early mortality is increased approximately two- to threefold in obese middle-aged people.[6] Obesity also interacts strongly with other risk factors for heart disease such as diabetes and smoking[7] – both common in people with psychiatric illnesses – and this further exacerbates the risks to health. Furthermore, some of the negative psychological consequences of obesity (Box 7.2) hinder successful recovery and rehabilitation from psychiatric illness. Therefore, the recognition and management of obesity are arguably two of the most

Table 7.1 World Health Organization classification of body mass index

Body mass index (kg/m²)	Category
< 18.5	Underweight
18.5–25	Healthy weight
25–30	Overweight
30–35	Grade 1 obese
35–40	Grade 2 obese
> 40	Grade 3 obese

Source: World Health Organization.[8]

Box 7.2 Common psychological and social associations of obesity

- Lower educational achievement
- Poorer employment opportunities
- Reduced income
- Reduced likelihood of forming relationships or marrying
- Teasing and bullying about weight
- Low self-esteem
- Depression
- Isolation and agoraphobia

important physical health challenges facing mental health teams.

Evaluation of the obese person

Successful restoration of healthy weight in those with obesity requires multidisciplinary assessment and sustained intervention. Whereas medical consequences of obesity may already be known, it is often appropriate that a doctor or a nurse with a special interest in obesity should be involved, at least in the initial assessment. Also essential are the services of a dietitian, physical trainer and sometimes a psychologist with a specific interest in eating behaviour. These multidisciplinary services are often available in a primary care setting or in specialist hospital-based clinics. Each person has their individual reasons for weight gain, and so the correct identification of these is an essential starting point to develop a successful long-term weight control strategy. For a comprehensive account of the evaluation and management of obesity, the reader is referred to specialist sources.[9]

Box 7.1 Physical health consequences of obesity

- Type 2 diabetes
- Hypertension
- Dyslipidaemia
- Cardiovascular disease
- Fatty liver
- Gallstones
- Gastro-oesophageal reflux
- Chronic back pain
- Osteoarthritis
- Polycystic ovary syndrome (female infertility and hirsutism)
- Malignant diseases (especially tumours of the gastrointestinal and female reproductive systems)
- Obstructive sleep apnoea
- Cor pulmonale
- Benign intracranial hypertension
- Venous stasis and ulceration
- Venous thromboembolism

The weight history

The weight history aims to uncover the factors that led to weight gain. It is useful to gain insight into when an individual first became overweight, since this often identifies the important causes. Many obese adults report that weight gain was already underway in the first decade of life, although weight gain in the teenage years and after childbirth in women are also commonly reported. In contrast, for others major changes in circumstances, lifestyle or employment, including reductions in physical activity and recreation, lead to progressive weight gain as adults. A variety of additional, and sometimes very specific factors commonly predispose people with psychiatric illnesses to weight gain, including:

- sedentary lifestyle
- poor diet

Weight management resources are best concentrated on those individuals who are motivated.

- emotional eating (often from stress or boredom)
- negative symptoms of schizophrenia and depression
- social isolation
- eating disorders
- excess alcohol consumption
- low income and lack of access to recreational activities
- interruptions in regular employment
- hospitalisation in a secure setting
- antipsychotic or antidepressant medication.

Childhood physical and sexual abuse is also not an uncommon feature coming to light in the history of adult obesity,[10] although the role of such factors is still not well understood.

It is also important to understand how patients view themselves and whether they see weight as a problem. Those who do not perceive any problem or who are unwilling to initiate change are likely to find interventions frustrating and futile.

The dietary history

Eating is an appropriate physiological response to hunger and the feeling of satiety should lead to the discontinuation of eating. Thus, eating in response to stress, loneliness or other emotions ('comfort eating'), even when feeling full, is inappropriate and is a common reason for weight gain. It is essential for dietary habits to be evaluated, ideally by a specialist dietitian. A variety of dietary behaviours often contribute to weight gain and the identification and correction of these is essential for successful weight loss. They include:

- eating in response to emotion and stress
- high intakes of snack foods or confectionery
- frequent take-away meals
- large portion sizes
- calorie-dense foods (high in fat and/or carbohydrate)
- non-diet soft drinks
- high intakes of alcohol
- omission of breakfast.

Many patients have major misconceptions of what constitutes a healthy diet.

Many patients have major misconceptions of what constitutes a 'healthy diet' and may never have known what this means. The dietary history is best captured with a simple self-completed food diary. Obese individuals are frequently found to consume excessive calories and to derive a disproportionate number of calories from energy-dense foods that are rich in fat and/or carbohydrate.

In addition to food choices, the characteristics of eating behaviour frequently explain weight gain. The frequency and size of meals, and the factors that are responsible for these, are of central importance. 'Hidden' calories obtained from alcohol and sugary drinks are important causes of weight gain for some. Abnormal eating may also occur at unusual times, including during the night, or covertly. Omission of breakfast is a common habit that predisposes to weight gain, probably due to overeating later in the day. Other social factors, such as reduced income as a result of mental illness, or institutional care, may contribute to poor diet, as healthier options such as fresh fruit and vegetables may be less easily available.

A trained dietitian can estimate daily calorie consumption from a food diary. In simple terms, an average-size man requires approximately 2500 kcal per day and a woman 2000 kcal per day to maintain a healthy weight. Sustained calorie intakes in excess of this, if not offset by a commensurate increase in physical activity, result in weight gain. The underreporting of food intake and the overestimation of physical activity are frequently observed in overweight and obese individuals. Many adults have attempted to lose weight by dieting at some point, and so it is highly relevant to explore previous attempts at weight loss and to identify the reasons for failure.

Physical activity

Physical inactivity is often apparent from the weight history and obese patients have usually led sedentary lives. Increased voluntary physical activity is always a key objective in order to realise long-term weight control. Overall duration of daily physical exertion is frequently too short and there is often avoidance of low-level physical exertion such as walking or using staircases. The physical exertion that is undertaken is frequently inadequate and contributes little to daily energy expenditure. People with psychiatric illness may have prolonged periods of unemployment that will further reduce opportunities for daily activity. The negative physical effects of depression also pose barriers to simple daily activity, the use of leisure facilities or participation in sports and activities.

When available, pedometers can be a simple way of assessing individual activity and can be used therapeutically to set daily goals and to motivate.

Medical aspects of obesity

Although relatively rare, there are some important medical conditions in which obesity and psychiatric illness can coexist:

- Hypothyroidism is a common, treatable cause of modest weight gain and can also result in depression.
- Cushing's syndrome has characteristics that include so-called 'moon face', a preponderance of abdominal fat and violaceous abdominal striae, thin skin, easy bruising, hypertension and type 2 diabetes mellitus, depression and occasionally psychosis.
- Hypopituitarism, although rare, may present with weight gain, due to deficiencies of thyroid stimulating hormone, growth hormone and gonadotrophins. Therefore, obesity and features of hypogonadism require investigation.

Other conditions that may cause obesity to coexist with mental health problems or intellectual difficulties include Prader–Willi syndrome, Kallmann syndrome and any conditions with structural brain lesions affecting the hypothalamic and limbic centres that control appetite and satiety.

With the exception of hypothyroidism, which is common, there is no need to routinely investigate for any of these conditions unless there is a clear clinical indication, in which case the patient should be referred for an endocrinology opinion.

Table 7.2 Effects of commonly used psychiatric medications on body weight

Drug	Effect on weight
Tricyclic antidepressants	Increase
Selective serotonin reuptake inhibitors	Decrease
Phenothiazines	Increase
Atypical antipsychotic medications	Increase
Valproate	Increase

Box 7.3 Relevant measures and routine investigations for an obese person

- Weight and height
- Body mass index (kg/m^2)
- Waist circumference
- Blood pressure
- Thyroid function tests
- Fasting plasma glucose or oral glucose tolerance test
- Fasting cholesterol and triglycerides
- Liver function tests
- Sleep study (if obstructive sleep apnoea is suspected)

While endocrine causes of obesity are uncommon, medication side-effects are much more frequently involved in the weight gain experienced by psychiatric patients (Table 7.2).

Obesity is a significant medical issue largely because of the diseases for which it represents a risk factor; these are described in detail elsewhere.[11] Obese persons are commonly more prone to type 2 diabetes mellitus, hypertension, cardiovascular disease and musculoskeletal problems and these should be specifically determined from the medical history.

Obstructive sleep apnoea is also common and enquiry should be made for the hallmark symptoms of snoring, apnoeic episodes during sleep and daytime sleepiness. Sometimes, family and friends may have greater awareness of these symptoms than the affected individual. Unfortunately, there is no satisfactory screening questionnaire for obstructive sleep apnoea with sufficient sensitivity, and so the decision to investigate rests on clinical suspicion. Clinical suspicion is greater for men with a marked central fat distribution. An affirmative response to the question 'Do you fall asleep during the day when you are not busy?' and the presence of a large neck circumference are both predictive of obstructive sleep apnoea.[12] Thus, in the medical assessment of the obese individual it is important to undertake some basic routine measurements (Box 7.3).

Physical examination

Examination of the obese person requires accurate documentation of weight (using industrial scales for

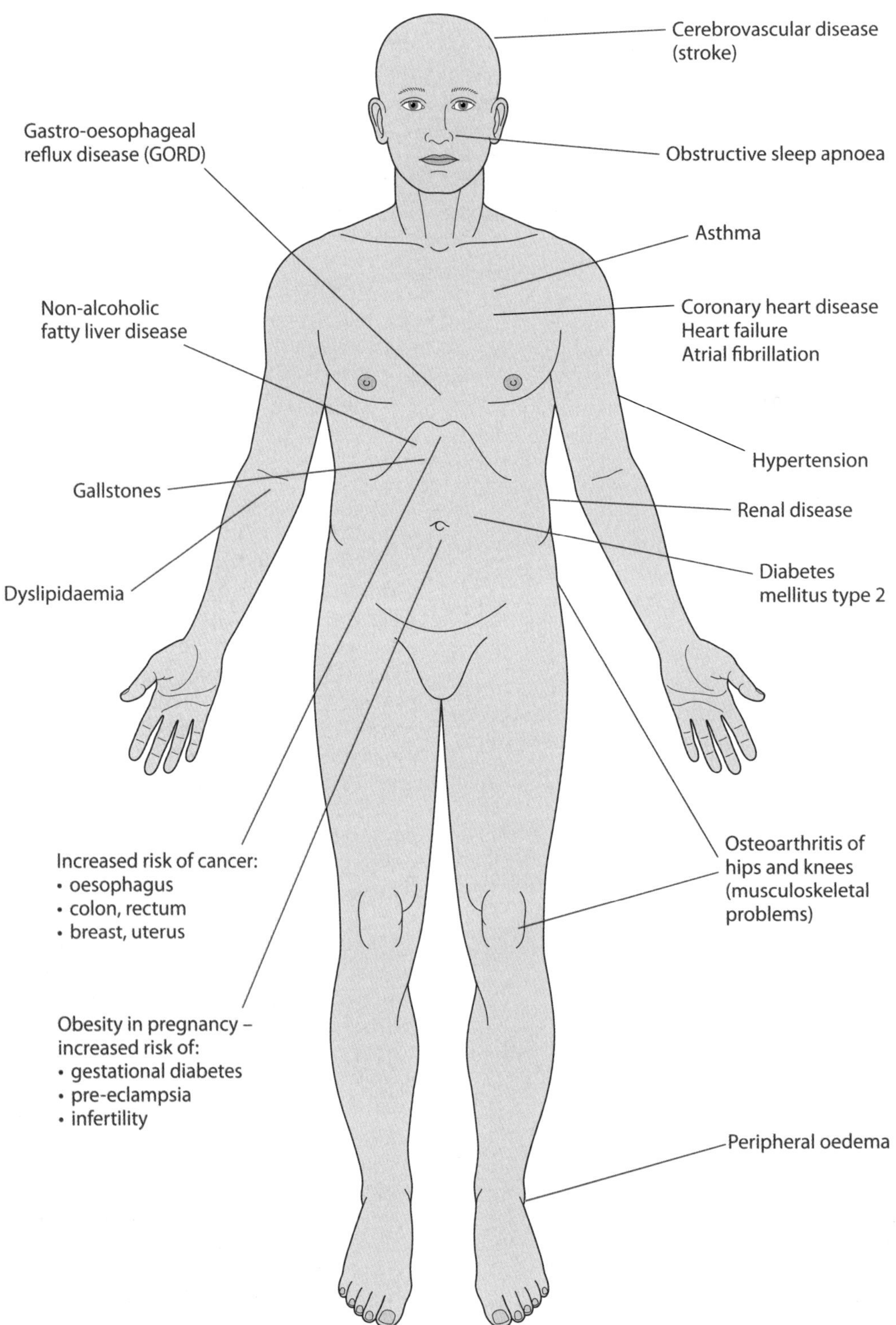

Fig. 7.1 Medical complications of obesity. [11]

very heavy patients), height and calculation of BMI. Blood pressure should be measured using a large-size blood pressure cuff to avoid overestimation. Waist circumference is often used as an additional measure of obesity, or more correctly fat distribution, since abdominal obesity is more strongly predictive of risk of diabetes and heart disease.[13] Thus, a waist circumference of over 94 cm in men and 80 cm in women indicates increased risks of heart disease and diabetes, with waist circumference above 102 cm in men or 88 cm in women carrying the highest risk.[14]

A full physical examination of cardiovascular and respiratory systems and abdomen is appropriate. Other complications such as joint deformities, cutaneous fungal infections, pressure sores and peripheral oedema may be observed in more severely obese individuals (Fig. 7.1).

Treating obesity in the community

It is appropriate to set target weights for patients that will both be realistic and convey a health benefit. Reducing excess weight by 10% brings about a significant reduction in cardiovascular morbidity, diabetes and risk of cancer. This degree of weight loss is a sensible goal for anyone who is overweight or obese, and equally so for those with psychiatric illnesses. The key features that have come to be seen as essential for a successful weight loss programme within a health service context are:

- multidisciplinary involvement
- combined dietary intervention and physical activity
- behavioural change
- goal setting
- frequent contact with a support team
- long-term support
- availability of bariatric surgery for severely obese individuals.

Benefits of a 10 kg-weight loss include:

- 20% reduction in total mortality
- 30% reduction in death due to diabetes
- 40% reduction in obesity-related cancer death
- reduced blood pressure and total cholesterol
- reduced joint and back pain
- improved lung function and reduced sleep apnoea.

Predictions based on Jung, 1997.[15]

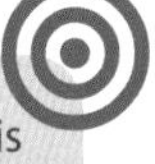

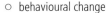

Weight loss of 10% is a sensible goal for anyone who is overweight or obese.

Dietary modification

The modest efficacy of dietary modification is well established.[16] There are innumerable diets that are promoted in non-medical literature and many well established commercial slimming clubs. The use of these resources is usually to be strongly encouraged. However, there is no evidence that any diet that excludes one specific macronutrient such as fat or carbohydrate is superior to any other over the long term. A dietitian is best placed to advise on dietary modification but it is important to recognise that for the majority of those with a BMI of greater than 40 kg/m^2 modifications of diet and exercise alone are unlikely to result in the achievement, let alone the long-term maintenance, of a healthy weight.

In commercial weight-management services three main types of diets are commonly employed:

- *Reduced-calorie diet.* Organisations such as WeightWatchers® typically combine a programme of reduced-calorie diet (deficient by around 500 kcal/day) with group support sessions and activity plans.
- *Reduced-carbohydrate diet.* Low-carbohydrate diets such as the 'Atkins diet' permit only small quantities of carbohydrate (less than 20 g per day) but unlimited fat and protein. The protein causes early satiety and the deficient carbohydrate depletes stored glycogen, necessitating fat metabolism and inducing a ketotic state. Thus, low-carbohydrate diets are sometimes known as ketogenic diets.
- *Very low-calorie diets* (VLCD). These contain less than 800 kcal/day and should be used only under medical supervision, for limited periods. They lead to weight loss of 1–2 kg/week but the weight loss is usually not sustained at 12 months. Thus, it has been shown VLCDs do not perform better in the long term than standard low-calorie diets.[17] Meal-replacement

diets are one specific technique for the delivery of VLCDs. These use high-protein drinks containing important vitamins and minerals, typically in place of two of the three daily meals, and this is an effective way to reduce overall daily calorie consumption. Such VLCDs offer a strictly defined diet, which helps some patients who struggle to gauge food choices and portion sizes. They are usually employed as a second-line treatment, when other approaches have failed, or if rapid weight loss is needed for a specific medical reason.

Physical activity

Physical exercise programmes alone have not been demonstrated to dramatically reduce weight unless they are extremely intense, and this is seldom realistic. However, exercise does reduce visceral fat and hence reduces overall risk of obesity-related health problems, as well as contributing to long-term healthy weight maintenance. Undoubtedly increased physical activity, when combined with dietary modification, can both reduce weight and improve fitness and overall well-being and so it is appropriate to agree realistic daily exercise targets with patients, starting with 30 minutes of brisk walking, and increasing as much as possible. It is important to recognise that exercise becomes increasingly difficult for more severely obese people and is limited by physical restrictions such as breathlessness and musculoskeletal pain, and by the embarrassment and social stigma experienced by obese people. Personal trainers offer personalised exercise plans and many local authorities facilitate group sessions in swimming pools and gyms to reduce embarrassment (see Chapter 8).

Drugs for weight loss

A number of medications have been used in weight management but only one – orlistat – is presently still licensed. Until recently, the cannabinoid (CB_1) receptor antagonist rimonabant and serotonin/noradrenaline reuptake inhibitor sibutramine were both available for weight loss. Unfortunately, rimonabant was withdrawn because it can exacerbate serious depression and sibutramine was withdrawn because of an increased risk of cardiovascular disease. These have been disappointing developments in this field and there is a pressing need for safe and effective new drugs for weight loss.

Orlistat can be prescribed to selected patients who have been unsuccessful at losing weight with diet and lifestyle modifications. Suitable recipients include those with a BMI of greater than 30 kg/m^2 or those with BMI greater than 27 kg/m^2 who have a medical complication that would benefit from weight loss, such as type 2 diabetes. The role of orlistat in weight management programmes has been discussed in recent guidelines on the management of obesity from the National Institute for Health and Clinical Excellence.[18]

Orlistat acts as an irreversible gastric and pancreatic lipase inhibitor and reduces absorption of dietary fat by around 30%. This determines its efficacy and side-effects. Those already taking a very low-fat diet will obtain little benefit. Those with excessive dietary fat will find it more efficacious but will suffer worse side-effects of oily rectal discharge, diarrhoea, abdominal discomfort and, most troublingly, faecal incontinence. These side-effects lead to non-compliance in many patients.

Overall, orlistat reduces weight significantly – by approximately 3% compared with placebo. It also improves glycaemic control and lipid profiles. A dietitian should be involved in the assessment and selection of patients for treatment with orlistat, in part because of the importance of dietary fat reduction.

Weight loss surgery

As the prevalence of those with a BMI greater than 40 kg/m^2 continues to increase, weight loss (bariatric) surgery is likely to become more commonplace. Bariatric operations are often classified as restrictive, malabsorptive or a combination of the two.

Bariatric surgery is an option of last resort for selected patients with a BMI greater than 40 kg/m^2, or 35 kg/m^2 with significant comorbidities such as type 2 diabetes or hypertension.[18] Patients should be fit for surgery, have a thorough understanding of what the surgery involves and must be highly committed to long-term specialist follow-up. Before surgery the patient should undergo an exhaustive multidisciplinary assessment.

There are detailed guidelines on the care of patients undergoing bariatric surgery.[19] It is a major undertaking for any patient and requires a high degree of long-term commitment to sustained dietary change and follow-up. Not surprisingly, the presence of a significant, active psychiatric disorder or drug or alcohol addiction have long been seen as contraindications to bariatric surgery, and so especially careful assessment is required in these cases.

There are two commonly performed types of bariatric surgery (Fig. 7.2), which are described in detail elsewhere:[9,19]

- *Laparoscopic adjustable gastric banding.* This operation restricts the stomach volume. The tightness of the gastric band can be adjusted by filling it with saline through a small subcutaneous port. Post-operatively the patient is able to tolerate only a few mouthfuls of solid food before the stomach fills and satiety is experienced. This helps to bring about a significant reduction in the size of portions and the pace of eating. After bariatric surgery, weight takes about 2 years to reach a new plateau. Weight loss with good compliance is excellent and sustained, with the majority of individuals typically able to lose around 30% of their starting weight. This is the safest available form of bariatric surgery, with an operative mortality of usually less than 1 in 2000.
- *Gastric bypass.* This procedure, also performed laparoscopically, disconnects the top of the stomach and divides the jejunum. A small pouch of stomach is re-anastomosed to the jejunum, bypassing the stomach and duodenum (see Fig. 7.2). The operation leads to weight loss by controlling portion sizes, and by reducing hunger and increasing satiety – probably by inducing additional hormonal changes in the gut. This procedure is more invasive than gastric banding, and has a perioperative mortality risk of around 1 in 200. Furthermore, it leads to long-term deficiencies in vitamins and minerals. Thus, micronutrients must be taken as lifelong supplements. Individuals with likely poor adherence to such supplementation are not good candidates for gastric bypass surgery. Weight loss is more rapid in the first year compared with gastric banding, although recent data suggest that long-term weight loss is similar with these operations.

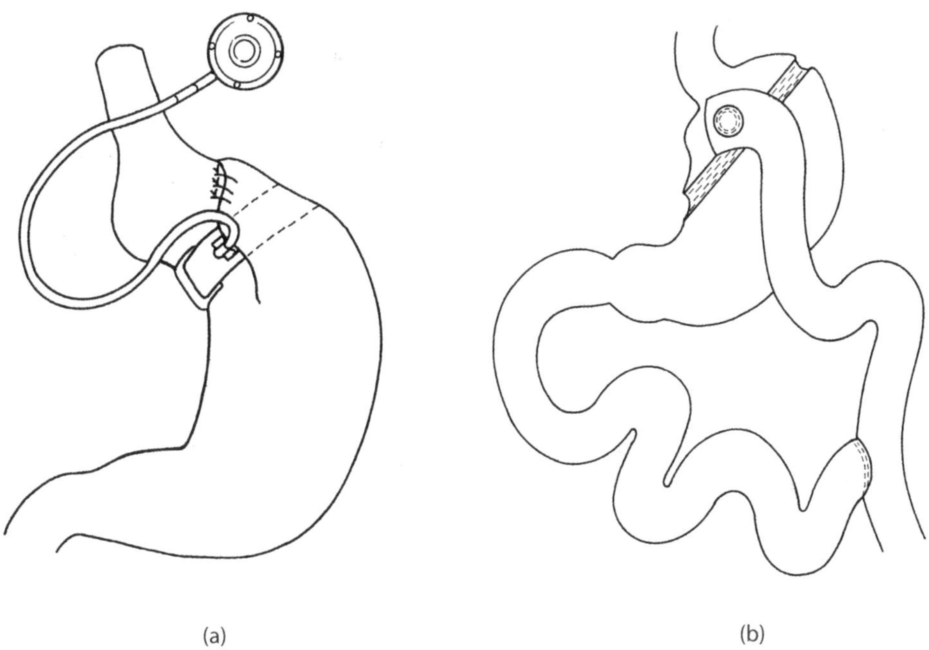

Fig. 7.2 Two common forms of bariatric surgery. (a) Adjustable gastric banding. An inflatable band is placed around and restricts the top of the stomach. The tightness of the band is adjusted with saline using a syringe and needle via a reservoir connected to a subcutaneous port. Weight loss results from control of food satiety and appetite. (b) Gastric bypass. The top of the stomach and jejunum are divided. The distal intestine is anastomosed to the residual stomach, bypassing the rest of the stomach and duodenum. Weight loss results from control of satiety, appetite and perhaps additional changes in gut hormones.

Although bariatric surgery is appropriate only for selected individuals, it is often a life-saving procedure for people who are severely obese, and indeed is the only treatment which increases life expectancy in this group.[20] If this treatment is considered, the patient should be referred to a clinic with the skills to undertake a full assessment of appropriateness and suitability.

Obesity in psychiatric in-patients

The recognition and treatment of obesity in in-patients with psychiatric illnesses are attracting increasing attention.[3] The same basic principles of assessment and treatment apply as described above. Encouragingly, it has been possible to achieve modest weight loss with in-patient educational programmes.[21] In fact, it is potentially easier to control the environment and choices of in-patients than of community patients, whose greater freedom of choice makes it difficult for them to adhere to weight loss programmes and to follow advice on diet and exercise. Therefore, subject to the agreement of the in-patient, it may be possible to modify diet and environment in a favourable way. In in-patient psychiatric units where obesity is a significant concern, it may be appropriate to make available healthier lifestyle options and enlist the assistance of professionals with an interest in this area of medicine.

When to refer for a specialist opinion on obesity

Appropriate specialist referral of individuals with obesity and psychiatric conditions will not usually differ from those with obesity alone. Most patients with mild to moderate obesity, so long as they are motivated and well supported, can be assessed and successfully treated by the non-expert. Patients with more severe obesity (BMI over 40 kg/m^2) are more likely to benefit from a specialist referral (Box 7.4).

Specialist weight management services are now far more widespread than they were in the past. Such services cater specifically for the needs of this patient group; for instance, they often provide specially adapted clinic access and seating areas suitable for extremely obese individuals. If extremely obese people (typically BMI over 50 kg/m^2) are to be referred to out-patient clinics or in-patient services, it is important that ambulance crews and relevant clinical staff are aware of the size of the person in advance, as special equipment and additional staff may be required for safe transfer and handling.

Depending on the nature of the problem, the specialist to whom the patient is best referred may be a dietitian, a psychologist, an endocrinologist with a special interest in obesity medicine, or all of these. A dietitian's assessment is usually an appropriate first option for a standard weight management evaluation. Depending on the nature of the problem, a clinical psychologist or eating disorder specialist may also need to be involved. For consideration of possible medical causes of more severe obesity and/or assessment of medical complications arising from obesity, referral to a physician with an interest in obesity is appropriate (depending on the problem, either a general practitioner with a special interest in obesity or an endocrinologist). If bariatric surgery is to be being considered, then a full multidisciplinary assessment is mandatory and this should be provided by the local bariatric surgical team.

Box 7.4 When to refer to specialist obesity services

- Failure of weight control
- Review of weight reduction strategies, including cognitive, motivational and behavioural approaches
- Uncertainty about the underlying cause of obesity
- Suspicion of an endocrine or other medical disorder
- Suspicion of an eating disorder (e.g. binge eating)
- Review of the role of antipsychotic drugs in weight gain
- Assessment of associated medical comorbidities (e.g. diabetes, cardiovascular disease, obstructive sleep apnoea)
- Assessment of severely obese individuals (BMI > 50 kg/m^2)
- Consideration of bariatric surgery

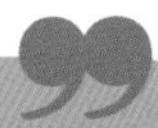

Summary

The physical health needs of people with psychiatric disorders have traditionally been neglected. Many people with psychiatric illnesses have low self-esteem and self-efficacy and these are common barriers to the maintenance of a healthy body weight. However, long-term physical health objectives for all adults, with or without psychiatric illnesses, include the achievement and maintenance of a healthy body weight through a healthy diet and regular exercise.

For in-patients, hospital environments can be made far more conducive to healthier body weight by optimising access to physical activities and a healthy diet. Mental health teams could broaden their traditional roles and responsibilities in order to take on more responsibility for lifestyle and the avoidance of physical health problems. It is unfortunate that the benefits of successful psychiatric treatments can be undermined by the negative physical health consequences of weight gain. It may be necessary to avoid or withdraw certain psychotropic drugs when they cause significant weight gain or other metabolic problems.

In the community, while some patients may be able to attend self-help slimming groups, professional assistance can often be accessed readily through primary care or specialist services.

Ultimately, there is no greater barrier to weight loss than a purposeless existence; motivation and hope are required in order to sustain behavioural change over many months. Mental health professionals are in a prime position to facilitate this.

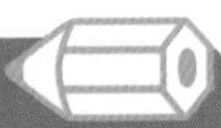

Learning points

- Psychiatric illnesses expose many people to increased risks of weight gain, as a result of long-term changes in lifestyle, environment and drug treatments. Obesity has strongly negative effects on physical and mental health and reduces life expectancy.
- Obesity is an important, avoidable and potential reversible risk factor for diabetes, hypertension, coronary heart disease, cancer and many other serious physical health problems.
- Obesity has a powerful negative impact on self-esteem and for some individuals is a dominating factor contributing to educational and social failure and depression.
- Obesity is commonly defined as body mass index (BMI) $>30\,kg/m^2$. Waist circumference over 94 cm in men and 80 cm in women also indicates increased risks of heart disease and diabetes; waist circumference over 102 cm in men and 88 cm in women indicates highest risk.
- The clinical obesity assessment is part of the traditional physical history and examination undertaken by psychiatrists. The aim is to identify causes of weight gain (so these can be addressed), important medical complications (which require medical investigation and management) and strategies for long-term weight control.
- The key components of the obesity assessment are a weight history, dietary history, medical history, physical examination, measurement of weight and height (with calculation of BMI) and blood pressure. Simple routine blood tests are appropriate but medical causes of obesity are rare and so most endocrine investigation is reserved for selected cases.
- Essential components of a weight control strategy are caloric restriction and increased physical activity. Long-term professional support is required. Orlistat is the only currently available weight loss drug and is suitable for some patients with high dietary fat intakes. Bariatric surgery is reserved for carefully selected individuals with severe obesity (usually BMI $>40\,kg/m^2$) when all other options have failed.
- The prevention, identification and management of obesity are legitimate concerns of mental health teams, who are best placed to address the needs of this patient group.

References

1 McElroy SL, Kotwal R, Malhotra S, *et al.* Are mood disorders and obesity related? A review for the mental health professional. *J Clin Psychiatry* 2004; **65**: 634–51.

2 McElroy SL, Frye MA, Suppes T, *et al.* Correlates of overweight and obesity in 644 patients with bipolar disorder. *J Clin Psychiatry* 2002; **63**: 207–13.

3 McIntyre RS. Managing weight gain in patients with severe mental illness. *J Clin Psychiatry* 2009; **70**: e23.

4 Newcomer JW. Metabolic considerations in the use of antipsychotic medications: a review of recent evidence. *J Clin Psychiatry* 2007; **68** (suppl 1): 20–7.

5 Newcomer JW. Second-generation (atypical) antipsychotics and metabolic effects: a comprehensive literature review. *CNS Drugs* 2005; **19** (suppl 1): 1–93.

6 Calle EE, Thun MJ, Petrelli JM, *et al.* Body-mass index and mortality in a prospective cohort of US adults. *N Engl J Med* 1999; **341**: 1097–105.

7 Manson JE, Colditz GA, Stampfer MJ, *et al.* A prospective study of obesity and risk of coronary heart disease in women. *N Engl J Med* 1990; **322**: 882–9.

8 World Health Organization. *Obesity: Preventing and Managing the Global Epidemic. Report of a WHO Consultation.* WHO Technical Report Series 894. WHO, 2000.

9 Kopelman P, Caterson I, Dietz W (eds) *Clinical Obesity in Adults and Children (3rd edn).* Wiley, 2009.

10 Gustafson TB, Sarwer DB. Childhood sexual abuse and obesity. *Obes Rev* 2004; **5**: 129–35.

11 Malnick SDH, Knobler H. The medical complications of obesity. *Quart J Med* 2006; **99**: 565–79.

12 Davies RJ, Ali NJ, Stradling JR. Neck circumference and other clinical features in the diagnosis of the obstructive sleep apnoea syndrome. *Thorax* 1992; **47**: 101–5.

13 Després JP, Lemieux I, Prud'homme D. Treatment of obesity: need to focus on high risk abdominally obese patients. *BMJ* 2001; **322**: 716–20.

14 National Obesity Forum. *Obesity Care Pathway Toolkit: Annexes 1 to 9.* NOF, 2005 (http://www.nationalobesityforum.org.uk/images/stories/care-pathway-toolkit/Toolkit_supporting_obesity_care_pathway_annexes_1_to_9__Feb_07_2006.pdf).

15 Jung RT. Obesity as a disease. *Br Med Bull* 1997; **53**: 307–21.

16 Avenell A, Brown TJ, McGee MA, *et al.* What are the long-term benefits of weight reducing diets in adults? A systematic review of randomized controlled trials. *J Hum Nutr Diet* 2004; **17**: 317–35.

17 Tsai AG, Wadden TA. The evolution of very-low-calorie diets: an update and meta-analysis. *Obesity (Silver Spring)* 2006; **14**: 1283–93.

18 National Institute for Health and Clinical Excellence. *Obesity: The Prevention, Identification, Assessment and Management of Overweight and Obesity in Adults and Children (Clinical Guidelines CG43).* NICE, 2006.

19 Mechanick JI, Kushner RF, Sugerman HJ, *et al.* American Association of Clinical Endocrinologists, the Obesity Society, and American Society for Metabolic and Bariatric Surgery medical guidelines for clinical practice for the perioperative nutritional, metabolic, and nonsurgical support of the bariatric surgery patient. *Obesity (Silver Spring)* 2009; **17** (suppl 1): S1–70.

20 Sjöström L, Narbro K, Sjöström CD, *et al.* Effects of bariatric surgery on mortality in Swedish obese subjects. *N Engl J Med* 2007; **357**: 741–52.

21 Lindenmayer JP, Khan A, Wance D, *et al.* Outcome evaluation of a structured educational wellness program in patients with severe mental illness. *J Clin Psychiatry* 2009; **70**: 1385–96.

8

Physical activity

Amy Pritty, Lisa Hart and Evelyn Goodwin

> Exercise can improve physical and mental well-being. Those with mental health problems may be restricted in what, and how much activity they can undertake, due to poor motivation or side-effects of psychotropic medication. In this chapter, guidance is given on the health benefits of exercise, removing barriers to exercise, what activities are available to improve fitness, how much exercise patients should undertake and what to monitor.

Introduction

There is a strong association between physical inactivity and the emergence of chronic diseases, including coronary heart disease, obesity, diabetes, hypertension, stroke and some cancers. The levels of physical activity and fitness status of psychiatric patients have been shown to be lower than those of the general population, leading to psychiatric patients having poorer health. Psychiatric patients in the community[1] and long-stay patients[2] are more likely to smoke tobacco, be obese, have diabetes mellitus and have a raised risk of coronary heart disease.

There is a positive relationship between physical activity and mental health in both clinical and non-clinical settings.[3] Exercise has the potential to improve a patient's physical and mental well-being simultaneously. Improved quality of life enhances the patient's ability to cope with and manage a mental health problem. Faulkner & Biddle have commented that, regardless of any mental health benefits, exercise should be promoted, since the physical needs of psychiatric patients are often unmet.[4]

Recommended physical activity

The Chief Medical Officer has recommended that adults should undertake daily at least 30 minutes of moderate-intensity physical exercise at least 5 days a week.[5] This can be achieved with short bouts of physical activity (of 10 minutes or more) interspersed throughout the day. A large proportion of psychiatric patients do not undertake sufficient activity to benefit their health.

Activity requirements

Professional instructors need to be trained to the level 2 gym instructor qualification or equivalent as a minimum.

The American College of Sports Medicine suggests that any good training programme will incorporate five major components:[6]

- cardiovascular fitness
- muscular strength
- muscular endurance
- flexibility
- motor skills.

One important factor that affects motivation to exercise is the use of psychotropic medication. This should not be seen as a barrier to exercise because there are several ways to engage an individual's interest in exercise and ways to adapt and develop new activities. Fitness interventions may need to be adapted, especially for those with *severe* mental disorders who are being treated with high-dose medication regimens.

All five components play a specific role in total fitness and well-being (Table 8.1). The most appropriate types of activity will often have to be adapted to meet the needs of the individual (or groups) taking part.

Activities should be graded according to individual needs and capabilities. The intensity of the activity (Table 8.2) should correspond to the recommendations and restrictions set out in an 'exercise prescription' (see case study 8.1 for an example). Activities need to progress gradually to allow for individual successes in achieving set aims and objectives. Breaking activities down into small structured segments affords continued interest and prevents boredom.

Table 8.1 Elements of and suggested activities for total fitness

Element of fitness to enhance	Suggested activities
Cardiovascular	Walking, jogging, running Swimming Cycling Racquet sports – tennis, badminton, table tennis Team games – football, cricket, rugby, volleyball, hockey, netball Cardiovascular equipment in gyms Aerobics Aqua aerobics Dancing Circuit classes
Strength and resistance	Weight training Resistance equipment machines Resistance bands Floor work, (body resistance work) Circuit training
Flexibility and relaxation	Stretch programmes Yoga Pilates Tai chi

Exercise sessions

Exercise sessions should comprise warm-up, training and cool-down activities.

Warm-up activities

The cardiovascular component of any exercise session should have a clear warm-up stage, to prevent injury to any major joint or muscle likely to be used in the work-out occurring as a result of being cold and unaccustomed to the exercise load. Instructors should aim to include:

- a clear structured plan from 'head to toe', to prevent any part of the body being missed
- basic shoulder rolls, side bends, trunk twists, knee raises and hamstring curls.

Each exercise should be performed for at least six repetitions. The range of movement should be progressively increased.

A basic stretching programme should be included in the warm-up, with individuals being encouraged to hold each stretch for at least 8–10 seconds. Stretches should target the muscles to be used in the main activity (Fig. 8.1). The total time spent in warming up, including stretches, should be 10–15 minutes.

The training zone

When moving onto the main component of the work-out, 'the training zone', the same principles and structure apply: break activities down into small sections to enable participation of people with different levels of ability, of those with medical conditions and of those taking medication.

Team sports can be broken down into skill sessions, focusing on the skills required to engage in the activity, which gives individuals time to practise and build confidence in engagement, rather than highlighting weaknesses.

Walking sessions can be enhanced by the addition of opportunities to engage in other fitness pursuits, such as the use of park benches to perform triceps dips and press-ups. During walking sessions, different speeds of pace can be used, as well as pedometers to record the total number of steps.

Case study 8.1 Example of a typical exercise prescription

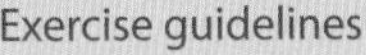

Exercise guidelines

Name: John Smith

Responsible clinician/general practitioner: James Paterson

NHS number: ********

Frequency: 5/7 times per week (aerobic activity), 2/3 times a week (light-resistance activity)

Intensity: Light–medium, type 1/2 activity

Time: 30 minutes, progressing to 1 hour

Type: Aerobic/weight management

Microcycle 1: Months 1–4. Heart rate 50–60% MHR (93–121 b.p.m.). RPE 5/6.5

Microcycle 2: Months 5–8. Heart rate 50–70% MHR (93–121 b.p.m.). RPE 5/7

Microcycle 3: Months 9–12. Heart rate 50–75% MHR (93–140 b.p.m.)

Warm-up: 10–15 minutes in duration, including mobilisation and stretches

Main section: 30 minutes in duration, but be aware that warm-up and cool-down times may be sufficient work-out time

Cool-down: 10–15 minutes in duration, including stretches after work-out

Recommended activities: Exercises should be rhythmic and incorporate large muscle groups. Type 1–2 activities to include walking, cardio and light-resistance work, swimming, yoga and pilates, skill training sessions

Restrictions on exercise: High-impact activity, high-intensity activity. Full weight-bearing activities. Contact team sports

Caution: If patient undertakes floor work, as medication side-effects include postural hypotension. Avoid exercise in hot, humid conditions because the patient is obese

Instructor advice: If patient experiences dizziness/chest pain, cool down and cease exercise. Focus on exercise to increase energy expenditure, reduce weight. Ensure adequate footwear is worn. Fluids should be freely available

Illnesses/injuries: Chest pain, mobility problems related to obesity

Family history: None significant

Waist measurement: 151 cm (high risk of developing coronary heart disease)

Fitness assessment (areas of concern): BMI – 47.1 kg/m^2 (morbidly obese),

body fat percentage – 43.7% (morbidly obese), blood pressure 142/82 mmHg (elevated systolic reading at time of taking)

Physical risk stratification: High

Medications: Citalopram, clozapine, tolterodine, desmopressin, simvastatin

Potential side-effects of medication*: Palpitations, tachycardia, postural hypotension, chest pains, nausea, dizziness, hypo-/hyperglycaemia, weight gain, muscle weakness

Date last amended: 13/07/2012m

*This list is an example of medication side-effects that may have an impact on exercise performance and/or response. Not all side-effects may occur.
BMI, body mass index; MHR, maximum heart rate; RPE, rating of perceived exertion

Table 8.2 Intensity of suggested activity

Intensity of exercise	Suggested activities
Level 1 – low intensity Participants should be warm enough to remove one layer of clothing, and experience a slight increase in breathing rate	Walking Active leisure activities Relaxation Floor activity Stretch programmes Yoga and pilates Tai chi
Level 2 – moderate intensity Participants experience a moderate increase in breathing rate	Swimming Cardiovascular and light resistance training Short tennis Sports skills sessions Volleyball Badminton
Level 3 – high intensity Participants experience a moderate to high increase in breathing rate All participants training at this level should have a good cardiovascular fitness and be engaging in regular activity	Contact team sports Football Heavy resistance training High-intensity cardiovascular work-out Spinning Running

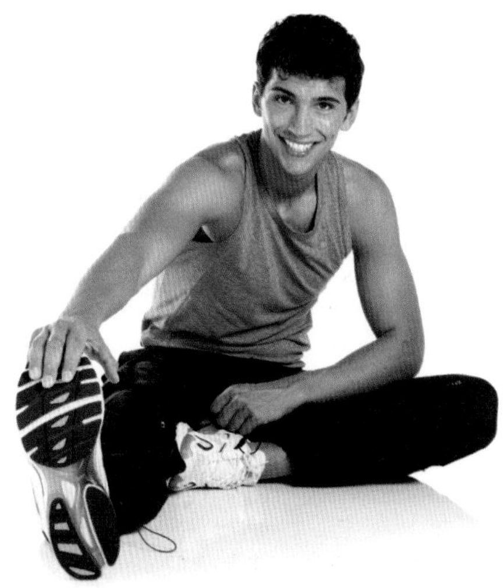

Fig. 8.1 Fitness stretching exercise.

Cool-down activities

The 'cool down' component should be of the same timescale as the warm-up session. Cool-down periods should always include a basic stretching programme that targets all the muscles that have been used. Each stretch should be held for a minimum of 20–30 seconds, as this helps to prevent muscle soreness and defines the end of the session.

Planning activities

When planning a programme of exercise, it is good practice to ensure that sessions target all five areas of exercise. Activities should be adapted to an individual's needs.

When planning any activity for an individual with a mental illness, the main consideration is the amount of time spent in the warm-up and cool-down phases. These sections of the work-out should be about

10–15 minutes in duration, and there may not be a specific 'training zone'. The side-effects of psychotropic medication and the severity of the mental disorder may have a negative impact on an individual's physical endurance and motivation to engage in any activity for prolonged periods and this will have a direct impact on the design and structure of the programme.

When designing strength and resistance training programmes, the focus needs to be on the *endurance* element of the training, rather than the *strength* element. This allows the individual to progress through the training programme at a level that can be comfortably maintained. Allowing for development of the training programme promotes adherence to it. It is advisable to use:

- smaller weights with lots of repetitions
- routines that are not too complicated or onerous.

People should have the opportunity to take ownership of the exercise session and to be able to work at an appropriate level, without feeling pressured to perform beyond their personal limits.

Flexibility training provides opportunities to develop breathing techniques, aiding sleep patterns, thus helping to minimise stress. It often requires very little equipment other than a warm environment and loose, comfortable clothing. As with any physical training, all movements can have different stages of progression, enabling individuals to engage at different levels of ability.

Physical activity programmes for those with a mental illness

For patients with mental health problems, the recommended guidelines for exercise are the same as those for 'apparently healthy individuals' (Table 8.3). If a person also suffers from a physical illness, then the recommendations appropriate for that illness apply. For patients with physical comorbidities, it is advisable to consult with an exercise professional with the qualifications to provide and develop an exercise prescription. Providers can be sourced through the YMCA FIT fitness industry training packages. Individuals also interested in mental health fitness training can find relevant training providers through YMCA FIT.

However, there are a number of considerations to take into account when planning exercise programmes aimed to enhance positive mental health:

- a significant amount of support is likely to be required throughout the exercise programme
- participants may be lacking in self-confidence, self-esteem and self-efficacy
- participants may feel isolated and out of place in an exercise setting
- participants will benefit from a continuity of staff, although without over-reliance on one or more particular staff members
- support structures from peers, carers or ward staff, particularly a key nurse, need to be in place
- the exercise programme must be flexible to allow for variations in a person's mental state.

Promoting participation

The following steps can be taken to promote the participation in an exercise programme of patients who have a mental illness:

- ensure sessions are fun, less technical, shorter and less intense
- take physical activity sessions to wards and familiarise patients with the activity
- provide suitable clothing for exercise, if patients do not have their own
- involve each patient's clinical team or carers, to help support the patient
- deliver sessions to small groups or provide individual support to increase confidence and enhance engagement.

There are a number of strategies that can be adopted to promote participation and increase motivation for patients suffering from mental illness (Box 8.1).

It is important that trainers also be aware that:

- a significant amount of staff support throughout the exercise programme is likely to be required in order to encourage adherence
- participants may be lacking in self-confidence, self-esteem and self-efficacy, and so programmes should be tailored to suit particular patients
- patients may feel isolated and out of place in an exercise setting when initially commencing a programme, so it is important to ensure that the patient feels fully supported
- the exercise programme needs to be flexible, due to the episodic nature of mental ill-health.

Table 8.3 Generally accepted exercise guidelines for apparently healthy individuals

Frequency	Intensity	Time
Aerobic activity (cardiorespiratory exercise)		
> 5 days of the week	Moderate	30–60 minutes per day (150 min per week)
> 3 days of the week	Vigorous	20–60 minutes per day (75 min per week)
> 3–5 days of the week	Combination (light–moderate may be beneficial for deconditioned individuals)	(<20 minutes per week for previously sedentary individuals can be beneficial)
Resistance		
2–3 days per week, 2–4 sets	Moderate–hard	8–12 reps for strength and power
	Very light–light	10–15 reps for strength in middle-aged /older adults beginning an exercise programme
	Light–moderate	15–20 reps for muscular endurance
Flexibility		
> 2/3 days per week (greatest gains occur when performed daily – full range of movement)	Stretch to the point of mild discomfort	10–30 seconds (most adults) 30–60 seconds (older individuals)

Adapted from American College of Sports Medicine evidence-based recommendations.[7] Reps, repetitions.

Barriers to participation in exercise programmes

Poor mental health is one of the greatest barriers to participation in exercise and physical activity, but some general barriers to participation apply to all, irrespective of mental state. There are two main types of barrier to exercise: personal and environmental (Table 8.4). To overcome these, exercise professionals should explain the benefits of exercise to patients to dispel any misconceptions and identify realistic, achievable goals.

Psychological barriers

Patients with mental health problems may have lost their motivation, enthusiasm and ability to enjoy life. Some may find it hard to get up, get dressed and maintain a daily routine, before even thinking about taking part in physical activity. Additionally, certain aspects of some mental illnesses include an inability to experience pleasure or to see beyond the condition. Patients may also find it difficult to concentrate on tasks and may be easily distracted. Fear of the unknown or a lack of

Box 8.1 Strategies to promote exercise programme participation by patients with mental illness

- Complete a 'physical activity readiness questionnaire' (PAR-Q) beforehand, to ascertain a patient's likes and dislikes
- Complete an assessment of the patient's readiness to change and motivation level, assessed through a series of questions directly related to motivations, likes and dislikes in relation to physical activity
- Combine activity sessions with an education programme which informs patients about the benefits of activity
- Work with the patient to develop the exercise programme and promote ownership of the plan
- Aim to ensure continuity of staff
- Incorporate support structures from ward staff, particularly the named nurse and peers, but do try to avoid over-reliance on one or more particular staff members
- Involve the patient's care team or mental health worker to support the patient

Table 8.4 Barriers to exercise

Barrier	Reason	Solution
Personal		
Fear of injury	Fear of incurring a lasting disability or aggravating old and current problems	*Educate* Start gradually and slowly build up. Always warm up and cool down. Being physically active means that patients are less likely to suffer from injuries
Poor health	Musculoskeletal ailments or chronic diseases such as diabetes may cause fear for patients	*Educate* Exercise will improve conditions, allowing the patient to be more active
Lack of motivation	Previous experiences can contribute to negative attitudes towards exercise	*Educate* Being more active will give the patient more energy. Ensure the patient has realistic expectations
Fatigue	Some medication and being overweight can lead to patients becoming easily tired	*Educate* Exercise improves energy levels and improves sleep patterns, so patients will not feel as tired
Isolation	Many patients do not want to exercise. Adherence to exercise programmes is often poor without social support	*Exercise in groups* to provide social support and work with link staff on wards
Lack of time	Patients may place work or therapy priorities ahead of physical activity	*Plan* Identify available time slots. Most patients have at least an hour a day to spend on exercise, and as exercise is a stimulant it leads to more productive use of time
Misconceptions	Patients may have a limited conception about exercise and previous experience may lead them to think that exercise is boring	*Educate and plan* Use a variety of diverse activities and promote fun while exercising
Not having appropriate clothing	Patient is unable to afford or access appropriate clothing	*Supply clothing* to patients where funds can be acquired
Environmental		
Lack of access	Limited facilities and access to facilities, shortage of staff	*Plan* Confirm venues and be flexible to allow exercise to take place in a variety of settings
Inclement weather	Restricts activities that patients can engage in outdoors	*Plan* Programmes need to be flexible to offer other options

To overcome barriers, exercise professionals should explain the benefits of exercise to the patients to dispel any misconceptions and identify realistic and achievable goals.

awareness of the potential benefits of physical activity may also be barriers.

Social barriers

Lack of support from peers may be an important social barrier. Patients may also find it difficult to communicate, and may be afraid of being in the company of others (social anxiety).

Physical barriers

Physical symptoms can be a barrier to exercise. These include lethargy, clumsiness and stiffness of joints or movements. Physiological responses to exercise naturally include sweating, increased breathing rate, increased heart rate, flushing and rise in body temperature, but these may all cause or be interpreted as anxiety. Low fitness levels may also be a barrier to exercise.

Medication barriers

The intake of (sometimes large) doses of psychotropic medication may have side-effects that impair an individual's ability to exercise.

Barriers due to physical illness

There are specific absolute contraindications to exercise:

- severely uncontrolled blood pressure in excess of 180/110 mmHg
- severely uncontrolled diabetes, epilepsy or asthma
- symptomatic sciatic pain flare-ups
- symptomatic rheumatic flare-ups
- uncontrolled tachycardia over 100 b.p.m.
- unstable angina
- febrile illness.

Physical activity programmes in the community

On leaving the in-patient setting, patients may have access to day-care facilities run by occupational therapists, who may provide a range of activities, including exercise and sport. The training requirements for staff delivering the exercise prescription should be the same as the training requirements for any staff delivering similar exercise sessions. Recreational, fitness and health promotion opportunities are also available in the community for psychiatric patients, including those shown in Box 8.2.

Box 8.2 Community-based recreational, fitness and health promotion opportunities for psychiatric patients

Recreational and fitness activities:

- golf
- canoeing
- skiing
- sailing
- windsurfing
- rock climbing
- hill walking
- rollerblading
- ice skating
- green gyms
- dog walking
- organised bike rides
- walking groups (e.g. www.ramblers.org.uk).

Health promotion activities:

- health and fitness advice
- weight management education
- smoking cessation
- drug/alcohol/substance misuse sessions
- physical health awareness and education
- mental health awareness and education
- dental hygiene
- personal hygiene.

Established projects

The 'Time to Change' campaign's 'Get Moving' project is a week of physical activity events to bring people together to 'challenge the mental health stigma and discrimination, and to promote the benefits of being active for mental wellbeing' (www.time-to-change.org.uk).

'Healthy Active Minds' run by the National Health Service and the Sports Trust in Edinburgh is a general practitioner (GP) referral scheme for patients suffering from mental health issues and aims to give participants an activity action plan with options for exercise in either a leisure or community setting (www.edinburghleisure.co.uk).

In the London borough of Bromley, the Active Lifestyles Exercise Referral Scheme is promoted through general practice surgeries for individuals with physical and mental health issues. The group provides structured gym sessions that promote a sense of wellness and fitness and of community and support for patients (www.mytimeactive.co.uk/health/improving-community-health/exercise-referral.aspx).

General practitioner referral schemes

Through these exercise referral schemes, an individual is referred to an exercise programme by a healthcare professional such as a GP. The schemes aim to increase an individual's activity level and target the prevention and management of existing medical conditions and illnesses, such as coronary heart disease, stroke, obesity, type 2 diabetes, arthritis and common mental health problems. They operate through local authorities and primary care trusts. It has been estimated that there are approximately 600 schemes running in England.[8]

Some sports centres operate a GP referral scheme, offering activities such as free swimming sessions and subsidised gym sessions, as well as weight management programmes. Patients are invited to an interview in a local sports or community centre with a fitness instructor who is a qualified GP referral fitness specialist, to discuss their needs and wants. Assessment and formulation of an exercise prescription will follow.

Health benefits of exercise

Exercise has the potential to influence a person's physical and mental health simultaneously.

Physical health

Physical activity not only contributes to well-being but is essential for good health. Physical activity, maintained throughout life, reduces the risk of:

- major chronic diseases, such as coronary heart disease, obesity and cancer by 50%
- premature death by 20–30%[5]
- stroke by 30–60%
- hypertension
- osteoporosis.

It also improves the management of asthma and diabetes, reduces cholesterol and aids weight loss.

Psychiatric patients, particularly those who are older or obese, have a higher prevalence of diabetes mellitus, epilepsy, respiratory disease and joint problems. Psychotropic medication may adversely affect cardiac function through conduction and rhythm disturbances, which can lead to sudden death.

Physical health issues in patients with mental health problems may be compounded by the adverse effects that prescribed medications have on cardiovascular health and body weight. Patients should be provided with practical strategies to maintain and improve their health, such as physical activity.

A strong association exists between physical inactivity and the emergence of chronic diseases. Physical activity has the potential:

- to reduce mortality, of all causes
- to prevent several chronic diseases
- to have a positive impact on existing chronic conditions
- to decrease morbidity
- to increase longevity and quality of life.

Benefits of exercise on those with physical disease

Coronary heart disease

Physical activity has been shown to play both a primary and a secondary role in the prevention of a cardiac event. Aerobic exercise training reduces the heart's demand for oxygen and increases cardiac efficiency; it can also decrease blood pressure, decrease heart rate response and increase myocardial blood flow.

Hypertension and peripheral arterial disease

Aerobic activity can aid the reduction of blood pressure and after a single session there is an acute reduction in blood pressure that can last 12 hours. Exercise can reduce coronary heart disease risk factors; regular moderate-intensity exercise will confer the greatest benefit.

Obesity

Engagement in regular physical activity increases total energy expenditure and increases resting metabolic rate. Activity will promote body fat metabolism while preserving lean mass and may reverse diet-induced suppression of basal metabolic rate. Regular activity will also be of benefit through improved weight management, increased physical work capacity and improved well-being.

Diabetes

Specific health benefits of exercise for diabetes are improved glucose control in type 2 diabetes. Exercise has an insulin-like effect that enhances the uptake of glucose even in the presence of insulin deficiency. It improves glucose tolerance and insulin sensitivity in type 1 and type 2 diabetes, decreases glycosylated haemoglobin and insulin requirements, and improves lipid profile.

Osteoporosis

Exercise which subjects the skeleton to ground force reaction is a determining factor of peak bone mass. Engagement in weight-bearing exercise can help maintain bone mineral density in postmenopausal women and can reduce the risk of developing osteoporosis in later life, if started in adolescence. It reduces the risk of falls in later life by strengthening muscles and improving balance and coordination skills.

Arthritis

In osteoarthritis, physical activity helps to reduce joint pain and stiffness, to increase flexibility, to maintain muscular strength and prevent deconditioning, to decrease pain, and to improve aerobic fitness. In rheumatoid arthritis, physical activity does not directly improve the disease process, but there are benefits from improved aerobic capacity, improved muscular strength, increased endurance, and improved joint mobility.

Back pain

Physical activity can help the management of back pain by increasing overall muscular strength and endurance, improving flexibility, improving bone mass, and increasing the strength of connective tissue.

Asthma

Specific activities to strengthen the respiratory muscles and also aerobic activity can help in the management of asthma by reducing the frequency of flare-ups and stabilising the disease. There can also be a reduced need for medication as lung function improves and strengthens.

Chronic obstructive pulmonary disease

Physical activity can improve the efficiency of breathing and oxygen transportation. It can also improve oxygen extraction, efficiency and endurance of the trained skeletal muscle. There is an improved level of exercise tolerance and a reduced incidence of breathlessness and fatigue, resulting in an improved quality of life.

Multiple sclerosis

The aim of engaging in physical activity is to maintain and improve physical functioning and fitness. This will help to reduce fatigue, increase strength and limit disability; it will also enhance psychological well-being

Benefits of exercise on those with mental illness

Research studies set in both clinical and non-clinical settings have found a positive relationship between physical activity and mental health and illness.[3] Studies have concluded that physical activity can be used as an aid to treatment for individuals suffering from mental health problems.

General mental health

Both acute and chronic exercise have been found to decrease mental health symptoms and a positive relationship between physical activity and psychological well-being has been confirmed in several large epidemiological studies. Aerobic exercise has been shown to have a positive effect on tension, vigour, depression, anger, fatigue and confusion, and there is evidence from experimental trials that exercise of moderate intensity has a positive effect on psychological well-being.

Depression

Epidemiological evidence suggests that physical activity is associated with a decreased risk of developing clinically defined depression; the strongest evidence has been reported by Craft and Landers, and Mutrie.[9,10] Both aerobic and resistance forms of exercise can be used to treat moderate or severe depression as an adjunct to standard treatment. Exercise can have effects similar to those of other psychotherapeutic interventions used in mental health services.

Anxiety and stress

Physical activity can produce modest reductions in anxiety.[3] A series of exercise sessions can reduce trait anxiety but even a 'one off' session has a favourable impact, independent of any physiological improvement in fitness. Single sessions can reduce short-term anxiety and physiological reactivity to psychosocial stressors, enhance a participant's recovery from stress and reduce long-term anxiety tendencies. Increased core temperature offers a short-term tranquillising effect as this increases noradrenaline, serotonin and dopamine levels, all of which have an effect on stress and its symptoms.

Schizophrenia

Exercise may be effective in treating symptoms of schizophrenia,[4] and physical activity can be a good strategy for coping with distressing symptoms. Patients with schizophrenia are subjected to long-term effects of antipsychotic medication and often have a history of high rates of substance misuse, yet much of their excess mortality is due to natural causes. A person with schizophrenia can expect to live 10 years less than someone without a mental health problem and around half of this excess mortality is caused by physical health problems;[11] regular bouts of physical activity can help alleviate these.

Fitness assessment

Assessment is the key to safe, effective, enjoyable exercise programming that matches personal goals to health needs.

Information about patients' health should be obtained before they take part in any form of physical activity, in order to identify any potential health risks. This information should include:

- medical history
- age and gender
- current illnesses or injuries
- knowledge of current fitness status
- medication, in particular, any medication that might affect blood pressure, cardiac function or blood sugar level.

All patients should complete a physical activity readiness questionnaire (PAR-Q)[a] and have a fitness assessment. Details of this should be recorded and the patient's current fitness status should be evaluated.

A fitness assessment is performed in order to assess a patient's current level of ability and to identify his or her fitness status; this assessment provides a baseline from which health-related exercise programmes can be developed. It also enables exercise professionals to prescribe exercise and activity appropriate to that individual. The results highlight areas of physical health and fitness that are outside normal parameters. Assessments enable staff to monitor and review progress on a regular basis.

A comprehensive fitness assessment and the equipment required are detailed in Table 8.5.

Table 8.5 Equipment required for a comprehensive fitness assessment

Assessment	Necessary equipment
Height	Height measure
Weight	Scales
Body mass index (BMI)	BMI chart/calculation
Body fat percentage	Body fat monitor
Waist measurement	Tape measure
Blood pressure	Sphygmomanometer and cuff
Resting pulse	Pulse oximeter/feel at radial pulse
Flexibility	'Sit and reach' box
Respiration rate	Stopwatch or similar (watch rise and fall of chest for 1 minute)
Grip strength	Dynamometer
Aerobic capacity	Heart rate monitor and ergomedic cycle

Measurement of height and weight

These measurements can be used to calculate the body mass index (BMI), which is height (best determined using a fixed wall height measure) in metres squared, divided by weight in kilograms (determined using approved scales). Standard tables are available in paper format or on line (www.bmi-calculator.net). The assessment helps to establish any existing or potential weight-related health problems.

Resting pulse

Measurement of the resting pulse by palpation helps to establish a satisfactory baseline in relation to the patient's age, medical condition and medication. People who are fit generally tend to have a lower resting heart rate. People who are unfit may have a heart rate above 100 beats per minute (b.p.m.). This measurement is a good indicator of a person's overall fitness.

Resting blood pressure

This provides a baseline. It is important that the patient is relaxed as anxiety can affect the outcome. Ideally, no less than two readings should be taken about 1 minute apart; electronic sphygmomanometers are available.

a. PAR-Q is a self-screening tool that can be used by anyone who is planning to start an exercise programme. It is often used by fitness trainers or coaches to determine the safety or possible risk of exercising for an individual based on their answers to specific health history questions.[12]

Aerobic capacity

This is the ability of the heart and lungs to supply the muscles with nutrients and oxygen and to remove waste products efficiently. It is a measure of stamina or endurance. Aerobic capacity is assessed using an ergo cycle (Fig. 8.2).

Exercise tolerance assessment

This assessment should take place before the other elements of the fitness assessment. It helps to identify any adverse cardiovascular or respiratory responses to exercise and acts as a measure of whether illnesses or medical conditions are affecting cardiovascular fitness. The assessment shows how well the patient copes with equipment use, and enables the setting of safe levels of exercise intensity within the fitness programme. Before the assessment, it is vital to ensure the patient is well enough and there are no absolute contraindications, such as elevated resting heart rate (above 100 b.p.m.), blood pressure above 180/110 mmHg, or any other uncontrolled comorbidity. The patient must have available any regular medication such as an asthma inhaler.

Any patient taking beta-blockers, calcium channel blockers, potassium channel activators or alpha blockers should be assessed using the Rating of Perceived Exertion (RPE) scale to enable the exercise professional to ascertain safe exercise tolerance, as these medications affect heart rate and response to exercise (Tables 8.6, 8.7).[12]

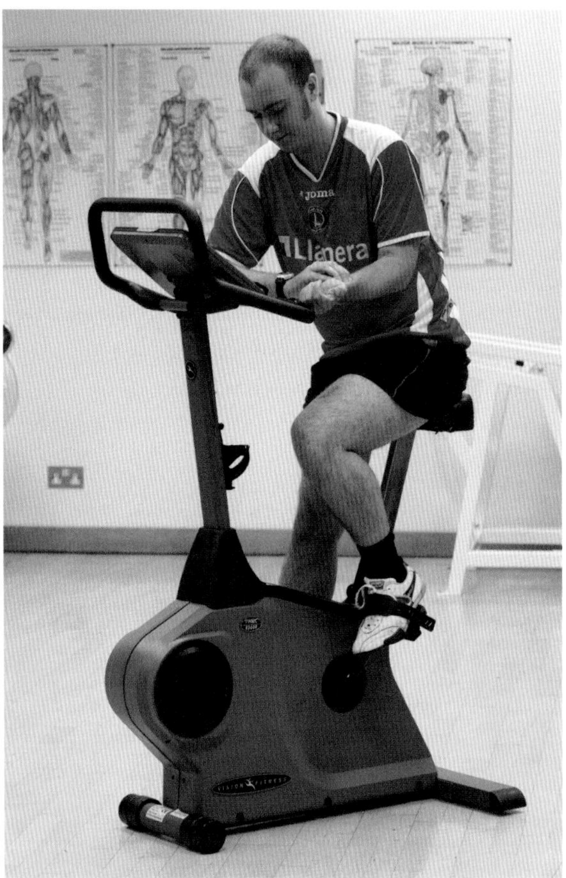

Fig. 8.2 An ergo cyle.

Body fat percentage

High percentages of body fat indicate obesity, which in turn increases the risk of heart disease, high blood pressure, diabetes, joint problems and other medical conditions (see Chapter 7, on obesity).

Waist measurement

Waist circumference is a good predictor of cardiovascular risk. Visceral fat is associated with an increased risk of cardiovascular disease and a waist measurement correlates with the amount of visceral fat.

The circumference of the waist, taken as the mid-point between the lowest rib and the iliac crest, should be measured while the individual is breathing out and the abdomen is relaxed.

Strength

The grip strength dynamometer assesses the ability of a muscle or muscle group to exert or resist a force. Strength as a fitness component is important because it is essential for support, posture and muscle tone. It is also important for patients in rehabilitation following an injury and contributes to all round fitness.

Flexibility

The 'sit and reach test' measures the flexibility of the lower back and hamstrings. It is carried out utilising a 'sit and reach' box. Individuals should perform the test in a

Table 8.6 Rating of perceived exertion (RPE) on a scale of 6–20

RPE	Description of intensity	Heart rate equivalent (b.p.m.)
6		60
7	Very, very light	70
8		80
9	Very light	90
10		100
11	Fairly light	110
12		120
13	Somewhat hard	130
14		140
15	Hard	150
16		160
17	Very hard	170
18		180
19	Very, very hard	190
20		200

Adapted from Borg, 1982.[13]

sitting position, feet and knees hip-distance apart. Feet are positioned on the edge of the box, and knees should be fully extended. Under control, the individual reaches forward and pushes the fingers along a table or box as far as possible, bending at the hips with the arms fully extended. The distance from the fingertips to the edge of the table represents the score for that person. Several attempts are allowed but a warm-up is essential.

Lung function

Peak expiratory flow, measured using a peak flow meter, is an objective measure of resting respiratory function. It gives an indication of the maximum rate of flow that a person can achieve. It can be used to help identify lung weakness or damage, smoking or asthma. More detailed information on lung function requires more complex hospital equipment.

Table 8.7 Rating of perceived exertion (RPE) on a scale of 1–10

RPE	Description of intensity	Percentage of MHR
1	No exertion at all	10%
2		20%
3	Light	30%
4		40%
5	Moderate	50%
6		60%
7	Hard	70%
8		80%
9		90%
10	Very hard, as hard as you could work	100%

Adapted from Borg, 1982.[13] MHR, maximum heart rate.

Appendices

(1) Resources and equipment

There are vast arrays of resources and equipment that can be acquired or accessed before exercise schemes can commence. They are listed in Table 8A.

(2) Qualifications of staff

An appropriate skill mix is required to deliver physical activity to patients on exercise referral schemes. To assess fitness and design programmes and exercise prescriptions, health and fitness instructors must have a degree in a health- and fitness-related field, or a GP referral qualification.

To facilitate programmes, instructors must have at least one of the following:

- National Pool Lifeguard Qualification
- NVQ coaching qualifications, level 2 or above
- swimming teaching qualifications
- an 'exercise to music' qualification, level 2 or above
- a gym instructor qualification, level 2 or above.

Other relevant qualifications include yoga and pilates.

Anyone can and should advocate brisk walking, but formalised exercise programmes should be left to exercise professionals, who have the experience and qualifications in working with high-risk populations. Exercise professionals who are members of the Register of Exercise Professionals (REPS) have competency in this area.

Table 8A Equipment for undertaking various exercise activities

Activity	Equipment
Gym	Upright and recumbent cycle; treadmills; rowers; steppers; cross-trainers; fixed-resistance machines; dumbbells; weights; resistance bands
Swimming	Swimming hats, suits, shorts; goggles; woggles (flotation aids); water weights
Ward-based activities	Curling set; parachute; flexi-balls
Team sports	Goal posts/nets; footballs; rugby balls; basketballs; badminton racquets, nets, shuttlecocks; rounders bats, posts, balls; cricket stumps; volleyball posts, nets, balls; table tennis nets, bats, balls; netball posts, balls; whistles
Other	Mats; music player and CDs; heart rate monitors; leaflets
Clothing	Trainers; jogging bottoms; t-shirts; swim-wear
Fitness assessment equipment	Scales; height measure; 'sit and reach' box; blood pressure monitor, sphygmomanometer; body fat monitor; grip strength dynamometer; ergo cycle; peak flow and cardboard mouth tubes; pulse oximeter; modified walk test tape

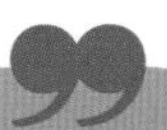

Summary

Psychiatric patients have been shown to be less physically active and have higher rates of comorbidities associated with both inactivity and obesity. Owing to their mental health problems, many patients do not engage in regular physical activity and are unaware of the physical and psychological health benefits that can be achieved. Health professionals working in either forensic or community settings face many challenges in encouraging patients to adopt a physically active lifestyle and to raise awareness of the health benefits of exercise.

Exercise can be utilised to assist in the management of several mental health and physical health conditions and exercise prescription can run alongside medication and psychological interventions.

It is essential that health professionals recognise the important role exercise interventions can play in targeting the growing physical healthcare problems of psychiatric patients.

All patients should have a physical assessment and a comprehensive physical fitness assessment by a trained fitness specialist and be encouraged to take part in some form of regular exercise or activity. This should focus on:

- cardiovascular fitness
- muscular strength
- muscular endurance
- flexibility
- motor skills.

It should take into account any potential limitation due to underlying physical or mental illness and drug treatment.

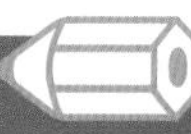

Learning points

- The five components of fitness that should be incorporated into training programmes for patients to gain maximum benefits are: cardiovascular fitness; muscular strength; muscular endurance; flexibility; motor skills.
- The intensity of the exercise should correspond to the recommendations and restrictions of the exercise prescription.
- Exercise sessions comprise warm-up, training and cool-down activities.
- A basic stretching programme should follow the warm-up.
- Activities should progress gradually.
- Breaking activities down into small structured segments promotes continued interest.
- Stretching that targets all muscles groups used in the exercise should follow the cool-down.
- In strength and resistance training programmes, the focus should be on the endurance component of the training, not the resistance component.
- Psychotropic medications may cause side-effects that impair an individual's ability to exercise.
- Fitness assessments are the key to designing safe, effective, enjoyable exercise programmes that match personal goals to health needs.
- Treatment with beta-blockers, calcium channel blockers, potassium channel activators and alpha-blockers may affect heart rate and response to exercise.
- The Rating of Perceived Exertion (RPE) scale should be used to enable the exercise professional to ascertain safe exercise tolerance for patients taking the above medications.
- A Physical Activity Readiness Questionnaire (PAR-Q) should be completed before patients start an exercise activity, to ascertain their likes and dislikes.
- Exercise which subjects the skeleton to a ground force reaction is an important factor in maintaining peak bone mass.

References

1 McCreadie RG; Scottish Schizophrenia Lifestyle Group. Diet, smoking and cardiovascular risk in people with schizophrenia: descriptive study. *Br J Psychiatry* 2003; **183**: 534–9.

2 Cormac I, Ferriter M, Benning R, *et al*. Physical health and health risk factors in a population of long-stay psychiatric patients. *Psychiatr Bull* 2005; **29**: 18–20.

3 Biddle SJH, Fox KR, Boutcher SH (eds). *Physical Activity and Psychological Well-being*. Routledge, 2000.

4 Faulkner G, Biddle SJH. Exercise and mental health: it's just not psychology! *J Sports Science* 2001; **19**: 433–44.

5 Department of Health. *At Least Five a Week. Evidence of the Impact of Physical Activity and Its Relationship to Health: A Report by the Chief Medical Officer*. Department of Health, 2004.

6 Haskell WL, Lee IM, Pate RR, *et al*. Physical activity and public health: updated recommendation for adults from the American College of Sports Medicine and the American Heart Association. *Circulation* 2007; **116**: 1081–93.

7 Garber CE, Blissmer B, Deschenes MR, *et al*. American College of Sports Medicine position stand: Quantity and quality of exercise for developing and maintaining cardiorespiratory, musculoskeletal, and neuromotor fitness in apparently healthy adults – guidance for prescribing exercise. *Med Sci Sports Exerc* 2011; **43**: 1334–59.

8 National Institute for Health and Clinical Excellence. *Four Commonly Used Methods to Increase Physical Activity* (Public Health Guidance, PH2). Chapter 1: Recommendations, 1.2: Exercise Referral Schemes. NICE, 2006.

9 Craft LL, Landers DM. The effects of exercise on clinical depression and depression resulting from mental illness: a meta analysis. *J Sport Exercise Psychology* 1998; **20**: 339–57.

10 Mutrie N. The relationship between physical activity and clinically defined depression. In *Physical Activity and Psychological Well-being* (ed S. J. H. Biddle, K. Fox, S. H. Boutcher): 46–62. Routledge, 2000.

11 Brown S, Birtwhistle J, Roe L, *et al.* The unhealthy lifestyle of people with schizophrenia. *Psychol Med* 1999; **29**: 697–701.

12 Quinn E. PAR-Q: The Physical Activity Readiness Questionnaire. About.com Sports Medicine 2008, 12 December (http://sportsmedicine.about.com/od/fitnessevalandassessment/qt/PAR-Q.htm).

13 Borg GAV. Psychological bases of perceived exertion. *Med Sci Sports Exerc* 1982; **14**: 377–81.

Physical health standards and examination

Michael Phelan and Bronwen Williams

People with mental disorders need high-quality physical healthcare. This chapter describes the standards for physical health services and the main topics to cover when taking a medical history. It suggests a structure for undertaking a physical examination and makes recommendations for the equipment needed on the ward for physical examinations.

Introduction

Mental health organisations and most mental health professionals now recognise the importance of the physical health of their service users. Nevertheless, in a busy world, with many competing demands, it is a topic that can still be neglected and never reach the top of a long list of priorities. Efforts to improve physical health can also be hampered by confusion over who is responsible, both on an organisational level and at the level of individual patient care.

This chapter will outline the importance of establishing agreed standards of care and then describe the minimum standards that should be expected in the areas of taking the medical history and physical examination.

Standards of physical healthcare

Standards offer clarity to patients about what they can expect and to staff about what is expected of them. The standards agreed within a large mental health NHS trust and subsequently published by the Royal College of Psychiatrists are shown in Box 9.1. They were written with the intention that they would establish a reasonable level of care that would be applicable across a range of service settings and patient groups. They were thought of as 'bronze level' standards that everyone should be achieving most, if not all, of the time. Some teams and units may well achieve more and set themselves more demanding or specific standards

Agreeing standards is only the first step in trying to improve the quality of care. It is also necessary to measure or audit performance against the agreed standards, and to identify any barriers to meeting them. The standards agreed by the Royal College of Psychiatrists are designed so that each item can be recorded and audited, to highlight where standards are not being achieved and help in the process of identifying the barriers to good physical healthcare.

Some of the potential barriers to providing physical healthcare within a mental health setting are listed in Box 9.2. Individual, organisational and environmental barriers can all be identified. The process of tackling some

Box 9.1 Physical health standards

(1) Initial physical assessment of in-patients

Physical examination

- All patients should have a comprehensive physical examination within 24 hours of admission
- If an examination is not possible (e.g. patient refuses or is too disturbed) the reason should be clearly stated in the notes and relevant observations documented (e.g. nutritional status, gait, abnormal movements)

Physical health review

- A full physical health review should be completed within 2 weeks of admission. This should include: details of past and present illnesses; a comprehensive symptom review; all current medication; health promotion history (including smoking, diet and exercise); details of health screening (e.g. dental care, cervical screening)
- It is recommended that this information is collected on a standard form, and an action plan agreed with the patient

Physical investigations

- Appropriate physical investigations should be completed during the first week of admission
- The results of physical investigations should be reviewed and filed in the notes

(2) Ongoing physical healthcare of in-patients

- Patients should have their weight and blood pressure recorded at least monthly
- Physical health review, examination and investigations should be repeated at least every 6 months
- Patients should have access to dental care, chiropody, a dietitian, physiotherapy, sexual healthcare and an optician

(3) Management of long-term physical illness of in-patients

- The symptoms, progress and treatment of long-term physical disorders (e.g. diabetes, hypertension and arthritis) should be reviewed with the patient and documented at least monthly by medical staff
- Long-term physical disorders should be reviewed by a general practitioner or hospital specialist at least every 6 months

(4) Health promotion for in-patients

- Patients should have easy access to appropriate written health promotion information
- Patients should have access to exercise, smoking cessation support and appropriate dietary advice

(5) Environment for in-patients

- Patients should be provided with appropriate food and drink to meet their nutritional, therapeutic and cultural needs
- Patients should have access to fresh air and exercise space
- A smoke-free environment should be provided
- Access to appropriate, clean, washing and toilet facilities should be maintained at all times

(6) Emergency care for in-patients

- Wards should have access to resuscitation equipment that is regularly maintained
- Wards should have ready access to emergency medical care
- A first-aid kit should be available on each ward

(7) Community physical health standards (enhanced care programme approach – CPA)

- Discharge summaries should include a section on physical health
- CPA care coordinators should liaise with patients' general practitioners every year to confirm that an annual physical health assessment has been conducted. If this is not possible, alternative arrangements should be found for patients to have a physical assessment
- CPA reviews should include a review of physical health needs and an agreed care plan to address identified needs
- Community patients should have access to appropriate community groups that support and encourage good physical health, such as walking groups, weight management sessions and healthy living groups

Source: Royal College of Psychiatrists, 2009.[1]

Box 9.2 Common barriers to the provision of good physical healthcare

Individual

Staff – lack of training/awareness

Patient – level of disturbance or unwillingness to participate

Organisational

Lack of prioritisation given to physical health

Lack of clarity over responsibilities

Interface between mental and acute medical care providers

Environmental

Lack of examination room or equipment

Lack of exercise facilities

Inaccessible radiology or pathology services

of these problems can be challenging and bring to light fundamental issues about current mental health services. On an individual level there are significant issues around the training of mental health staff and the relative paucity of physical health training that the majority of mental health professionals receive. On an organisational level the separation between mental health and acute services does not encourage a holistic approach to individual patient care. Numerous environmental issues can also hamper progress. The rest of this chapter will focus on two key areas to which the standards apply – taking a physical health history and physical examinations.

Taking a physical health history in psychiatry

All doctors are taught that careful history-taking is the cornerstone of good medical care. For most patients the story they tell, and the symptoms they describe, will provide the basis of a provisional diagnosis, which will then be confirmed by physical examination and investigations. This basic tenet of medical practice was demonstrated by Hampton *et al.*[2] in a study of medical out-patients: 83% of diagnoses could be made from the patients' history and 9% from examination. In mental health settings, this fundamental principle must never be forgotten, and in some cases it needs to be re-learnt.

Although psychiatrists take pride in their ability to listen and communicate with their patients, evidence suggests that this ability is not used when dealing with physical health issues. A study by Osborn & Warner[3] showed that whereas junior psychiatrists completed a physical examination on most in-patients, it was rare for them to have completed and documented a physical health assessment. There are obvious reasons why it can be difficult, or even at times impossible, to obtain a good medical history from patients when they are first admitted to an acute psychiatric ward: principally disturbance or lack of cooperation. When this happens it is obviously essential that it is documented and further attempts should be made when the patient is more settled.

Taking the physical history and physical health assessments should be viewed as a continuous process throughout a patient's contact with services. After an initial screening, in-patients should be regularly asked about physical symptoms, especially when medication is being changed or if they have an underlying medical condition. Similarly, out-patients should routinely be asked about their general physical health, and more specific and detailed questions should be asked when appropriate.

The content of a medical history will always be a balance between brevity and completeness, and there will always be room for professional judgement about what needs to be asked and when it should be asked. In most situations the following seven areas need to be considered.

(1) Family history. Patients should be specifically asked about disorders known to have a significant genetic component, such as ischaemic heart disease, diabetes, hypertension and autoimmune disorders. This may highlight patients who have an increased risk of specific conditions and may also bring to light fears that patients may have about their own health, especially if relatives have died young.

(2) Medical history. Past conditions may have relevance to current symptoms and disabilities and help staff understand how a person responds to physical illness, and any relationship between the physical and mental disorders. Patients need to be specifically asked about allergies. They may mention long-standing conditions or recurrent disorders such as hypertension or tuberculosis, which may have recently been overlooked because of their mental health concerns.

(3) Current illnesses and disabilities. There can be a tendency for doctors to ask about diagnosed illnesses and to ignore disabilities. Questions about eyesight, hearing, swallowing difficulties and mobility may

highlight important needs, which can often be met relatively easily, such as replacement glasses or dentures.

(4) Current medication. It is essential that prescribed and over-the-counter medication is recorded. The importance of medicines reconciliation (checking medication details from more than one source) and the key role that hospital pharmacists can play in reducing errors has been highlighted by the National Institute for Health and Clinical Excellence.[4] Consideration must be given to the potential interactions of any medications (including any psychotropic drugs). It is good practice to review all medications, as patients may still be taking some that are in fact no longer required. An accurate list of prescribed medication may also indicate a previously diagnosed physical illness not mentioned by a patient. Patients need to be asked about their adherence to prescribed treatment; erratic compliance is not a problem limited to psychiatric medication.

(5) Habits and lifestyle. Initial screening questions should ask about smoking habits, alcohol consumption, recreational drug use, diet, exercise, sexual activity/ dysfunction and safe-sex practices and, if relevant, contraception. For most patients such questions will reveal at least some areas where interventions have the potential to improve their physical health.

(6) Health screening. Many patients struggle to access recommended routine health screening and mental health staff have an important role to play in helping patients do so. All should be asked about their last dental and optician visit, and when they last had their blood pressure, urine and lipids tested. Female patients should be asked about cervical screening (recommended every 3 years for ages 25–49 and every 5 years for ages 50–64) and mammography (recommended every 3 years for ages 50–70). Patients at risk – through a history of diabetes, ischaemic heart disease, stroke, chronic obstructive pulmonary disease (COPD), asthma, immunocompromise or age over 65 – should be asked about seasonal influenza and pneumococcal vaccination and offered these in the in-patient setting. Patients at risk from blood-borne viruses (e.g. intravenous drug users and health workers) should be asked about hepatitis B status and vaccination.

(7) Symptoms. Patients may not spontaneously mention physical symptoms, especially if they are long-standing or perceived as embarrassing. It is therefore important that specific questions are asked about each body system.

The standard psychiatric history usually covers some but not all of this. Medical history usually covers smoking and alcohol. It is far less likely that patients will be asked in detail about physical symptoms and when they last went to the dentist. To encourage and remind doctors to ask about areas that have traditionally been neglected, it can be helpful to introduce standardised forms. This helps to ensure that all relevant questions are asked, and that the answers are clearly documented. The Physical Health Check (PHC) is an example of a tool that was developed to encourage a systematic approach to the assessment of patients' physical health needs by doctors and other mental health professionals[5] (available from www.rethink.org).

Regardless of whether specific forms are used, it is essential that physical health issues are clearly documented in the patient record. For clarity, this should be in a specific section of the patient's file or computer record and should include the outcome of what patients have been told and action plans that have been agreed. If patients are unhappy about answering questions or refuse further examination or investigation, this needs to be recorded.

It is essential that there is good communication between the mental health team and the patient's general practitioner (GP), so that the GP is made aware of any relevant issues, and that duplication is avoided. Information about physical health should be included in discharge summaries and out-patient letters (see Chapter 3 on general practice). Further information on taking a physical health history is available in Phelan & Blair.[6]

Physical examinations in psychiatry

Alongside a good physical health history, a physical examination is essential in acute psychiatric care, other in-patient settings and in some out-patient settings. A physical examination will supplement information already obtained from the patient and other sources, but may also reveal previously undetected clinical signs and pathology. This may be because of a lack of symptoms (as in hypertension) or because the patient has been unable to tell others about the symptoms due to communication difficulties.

It is generally agreed that all patients should have a comprehensive physical examination within 24 hours of admission. Patients do, however, have the right to refuse, and if they do so, or if the patient is too disturbed to be examined, this should be clearly documented in the patient record alongside any relevant observations

Box 9.3 Recommended medical equipment for psychiatric wards

- Examination couch
- Disposable gloves
- Weighing scales
- Height measure
- Thermometer
- Urinalysis sticks
- Urine drug screen
- Alcometer
- Pulse oximeter
- Stethoscope
- Sphygmomanometer
- Tendon hammer
- Tuning fork (256 Hz)
- Ophthalmoscope and auroscope
- Neurological testing pins
- Snellen chart

Adapted from Garden, 2005.[7]

noted. There is also an argument for offering a second physical health review (including an examination) within 2 weeks of admission, at a time when patients are less psychologically distressed and are more familiar with their surroundings.

The examination

Whenever possible, the examination should take place in an appropriate, private environment. The equipment required for a comprehensive examination is listed in Box 9.3. It is essential to expose the patient adequately and, as patients with mental illness are often prone to self-neglect, all outer garments should be removed, while maintaining patient's dignity.

Inspection

It could be argued that observation is the most important part of the physical examination, and it is often all that the clinician is able to do when examining an acutely disturbed patient. Box 9.4 lists some of the important clinical signs to look out for in patients with an acute psychiatric disorder. Observation starts as soon as the clinician meets the patient:

- Assess the patient's general appearance, including demeanour, nutritional status, state of hydration, personal hygiene, the nature and state of clothing.
- Observe any abnormality in gait, posture, movement or facial expression.
- Identify any abnormalities in skin complexion, hair texture and distribution, and odours.
- Measure weight and height and calculate body mass index (weight in kilogrammes divided by height in metres squared). Record these measurements at least monthly as part of the ongoing physical healthcare of psychiatric in-patients.
- Measure waist circumference – obesity and insulin resistance are a major concern in psychiatric patients.
- Check body temperature – usually raised with infection and neuroleptic malignant syndrome (with muscle rigidity).
- Inspect the oral cavity, as psychiatric patients are known to have poor dentition and reduced access to dental care.[8]

> A chaperone is essential if there is a gender difference between patient and psychiatrist, if the patient is acutely disturbed or if the patient is under the influence of illicit drugs or alcohol.

Palpation

Palpation covers the following points (Fig. 9.1):

- Starting with the hands, check skin temperature, texture and sweating.
- Look for clubbing and peripheral stigmata of chronic liver disease.
- Examine the nails for excess biting (indicating anxiety), nicotine staining, leukonychia, koilonychia, splinter haemorrhages (indicating vasculitidies or bacterial endocarditis) and onycholysis.
- Palpate the cervical, axillary and inguinal lymph glands – generalised or local enlargement may indicate tuberculosis, lymphoma, HIV infection or occult malignancy and requires further investigation. If a thyroid mass or goitre is noted, it is sensible to examine the patient's thyroid status more fully and auscultate for a thyroid bruit.

Cardiovascular system

- Observe in particular for signs of hyperlipidaemia – palmar or tendon xanthomas, corneal arcus and xanthelasma. This is particularly relevant if the patient is taking antipsychotic medication.

Box 9.4 Physical signs associated with common mental health problems

Depression

- Low body mass index (BMI) (from chronic self-neglect)
- High BMI (from over-eating or as a side-effect of medication)
- Vitamin deficiencies (from chronic self-neglect):

  B1 – Wernicke-Korsakoff syndrome

  B12 – Glossitis, angular cheilosis, dementia, peripheral neuropathy

  A – Night blindness, dry and atrophied skin

  D – Rickets and osteomalacia

  E – Haemolysis, spinocerebellar degeneration, peripheral neuropathy

  K – Bleeding, bruising
- Psychomotor retardation
- Catatonia
- Monotonous speech
- Apathy, poverty of facial expression, poor eye contact
- Amenorrhoea
- Constipation

Anxiety

- Tremor
- Dry mouth, frequent swallowing
- Sweating
- Tachycardia
- Dilated pupils
- Hyperventilation

Hypomania

- Psychomotor agitation
- Low BMI (despite increased appetite)
- Involuntary movements (from lithium toxicity)
- Increased desire for sexual activity
- Loud, pressurised speech

Schizophrenia

- High BMI (from negative symptoms or as a side-effect of antipsychotic medication)
- Parkinsonism (as a side-effect of certain antipsychotic medications)
- Tremor
- Poverty of facial expression
- Tardive dyskinesia (side-effect of typical antipsychotic medication)
- Catatonia
- Photosensitivity rash (side-effect of chlorpromazine)

Anorexia nervosa

- Low BMI
- Abnormal hair distribution (lanugo, diffuse alopecia)
- Dry skin
- Amenorrhoea
- Cardiac arrhythmias and syncope
- Teeth problems and poor oral hygiene (as a result of purging, e.g. vomiting)
- Hypotension
- Hypothermia and increased sensitivity to cold

Borderline personality disorder

- Self-cutting marks
- Tattoos
- Marked emotional instability

Dementia

- Low BMI (from chronic self-neglect)
- Vitamin deficiencies (see above)
- Cerebrovascular disease
- Previous cerebrovascular accident or transient ischaemic attack or other risk factors
- Signs of hypothyroidism

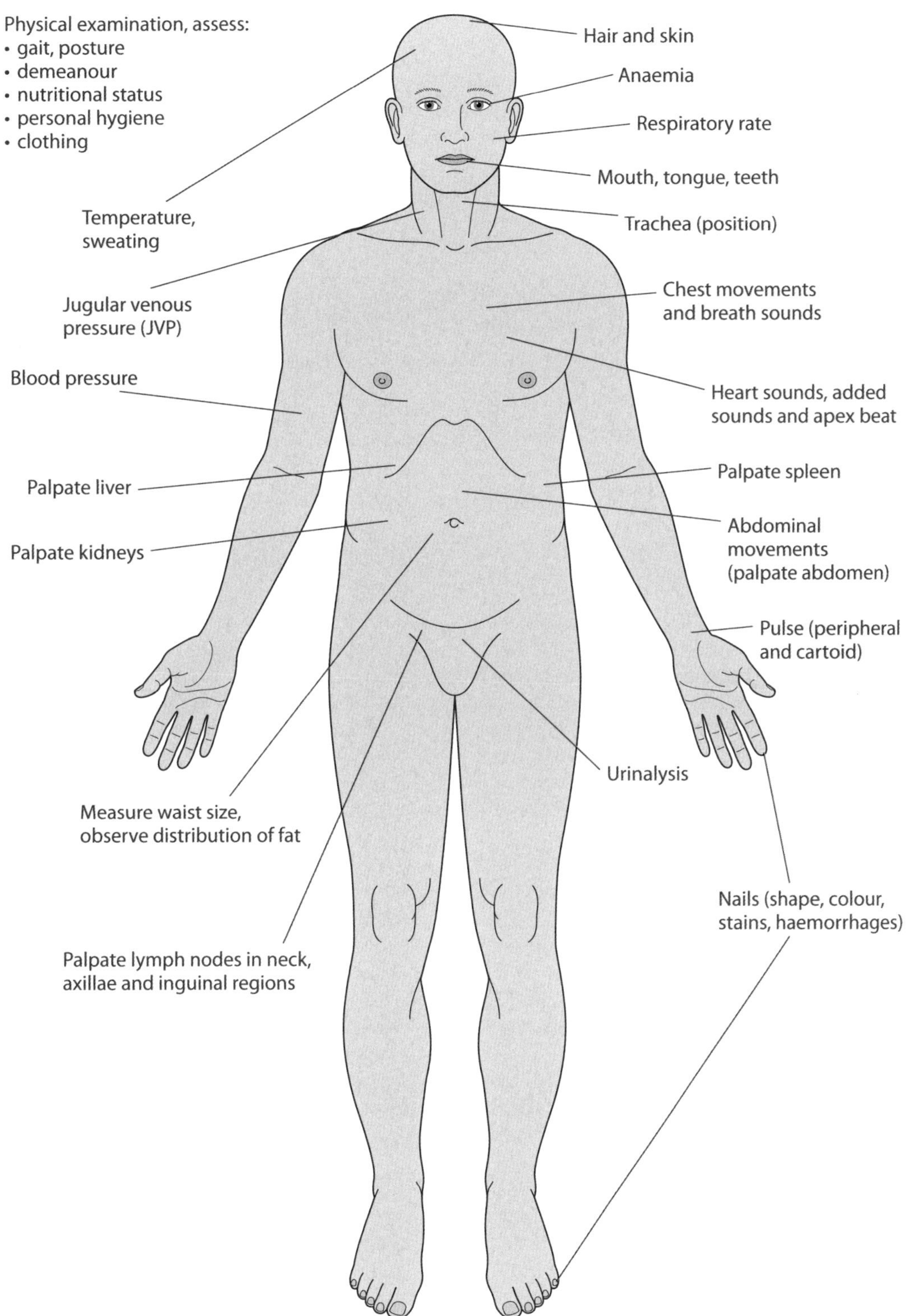

Fig. 9.1 Physical examination (more detailed information is given in the text).

Table 9.1 Possible psychiatric causes of abnormal blood pressure reading

Abnormality	Possible cause
Hypertension	Heightened arousal on admission Psychotropic medication (e.g. venlafaxine, clozapine) Hyperthyroidism Phaeochromocytoma Renal disease
Hypotension	Anorexia nervosa Addison's disease
Postural hypotension	Diabetes Autonomic dysfunction Psychotropic medication Dementia with Lewy bodies

- Palpate the radial pulse for rate, rhythm, volume and character. If the pulse is irregular it is important to identify the nature of the irregularity, usually by undertaking electrocardiography (ECG), as atrial fibrillation can be associated with hyperthyroidism, stroke and vascular dementia. Ventricular ectopic beats and prolongation of the QT interval (usually corrected or QTc interval) can be associated with psychotropic medication.
- Measure the blood pressure – Table 9.1 illustrates some relevant psychiatric conditions and associations.
- Examine the jugular venous pressure and waveform at 45° just above the clavicle, as this provides valuable information regarding the patient's fluid status and cardiac function. Pulse rate elevation is a valuable sign of raised right atrial pressure.
- Palpate the apex beat while the patient is sitting forwards and note any displacement, the character of the impulse, heaves and thrills.
- Listen to the heart for the first and second heart sounds – you might also hear a pericardial rub (a squeak in time with the heart beat) or a murmur.
- Ausculate for carotid bruits, especially in elderly patients in whom vascular dementia is suspected.
- Palpate peripheral pulses to exclude ischaemia, especially in patients with peripheral vascular disease and patients who misuse intravenous drugs.

Respiratory system

- Observe the following in particular:
  - respiratory rate
  - the chest wall for symmetrical movements and abnormalities of the chest wall.
- Palpate for tracheal displacement by an enlarged thyroid mass, mediastinal mass – such as lymphoma or carcinoma – or lung pathology such as collapse, fibrosis or pleural effusion
- Palpate for symmetrical chest expansion.
- Percuss the chest wall and compare resonance over equivalent areas of the chest wall.
- Ausculate the lungs alternately, comparing each side for wheeze (especially in the heavy smoker), crackles, crepitations and bronchial breathing.
- If available, measure oxygen saturation using pulse oximetry and follow up any abnormal findings with a chest X-ray, if indicated.

Gastrointestinal system

Position the patient comfortably supine with arms either side of the abdomen in order to relax the muscles of the anterior abdominal wall. Then examine the abdomen as follows.

- Observe the shape and symmetry of the abdomen for distension, visible peristalsis, surgical scars, dilated abdominal veins or caput medusae that occur with liver cirrhosis.
- Palpate the abdomen lightly at first and then deeply for tenderness and masses, observing the patient's face for any grimace indicative of pain.
- Palpate the liver, gall bladder, spleen and kidneys for size, shape and tenderness.
- Percuss the liver and spleen individually and if the abdomen is distended percuss for shifting dullness.
- Rectal examination is not routinely carried out in psychiatric practice unless clinically indicated.
- Complete the examination with urinalysis if the patient has renal impairment, lithium treatment, symptoms of urinary infection, or suspected diabetes.

A new-onset heart murmur heard in the context of pyrexia and intravenous drug misuse should alert the clinician to the possibility of bacterial endocarditis.

Summary

People with mental health problems are known to have a high level of morbidity due to physical illness, creating a need for high-quality physical healthcare in this population. The minimum expected standards of care should be achievable not only in the acute in-patient setting but also in other in-patient and out-patient contexts. These standards for physical healthcare have been set out to provide clarity and transparency for both healthcare professionals and service users regarding the responsibility of the psychiatrist in general physical healthcare. As medical practitioners, psychiatrists have an integral role in the management of physical as well as mental healthcare. They should aim to understand the complex interaction between mental and physical health and use this in the prevention, detection and treatment of general health problems, so providing a service that meets both mental and physical healthcare needs.

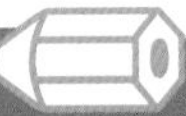

Learning points

- Agreeing standards of care will clarify expectations for staff and patients.
- There are multiple barriers to achieving good physical healthcare.
- Taking a physical history is at least if not more important than performing a physical examination.
- The physical health of in-patients should be reviewed on a regular basis, not just at the time of admission.
- Potential physical symptoms need to be asked for specifically.
- There must be good communication between the mental health team and the GP if the patient's physical health is to be managed effectively
- Adequate and well-maintained medical equipment must always be available for physical examinations.
- Inspection is probably the most important aspect of physical examination, and at times will be all that is possible.
- Be aware of important clinical signs in patients with mental health problems (Box 9.4, p. 106) and look for them routinely on physical examination.
- Atypical antipsychotic medication can cause hyperlipidaemia and insulin resistance and these need to be routinely monitored for on physical examination.
- The Physical Health Check is a useful tool designed for use by mental health professionals to improve the monitoring of physical health in people with mental illness.

Neurological examination

This is discussed in detail in Chapter 10.

References

1 Royal College of Psychiatrists. *Physical Health in Metal Health.* RCPsych, 2009.

2 Hampton JR, Harrison MJE, Mitchell JR. Relative contribution of history taking, physical examination and laboratory investigations to diagnosis and management of medical outpatients. *BMJ* 1975; **272**: 486–9.

3 Osborn D, Warner J. Assessing the physical health of psychiatric patients. *Psychiatr Bull* 1998; **22**: 695–7.

4 National Institute for Health and Clinical Excellence. *Technical Patient Safety Solutions for Medicines Reconciliation on Admission of Adults to Hospital.* NICE, 2007.

5 Phelan M, Stradins L, Amin D, *et al*. The Physical Health Check: a tool for mental health workers. *J Mental Health* 2004; **13**: 277–84.

6 Phelan M, Blair G. Medical history-taking in psychiatry. *Advances in Psychiatric Treatment* 2008; **14**: 1–6.

7 Garden G. Physical examination in psychiatric patients. *Adv Psychiatr Treat* 2005; **11**: 142–9.

8 Mirza I, Day R, Phelan M, *et al*. Oral health of psychiatric in-patients. *Psychiatr Bull* 2001; **25**: 143–5.

10

The neurological examination

Adrian Wills

The ability to perform a neurological examination should be part of the medical skills retained by a psychiatrist. This chapter describes how to conduct a neurological examination. It outlines the methods for assessing each component of the neurological examination, including how to assess cognitive function. It also gives tips on how to spot factitious neurological symptoms.

Introduction

Patients with psychiatric disorders are just as likely to develop neurological disease as those without. In addition, a number of medications used in psychiatric practice have neurological side-effects. A few patients have an underlying neurological explanation for their psychiatric presentation. Thus, the ability to perform a neurological assessment is one of the clinical skills required by doctors in psychiatric practice.

The neurological examination can be mastered only by repetition. Its main components are detailed here, with some indication of their clinical utility. Specific reference is made to various psychiatric presentations.

All patients should have a general physical examination (cardiac, respiratory, abdominal, as set out in Chapter 9). Blood pressure and weight should be recorded as well as urinalysis if possible. It is important to establish handedness (virtually all right-handers are left-hemisphere dominant, as are many left-handers).

Cranial nerve assessment

How thorough the examination of cranial nerves (Fig. 10.1) can be will depend on having a variety of basic equipment (essential) and a cooperative patient. If you suspect serious disease on the basis of a limited clinical examination, urgent referral to a specialist may be warranted. A detailed description of how to test each cranial nerve is beyond the scope of this book; many basic student textbooks can provide this information.

Cranial nerve I (olfactory nerve)

Failure of the sense of smell (anosmia) may be seen in sinus disease (most common), following head injury and as a consequence of tumours in the frontal lobe, particularly olfactory groove meningiomas (rare).

It is unlikely that smell bottles will be available; commonly available items may be substituted as a test of smell, such as perfume, disinfectant or fruit.

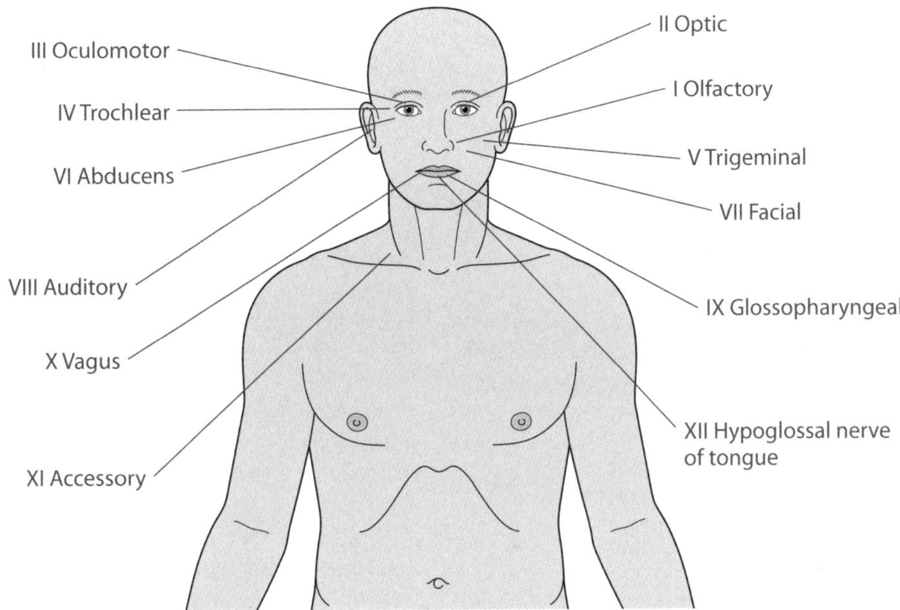

Fig. 10.1 Cranial nerves.

Cranial nerve II (optic nerve)

This requires an assessment of visual acuity, examination of the fundus, visual fields and response to light.

- Formal assessment of visual acuity requires a Snellen chart (p. 52). If one is available, patients who normally wear glasses should use them for the test. If no chart is available, check near vision with a newspaper and distance vision with any wall-hung sign. Unilateral visual loss may reflect:
  - ocular defects (cataracts, glaucoma)
  - optic nerve pathology (frontal tumour, demyelination).
- If you have an ophthalmoscope *and* have a cooperative patient, look for evidence of:
  - optic disc swelling (papilloedema)
  - optic atrophy (if unilateral consider frontal tumour, if bilateral – toxic ambylopia induced by alcohol or vitamin deficiency [B12, thiamine]).
- Perform visual field assessment, comparing your own with the patient's, by confrontation technique. Any loss of vision, however small, of new onset warrants a referral for investigation.
- Both pupils should constrict when light from a torch is shone in the eye. Failure to do so may indicate optic nerve damage on one side or loss of the consensual reflex.
- Check the accommodation reflex. The pupil should change size as the eye focuses on near and then far objects.

Patterns of pupillary abnormality include: unilateral small regular pupil with mild ptosis (Horner's syndrome); unilateral dilated pupil (optic nerve or oculomotor nerve lesion); small irregular pupils which accommodate but do not react to light (Argyll–Robertson treponemal disease); a large pupil which barely reacts to light, but with a brisker accommodation reflex (Adie pupil); bilateral dilated pupils with failure of vertical gaze (Parinaud's syndrome – midbrain lesion); and an oval pupil with poor reaction to light (glaucoma).

Cranial nerves III, IV and VI

The oculomotor, trochlear and abducens nerves work as a functional unit.

- Ask about double vision.
- Test eye movements using a target moving in an 'H' pattern. In third-nerve palsy (aneurysm), one eye is 'down and out' with a dilated pupil and complete ptosis. In fourth-nerve palsy, the eye cannot look down. Sixth-nerve palsy (arising in the context of raised intracranial pressure, diabetes, after a head injury) results in a failure of abduction.

- Look for nystagmus. If it is present in the horizontal plane, it is usually due to labyrinthine disease; if in the vertical, suspect brain-stem pathology.

Cranial nerve V (trigeminal nerve)

This has both motor and sensory components. For the motor component, ask the patient to open and close the mouth (jaw deviation suggests dysfunction of cranial nerve V). A brisk jaw jerk may indicate a lesion above the mid-brain (arising from cerebrovascular disease or motor neuron disease). The sensory component can be tested with cotton wool – cranial nerve V supplies the skin over the face – and the corneal reflex.

Cranial nerve VII (facial nerve)

This supplies the upper and lower face and gives the ability to raise the eyebrows and smile. The upper face has bilateral cortical input, so a lower motor neuron lesion causes complete palsy, known as Bell's palsy – with ear pain, hyperacusis (stapedius) and loss of taste in the anterior two-thirds of the tongue (corda tympani). A lower motor neurone pattern may also be caused by an ipsilateral pontine lesion. An upper motor neuron lesion (from stroke or tumour) leads to relative sparing of the upper face.

Cranial nerve VIII (auditory nerve)

Whisper in each ear. Unilateral sensorineural deafness should be considered as caused by an acoustic neuroma until proven otherwise. Refer for an ear, nose, throat (ENT) opinion. Conductive deafness can be easily differentiated by using a vibrating tuning fork held adjacent to ear and then is placed on the mastoid (air conduction is louder than bone conduction in normal hearing and sensorineural deafness, vice versa in conductive deafness). If an auroscope is available use it!

Cranial nerve IX (glossopharyngeal nerve)

Test palatal sensation with orange stick.

Cranial nerve X (vagus nerve)

Ask the patient to say 'aah'; look for palatal deviation (away from lesion).

Cranial nerve XI (accessory nerve)

Shrug shoulders.

Cranial nerve XII (hypoglossal nerve)

Look for wasting of the tongue and fasciculation (motor neuron disease), ask patient to protrude tongue (deviates towards lesion). Slow tongue movements without wasting imply spasticity (motor neuron disease, widespread cerebrovascular disease). Severe involuntary tongue and facial movements are most often seen in tardive dyskinesia (due to psychotropic medication).

Dysphonia implies a disorder of the vocal cords. The voice has a hoarse or whispering quality. There may be impairment or alteration of a voluntary cough. Refer to an ENT specialist.

Dysarthria or impaired articulation has many non-neurological causes, such as mouth ulcers. Neurological disease affecting the cerebellum, extrapyramidal system or laryngeal musculature (upper or lower motor neuron in nature) may cause various forms of dysarthria.

'Cerebellar speech' is mimicked by drinking too much alcohol. A nasal tone is heard in bulbar palsies, while a guttural or growling ('Donald Duck') voice is often associated with emotional incontinence and a brisk jaw jerk and is seen in a pseudobulbar palsy. Quiet, monotonous and indistinct speech occurs in extrapyramidal speech; there may also be an acquired stammer. Asking the patient to say 'p', 't' and 'k' will test the lip, tongue and palatal dexterity, respectively.

Examination of the limbs

Inspect for wasting or fasciculation (twitching of muscles). Ask the patient to hold the arms outstretched

Box 10.1 The Medical Research Council (MRC) scale of muscle power

0 No movement
1 Flicker of movement
2 Movement with gravity eliminated
3 Movement against gravity
4 Weak
5 Normal power

Source: Collin & Wade, 1990.[1]

with palms facing the ceiling to observe pronator drift (seen in mild pyramidal weakness). Power should be documented using the Medical Research Council (MRC) scale (Box 10.1). Look for postural tremor.

Upper limbs

Tone should be described as increased or normal. A spastic (pyramidal) increase in tone is best assessed by rapid flexion/extension movements at the elbow (called 'clasp knife', as the limb seems to suddenly give way). Extrapyramidal increases in tone can be demonstrated at the wrist by slow flexion/extension movements. Cog-wheeling has a ratcheting quality, whereas in 'lead pipe' rigidity the increased tone is unchanged throughout the range of passive movement. 'Gegenhalten', seen in patients with dementing disorders, describes an inability to relax, where it feels as though the patient is deliberately trying to frustrate the examiner.

The muscle examination should include:

- shoulder abduction
- elbow extension and flexion
- wrist and finger extension
- finger flexion and abduction
- thumb abduction.

Table 10.1 indicates the roots and nerve supply of the muscles tested.

Checking the deep tendon reflexes follows next: biceps, triceps and supinator. Finger flexion jerks may indicate an upper motor neuron lesion but can also be observed in anxious patients. If asymmetrical, this sign is likely to have added significance (see Table 10.2). Hoffman's sign (flicking of the distal thumb, leading to flexion of the fingers) is also suggestive of an upper motor neuron lesion.

The grading system for deep tendon reflexes is presented in Box 10.2.

Reinforcement can be obtained by jaw clenching or Jendrassik's manoeuvre (the patient links hands and pulls). Deep tendon reflexes may also be inverted whereby the tested reflex is absent but there is spread to a lower level; for example, testing the biceps reflex may elicit finger flexion, not elbow flexion. This indicates a

Table 10.2 Main deep tendon reflexes

Reflex	Nerve	Root
Biceps	Musculocutaneous	C5/6
Supinator	Radial	C5/6
Triceps	Radial	C7
Finger flexors	Median/ulnar	C8
Knee	Femoral	L3/4
Ankle	Tibial	S1/2

Box 10.2 Grading system for deep tendon reflexes

Absent = 0
Present with reinforcement = +/-
Depressed = +
Normal = ++
Increased = +++

Table 10.1 Movements of the upper limb and nerve roots

Limb movement	Muscle tested	Nerve	Root
Shoulder abduction	Deltoid	Axillary	C4/5
Elbow extension	Triceps	Radial	C7
Elbow flexion	Biceps	Musculocutaneous	C5/6
Wrist extension	Extensor carpi	Radial	C8
Finger extension	Extensor digitorum	Posterior interosseous	C8
Finger flexion	Long flexors	Median/ulnar	C8
Index finger abduction	First digital interosseous	Ulnar	T1
Thumb abduction	Abductor pollicis brevis	Median	T1

lower motor neuron lesion at the level of the reflex but an upper motor neuron lesion below.

The main superficial reflexes include the abdominal (upper-T8/9, lower-T10/11), cremasteric (L1/2) and anal (S4/5). These are absent in some upper motor neuron syndromes.

Coordination

Coordination can be assessed in several ways:

- Ask the patient to perform a rhythmical hand-tapping task (this will be impaired in cerebellar disease).
- Ask the patient to perform the finger–nose test. Missing the target (past pointing) or an intention tremor (whereby amplitude increases as the finger nears the target) is a hallmark of cerebellar disease.
- Classical pill-rolling tremor, virtually diagnostic of idiopathic Parkinson's disease or drug-induced Parkinsonism, is a low-frequency resting tremor that may also affect the chin, lips, legs and trunk, can be markedly increased by stress or emotions, and is also evident when walking.

Lower limbs

Assess tone by rapid, passive flexion of the patient's hip and knee; feel for the spastic 'catch', which accompanies pyramidal disorders. Clonus is best demonstrated by rapid ankle dorsiflexion: push the sole of the foot briskly upwards and maintain pressure; greater than four downward beats is pathological.

Observe for wasting/fasciculations but also isolated tremor of the lower limb, which is strong evidence for idiopathic or drug-induced Parkinson's disease. Assess the power of hip flexion/extension, knee flexion/extension and ankle plantar and dorsiflexion.

Elicit the knee and ankle reflexes next; nerve roots are shown in Table 10.3. Elicit the plantar response by gently scraping an orange stick along the lateral border of the sole and then turn it medially to finish below the first metatarsal. An *extensor plantar response* is always pathological in any patient over the age of 12 months.

Finally, assess the gait and perform Romberg's manoeuvre by asking the patient to stand for 30 seconds with the feet slightly apart and eyes closed. This should be recorded as positive only if the patient would fall without the intervention of the examiner.

> The history is the mainstay of accurate neurological diagnosis.

Sensory examination

The sensory examination follows next. It is often not time efficient to map out all the sensory modalities of pinprick, light touch, temperature and joint position/vibration sense. The following are of more practical use:

- Use a pin. A sensory level indicates a spastic paraparesis.
- Complete hemisensory loss with differential vibration sense either side of the midline at the sternum suggests a functional disorder.

Table 10.3 Lower limb movements and nerve roots

Limb movement	Muscle tested	Nerve	Root
Hip flexion	Iliopsoas	Femoral	L1, 2
Hip adduction	Hip adductors	Obturator	L5, S1
Hip extension	Gluteals	Internal gluteal	L5, S1
Knee extension	Quadriceps	Femoral	L2, 3
Knee flexion	Hamstrings	Sciatic	L5, S1
Foot dorsiflexion	Tibialis anterior	Deep peroneal	L5, S1
Foot plantar flexion	Gastrocnemius	Tibial	S1, 2
Foot inversion	Tibialis posterior	Tibial	L4, 5
Foot eversion	Peroneus longus	Superficial peroneal	L5, S1
Hallux dorsiflexion	Extensor hallucis longus	Deep peroneal	L5, S1

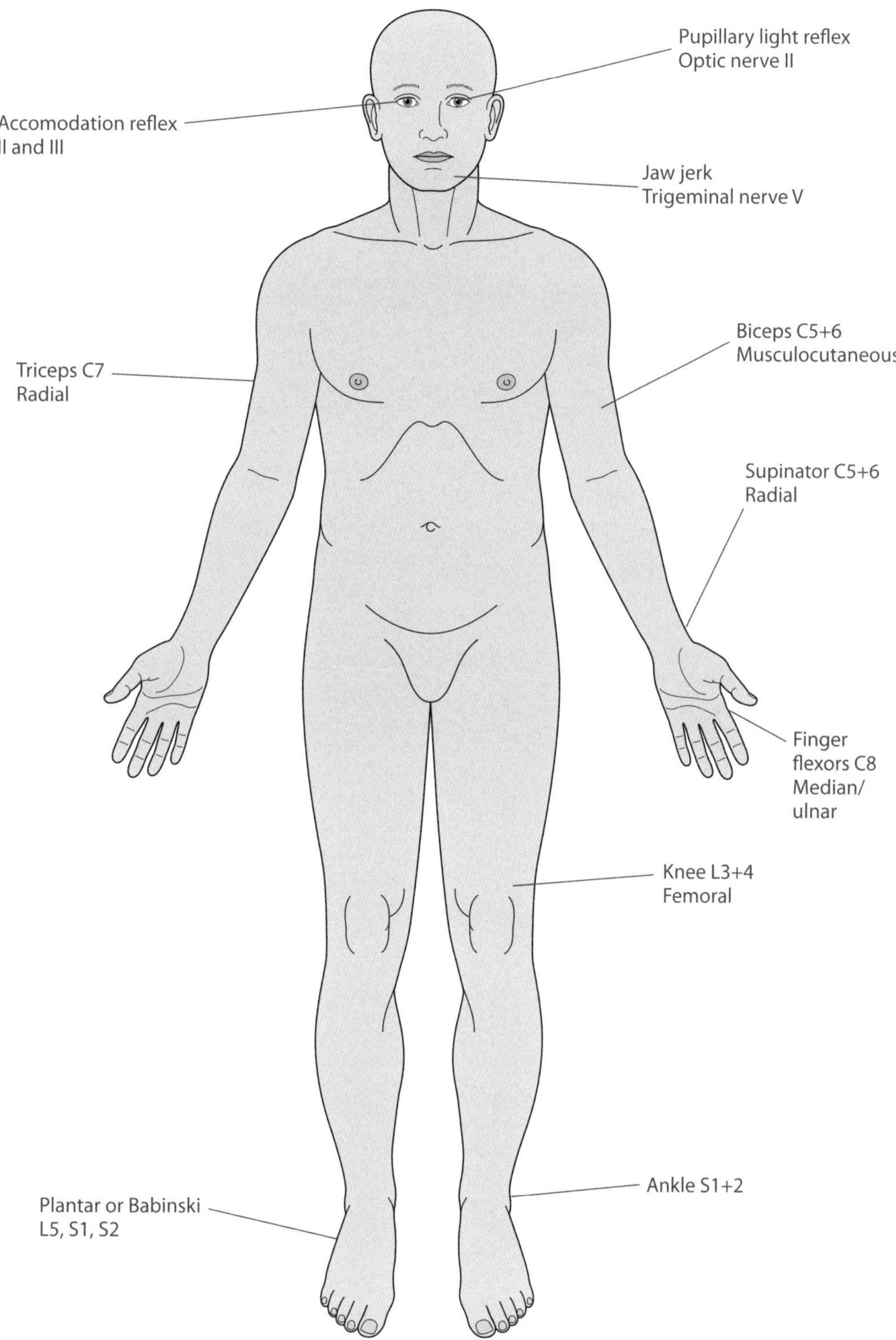

Fig. 10.2 Reflexes (with nerve and root).

Table 10.4 Disturbances of gait commonly encountered in psychiatric practice

Type of gait	Description	Common causes
Gait apraxia	Small, shuffling steps	Small-vessel disease; hydrocephalus
Parkinsonian	Shuffling; loss of arm swing	Idiopathic or drug-induced Parkinson's dise
Spastic paraparesis	Stiff, like walking through mud	Cord lesion; parasagittal lesion
Myopathic	Waddling	Muscular dystrophy
Foot drop	Foot slapping	Neuropathy
Spastic monoplegia	Exaggerated circumduction of hip	Stroke
Cerebellar ataxia	Wide based; 'drunken'	Any cerebellar pathology
Sensory ataxia	Wide based; foot slapping; deteriorates with eye closure	Subacute combined degeneration of the co

- Romberg's positive may be due to loss of sense of joint position and vestibular pathology; cerebellar pathology usually does not cause Rombergism.

The reflexes are indicated in Fig. 10.2.

Gait

The various gait disturbances encountered in clinical practice are shown in Table 10.4.

Movement disorders in psychiatric patients

Signs of Parkinson's disease are the tetrad of:

- pill-rolling tremor
- bradykinesia (an essential feature of the diagnosis)
- rigidity
- loss of postural reflexes.

These four are almost always due to medication or idiopathic Parkinson's disease (p. 181). Even newer antipsychotic medications can cause Parkinsonism. Other causes include valproate (used in epilepsy but also used as a mood stabiliser), anti-emetics and vestibular sedatives, selective serotonin reuptake inhibitors (SSRIs), methylphenidate (used in attention-deficit disorder), lithium (although this is controversial) and phenelzine.

Akathisia or restlessness is usually caused by neuroleptics, but consider lithium, SSRIs and the mood stabiliser carbamazepine.

Myoclonus (brief shock-like jerks that are non-suppressible) may be due to lithium toxicity or clozapine toxicity.

Tremor – may also be due to drugs such as lithium and valproate.

Tardive dyskinesia is a florid grimacing/chewing movement of face and tongue associated with the older antipsychotic medications, particularly when used long term.

Chorea is a continuous writhing or jerky movement, which may look like excessive fidgetiness. The involuntary movements can be incorporated into semi-purposeful routines. Causes include psychotropic medication, anticonvulsants, cocaine, amphetamines, lithium and opiates. If associated with dystonia (abnormal posturing caused by co-contraction of agonist and antagonist muscles), this is usually labelled as a dyskinesia and is most often induced by psychotropic medication or L-dopa.

Tics, which are complex motor or vocal stereotypies, can be voluntarily suppressed temporarily. Tics are sometimes more evident when the patient is unaware of being observed. Tics can occur in isolation or as part of a more generalised disorder, such as Tourette syndrome.

In complex movement disorders, consider psychotropic medications.

Cognitive examination

The Mini-Mental State Examination (see Box 10.3) is a useful but rather insensitive examination, particularly with frontal lobe disorders. The Addenbrooke's Cognitive Examination (www.stvincents.ie/dynamic/

File/Addenbrookes_A_SVUH_MedEl_tool.pdf) is more comprehensive but is more time-consuming to administer.

Differentiating between dementia and pseudodementia

The presence or absence of primitive reflexes can be useful in differentiating between dementia and pseudodementia (Table 10.5).

Language

Dysphasia and aphasia are defined as impairment in the production of language and either usually implies cortical dysfunction.

The classification of dysphasia can be complex but the principal division is twofold:

- receptive or Wernicke's dysphasia, in which the patient sounds fluent but is nonsensical and has poor comprehension
- expressive or Broca's dysphasia, in which the patient is often agrammatical and hesitant but comprehension is usually preserved.

To determine whether or which the patient has dysphasia, the psychiatrist can ask the patient to follow one or more step commands, to test comprehension. Repetition can be useful. For example, the response to 'Say after me, "no ands, ifs or buts"' is usually impaired in Broca's and Wernicke's aphasia. It can be difficult to differentiate the speech disorder of schizophrenia ('word salad') from Wernicke's aphasia. If repetition is impaired in isolation, this suggests a lesion in the arcuate fasciculus connecting Broca's and Wernicke's areas. Reading and writing are often impaired (dyslexia/dysgraphia) in tandem, but there are many patients with a severe expressive dysphasia where reading from a text is virtually perfect.

Box 10.3 Features of the Mini-Mental State Examination

The MMSE tests orientation (for time and place), registration (ability to repeat the names of three objects), attention and calculation (counting backwards by seven), recall (ability to recall the names of the three objects), language (reading and writing), and copying a complex drawing, with points being allocated for correct responses.

The maximum score is 30. Sequential tests can be used to check for decline in cognitive function. A score of < 25 may suggest a dementing process but depressive pseudodementia and acute confusional states may cause diagnostic difficulty.

See: Folstein *et al*, 1975.[2]

Table 10.5 Tests of primitive reflexes to differentiate between dementia and pseudodementia

Reflex	How elicited	Result indicative of dementia, as opposed to pseudodementia
Snout reflex	Apply gentle pressure over nasal philtrum	Observe lips puckering. This is probably the most specific test
Sucking reflex	Place a spatula in the patient's mouth	Patient sucks spatula
Rooting reflex	Gently stroke the side of the face	The head turns to the same side
Palmo-mental reflex	Stimulation of the thenar eminence	Involuntary contraction of mentalis
Grasp reflex	Apply distally moving deep pressure over part of the palmar surface	An instinctive grasp reaction can be seen, where progressive closure of the hand occurs on contact with the palm
Brisk pout reflex	Tapping around the mouth	Closure of the mouth with pouting of the lips is non-specific and can occur in many upper motor neuron lesions and may be associated with a prominent jaw jerk

The Test Your Memory (TYM) test is said to have excellent specificity (86%) and sensitivity (93%) in the diagnosis of Alzheimer's disease (easily the commonest cause of dementia). It can be self-administered by patients.[3] The TYM can be obtained online by health professionals (www.tymtest.com/the-tym-test.html).

A number of rarer aphasic syndromes are described in neurological textbooks.

Lobar function and memory

The following tests of frontal lobe function can be performed at the patient's bedside.

- *Cognitive estimates* – for example, 'How far is it to Paris?' You will need to take into account the educational background of the patient. Using the spouse as a control subject *may* be helpful.
- *Verbal fluency* – for example, 'Say as many words as possible in 60 seconds beginning with the letter "p"'. Normal people usually manage to say 17 or more. Alternatively one can ask the patient to name as many different animals as possible (normal >21).
- *Luria's three-step sequence.* This is a series of complex motor tasks to assess recruitment of association motor cortices. The sequence is palm flat, palm vertical and then make, a fist usually on a desk top.
- *Modified 'Stroop' test.* In the classic test, the word 'green' may be printed in red ink and the participant is required to respond to the *ink colour* rather than the *word.* A modification of this is to present photographs on different coloured backgrounds and ask the patient to respond to the background colour. Reaction time is measured as an index of any interference in processing introduced by the patient's reaction to the photographic image content.
- *Perseveration* is demonstrated by the examiner holding out a hand and observing that the patient will repetitively attempt to perform a handshake.
- *Utilisation behaviour* is a form of environmental dependency. If, for example, the patient is given a pair of glasses, he or she will put them on. If another pair is offered, these will be worn likewise, and so on.
- *Dyspraxia* is an inability to perform a complex sequence of movements, where the command has been understood, and in the absence of significant motor or sensory deficits. Ask the patient to copy certain hand positions or mime an action to test this. Impairment usually implies dysfunction of the contralateral parietal lobe. Dressing and constructional dyspraxias (e.g. copy a five-pointed star) are seen in non-dominant parietal lobe impairment. Ideational dyspraxia has been used to describe an inability to use real objects, although mimicry is retained. The inability to carry out motor acts to command has been referred to as 'ideomotor dyspraxia'. Both conditions are seen after left hemisphere damage as well as in generalised neurodegenerative processes such as cortico-basal degeneration.
- *Agnosia* implies non-recognition and may be visual, tactile or auditory. Placing a familiar object in the person's hand while their eyes are closed may test for tactile agnosia; the pathology is usually in the contralateral parietal lobe. Visual agnosias include prosopagnosia, which implies an inability to recognise familiar faces; this is commonly associated with bilateral lesions of the parieto-occipital regions. *Anosagnosia* is a denial of impairment, as seen in Anton's syndrome.
- *Memory* is an example of a distributed cognitive function. Various classifications are used including long/short term, episodic/semantic, retrograde/anterograde and visual/verbal. It is important to remember that digit span is not a test of memory, but rather of alertness (patients with Korsakoff's psychosis often have preserved digit span). The duration of anterograde amnesia (post-traumatic) may be a useful indicator of the severity of a head injury.

Brief neurological assessment (excluding cognition)

There may be times when full, formal assessment of neurological function is difficult or impossible. Below is described the briefest clinical neurological assessment you can perform:

- fundoscopy (observe pupillary reactions)
- eye movements
- visual fields
- smile

- raise eyebrows
- shrug shoulders
- stick out tongue
- hold arms outstretched with palm facing ceiling and eyes closed
- shoulder abduction
- pretend to play piano
- hip flexion
- ankle dorsiflexion
- reflexes (triceps, biceps, knee, ankle)
- plantars
- watch patient walk.

How to spot factitious neurological symptoms

Functional neurological symptoms are common but malingering as an underlying mechanism is relatively rare. Fabricating physical symptoms usually has a motive of some form of 'gain'. Malingering and factitious disorder both differ from somatoform disorders (e.g. hypochondriasis, conversion disorder, pain syndrome) in that the former are voluntarily produced while the latter are not.

Factitious disorder and malingering occasionally occur together, while concurrent factitia and somatoform disorders are rare. Recognising the differences in these complex presentations and learning the management of factitia can reduce the risk of iatrogenic complication and avoid unnecessary costs and medico-legal repercussions.

Factitious illness may have a broad spectrum of presentations. In its milder form there may be only a slight exaggeration of physical symptoms. The most extreme and dramatic form is *Munchausen syndrome*; this can include extensive travel and the seeking of multiple invasive procedures and operations, sometimes with serious risk to life. Impersonation and fabrication often accompany Munchausen syndrome.

The fabrication of illness may involve:

- physical methods – a measuring device such as a thermometer can be used to cause alarm
- self-harm, which may include major trauma, complaints of swelling and delayed wound healing
- muscle paralysis, weakness or disorder of gait, which can be readily mimicked
- over-exercise
- drug overdose
- the feigning of blindness or deafness
- complaints of 'chronic pain'
- the reporting of a false history, such as describing a diagnosis of epilepsy or cardiac arrest
- taking psychotropic medication to mimic tremor.

Detection is more difficult in those who do have a coexisting organic illness.

When to suspect a factitious disorder

Suspect a factitious disorder if:

- there are discrepancies between the alleged complaint and objective findings
- the presentation is dramatic, 'heroic' or atypical, or signs keep changing, or are inconsistent and vague
- multiple complaints are made over a prolonged period without a clear diagnosis being made
- multiple admissions have been made to various hospitals in different cities
- there is a lack of cooperation with diagnostic evaluation and in adherence to prescribed treatment
- signs appear when the patient is aware of being observed, or when experienced staff are known to be away or when records are difficult to access (e.g. in the accident and emergency department, during holidays, late on a Friday afternoon)
- a 'textbook' description is given of the illness and/or the patient has an unusual grasp of medical terminology or is employed in a medically related field
- the patient has borderline personality disorder, a history of lying or the pattern of lying is 'fantastic' (*pseudologia fantastica*)
- the patient is known to engage in other forms of attention-seeking behaviour
- the patient accepts with equanimity the discomfort and risk of diagnostic procedures or surgery.

Detection

Some features at presentation which are unusual in *organic cases* include:

- the history contains vague and inconsistent details, although possibly superficially plausible
- symptoms or behaviours only present when the patient is being observed
- long medical record with multiple admissions at various hospitals in different cities

- admission circumstances that do not conform to an identifiable medical or mental disorder
- the patient has few or no visitors despite giving a history of holding an important or prestigious job or a history that casts the patient in a heroic role
- substance misuse, especially of prescribed analgesics and sedatives
- the patient is controlling, hostile, angry, disruptive, or attention-seeking behaviour occurs during hospitalisation
- fluctuating clinical course, including rapid development of complications or a new pathology if the initial workup findings prove negative
- giving approximate answers to questions, usually occurring in factitious disorder with predominantly psychological signs and symptoms such as Ganser syndrome, which is characterised by giving approximate answers to questions (e.g. 'How many legs does a cat have?' Answer 'Three').

However, it is worth remembering that some of these features may be present in patients with organic illness (see Table 10.6 for differentiating organic and non-organic complaints). .

Factitious disorders are described in Chapter 28 (Liaison psychiatry). Features of chest pain that are unlikely to be organic are desribed on p. 148. Psychogenic movement disorders are described in p. 181.

Before making a diagnosis of factitious disorder consider obtaining a second opinion from an experienced colleague.

Most patients with orthostatic tremor (a very rare condition) are given an initial psychological or psychiatric diagnosis. As a consequence the period between symptom onset and correct diagnosis is often a matter of years

'Hard' symptoms and signs in psychiatric patients

The presence of certain signs and symptoms should alert psychiatrists to the presence of *serious underlying neurological illness* but must always be interpreted in the context of the patient's history. These include:

- weight loss without anorexia
- dysarthria
- papilloedema or optic atrophy
- dysphagia, particularly for liquids (narrowing of the oesophagus is usually a fairly gradual process, and with mechanical dysphagia solids tend to 'stick' and liquids tend to slip down more easily)
- unilateral deafness
- muscle wasting
- extensor plantar response
- visual hallucinations
- indifference to cognitive deterioration (patient denies problem, partner very concerned).

Table 10.6 Differentiating organic from non-organic weakness

Clinical sign	Cause
Pronator drift (tendency for the outstretched, supinated arms to pronate when the eyes are closed)	Organic
Hoover's sign (inability to extend hip to command but extension clearly present when testing contralateral hip flexion)	Non-organic
For a patient with 'paralysis', drop their hand on their face; the hand misses face due to self-generated avoidance	Non-organic
Patient walks into consulting room but cannot flex hip(s) against gravity (MRC grade 3 or less)	Non-organic
Associated reflex change and/or extensor plantars	Organic
Differential vibration sensation at midline (sternum/forehead)	Non-organic

Epilepsy and non-epileptic attack disorder

Chapter 14 (Neurological disorders) includes information about epilepsy and the differentiation from non-epileptic seizures (see Table 14.1, p. 180).

Distinguishing seizures from non-epileptic attacks (pseudoseizures)

Non-epileptic attack (NEA) is a descriptive term for a group of psychogenic disorders. It refers to paroxysmal events that can be mistaken for, but are not due to, an epileptic disorder. Non-epileptic attack is most commonly caused by dissociation but personality disorder may coexist. Up to one-fifth of patients who present to epilepsy clinics with 'seizures' do not have epilepsy. The majority of such patients suffer from psychologically mediated episodes. The female:male ratio is over 4:1. There is often a background history of medically unexplained symptoms and physical or sexual abuse. Non-epileptic attack and epilepsy coexist in up to 30% of patients, so diagnosis can be challenging (video-telemetry is the 'gold standard' diagnostic test).

Features suggesting NEA include:

- prolonged duration
- non-stereotyped attacks
- the presence of provoking factors such as emotional upset
- violent thrashing movements, pelvic thrusting, gaze aversion, forced eyelid closure

Lateral tongue biting is highly suggestive of epilepsy.

Measurement of the prolactin level, if performed within 20 minutes of the 'seizure', can be useful, as it rises to more than three times baseline in tonic–clonic or complex partial seizures, but the test is somewhat non-sensitive and non-specific.

After a mean follow-up of 3 years about two-thirds of NEA patients continue to have dissociative seizures and more than half remain dependent on social security.

> EEG is relatively unhelpful in differentiating epilepsy from other causes of altered awareness.

Which patients should psychiatrists refer to neurology services?

Patients with the following conditions should usually be referred:

- epilepsy or seizures (organising an electro-encephalogram (EEG) before referral is rarely helpful)
- young-onset dementia.
- 'psychosis' with abnormal neurological signs (again, EEG is rarely helpful)
- complex movement disorders unexplained by psychotropic medication.
- recent onset of muscle weakness and/or difficulty walking
- seizures of recent onset
- visual hallucinations.

Assessment of depressed consciousness

The Glasgow Coma Score (GCS) is most useful, particularly in communicating information to other physicians (see Chapter 4, p. 36, for a full version of the scale).[4] It is scored between 3 and 15, based on assessment of:

- best eye response (scores up to 4)
  - no eye opening
  - eye opening to pain
  - eye opening to verbal command
  - spontaneous eye opening
- best verbal response (scores up to 5)
  - no verbal response
  - incomprehensible sounds
  - inappropriate words
  - confused
  - orientated
- best motor response (scores up to 6).
  - no motor response
  - extension to pain
  - flexion to pain
  - withdrawal to pain
  - localising pain
  - obeys commands.

References

1 Collin C, Wade D. Assessing motor impairment after stroke: a pilot reliability study. *J Neurol Neurosurg Psychiatry* 1990; **53**: 576–9.

2 Folstein M, Folstein S, McHugh PR. Mini-Mental State: a practical method for grading the cognitive state of patients for the clinician. *J Psychiatr Res* 1975; **12**: 189–98.

3 Brown J, Pengas G, Dawson K, Brown L, Clatworthy P. Self administered cognitive screening test (TYM) for detection of Alzheimer's disease: cross sectional study. *BMJ* 2009; **330**: b2030.

4 Teasdale G, Jennett B. Assessment of coma and impaired consciousness: a practical scale. *Lancet* 1974; **ii**: 81–3.

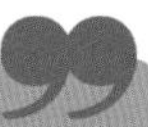

Summary

The neurological examination is an essential part of patient assessment but should be interpreted only in light of the history, barring artificial circumstances such as in postgraduate examinations. With practice, the full examination could be performed in 30 minutes, whereas the brief assessment described above should take 5 minutes or less. As with any skill, practice makes perfect!

Learning points

- The neurological examination can be mastered only by repetition.
- With practice, a brief screening examination can be completed in less than 5 minutes.
- Remember to assess the cranial nerves and gait.
- Abnormalities of speech are usually dysphasic, dysarthric or dysphonic; the last is most often caused by a vocal cord palsy.
- Movement disorders are extremely common in psychiatric patients.
- Many drugs used in psychiatric practice have neurological side-effects, which can persist for many months after drug cessation.
- 'Red flag' neurological symptoms include visual hallucinations, dysphagia for liquids and unilateral sensori-neural deafness.
- 'Red flag' signs include extensor plantars and prominent ('barn door') fasciculation.
- Non-epileptic attack disorder is common and can be difficult to distinguish from genuine epilepsy (refer the patient to a neurologist).
- Organising investigations before referral (especially electroencephalography) is rarely helpful.
- The Glasgow Coma Score (GCS) remains the most useful measure of consciousness.

11

Medico-legal aspects of treating patients with mental disorders and learning disabilities

Kate Hill and Joanne Haswell

Written by experts in the law in England and Wales, this chapter provides an overview of the legal aspects of treating people with mental disorders and physical conditions. It covers the assessment of mental capacity, as well as the factors to consider when treating the physical health conditions of adults who lack mental capacity.

Introduction

The law can seem very complicated at times. Clinicians frequently feel the law is obstructive; that if they were to do everything the law required they would see one patient every 6 months; and that their hands are frequently tied by red tape and section numbers.

Sometimes these are valid complaints. Sometimes, however, the clinician has forgotten that much of the law is based on common sense principles. More often than not, far from being an obstacle, the law can offer a methodology to follow when things get tough.

This chapter is very much an overview of the law in England and Wales. It would be impossible to cover every scenario and every legal nuance in such a limited space; for example, it does not cover the treatment of children. As always, clinicians are advised to seek legal advice before acting on any of the information contained in this book.

Treating mental health patients for physical conditions

People with mental disorders or learning disabilities who require treatment for a physical condition that is not a symptom or causative of a mental disorder must be approached in exactly the same way as people who have a physical illness but do not have a mental disorder or learning disability.

The rules for the management of people with mental disorders who require treatment for a physical illness *unrelated* to that mental disorder are relatively straightforward. If a person with a mental disorder requires treatment that does not fall within the definition of treatment for mental disorder within the meaning of the Mental Health Act 1983, then he or she must be treated:

- in accordance with the common law principles of informed consent
  or
- under the Mental Capacity Act 2005.

The following chart (Fig. 11.1) gives an overview of the legal principles.

To keep things simple, consider treating physical illness in a patient with mental disorder as falling into two categories:

- the physical illness IS related to their mental disorder
- the physical illness IS NOT related to their mental disorder; this can be further subdivided as follows:
  - treating people who HAVE CAPACITY to make a treatment choice
  - treating people who LACK CAPACITY to make a treatment choice.

Treating those with mental disorders for physical conditions related to their mental disorder

If a patient (who is detainable) requires treatment for a physical condition which is connected to his mental disorder, then he may be treated under the provisions of the Mental Health Act. The treatment must fall within the definition of medical treatment for a mental disorder (Box 11.1, 11.2).

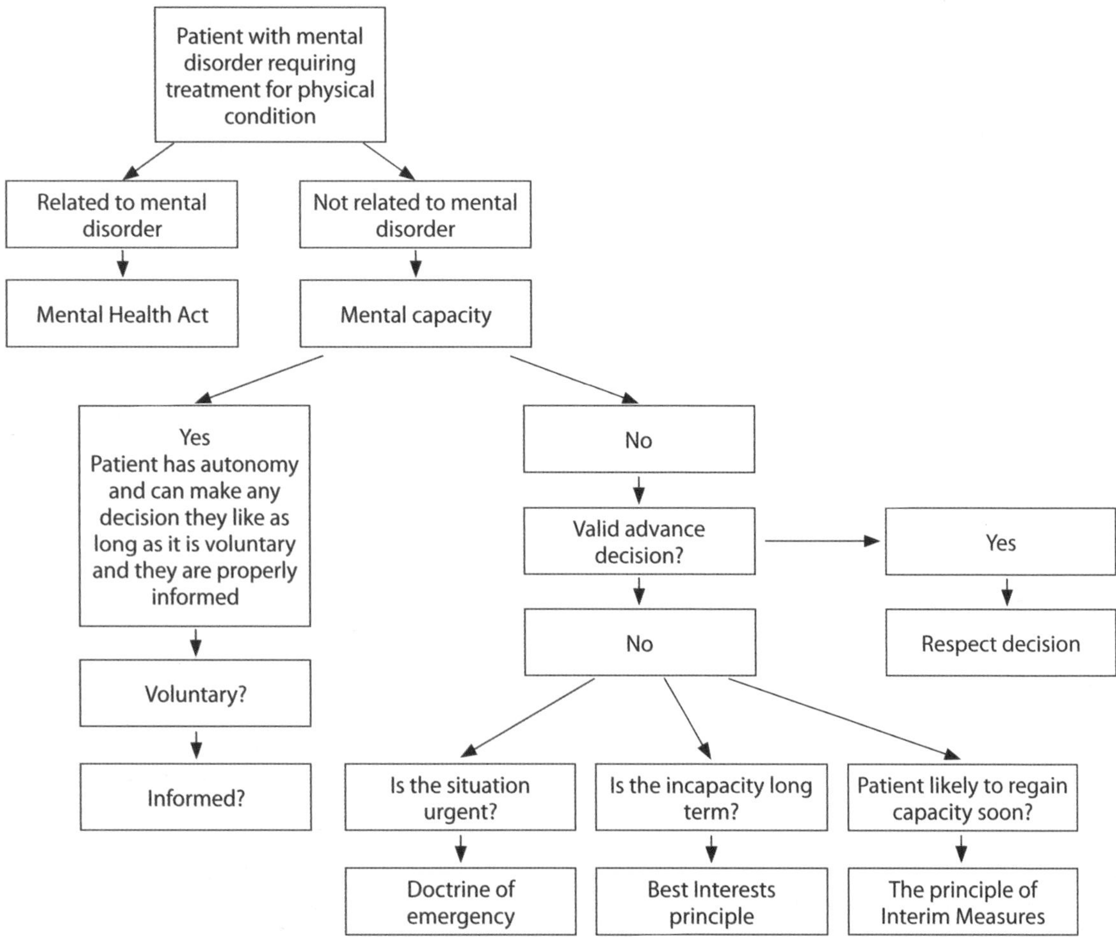

Fig. 11.1 Overview of the legal principles for the management of people with mental disorders who require treatment for a physical illness unrelated to that mental disorder.

Box 11.1 Definition of medical treatment for a mental disorder

Medical treatment for a mental disorder means treatment which is for the purpose of alleviating or preventing a worsening of, a mental disorder or one or more of its symptoms or manifestations – see *Code of Practice*, Mental Health Act 1983 section145(4), (as revised 2008)

The Mental Health Act 1983 provides for the compulsory detention of mentally disordered patients. It also provides a framework, in Part IV, for the treatment of non-consenting patients.

Section 57

Briefly, patients must be capable of giving *and* give their consent to these interventions and the treating clinician must first consult with two other professionals (one of which shall be neither a nurse nor a doctor and neither of which shall be the patient's responsible clinician) before proceeding with treatment.

Section 58 applies to medication and sets out the certification and consultation requirements when treating a patient for longer than 3 months and only applies to detained patients.

In summary, unless the treatment is urgent and covered by section 62 (see below), the patient should not be treated unless he is capable of giving, and has given his consent or, if he is not capable of giving consent, an independent doctor has certified (if the treatment is being given after three months) that fact and that the treatment is appropriate.

Section 62 provides that the rules set out in section 57 and 58 do not apply in urgent situations. Where the situation *is* urgent, treatment which is

- immediately necessary to save a patient's life
- intended to alleviate suffering or to prevent a serious deterioration
- not irreversible or hazardous

may be given as long it is a proportionate intervention to prevent a patient from behaving violently or being a danger to himself or others, subject to certain qualifications. Electroconvulsive therapy (ECT) may be given under this section; ECT is otherwise covered by section 58A.

Treatment of a patient with a Community Treatment Order is outside the scope of this chapter.

Section 63 provides that treatment that does not fall within the remit of section 57, 58 and section 58A can be given without consent as long as it is medical treatment for a mental disorder.

Box 11.2 Interpretation of the Mental Health Act 1983

145.—(1) In this Act, unless the context otherwise requires...

'medical treatment' includes nursing, psychological intervention and specialist mental health habilitation, rehabilitation and care (but see also subsection (4) below)...

(4) Any reference in this Act to medical treatment, in relation to mental disorder, shall be construed as a reference to medical treatment the purpose of which is to alleviate, or prevent a worsening of, the disorder or one or more of its symptoms or manifestations...

What constitutes medical treatment for mental disorder

A leading case on this subject is *B v Croydon* 1995 (Box 11.3).[1]

In summary, where a refusal to eat is a symptom of the patient's disorder, feeding will fall within the definition of treatment for mental disorder.

Further forms of physical intervention which *may* fall within the definition of medical treatment for mental disorder include:

- the monitoring of the blood of a patient on clozapine because the monitoring is an essential adjunct to the main treatment
- assisting a patient to bathe where the patient's refusal to address personal hygiene is deemed to be a symptom of the mental disorder
- treating a patient with thyroxine where a psychosis has developed as a result of hypothyroidism
- feeding a patient with anorexia nervosa via a nasogastric tube
- treatment with intravenous fluids where a patient stops eating and drinking due to severe depression, which in turn leads to severe dehydration.

If you are in any doubt as to whether the proposed treatment is treatment for, or related to, a mental disorder, seek legal advice.

Box 11.3 The case of *B v Croydon* 1995

A patient was suffering from a borderline personality disorder coupled with post-traumatic stress disorder. She had a history of self-harming. The only treatment for her condition was psychoanalytic psychotherapy. She was detained under section 3 of the Mental Health Act 1983. She began to refuse food and her weight dropped to such a low level that it was felt that she should gain weight before resuming therapy. She did gain weight when initially threatened with tube feeding but eventually her weight dropped again. The threat of tube feeding was used again, upon which the patient sought an injunction to restrain the team from force-feeding her.

Although the patient had voluntarily started to eat by the time of the hearing, it was nonetheless held that tube feeding did constitute treatment for mental disorder within the meaning of section 63. This meant that the patient could have been fed by nasogastric tube not withstanding her refusal to consent to the treatment.

The Court of Appeal held that

- a range of acts 'ancillary' to the patient's core treatment will fall within the definition 'medical treatment'
- treatment is 'ancillary' if it is nursing and care 'concurrent with the core treatment or as a necessary pre-requisite to such treatment or to prevent the patient from causing harm to himself or to alleviate the consequences of the disorder' (per Hoffman J 687) and
- relieving the symptoms of the mental disorder is just as much a part of treatment as relieving its underlying cause.

Source: [1995] 1 All ER 683 (page 683, 1st volume, *All England Law Reports*).

Treating those with mental disorders for physical conditions not related to their mental disorder

When a patient has a physical condition requiring treatment and that condition is not related to his mental disorder, he must be treated in the same way as someone without a mental disorder.

The next steps will be determined by whether or not the patient has capacity, according to the Mental Capacity Act 2005.

A detained patient cannot be forced to have any treatment that is unrelated to his mental disorder unless he lacks capacity, in which case, treatment may be possible under the Mental Capacity Act *not* the Mental Health Act.

Box 11.4 The case of *Re:C*

The case concerned a patient with chronic schizophrenia at a high secure hospital, who thought (wrongly) that he was a famous doctor with fantastical abilities. The patient developed a gangrenous foot. It was felt that if the foot was not amputated the patient's chances of survival were as low as 15%. The patient refused amputation, saying he would rather die with all of his limbs intact and that, in any event, God did not want him to have the surgery.

The clinical team were concerned the patient's mental illness was affecting his ability to make the decision so the matter went to a court hearing where it was held that the patient did have capacity since he:

- was able to retain the information long enough to make a decision
- was able to understand it, having had it explained to him in a clear way
- believed the information, or to put it another way, he was orientated in reality with regard to his gangrene and his chances of recovery if he refused the amputation
- was able to weigh up the information and make a decision.

An injunction was granted preventing amputation. Conservative treatment was effective and the patient lived to tell the tale.

Source: [1994] 1 All ER 819 (page 819, 1st volume, *All England Law Reports*).

Mental capacity assessments

The Mental Capacity Act 2005 codified the test for capacity that must be used (see below). The capacity test has its origins in the case of Re:C (Box 11.4).[2] A capacity assessment must be done if there is a possibility that the patient's decision-making ability might be compromised in some way.

Patients have the right to make decisions that other people think are unwise. An irrational decision is only evidence of one aspect of incapacity. A doctor must measure a patient's ability to weigh up or process the information specific to the treatment in question.

People have different beliefs and principles. Some might think the patient's decision to choose death over amputation as in the Re:C case was illogical. However the Court decided that the patient was capable of processing the information about his condition and the proposed treatment options and applying it to his own life and principles.

Compare him, however, with a self-harming patient who refuses a blood transfusion despite having dangerously low haemoglobin levels. The reason she gives for refusing is that she believes that blood is evil and makes her do evil things and that the less blood she has in her body the less likely she is to do evil things. It would probably be reasonable to conclude that this was an *irrational decision* in the extraordinary sense and thus the doctor might conclude the individual lacks capacity.

The doctor might also want to consider whether the 'irrational decision' is linked to, or is a result of, the patient's mental disorder e.g. a refusal to eat might be manipulative behaviour symptomatic of personality disorder or it could be a political protest.

The Two Stage Capacity Test

A patient is deemed to lack mental capacity if he is unable to make the decision in question because of impairment or disturbance in the functioning of his mind or brain. In particular, the statute states that, a person lacks capacity in relation to a matter if at the material time he:

1 is unable to make a decision for himself in relation to the matter – because of an impairment of, or a disturbance in the functioning of, the mind or brain. It does not matter whether the impairment or disturbance is permanent or temporary (Mental Capacity Act 2005 Section 2);
   and
2 is unable to make a decision for himself because he cannot:
   - understand the relevant information AND/OR
   - retain that information AND/OR
   - use or weigh that information to reach a decision AND/OR
   - communicate his decision through speech, sign language or any means (Mental Capacity Act 2005 Section 3).

A person should not be regarded as unable to understand relevant information if he is able to understand an explanation given in a way appropriate to his circumstances (such as simple language, visual aids or any other means).

A person is not to be regarded as unable to retain information if he is able to retain the relevant information for a short period only.

Information relevant to a decision includes (but is not limited to) information about the reasonably foreseeable consequences of deciding one way or another, or failing to make the decision.

Capacity is decision-specific; a higher level of capacity is required for more serious decisions.

You should always have a view as to whether your patient has capacity or not. If it is not clear whether the patient has mental capacity for the decision being made, then a second opinion should be sought. If both clinicians are uncertain, then an independent psychiatrist and/or a lawyer should be contacted. The expression 'sitting on the fence' is used for those who are undecided and 'the fence' is not a good place to be when it comes to capacity assessments!

The standard of proof when assessing capacity

The standard of proof is the *balance of probabilities*, so when assessing capacity, doctors should ask 'is it more likely than not that this person has/does not have capacity?'

Responsibility for capacity assessments

The person responsible for the capacity assessment is the person who is going to be carrying out the proposed treatment, examination or test. If a psychiatrist is asked for an opinion by, for example, a surgeon, the psychiatrist does not assume overall responsibility for the assessment of the patient's capacity to consent to surgery – the psychiatrist acts in an advisory capacity only.

You should always have a view as to whether your patient has capacity or not. If it is not clear whether the patient has mental capacity for the decision being made, then a second opinion should be sought.

Documentation of capacity assessments

Any assessment of mental capacity should be fully documented in the patient's notes. It is not enough to record 'patient has mental capacity'; you must record how you came to that conclusion.

The British Medical Association has published advice on the assessment of mental capacity. Useful references are *The BMA Consent Tool Kit Fifth Edition*, 2009 and *Mental Capacity Act Tool Kit*, 2008.

If a patient has fluctuating capacity, for example someone with dementia who has lucid or 'good' days, consider obtaining an advanced statement from them on a 'good' day. More information on advance decisions and advanced statements is available later in this chapter as well as from your local trust policy (every trust should have one) or *Code of Practice Mental Health Act 1983* Chapter 9.

Treating patients with capacity

If you decide that your patient *does have capacity* and is presenting with a physical condition *not related to the mental disorder*, the patient must be taken through the informed consent process.

If a doctor treats a patient who has capacity against the individual's wishes, or without first obtaining proper informed consent, he can be disciplined by his employer, sued through the civil courts and can be erased from the medical register. Patients with capacity have autonomy and can make any decision they wish, even if the decision results in their death

- as long as the decision is voluntary
  and
- the individual is properly informed about the proposed treatment and its risks and benefits and any alternative treatment.

Healthcare professionals must therefore make sure that patients are not coerced in any way as duress can vitiate consent. This includes coercion from healthcare professionals, family, friends and carers, as well as other service users.

The duty to inform patients must not be underestimated. Patients are entitled to and must receive information about the

- risks of
- benefits of
- alternatives to, and (together with the risks and benefits of each alternative)
- material information

  about the proposed treatment.

Material information is information that the patient would be likely to attach significance to because of their unique personality and circumstances, such as their job, home circumstances and personality which may require establishing whether

- the patient is able to take time off work without making prior arrangements
- their job involved driving
- weight is a significant concern.

Patient information leaflets, if used properly, can help to document discussions about informed consent. For example, assuming the patient information leaflet is a comprehensive one covering risks, benefits and alternatives, the clinical records could be documented as follows:

> 'Went through the (named) patient information leaflet. In particular, I emphasised the fact that Mr Brown, a taxi driver, would not be able to drive while taking this medication. Mr Brown asked the following questions [insert questions and answers given]. He said he wanted to proceed with the treatment and the reason he gave for wanting to go ahead was as follows [quote patient verbatim]'.

Remember that patient information leaflets are generic and it may be necessary to supplement or emphasize the information contained in the document.

Treating patients who lack capacity

If it is decided, after conducting an assessment, that a patient lacks capacity, treatment for a physical condition can still be provided but this will *not* be with the consent of the patient, since a patient who lacks capacity cannot give valid consent. Instead patients who lack capacity are treated under the doctrine of emergency or the best interests principle.

Urgent treatment: the doctrine of emergency

Patients may be treated in emergency situations where it is not possible for them to give consent (perhaps because they are unconscious or in considerable pain).

The legal principle is that patients may be treated provided that:

- it is a defined emergency
- the treatment is to prevent a serious deterioration in the patient's physical or natural condition
- no treatment is given beyond the point of crisis.

Often the preliminary emergency treatment has the effect of not only addressing the *physical problem* but also addressing the *lack of capacity*. For example, treating a urinary tract infection may resolve confusion and end non-compliance. Once the patient has regained capacity, the patient should of course be involved fully in their on-going treatment as they are now *capacitous* (Case study 11.1).

Any treatment which falls outside this definition must be administered under the doctrine of best interests.

Non-urgent treatment: the doctrine of best interests

The principle which applies in non-urgent situations is the doctrine of best interests. This doctrine, set out in the Mental Capacity Act 2005, enables doctors to treat a patient who lacks capacity as long as the treatment is in his or her best interests. The doctrine of best interests has three stages:

1 identify all the options; in most cases there will be several but there will always be at least two- do something or do nothing;

2 'Profile the patient';

   a assess the patient's past and present ascertainable wishes including any advance decision or statement made.

   b consult interested parties where appropriate and practicable to do so (involve the Independent Mental Capacity Advocacy (IMCA) service for serious interventions where the patient has no family or friends). If it is not practicable or appropriate to consult certain interested parties, document reasons for the decision in the notes;

   c consider other factors such as spirituality or religion, social network etc.

3 Pick the option that best suits the patient's circumstances and is 'proportionate' giving reasons why you have and reasons why you have rejected other options.

'Proportionality' can be explained simply as follows: do not take a sledgehammer to crack a nut. For example, a carer may need to hold a person's arm when crossing the road to stop the individual from being run over but it would be disproportionate to stop the person from going outside at all.

Case study 11.1 Emergency treatment of a psychiatric patient

A community patient who had consumed a quantity of alcohol and painkillers falls down a railway embankment sustaining multiple injuries. She is brought to the accident and emergency department but refuses treatment.

A clinician may not force treatment of any sort on a patient who has capacity unless that treatment falls within the scope of the Mental Health Act 1983 (discussed earlier in this chapter). Or if the doctor suspects that the patient's decision-making ability might be compromised, they must do a capacity assessment and decide;

1 if, on balance of probabilities, the patient has an impairment/disturbance in the mind/brain;

2 if that impairment has affected the patient's ability to retain or understand the information, or her ability to use or weigh that information to make a decision on whether to accept life-saving treatment. If so, then emergency treatment to prevent a serious deterioration in physical or mental wellbeing (but no treatment past the point of crisis) could and should be carried out.

Restraint

Healthcare professionals are entitled to use 'restraint' to treat under the doctrine of emergency and the doctrine of best interests.

Restraint is defined in the Mental Capacity Act 2005 as:

- the use of force or the threat of force to make someone do something they are resisting;
  OR
- restricting someone's freedom of movement, whether they are resisting or not.

Restraint is appropriate and does not require special authorisation if it:

- is used to prevent harm to someone who lacks capacity;
- falls short of a deprivation of liberty;
- is a proportionate response to the likelihood and seriousness of harm.

Deprivation of liberty

Where the use of restraint can be said to amount to a deprivation of liberty, healthcare professionals must apply for authorisation to undertake the acts that constitute the deprivation. These *Deprivation of Liberty Safeguards (DOLS)* are enshrined in the amended Mental Capacity Act 2005 and were prompted by the case of Bournewood, *HL vs United Kingdom* 2004 (Box 11.5).[3]

Box 11.5 The Bournewood Case

A man with autism lacked capacity to decide whether or not he should be admitted to hospital. His carers wanted to remove him from hospital but their request was refused by the hospital who continued to treat him on an informal basis, i.e. not under the Mental Health Act 1983 which meant that there was no right of appeal or right to a second opinion.

The European Court considered the case and had to decide two things:

- whether there had been a deprivation of liberty or just an appropriate use of restraint;
- if there had been a deprivation of liberty, whether this deprivation of liberty had taken place in accordance with a procedure prescribed by law.

The Court held that there had been a deprivation of liberty and that there was no procedure prescribed by law. The Government in England responded to this ruling by introducing Deprivation of Liberty Safeguards (DOLS), a procedure prescribed by law for depriving patients who lack capacity, and are not detained, of their liberty.

Source: *HL v. UK* 45508/99 (2004) ECHR 471.

There is no nice neat list of acts that will (or will not) constitute a deprivation because the European Court said:[3]

> 'to determine whether there has been a deprivation of liberty the starting point must be the specific situation of the individual concerned and account must be taken of a whole range of factors arising in a particular case such as the type, duration, effects and manner of implementation of the measure in question. The distinction between a deprivation of and a restriction upon liberty is merely one of degree or intensity and not one of nature or substance'

Whether an act or series of acts moves beyond restraint to become a deprivation is therefore a question of fact. Common sense will take a healthcare professional a long way in recognising the difference.

Advance decisions

An advance decision is a decision made by a capacitious adult which states that if, in the future at a time when the person lacks capacity and in specified circumstances, certain treatment is proposed, the treatment is not to be carried out or continued. An advance decision is therefore an *advance refusal*, such as a refusal to have a blood transfusion on religious grounds.

Advance decisions do not need to be witnessed and signed by the patient in order to be valid unless they relate to life sustaining treatment.

For information on the validity and applicability of advance decisions, see section 24 onwards of the Mental Capacity Act 2005. If the validity of an advance decision is unclear, seek legal advice.

Court of Protection

The Court of Protection created by the Mental Capacity Act 2005 has a comprehensive jurisdiction over the health and welfare and financial affairs of people who lack capacity.

The Court of Protection may make orders such as:

- declarations as to mental capacity
- declarations as to best interests (single orders)
- appointment of a deputy
- declarations as to validity of lasting powers of attorney
- orders relating to financial matters (single orders)
- declaration as to the lawfulness or otherwise of any act done, or yet to be done, in relation to a patient
- declaration as to the existence, validity and applicability of advance decisions.

Lasting Powers of Attorney

The Mental Capacity Act 2005 created a new Lasting Power of Attorney which can be used to assign to another person the right to make decisions on a patient's behalf relating to:

- health
- welfare
- property
- money.

The Attorney must always act in the best interests of the donee, i.e. the patient.

The format of a lasting power of attorney is set out in Schedule 1 Part 1 of the Mental Capacity Act 2005. The forms and guidance can be found on the Office of the Public Guardian website (www.publicguardian.gov.uk).

Single Orders or Deputies

If a doctor is faced with family members who all have different and strong views, he could consider obtaining a single order from the Court of Protection to resolve the dispute.

If a patient has not appointed someone to make healthcare decisions on their behalf by way of a lasting power of attorney, the Court of Protection may appoint a 'deputy' who is likely to have some relationship to the patient. However, the deputy's appointment is likely to be very limited in scope and duration. Deputies are likely to be appointed in rare cases, for example 'where there is a dispute between family members as to who has the patient's best interests at heart and where the patient has chronic and/or degenerative health problems calling for repeated assessments and decisions by doctors and carers' (Government response to recommendation 54 of the Joint Committee's report, www.parliament.the-stationery-office.com). If there is a lasting power of attorney, any disputes must be resolved by way of single order of the court rather than by the appointment of a deputy.

Independent Advocates

The Mental Capacity Act 2005 set up a service called the Independent Mental Capacity Advocate (IMCA) to help those with no family or friends. Doctors have a duty to contact an IMCA if there is no one they can involve in a best interests assessment.

Public Guardian

The Public Guardian is in charge of the Office of the Public Guardian that will help the Court of Protection by looking after the applications and paperwork for Lasting Powers of Attorney and Deputies. Additionally they monitor the work of the Deputies and work with the police and social services if it is suspected a vulnerable person is being abused.

Court of Protection Visitors

The Lord Chancellor can appoint 'special visitors' who are clinicians and 'general visitors' who are not clinicians; their role is to carry out visits and provide independent reports on matters relating to the exercising of powers under the Mental Capacity Act 2005. Special visitors will have powers to see and take copies of medical records and to see the patient in private.

Information-sharing

The principles of informed consent apply to information sharing, so if a patient has capacity, the doctor should seek consent to share information. If the individual lacks capacity, in urgent situations information should only be shared if it is immediately necessary to do so. In non-urgent situations, apply the 'best interests' principle to information sharing.

Additionally it is important to be familiar with the Caldicott principles and the Data Protection Act 1998.

The Caldicott principles

These are:

- justify the purpose(s) of using confidential information;
- only use it when absolutely necessary;
- use the minimum that is required;
- access should be on a strict need-to-know basis;
- everyone must understand his or her responsibilities;
- understand and comply with the law.

Data Protection Act 1998

Eight data protection principles form the core of the Act. These apply to everyone who effectively handles information including doctors, unless relevant exemptions are obtained. Data must be:

- obtained and processed lawfully and fairly;
- held for the lawful purposes described in the data user's register entry;
- adequate, relevant and not excessive;
- accurate and up to date;
- kept only as long as necessary;
- respectful of the rights of data subjects;
- surrounded by proper security and disclosed only to those people described in the register entry;
- transferred only to countries inside the European Economic Area unless that country can ensure adequate protection for the rights and freedoms of the data subject.

If an individual is unsure about when information can be shared lawfully, ask for help, particularly so if there are concerns about communicating information about a patient to a family member. Independent practitioners who hold sensitive personal data should notify the Information Commissioner and register under the Data Protection Act.

Sharing information with the police

Information should not normally be shared with the police without speaking to a senior colleague and a defence organisation. There are times when information can be shared 'in the public interest', however this is a complex area. It is important to obtain legal advice from a lawyer with expertise in this area and to keep comprehensive records (Box 11.6).

Standards

The actions and omissions of doctors are measured by the Bolam test as amended by Bolitho (Box 11.7). If a doctor can show that he or she acted in accordance with Bolam as amended by Bolitho, he or she will not be deemed negligent.

Box 11.6 How to obtain legal advice

There are several ways. Contact:

- your in-house legal department – every trust and private organisation has its own firm(s) of solicitors. You must obtain permission before contacting solicitors as they can be very expensive; or
- the medical director; or
- your medical defence organisation, which you are strongly advised to join, whether or not your employer provides indemnity as these organisations protect your interests which may differ from the interests of your employer. Defence organisations can be contacted 24 hours a day.

Box 11.7 The Bolam and Bolitho cases

Bolam vs. Friern Hospital Management Committee 1957

A depressed patient was treated with electroconvulsive therapy without manual restraint or sedation. It was shown that this was an approach adopted by others and so the court held that the doctor, since he was acting in accordance with a practice accepted as proper by a responsible body of medical opinion, was not negligent.

[1957] 1 WLR 582.

Bolitho vs City and Hackney HA 1997

A child with croup suffered a cardiac arrest and severe brain damage after the on-call doctor failed to attend. It was claimed that intubation would have prevented the damage. The on-call doctor said she would not have intubated and her expert witness agreed. However, the court said that the body of medical opinion relied upon must have a logical basis: 'the Judge, before accepting a body of medical opinion as being responsible, reasonable or respectable, will need to be satisfied that, in forming their views, the experts have directed their minds to the question of comparative risks and benefits and reached a defensible conclusion on the matter'.

[1997] 4 ALLER 771.

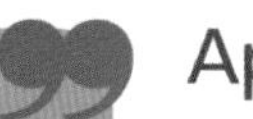

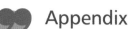

Summary

A person with a mental disorder/learning disabilities and a physical condition must be treated in the same way as a person without a mental disorder. Always have a view on whether the patient has capacity to make a decision. Decisions as to capacity and the consequences of that decision should be meticulously documented. Healthcare records should contain a doctor's rationale and not just the actions taken. Far from being an obstacle, the legal framework can actually help doctors document their work in a way that demonstrates their actions and omissions were responsible, reasonable and logical. This is, after all, the standard of care expected of a doctor in all matters.

Appendix

Relevant sections of the Mental Health Act 1983 are reproduced below.

Treatment requiring consent and a second opinion

57.—(1) This section applies to the following forms of medical treatment for mental disorder—

(a) any surgical operation for destroying brain tissue or for destroying the functioning of brain tissue; and

(b) such other forms of treatment as may be specified for the purposes of this section by regulations made by the Secretary of State.

Learning points

- A person with a mental disorder or learning disability who requires treatment for a physical condition that is not a symptom or causative of a mental disorder must be approached in exactly the same way as a person who has a physical illness but does not have a mental disorder or learning disability.
- If a person with a mental disorder requires treatment that does *not* fall within the definition of treatment for mental disorder within the meaning of the Mental Health Act 1983, then he or she must be treated in accordance with the common-law principles of informed consent, or under the Mental Capacity Act 2005, if the patient is over 16 and lacks mental capacity.
- If a patient who is detainable requires treatment for a physical condition which is connected to a mental disorder, then the patient may be treated under the provisions of the Mental Health Act 1983.
- A detainable patient cannot be forced to have any treatment that is unrelated to a mental disorder unless the patient lacks mental capacity, in which case treatment may be possible under the Mental Capacity Act 2005, not the Mental Health Act 1983.
- Patients have the right to make decisions that other people think are unwise. An irrational decision is only evidence of one aspect of incapacity.
- The standard of proof for mental capacity is the balance of probabilities.
- The person responsible for the capacity assessment is the person who is going to be carrying out the proposed treatment, examination or test.
- Carefully document the rationale used to reach the decisions made about a person's mental capacity as well as the actions taken.
- If a doctor treats a patient who has mental capacity against the individual's wishes, or without first obtaining proper informed consent, the doctor can be disciplined by their employer, sued through the civil courts and erased from the medical register.
- The authors strongly recommend that the doctors join a medical defence organisation, whether or not their employer provides indemnity, as these organisations protect the doctor's interests, which may differ from the interests of their employer.

(2) Subject to section 62 below, a patient shall not be given any form of treatment to which this section applies unless he has consented to it and—

(a) a registered medical practitioner appointed for the purposes of this Part of this Act by the regulatory authority (not being the responsible clinician (if there is one) or the person in charge of the treatment in question) and two other persons appointed for the purposes of this paragraph by the regulatory authority (not being registered medical practitioners) have certified in writing that the patient is capable of understanding the nature, purpose and likely effects of the treatment in question and has consented to it; and

(b) the registered medical practitioner referred to in paragraph (a) above has certified in writing that it is appropriate for the treatment to be given.

(3) Before giving a certificate under subsection (2)(b) above the registered medical practitioner concerned shall consult two other persons who have been professionally concerned with the patient's medical treatment but, of those persons—

(a) one shall be a nurse and the other shall be neither a nurse nor a registered medical practitioner; and

(b) neither shall be the responsible clinician (if there is one) or the person in charge of the treatment in question.

(4) Before making any regulations for the purpose of this section the Secretary of State shall consult such bodies as appear to him to be concerned.

Treatment requiring consent or a second opinion

58.—(1) This section applies to the following forms of medical treatment for mental disorder—
- (a) such forms of treatment as may be specified for the purposes of this section by regulations made by the Secretary of State;
- (b) the administration of medicine to a patient by any means (not being a form of treatment specified under paragraph (a) above or section 57 above or section 58A(1)(b) below) at any time during a period for which he is liable to be detained as a patient to whom this Part of this Act applies if three months or more have elapsed since the first occasion in that period when medicine was administered to him by any means for his mental disorder.

(2) The Secretary of State may by order vary the length of the period mentioned in subsection (1)(b) above.

(3) Subject to section 62 below, a patient shall not be given any form of treatment to which this section applies unless—
- (a) he has consented to that treatment and either the approved clinician in charge of it or a registered medical practitioner appointed for the purposes of this Part of this Act by the regulatory authority has certified in writing that the patient is capable of understanding its nature, purpose and likely effects and has consented to it; or
- (b) a registered medical practitioner appointed as aforesaid (not being the responsible clinician or the approved clinician in charge of the treatment in question) has certified in writing that the patient is not capable of understanding the nature, purpose and likely effects of that treatment or being so capable has not consented to it but that it is appropriate for the treatment to be given.

(4) Before giving a certificate under subsection (3)(b) above the registered medical practitioner concerned shall consult two other persons who have been professionally concerned with the patient's medical treatment but, of those persons—
- (a) one shall be a nurse and the other shall be neither a nurse nor a registered medical practitioner; and
- (b) neither shall be the responsible clinician or the approved clinician in charge of the treatment in question.

(5) Before making any regulations for the purposes of this section the Secretary of State shall consult such bodies as appear to him to be concerned.

Urgent treatment

62.—(1) Sections 57 and 58 above shall not apply to any treatment—
- (a) which is immediately necessary to save the patient's life; or
- (b) which (not being irreversible) is immediately necessary to prevent a serious deterioration of his condition; or
- (c) which (not being irreversible or hazardous) is immediately necessary to alleviate serious suffering by the patient; or
- (d) which (not being irreversible or hazardous) is immediately necessary and represents the minimum interference necessary to prevent the patient from behaving violently or being a danger to himself or to others.

(1A) Section 58A above, in so far as it relates to electro-convulsive therapy by virtue of subsection (1)(a) of that section, shall not apply to any treatment which falls within paragraph (a) or (b) of subsection (1) above.

(1B) Section 58A above, in so far as it relates to a form of treatment specified by virtue of subsection (1)(b) of that section, shall not apply to any treatment which falls within such of paragraphs (a) to (d) of subsection (1) above as may be specified in regulations under that section.

(1C) For the purposes of subsection (1B) above, the regulations—
- (a) may make different provision for different cases (and may, in particular, make different provision for different forms of treatment);
- (b) may make provision which applies subject to specified exceptions; and
- (c) may include transitional, consequential, incidental or supplemental provision.

(2) Sections 60 and 61(3) above shall not preclude the continuation of any treatment or of treatment under any plan pending compliance with section 57, 58 or 58A above if the approved clinician in charge of the treatment considers that the discontinuance of the treatment or of treatment under the plan would cause serious suffering to the patient.

(3) For the purposes of this section treatment is irreversible if it has unfavourable irreversible physical or psychological consequences and hazardous if it entails significant physical hazard.

Electro-convulsive therapy, etc.

58A.—(1) This section applies to the following forms of medical treatment for mental disorder—

(a) electro-convulsive therapy; and

(b) such other forms of treatment as may be specified for the purposes of this section by regulations made by the appropriate national authority.

(2) Subject to section 62 below, a patient shall be not be given any form of treatment to which this section applies unless he falls within subsection (3), (4) or (5) below.

(3) A patient falls within this subsection if—

(a) he has attained the age of 18 years;

(b) he has consented to the treatment in question; and

(c) either the approved clinician in charge of it or a registered medical practitioner appointed as mentioned in section 58(3) above has certified in writing that the patient is capable of understanding the nature, purpose and likely effects of the treatment and has consented to it.

(4) A patient falls within this subsection if—

(a) he has not attained the age of 18 years; but

(b) he has consented to the treatment in question; and

(c) a registered medical practitioner appointed as aforesaid (not being the approved clinician in charge of the treatment) has certified in writing—

(i) that the patient is capable of understanding the nature, purpose and likely effects of the treatment and has consented to it; and

(ii) that it is appropriate for the treatment to be given.

(5) A patient falls within this subsection if a registered medical practitioner appointed as aforesaid (not being the responsible clinician (if there is one) or the approved clinician in charge of the treatment in question) has certified in writing—

(a) that the patient is not capable of understanding the nature, purpose and likely effects of the treatment; but

(b) that it is appropriate for the treatment to be given; and (c) that giving him the treatment would not conflict with—

(i) an advance decision which the registered medical practitioner concerned is satisfied is valid and applicable; or

(ii) a decision made by a donee or deputy or by the Court of Protection.

(6) Before giving a certificate under subsection (5) above the registered medical practitioner concerned shall consult two other persons who have been professionally concerned with the patient's medical treatment but, of those persons—

(a) one shall be a nurse and the other shall be neither a nurse nor a registered medical practitioner; and

(b) neither shall be the responsible clinician (if there is one) or the approved clinician in charge of the treatment in question.

(7) This section shall not by itself confer sufficient authority for a patient who falls within section 56(5) above to be given a form of treatment to which this section applies if he is not capable of understanding the nature, purpose and likely effects of the treatment (and cannot therefore consent to it).

(8) Before making any regulations for the purposes of this section, the appropriate national authority shall consult such bodies as appear to it to be concerned.

(9) In this section—

(a) a reference to an advance decision is to an advance decision (within the meaning of the Mental Capacity Act 2005) made by the patient;

(b) 'valid and applicable', in relation to such a decision, means valid and applicable to the treatment in question in accordance with section 25 of that Act;

(c) a reference to a donee is to a donee of a lasting power of attorney (within the meaning of section 9 of that Act) created by the patient, where the donee is acting within the scope of his authority and in accordance with that Act; and

(d) a reference to a deputy is to a deputy appointed for the patient by the Court of Protection under section 16 of that Act, where the deputy is acting within the scope of his authority and in accordance with that Act.

(10) In this section, 'the appropriate national authority' means—

(a) in a case where the treatment in question would, if given, be given in England, the Secretary of State;

(b) in a case where the treatment in question would, if given, be given in Wales, the Welsh Ministers

Treatment not requiring consent

63. The consent of a patient shall not be required for any medical treatment given to him for the mental disorder from which he is suffering, not being a form of treatment to which section 57, 58 or 58A above applies, if the treatment is given by or under the direction of the approved clinician in charge of the treatment.

References to legislation

Legislation is covered by the Open Government Licence: www.nationalarchives.gov.uk/doc/open-government-licence

Recommended reading

Department of Health. *Code of Practice Mental Health Act 1983*. TSO (The Stationery Office), 2008.

Department of Health. *Mental Capacity Act 2005 Code of Practice*. TSO (The Stationery Office), 2007.

Kwong Q, O'Brien A, Hill K, *et al*. *Medical Communication Skills and The Law Made Easy*. Elsevier, 2009.

Jones R. *Mental Health Act Manual (15th edn)*. Sweet and Maxwell, 1996.

Jones R. *Mental Capacity Act Manual (5th edn)*. Sweet and Maxwell, 2012 (in press).

Recommended websites

Mental Health Law online (www.mentalhealthlaw.co.uk). This provides details of both legislation and case law relating to all aspects of mental health practice.

One Crown Office Row (www.1cor.com/news) is a barristers chamber's website which provides information on recent case law.

Three Serjeant's Inn (www.3serjeantsinn.com/medical_treatment_decisions_and_the_law) is a barristers chamber's website which provides information on medical and mental health case law.

RadcliffesLeBrasseur (www.rlb-law.com/bulletins-and-briefings/mental-health-law-briefings.asp) provides briefing papers on recent mental health and care homes law updates.

Section II

Medical specialties

12

Cardiovascular disease

David Gray

Cardiovascular diseases are more common in people with mental disorders. This chapter describes the assessment of cardiovascular diseases, how to reduce cardiovascular risks and the management of hypertension. Practical guidance is given on the management of cardiovascular symptoms. Standards for electrocardiographic monitoring of patients taking psychotropic medication are outlined and tips are given on when to refer a patient to a cardiologist.

Introduction

Cardiovascular disease presents with a limited range of symptoms. General practitioners (GPs) are well equipped to recognise and manage these but many people with mental health problems may not have ready access to primary care services. Many symptoms can be managed in the community by the psychiatric team and the team may need to act as 'surrogate GPs' for those patients without easy access to primary care. A working knowledge of common symptoms, how to deal with them and when to refer patients for specialist assessment greatly improves the quality of care and quality of life of those with vascular disease.

Cardiovascular disease is the biggest cause of premature mortality in the Western world[1] and through its various manifestations, such as angina, rhythm abnormalities and heart failure, it consumes a large proportion of health service resources and impacts adversely on an individual's and a nation's economy through lost working hours. Those with mental illness are often at increased risk of developing cardiovascular disease because of their medication and more restricted lifestyle; many also often have fewer opportunities to receive advice on preventing ill health than the wider general public (as discussed in other chapters).

Assessment of cardiovascular risk and risk reduction

The concepts of 'cardiovascular risk assessment' and the existence of 'cardiovascular risk factors' were first described over 50 years ago in a report of the Framingham study, a long-term epidemiological study (Box 12.1).

Framingham identified some risk factors amenable to influence:

- total cholesterol and high-density lipoprotein (HDL) cholesterol
- blood pressure
- smoking status
- physical inactivity
- body weight (notably obesity)
- diabetes mellitus.

Box 12.1 The Framingham Study

In the USA in the 1940s, young men and women were dying prematurely from vascular disease. To ascertain what might be the underlying cause, a long-term community epidemiological study, the Framingham study, was begun in 1948. Over 5000 residents of the Massachusetts town of Framingham volunteered to have their health monitored, at intervals, for life. All study participants had a wide range of biochemical and physiological variables measured at intervals. As a result, several specific characteristics were identified, subsequently designated *cardiovascular risk factors*, which were found to increase the risk of developing vascular disease. From these, statistical techniques were used to develop a model which would provide clinicians and patients with an estimate of future cardiovascular risk. The Framingham risk scoring system has been widely adopted around the world.

Further details are available on the Framingham Study website (www.framinghamheartstudy.org).

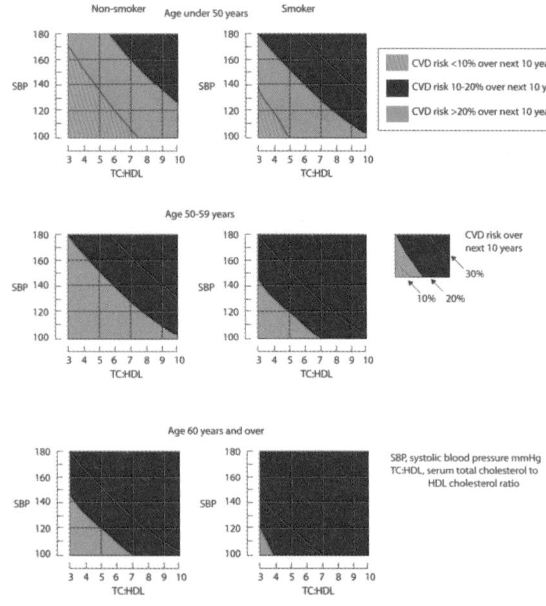

Fig. 12.1 An example of a cardiovascular risk calculator for non-diabetic men. Source: *Joint British Societies' Guidelines on Prevention of Cardiovascular Disease in Clinical Practice*. Reproduced with permission.

It also identified some that were immutable:

- age
- gender.

From these, a scoring system was devised indicating the risk of developing cardiovascular disease in the subsequent 10 years. Several *interactive* models are available online; on these websites (Box 12.2), individual personalised data can be directly entered and a risk score returned.

Simple tabular, non-interactive versions such as that shown below[2] are also available (Fig. 12.1), as is a version in the *British National Formulary* (BNF).[3]

The Framingham set of factors has been found to overestimate risk in some populations and to underestimate it in others.[4] Alternative scoring systems have been developed that purport to provide a more accurate estimate of risk appropriate to a UK population. These include QRISK® (http://qrisk.org), which was derived from 15 years' data from UK practices, and ASSIGN (http://cvrisk.mvm.ed.ac.uk/calculator.htm), which includes social deprivation as a risk factor.

It is important not to lose sight of what the Framingham study identified: the risk factors associated with the development of cardiovascular disease, with the 'predictive model' a statistical offshoot of the project. But any risk score is simply a 'best guess' of the likelihood of developing cardiovascular disease. Generally, the higher the score, the greater is the risk, but, for example, a 20% 10-year risk of developing cardiovascular disease can also be interpreted as an 80% 'risk' of *not* developing cardiovascular disease.

Since the results of the Framingham study were published, many more risk factors have been identified. A few are shown in Box 12.3. However, none features in the currently available scoring systems. For most purposes, the Framingham risk score provides a *reasonable* risk estimation for *most* populations.

Box 12.2 Interactive websites to estimate cardiovascular risk

- Framingham Heart Study: www.framinghamheartstudy.org
- Risk assessment tool for estimating 10-year risk of developing hard coronary heart disease (i.e. myocardial infarction and coronary death): http://hp2010.nhlbihin.net/atpiii/calculator.asp?usertype=prof
- Primary Cardiovascular Risk Calculator: www.patient.co.uk/doctor/Primary-Cardiovascular-Risk-Calculator.htm

A minimum standard for assessing cardiovascular risk in patients with psychiatric disease

All patients should be assessed for reversible risk factors when first referred for psychiatric assessment or on admission to a secure psychiatric unit and the findings recorded prominently in the patient record.

If the patient is *not* known to have vascular disease, that is, the patient has not had a heart attack, stroke, transient ischaemic attack (TIA) or peripheral vascular disease, a Framingham risk score should be obtained (see below) and recorded. Once cardiovascular risk factors have been identified, lifestyle and medication to minimise this risk should be discussed with the patient. This is particularly important for patients with psychiatric disorders, as they may not have ready access to general practice preventive and screening services, taken for granted by the general population.

If the patient has vascular disease, it is still important to identify risk factors, as survivors of a vascular event are at high risk of having another event. Everyone should be offered advice on lifestyle and appropriate drug treatment to reduce this risk. Note that it is *not* necessary to establish a risk score for a patient known to have vascular disease, as the risk of a second or subsequent event is already high in this population.

Box 12.3 Vascular risk factors identified since the results of the Framingham study were published

- Fibrinogen
- Family history
- Left ventricular hypertrophy
- Obesity
- Lipoprotein a
- Exercise
- Oestrogen use
- Glucose intolerance
- Behavioural factors
- Alcohol consumption
- Homocysteine
- Ethnicity
- Inflammatory markers – C-reactive protein
- Serum triglycerides
- Psychosocial factors
- Small low-density lipoprotein particles

- Primary prevention. Individuals have no history of vascular disease; a risk score should be estimated.
- Secondary prevention. Individuals have a history of angina, heart attack, stroke, transient ischaemic attack or peripheral vascular disease; no risk estimate is necessary but lifestyle advice and drug treatment to reduce vascular risk should be commenced.

Reducing vascular risk

Disease prevention can be:

- *primary* – this applies to individuals with no history of vascular disease
- *secondary* – this applies to individuals who already suffer from a vascular disease or who have had a vascular event.

It is important to be aware that the risk calculator is a tool for *primary prevention*; those who already have vascular disease do not need a risk score – they are considered to be at risk of disease progression and warrant intervention to reduce all individual risks as a matter of routine.

Vascular risk in patients with diabetes mellitus

Individuals with diabetes mellitus are at particularly high risk of developing cardiovascular disease.[5] Deaths from coronary heart disease (CHD) are increased twofold in diabetic men relative to non-diabetic men, while among women there is an even greater excess of death from CHD: diabetic women are at fourfold higher risk compared with non-diabetic women.[6] Consequently, diabetes is considered as 'heart-disease equivalent', so estimating a risk score is *not* appropriate. All existing cardiovascular risk factors must be treated, as the impact of an increasing number of risk factors is greater in those *with* than in those *without* diabetes.[7]

Primary prevention: the practicalities

Who to evaluate

A risk score should be estimated for any patient aged 40–74 years without, but likely to be at high risk of, cardiovascular disease.[8] In practical terms, this means everyone over 40.

Using the Framingham risk table

Start by collating the necessary information. Typically, these are:

- gender
- age in years
- systolic blood pressure
- total serum cholesterol, in mg/dl (most UK laboratories use mmol/l; multiply by 39 to convert from mg/dl to mmol/l; to convert mmol/l to mg/dl, divide by 39)
- high-density lipoprotein (HDL) and low-density lipoprotein (LDL) cholesterol levels
- current smoking habit ('yes' or 'no').

The systolic blood pressure used should be the *pre-treatment* level, but if this is not available clinical judgement can be used to estimate the score. For example, a patient on three antihypertensive drugs is likely to have had a higher blood pressure, and hence higher risk score, than a patient on a single drug.

The overall score from these main factors should be adjusted for known 'risk enhancers' which do not feature in risk scoring systems:

- family history of premature vascular disease, defined as a male first-degree relative aged under 55 or a female first-degree relative under 65 – increase risk score by a factor of 1.3
- family history of premature vascular disease in more than one first-degree relative – increase risk score by a factor of 1.5–2.0
- ethnicity – increase risk score by a factor of 1.4 in men of South Asian origin.

The following also increase risk but adjustment is not recommended for these:

- raised triglyceride levels (greater than 1.7 mmol/l)
- women with premature menopause
- impaired glucose tolerance (but patient not yet suffering from diabetes)
- chronic renal disease
- socioeconomic factors
- autoimmune disease.

Alcohol consumption, body mass index (BMI), fasting blood glucose level, renal function, liver function and thyroid function and the presence of left ventricular hypertrophy should also be recorded. They are not required for risk estimation but they will help identify any adverse metabolic effect of medication.

To generate a risk score (i.e., a 'best guess' of the risk of developing a heart attack or dying from vascular disease in the next 10 years) each factor is entered into the preferred scoring system or computer program. The risk score should be documented prominently in the patient's notes.

> The Framingham risk score is intended as an aid in *primary prevention* only. It is *not* appropriate for those who have a history of cardiovascular or cerebrovascular disease.

When not to use the Framingham risk score

Some patients are at high risk of CHD as the result of:

- familial hypercholesterolaemia (FH), which is caused by inherited mutations in various genes that affect cholesterol metabolism (suspect FH if total cholesterol exceeds 7.5 mmol/l and make enquiries about family members)
- type 2 diabetes.

It is *not* appropriate to use the Framingham system in these patients but patients should have a full assessment and lifestyle and drug interventions to reduce risk.

What to do for patients with a risk score of over 20%

General practitioners generally take a risk of 20% as an important threshold. For patients with a risk score over that threshold, current guidance[9] recommends the following as part of the management strategy for primary prevention:

- advice on lifestyle change should be given
- all modifiable risks should be addressed –
  - hypertension and diabetes should be reduced to 'target' levels (see below)
  - obesity, inadequate exercise, smoking and alcohol consumption should be tacked
- secondary causes of hypercholesterolaemia should be addressed – nephropathy, myxoedema, excess alcohol consumption
- a statin 'should be initiated with simvastatin 40 mg'.

Note that, unlike secondary prevention (see later), there is no 'target' level for cholesterol; aiming for secondary prevention targets is a good start but ideally total cholesterol and LDL cholesterol should be reduced as much as possible.

What to do for patients with a risk score of less than 20%

It would be negligent to ignore a blood pressure consistently at, for example, 220/130 mmHg or a total cholesterol level of 10 mmol/l just because the *overall* risk score was estimated as less than 20%. Individual risk factors must be addressed through lifestyle advice, and where necessary drug treatment, to reduce risk, as this will inevitably increase with time due to advancing age.

What to do for patients with a risk score very close to, but less than, 20%

The Framingham risk score is imperfect – it is an *estimate* – so clinicians should not stick rigidly to an absolute threshold of 20%. Individual risk factors should be addressed through lifestyle advice, and where necessary drug treatment, to reduce risk.

What to do with a patient with a single risk factor that is particularly high

Irrespective of the risk score, treat patients aggressively if their blood pressure is over 160/90 mmHg, if they have poorly controlled diabetes mellitus ($HbA1_c$ >6%) or their cholesterol level is >7.5 mmol/l, which suggests FH.

Management of abnormal lipids

The National Institute for Health and Clinical Excellence (NICE) recommends that 'before offering lipid modification therapy for primary prevention, all other modifiable risk factors should be considered and their management optimised if possible'.[9] Treatment to lower cholesterol is recommended if the 10-year risk exceeds 20%. The preferred statin is simvastatin 40 mg. Statins are generally well tolerated, causing predominantly muscle aches and pain; if these occur, change to atorvastatin 40 mg or rosuvastatin 10 mg. There is no published interaction with antipsychotic drugs.

Optimal and treatment levels for risk factors

Optimal levels suggested by the British Hypertension Society (http://bhsoc.org) are shown below in the section on 'Management of hypertension'. All patients should be advised about lifestyle factors, including:

- smoking cessation
- regular exercise lasting at least 15–30 minutes a day
- BMI within the range 21–25 kg/m^2.

Those with diabetes should have 'good' glucose control, as measured by $HbA1_c$, which almost equates to glucose levels, so aim for $HbA1_c$ of 6.5% or below. Control can be eased for those with a tendency to hypoglycaemia ($HbA1_c$ of 7%).

The 'lower the better' is the general view regarding cholesterol levels but expert consensus[2,10] suggests the aim should be for a total cholesterol of 4 mmol/l *and* LDL cholesterol of 2 mmol/l.

Aspirin and primary prevention

Aspirin can cause internal bleeding even at low doses[11] and the risk with the use of aspirin as a primary preventive measure exceeds any benefit in terms of reducing vascular disease.[12] It is best avoided.

Reducing risk of recurrent vascular disease – secondary prevention

For those who have vascular disease, lifestyle advice is just as important as in primary prevention. If an individual has evidence of coronary disease (myocardial infarction or angina), drug treatment should include a beta blocker, ACE inhibitor (angiotensin-converting enzyme inhibitor), aspirin and a statin. The general practice Quality and Outcomes Framework[13] (see Chapter 3) audit targets for cholesterol are:

- total cholesterol below 5 mmol/l
- LDL cholesterol below 3 mmol/l.

Specialist bodies[2] recommend lower than this:

- total cholesterol below 4 mmol/l
- LDL cholesterol below 2 mmol/l.

Management of hypertension

Blood pressure is a biological variable whose control is strictly regulated. Generally, the higher the blood pressure, the greater is the risk of myocardial infarction, stroke, renovascular disease and blindness. The British Hypertension Society recommends that all adults should have their blood pressure measured at least at 5-yearly intervals (http://guidance.nice.org.uk/CG/Wave2/14).

Investigations

Hypertension is usually an 'older' person's disease. An underlying cause should be sought if the patient:

- is aged under 40
- is treatment resistant
- has a family history of hypertension or stroke, when relatives were under the age of 50
- has hypernatraemia or hypokalaemia
- has abnormal renal function.

Determine if there is evidence of existing harm, that is, 'target organ' or 'end-organ' damage – look for evidence of stroke or TIA, angina or heart attack, renal disease, peripheral vascular disease and retinopathy.

Look for renal disease using estimated glomerular function (eGFR; now routinely reported when urea and electrolytes are requested) and ultrasound, 24-hour urinary vanillylmandelic acid (VMA) and cortisol levels; and monitor the potential effects of therapy – urea, creatinine and electrolyte, cholesterol and glucose levels, electrocardiography (ECG), presence of blood and protein in urine.

Patients with established hypertension may need to be investigated if their normally well-controlled (though high) blood pressure becomes more difficult to control.

Management

The aim of treatment is to reduce the risk of end-organ damage. Controlling blood pressure is usually straightforward. Advise anyone with high, borderline or high normal blood pressure (the classification is set out in Table 12.1) on lifestyle modifications. If blood pressure is persistently above target on three occasions, initiate antihypertensive drug therapy. Most people with high blood pressure require at least two antihypertensive drugs to achieve target levels; fixed drug combinations may be helpful in aiding compliance and reducing 'tablet burden'.

Table 12.1 Classification of blood pressure

	Blood pressure (mmHg)
Optimal	120/80
Normal	130/85
High normal	130–139/85–89
Mild hypertension	140–159/90–99
Moderate hypertension	160–179/100–109
Severe hypertension	>180/>110
Isolated systolic hypertension	140–159/<90

Current guidelines[14] suggest the following for patients with hypertension:

- aged under 55 – an ACE inhibitor; for example lisinopril or ramipril) or, if not tolerated, an angiotensin receptor antagonist (ARB; for example losartan or candesartan); if blood pressure is not controlled, add a calcium channel blocker or thiazide diuretic;
- aged 55 or over, or Black patients of any age (defined as of African or Caribbean descent, and not mixed race, Asian or Chinese) – initiate either a calcium channel blocker (such as amlodipine or diltiazem) or a thiazide diuretic (such as bendroflumethiazide); if not controlled, add an ACE-I (or ARB)
- if a third drug is required, use an ACE-I (or ARB) plus calcium channel blocker plus thiazide
- if blood pressure is not controlled on three different drugs, specialist referral is recommended.[15]

Other medications for hypertensive patients

All patients should be prescribed the following:

- aspirin 75 mg daily, unless contraindicated, if the patient is aged over 50 years
- a statin if the 10-year risk of cardiovascular disease exceeds 20% – if for secondary prevention, use a sufficient dose to reach targets of
  - total cholesterol less than 4 mmol/l or
  - LDL less than 2 mmol/l or
  - 25% reduction in total cholesterol or 30% reduction in LDL (whichever is the greater).

Threshold for starting drug treatment for hypertension

Initiate drug treatment in all patients with:

- sustained systolic blood pressure ≥160 mmHg or sustained diastolic ≥100 mmHg despite non-pharmacological measures
- sustained systolic blood pressure of 140–159 mmHg or diastolic of 90–99 mmHg if target organ damage is present, or there is evidence of established cardiovascular disease or diabetes, or 10-year cardiovascular disease risk ≥20%.

For most patients, aim for systolic ≤140 mmHg and diastolic ≤85 mmHg. For patients with diabetes, renal impairment or established cardiovascular disease a lower target, of ≤130/80 mmHg, is recommended. When using ambulatory blood pressure readings, use mean daytime pressures, expected to be about 10/5 mmHg lower than an 'office' equivalent for both thresholds and targets. If home readings of blood pressure are used, use the same adjustment of 10/5 mmHg.

Lifestyle measures

- Maintain normal weight for adults (body mass index 20–25 kg/m^2).
- Reduce salt intake to < 100 mmol/day (< 6 g NaCl or < 2.4 g Na^+/day).
- Limit alcohol consumption to ≤3 units/day for men and ≤2 units/day for women.
- Aerobic physical exercise (brisk walking rather than weight-lifting) for ≥30 minutes per day, ideally most weekdays but at least 3 days a week.
- At least five portions a day of fresh fruit and vegetables.
- Reduce intake of total and saturated fat.

When to refer to hospital or specialist

Urgent treatment in hospital is needed with:

- accelerated hypertension (severe hypertension and grade III–IV retinopathy)
- particularly severe hypertension (> 220/120 mmHg)
- impending complications (e.g. TIA, left ventricular failure).

Seek a specialist opinion when:

- blood pressure cannot be controlled by three drugs
- blood pressure is difficult to control
- an underlying cause is suspected
- blood pressure is unusually variable
- blood pressure is thought to be 'white coat'
- hypertension is present in pregnancy
- hypertension is present in those who may have an underlying or 'secondary' cause.

Possible underlying causes

The history or examination may suggest an underlying cause, such as:

- hypokalaemia, with increased or high normal plasma sodium (Conn's syndrome)
- elevated serum creatinine
- proteinuria or haematuria
- sudden onset or worsening of hypertension
- resistance to a multiple drug regimen (three or more drugs)
- young age (any hypertension < 20 years; hypertension needing treatment < 30 years).

Therapeutic problems

Therapeutic problems encountered in the management of hypertension include:

- multiple drug intolerance
- multiple drug contraindications
- persistent non-adherence or non-compliance.

Detailed advice on hypertension is available at the British Hypertension website.[16,17]

Common cardiovascular symptoms

The commonest cardiac conditions encountered are chest pain, breathlessness and palpitations. These may occur singly or in any combination.

Chest pain

Chest pain can arise in almost any structure in the chest. As a result, there are many *potential* causes (Table 12.2).

Decide first if the pain is potentially life-threatening. This is typically pain that 'sounds' cardiac, with characteristic features. The patient can be asked the questions in Table 12.3.

Knowing your patient may be helpful – some patients will report every minor ailment, but if a stoical patient reports chest pain, assume there is genuine cause until disproven.

Angina does not start *de novo*. Patients may have several risk factors. Physical examination may be normal.

What action should be taken?

It is safest to assume that a cardiac cause until proven otherwise. Record a 12-lead ECG:

- Normal ECG does not exclude a cardiac cause of pain but it should at least ease your panic; if you suspect

Ask about vascular risk factors in anyone who develops symptoms of angina.

Table 12.2 Potential causes of chest pain

Type/area of pain	Possible cause
Cardiovascular	*Unstable angina* and *myocardial infarction*
	Aortic dissection
	Pericarditis
	Cardiac dysrhythmia
	Stable angina
Pulmonary	*Pulmonary embolism*
Pneumonia	*Haemothorax and pneumothorax*
	Pleurisy
Gastrointestinal	Gastro-oesophageal reflux disease
	Hiatus hernia (which may not accompany gastro-oesophageal reflux disease)
	Peptic ulcer disease
Chest wall	Costochondritis
	Fibromyalgia
	Herpes zoster ('shingles')
Psychological	Panic attack
	Anxiety
	Depression
	Somatisation disorder
	Hypochondria
Others	Hyperventilation
	Da Costa's syndrome
	Bornholm disease

Potentially life-threatening causes are shown in *italics*.

a pulmonary embolism – the ECG may be normal sinus rhythm, sinus tachycardia, atrial fibrillation (Fig. 12.5) or (classically) S1Q3T3 pattern – give oxygen and dial 999.

- An ST segment depression implies myocardial ischaemia (Fig. 12.2).
- ST segment elevation usually indicates a heart attack. Give aspirin 300 mg orally, chewed and swallowed; dial 999 for an emergency ambulance. If facilities are available, establish venous access, give morphine 5–10 mg with an anti-emetic (e.g. cyclizine) and position a defibrillator close by in case ventricular fibrillation develops (Fig. 12.3). Do not rely on the ECG alone to make the diagnosis of heart attack as 'classic' ECG changes may take several hours to occur.
- A very slow heart rhythm may indicate heart block, sinus bradycardia, 'slow' atrial fibrillation or complete heart block (Fig. 12.4), causing a reduction in coronary blood flow and a fall in blood pressure.
- A fast heart rhythm may be a sinus tachycardia in response to anxiety, an irregular rhythm of atrial fibrillation or a potentially fatal ventricular tachycardia or fibrillation (Fig. 12.5).

Table 12.3 Questions to ask a patient with chest pain

Question	Relevance
Did it come on slowly or suddenly?	Sudden onset of severe pain usually arises from tubes that become blocked, like the coronary artery in heart attack, or burst internally, as in aortic dissection (the pain is often described as a 'tearing' pain in the interscapular region) or pulmonary embolus (usually accompanied by breathlessness, tachycardia and haemoptysis; it hurts to breathe in deeply)
What does the pain feel like?	Angina pain is often a 'crushing' sensation, 'heaviness', 'pressure on the chest' or a 'tight band around the chest'
Where is the pain?	Angina pain may be felt anywhere in the chest but is predominantly around the chest
Does it hurt anywhere else?	Angina pain may radiate down the left arm, or to the neck or teeth
What brings the pain on?	Physical exertion may make the pain worse
Is anything else wrong?	Patients usually report associated features such as difficulty in breathing and feeling sick; in a heart attack, there may be a feeling of 'impending doom'
Does it change when you sit forward?	Pain from the pericardium is usually considerably easier on sitting upright
Does it ease with glyceryl trinitrate (GTN)?	Glyceryl trinitrate is usually effective in angina and infarction

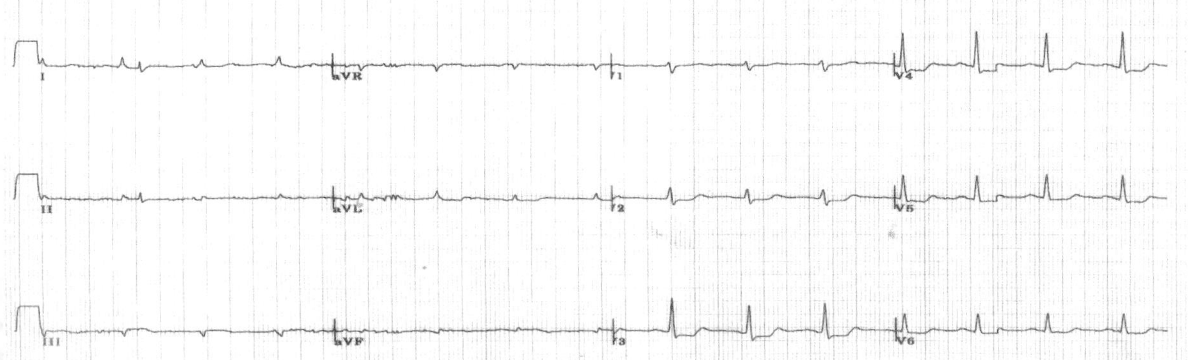

Fig. 12.2 ST depression V2 to V6: myocardial ischaemia.

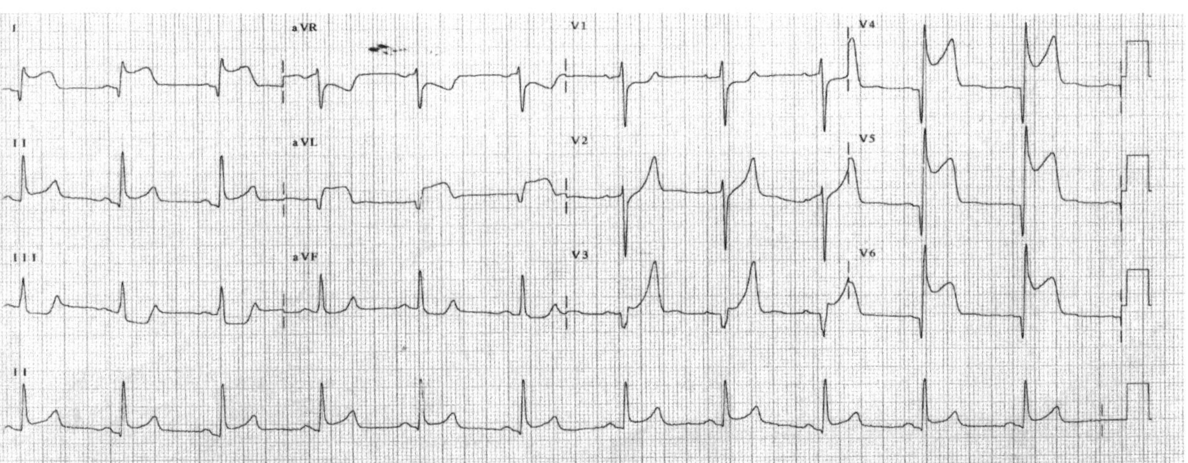

Fig. 12.3 ST elevation leads I, aVL and V3 to V6: acute myocardial infarction.

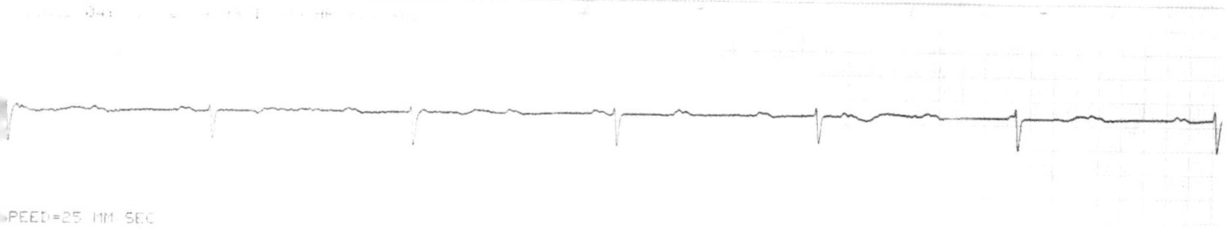

Fig. 12.4 Slow heart rhythm of complete heart block – P waves bear no relationship with QRS complexes.

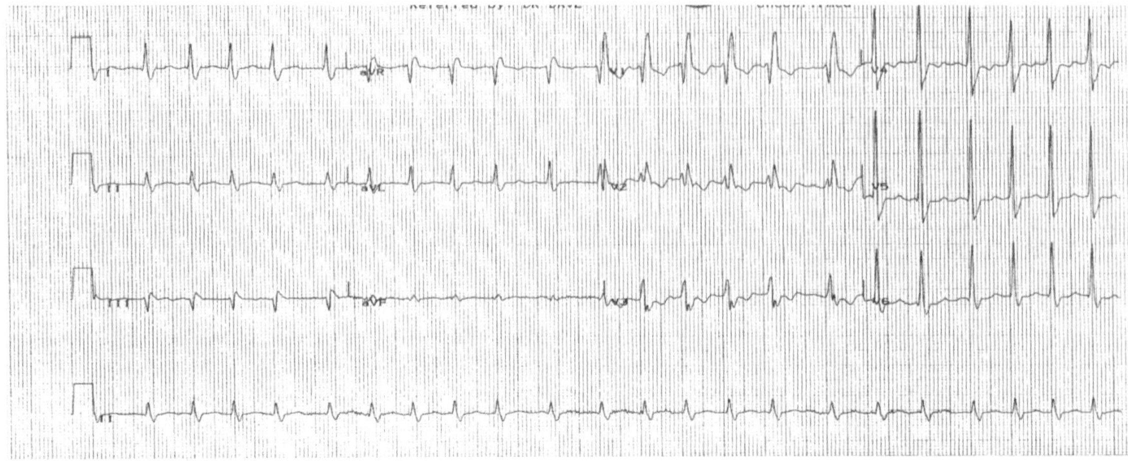

Fig. 12.5 'Fast' atrial fibrillation – a narrow complex tachycardia with irregular rhythm.

How do you know if the pain is genuine?

In short, detecting the *sham* patient can be difficult. Symptoms in a patient known to have coronary disease can be precipitated by anxiety, unusual exertion or even deliberate omission of anti-anginal medication. If the patient is known to have coronary disease, the pain must be taken seriously. With genuine pain, the body's usual stress response, the sympathetic nervous system's 'fight or flight' reaction kicks in, so:

- look for pallor, nausea, tachycardia and sweating
- watch for non-verbal clues such as the patient clenching a fist in front of the sternum
- do an ECG – cardiac pain may be evident as
  - ST depression (suggestive of myocardial ischaemia – see Fig. 12.2) and give GTN sublingually; the pain frequently settles quickly though may recur quickly
  - ST elevation (suggestive of an acute myocardial infarction – see Fig. 12.3)
  - an abnormal rhythm such as atrial fibrillation (if this occurs in a patient normally in sinus rhythm it may indicate a heart attack).

Do not worry if you cannot interpret the ECG: modern automated equipment provides an interpretation for you. These tend to overdiagnose problems but this means *safety first.*

Beta blockers or calcium channel blockers, prescribed for hypertension, some rhythm disturbances and angina, may mask pain and tachycardia. If genuine angina, sublingual GTN is usually effective in minutes, though pain may recur.

There is at present no readily available biomarker that can be reliably used to detect myocardial ischaemia at the bedside. Current markers may take many hours to appear in the bloodstream, so hospital admission is necessary.

The pain is *unlikely* to be cardiac if:

- it occurs on bending or flexing the spine or is mimicked by pressure on the chest wall – this is likely to be musculoskeletal
- it is *localised* and the patient indicates the site by pointing with one finger (the 'pointing sign') – in fact such pain is *never* cardiac
- it is severe when the patient is lying and eased when the patient sits forward – such pain is likely to be due to pericarditis.

Breathlessness

How do you know if the breathlessness is genuine?

As with cardiac pain, this can be difficult. If respiratory rate is normal (about 14–16 breaths/min), there are no signs of distress and pulse oximetry is normal, symptoms are likely to be factitious.

A normal ECG does not exclude a heart attack or angina.

When to take things seriously

Bad signs are any reduction in PaO_2 (oxygen levels assessed by pulse oximetry), inability to talk due to breathlessness, lower than usual blood pressure, fever, pain on inspiration and accompanying dizziness or chest pain.

Palpitations

The patient may complain of awareness of a 'fast heartbeat' or a 'missed heartbeat', sudden onset of a racing heartbeat (like tripping a switch), an erratic heartbeat or a feeling of 'light-headedness' or 'dizziness'.

What are palpitations?

They mean different things to different people, so you need to establish, as precisely as you can, what the patient means – 'fluttering', 'thumping in the chest', 'missed beat', 'racing heartbeat' and 'I can feel my heart beat' are commonly used expressions. Ask the patient to tap out the heartbeat on the desk – an irregular heartbeat or a 'missed' beat will become obvious. A significant arrhythmia is usually accompanied by a change in blood pressure and hence cardiac output, so common symptoms are dizziness and breathlessness.

Common problems

- *Ectopic beats.* Awareness of the heartbeat usually involves an ectopic beat, that is, an extra beat, followed by a pause and then a forceful beat.
- *Sinus tachycardia.* This is a fast heartbeat, which can be induced by feeling anxious or angry
- *Atrial fibrillation.* This is one of the commonest arrhythmias. It usually occurs against a background of hypertension, diabetes or coronary disease, although it can be due to an 'electrical short circuit'.

Much less common is ventricular tachycardia, where the cardiac rate is fast and the QRS complexes are much broader than normal (more than three squares, or 120 ms; see Fig. 12.6) – this is a life-threatening arrhythmia that requires immediate transfer to the nearest emergency department.

When to take things seriously

Any cardiac rhythm that is accompanied by chest pain, breathlessness or dizziness cannot be ignored – these are indicators that cardiac output has fallen.

If the pulse is erratic, and especially if it is *fast* and erratic, the most likely diagnosis is 'fast' atrial fibrillation and urgent action is needed.

If the pulse is much faster or slower than routinely observed and cannot be explained by drug therapy, do an ECG to look for heart block, 'slow' or 'fast' atrial fibrillation and supraventricular and ventricular tachycardia.

Assessment of the patient with cardiovascular symptoms

Some basic cardiac investigations can be organised quickly and simply, although their interpretation may

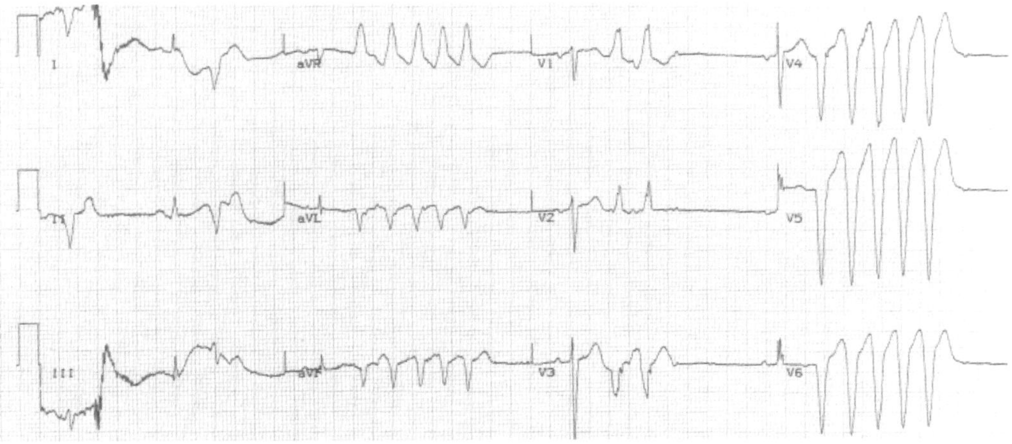

Fig. 12.6 Ventricular tachycardia.

require some skill and training. These are briefly described below, with a note of the level of skill (and type of staff) required to conduct and interpret the tests.

An exercise test is more reliable as an indicator of *prognosis* than *diagnosis*.

Electrocardiography (ECG)

The ECG detects changes in electrical activity, with elaborate electronics to filter out skeletal muscle activity, which masks underlying cardiac activity. Self-adherent electrodes applied to specific locations on the skin record the electrical activity of the heart. Correct lead placement is essential to avoid a wrong interpretation. Many ECG machines have embedded computer software to provide an analysis, although these are not perfect.

The ECG is most useful for identifying the cardiac rhythm and determining the timing of specific ECG intervals such as the QT interval (see below). It can be used to indicate any damage to heart muscle from a heart attack.

Many antipsychotic medications have an adverse effect on various ECG parameters, in particular prolonging the QT interval, putting patients at risk of potentially fatal heart rhythms.

- Skill level of operator – basic training needed in electrode placement.
- Skill level of interpreter – interpretive skills can be readily acquired with practice.

Exercise electrocardiography

Gradual occlusion of the coronary arteries may lead to *stable angina* with symptoms on exertion. ECG and blood pressure are monitored with the patient on a treadmill or fixed bicycle. A predetermined protocol is followed, with gradually increasing physical effort, faster heart rate and so increased cardiac work. The test is considered 'positive' if chest pain is reproduced or the ECG shows characteristic changes suggestive of cardiac ischaemia. The test is more reliable as an indicator of *prognosis* than *diagnosis*.

- Skill level of operator – needs training in technique and in cardiac resuscitation.
- Skill level of interpreter – interpretive skills can be readily acquired with practice.

Alternatives to exercise testing

Where exercising is difficult, for example for patients who are obese or otherwise relatively immobile (perhaps limited by arthritis), ischaemia can still be demonstrated using echocardiography, thallium scanning and magnetic resonance imaging techniques. These will be organised by the cardiologist where necessary.

- Skill level of operator – usually requires a physician and cardiac physiologist.
- Skill level of interpreter – usually consultant or trained/trainee registrar.

Coronary angiogram

During this test, a tube is passed under local anaesthetic to the coronary arteries and a contrast agent is injected. Imaging then reveals the coronary anatomy. At present, this is the only test that defines anatomy adequately enough for coronary revascularisation (coronary angioplasty or coronary artery bypass surgery), though other imaging techniques are being developed. It is invasive and there is a 1 in 1000 risk of death, heart attack, stroke or vascular damage.

- Skill level of operator – requires a team of highly trained staff.
- Skill level of interpreter – usually consultant or trained/trainee registrar.

Echocardiography

This uses ultrasound to create two-dimensional images of the heart. Three-dimensional imaging has been developed but is not widely available. The test provides a wealth of information about the size and shape of the heart, its pumping capacity (left and right ventricular function and dimensions), the extent and location of any damaged areas and the function of the heart valves. Transthoracic echocardiography is non-invasive and risk-free, but a clear image is difficult to obtain for some individuals, especially those with chronic lung disease or obesity. Better views can often be obtained using trans-oesophageal echocardiography.

- Skill level of operator – high (usually a cardiologist or cardiac physiologist).
- Skill level of interpreter – interpretive skills can be readily acquired with practice.

Suspected rhythm abnormalities

A variety of tests are available to record the heart rhythm when an individual is aware of 'palpitations'. Ambulatory continuous electrocardiography recording ('24 hour tape' or Holter recorder), usually over 24–48 hours, is appropriate if palpitations occur most days. A patient-activated device (cardiac memo) is useful when palpitations occur less frequently. A REVEAL™ device implanted superficially over the left chest wall is reserved for those whose symptoms are very infrequent or cause syncope.

- Skill level of operator – high.
- Skill level of interpreter – high (interpretation requires a trained cardiac physiologist).

Cardiac computed tomography

Multiple radiographic images are computer-integrated to generate cross-sectional views. Computed tomography (CT) angiography exposes an individual to roughly the equivalent of several hundred chest X-rays. Nonetheless, it may become the investigation of choice in future, as it has the potential to investigate both cardiac anatomy and cardiac physiology.

- Skill level of operator and interpreter – high (radiologist to conduct test and interpret images).

Cardiac magnetic resonance imaging

This images the heart using a powerful magnetic field, radio-frequency pulses and a computer to produce detailed pictures of the heart.

- Skill level of operator and interpreter – high (radiologist to conduct test and interpret image).

Management of specific problems

Angina

Most patients' symptoms can be ameliorated using a cocktail of medication that may include:

- a short-acting nitrate (note that GTN tablets expire 8 weeks after opening the bottle, whereas GTN spray lasts much longer)
- a long-acting nitrate (e.g. isosorbide mononitrate)
- a calcium channel blocker (e.g. amlodipine, diltiazem or verapamil)
- a beta-blocker (e.g. atenolol)
- a potassium channel opener (e.g. nicorandil)
- other types (e.g. ivabradine, ranolazine).

These can be co-prescribed. Check the BNF for possible interactions.

When symptoms cannot be controlled or quality of life is adversely affected, appropriate patients may be offered coronary angiography to ascertain coronary anatomy prior to revascularisation through percutaneous coronary angioplasty ('balloon stretch') or coronary artery bypass surgery.

Left ventricular dysfunction/heart failure

Patients should have appropriate treatment of all cardiovascular risks. Symptomatic improvement can be anticipated in response to medical treatment with:

- ACE inhibitors (e.g. lisinopril)
- diuretics (e.g. furosemide, which must be used only in sufficient dose to reduce excess fluid – usually ankle oedema)
- a beta-blocker (a carefully titrated low-dose beta-blocker reduces the sympathetic drive that occurs in heart failure).

Spironolactone has been shown to reduce the need for hospitalisation, but has no impact on symptoms.

For those who do not respond, appropriate patients may be offered cardiac resynchronisation therapy (clever pacemaker technology to make the left and right ventricles work in harmony), coronary artery surgery or cardiac transplant.

Palpitations

Most cardiac dysrhythmia can be controlled with medication that may include:

- beta-blockers
- flecainide
- amiodarone (although it has a long list of potential long-term adverse effects)
- digoxin
- verapamil and diltiazem.

There are also other drugs, but these are usually prescribed by a cardiologist.

Appropriate patients may be offered electro-physiological study to identify and ablate (destroy) the

Generally, the longer the QTc interval, the greater is the risk. A clinically significant cut-off is taken to be 500 ms.

source of the arrhythmia. An implantable cardioverter defibrillator may be used for potentially fatal dysrhythmia such as ventricular tachycardia or fibrillation.

Slow heart rate

A pacemaker implant is very effective at restoring cardiac rate. Battery life is about 7–10 years and unit replacement is straightforward.

Relevance to psychiatric patients

Psychiatric patients, especially those prescribed antipsychotic medication, face additional vascular risks compared with the normal population. Their care needs to balance effective treatment for both physical and psychiatric illness. Where treatment for both is essential, determine which has priority and minimise the risk attributable to other illnesses. This is particularly important with psychotropic medication in patients with concomitant rhythm disorders.

There is an increased risk of ventricular arrhythmias when some antipsychotic medications that prolong the QT interval (see below) and some antidepressants are co-prescribed with anti-arrhythmic drugs. The BNF carries an extensive list in Appendix 1: Interactions.

For drugs that prolong the QTc interval, the reader is referred to the website 'sudden arrhythmic death syndrome' (www.sads.org.uk/drugs_to_avoid.htm).

Monitoring of long QT in psychiatric patients

The QT interval on the ECG measures the time for depolarisation (muscle contraction) and repolarisation (recovery of muscle ready for the next contraction); this is usually no more than 400 ms in a man and 430 ms in a woman.

The QT interval is normally corrected to a heart rate of 60 beats/min and is known as the QTc interval. Prolongation of the QTc interval increases the risk of cardiac dysrhythmia, which may cause palpitations and fainting and potentially lead to sudden death due to ventricular tachycardia, torsades de pointes (a form of ventricular tachycardia) and ventricular fibrillation.

Inherited varieties of 'long QT syndrome' are well described but acquired long QT is much more common, as a result of medication and low serum potassium or magnesium levels.

Many antipsychotic drugs prolong QTc, including the atypical antipsychotic medication clozapine, phenothiazines such as chlorpromazine and butyrophenones such as haloperidol.

Patients with schizophrenia are at particular risk of sudden death. The reasons for this are probably multiple, involving negative health habits, disease and treatment-induced metabolic disorders with consequent increased risk of cardiovascular disease, medication-induced prolongation of the QTc interval, serious ventricular arrhythmias, as well as autonomic dysfunction with low heart rate variability and decreased baroreflex sensitivity. The risks may increase substantially with antipsychotic medication. While a response to antipsychotic medication is highly idiosyncratic, routine ECG monitoring may identify susceptible individuals.

On admission to psychiatric care, record an ECG *and* check electrolyte levels to establish a baseline and to check for existing cardiac contraindications to future treatment. These tests should be repeated under any of the following circumstances.

- If a patient on an antipsychotic medication experiences a collapse, dizziness, palpitations or erratic or fast heartbeat. Ventricular extrasystoles not previously documented should precipitate a review of and reduction in dose of the antipsychotic medication; self-limiting clozapine-associated resting tachycardia affects 25% of patients during drug titration, but should be taken seriously if it persists, especially if the tachycardia is accompanied by a fever, onset of breathlessness or palpitations, as these symptoms may herald a myocarditis or cardiomyopathy, warranting urgent cardiological referral for echocardiography and urgent review of treatment with clozapine.
- Before initiating an antipsychotic medication. Check an ECG when steady state has been achieved and at monthly intervals afterwards, or when clinically indicated and at times of intercurrent illness.
- Before increasing the dose of antipsychotic.
- When giving intravenous medication (if clinically feasible).

- If a patient taking an antipsychotic medication is found to have a low serum potassium or magnesium (the normal range is 3.5–5.5 mmol/l or mEq/l).
- Before a second antipsychotic medication is introduced.
- Before another drug known to prolong the QT interval, such as an antihistamine or erythromycin antibiotic, is prescribed (see: www.longQT.com for a comprehensive list).

Clinicians should be aware that antipsychotic medication should be used with caution, and in the lowest clinically effective dose, in those with known cardiovascular disease and in the elderly.

Standards for ECG monitoring of patients on psychotropic medication

The baseline ECG

All patients under psychiatric care should have a resting 12-lead ECG on referral or on admission to a psychiatric facility or before initiating or changing dose or type of psychotropic medication. This should be repeated annually or more frequently if clinically indicated.

The ECG can be used as a baseline against which to compare future ECGs. Each ECG should be reviewed to look for:

- evidence of a previous myocardial infarction – Q waves, inverted T waves, left bundle branch block or development of right bundle branch block *de novo*, with symptoms
- evidence of a cardiac dysrhythmia such as atrial fibrillation
- QT interval – because this is heart rate-dependent, most ECG machines will calculate this automatically as the rate-corrected (QTc) interval. This should be noted and documented. A prolonged QTc interval increases the likelihood of a potentially fatal cardiac dysrhythmia. Some psychotropic drugs may prolong the QTc, as described earlier.

Other indications for the ECG

An ECG should be recorded:

- if an antipsychotic medication is being considered, particularly in high dosage[18] (this may be one drug above BNF limits or two drugs in combination that exceed their combined percentage of BNF limits)
- a few weeks after starting antipsychotic medication, when steady state has been achieved, and every 3 months in the early stages of high-dose treatment
- if parenteral antipsychotic medication is given for emergency tranquillisation during an episode of acute violence
- when considering prescribing pimozide or haloperidol (special precautions also pertain for sertindole, as described in the drug's summary of product characteristics)
- if the patient receiving the medication has a history of cardiovascular disease
- at times of acute medical illness, especially if changes to medication are made
- when medication that may interact with existing therapy is introduced
- if the patient experiences symptoms such as syncope or 'fits' that could be due to arrhythmia.

It is also important to check urea and electrolyte levels, particularly plasma potassium, especially in patients at higher risk of electrolyte abnormalities (e.g. those with anorexia nervosa or dehydration or those who are taking diuretics).

When to consult a cardiologist

For many clinical questions, a telephone call to a 'friendly' cardiologist may suffice to resolve a concern. An ECG can often be faxed or emailed for an opinion.

Severe chest pain with ECG changes suggestive of a myocardial infarction is a medical emergency.

If a referral is necessary, the referring doctor should provide:

- a detailed history (as the patient may be more communicative with a familiar face than with a stranger)
- a statement regarding the likelihood that the patient is sufficiently cooperative to accept appropriate investigations
- current medication and doses of both psychiatric and medical drugs, whether used regularly or intermittently
- if available, a set of laboratory and imaging results (full blood count, urea and electrolytes, recent ECG and chest X-ray, glucose and lipid levels, thyroid function test).

Chest pain

- Refer to cardiology if there is a likelihood of myocardial ischaemia.

- Initiate simple treatment – a short-acting nitrate (GTN) and a long-acting nitrate daily (imdur – isosorbide mononitrate – or equivalent) are safe and effective for symptom relief; aspirin for secondary prophylaxis.
- Determine cardiovascular risk profile and risk score.

If symptoms are *atypical* (i.e. are not related to exercise or are triggered by food or emotion and stress), consider non-cardiac causes of chest pain.

Breathlessness

- Refer to cardiology if you have excluded pulmonary disease and symptoms suggest cardiac failure. Heart failure is very *unlikely* if the ECG is normal. The B-type natriuretic peptide (BNP) level will be abnormal.
- Initiate simple treatment – a loop diuretic (furosemide) daily and an ACE inhibitor (such as ramipril)
- Determine cardiovascular risk profile and risk score.

Palpitations

- Refer to cardiology if symptoms suggest a serious dysrhythmia. If it is associated with chest pain, breathlessness or dizziness, it warrants urgent admission.
- Refer to cardiology if a previously regular pulse becomes irregular, rapid or very slow.

Syncope or pre-syncope

A detailed history is even more important here. Comments from an observer may be pivotal. Postural symptoms are often induced by medication.

- Refer to cardiology if dizziness occurs in patient with:
  - a known cardiac history such as angina or heart failure
  - a heart murmur
  - a cardiac arrhythmia.

Abnormalities on ECG

Most ECG machines will provide an interpretation. Sometimes this will be correct.

- Refer to cardiology if the cardiac rate is below 60 or above 100 beats/min. Arrange emergency admission if:
  - there is chest pain, breathlessness or dizziness
  - the ECG suggests complete heart block or ventricular tachycardia
- If the QTc is prolonged, the patient generally responds to lowering of the dose of antipsychotic medication, reducing the risk of a serious ventricular dysrhythmia.

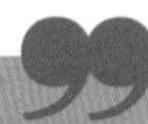

Summary

Patients with psychiatric disorders are at increased risk of developing cardiovascular disease. Because they may not have ready access to the services of a family doctor, they may not benefit from risk assessment and risk reduction strategies that those without psychiatric conditions take for granted. The mental health team may need to act as surrogates for the primary care team.

If a patient does report symptoms of chest pain, breathlessness or palpitations, it is helpful if someone on the mental health team has a working knowledge of cardiac disease and has access to a cardiologist prepared to help with the interpretation of ECGs and to give advice on disease management .

References

1 World Health Organization. Cardiovascular diseases (www.who.int/topics/cardiovascular_diseases/en).

2 British Cardiac Society, British Hypertension Society, Diabetes UK, *et al.* Joint British Societies' guidelines on prevention of cardiovascular disease in clinical practice. *Heart* 2005; **91** (suppl v): v1–52.

3 Joint Formulary Committee. *British National Formulary.* British Medical Association and Royal Pharmaceutical Society, various years (http://bnf.org/bnf/index.htm).

4 Empana JP, Ducimetiere P, Arveiler D, *et al.* Are the Framingham and PROCAM coronary heart disease risk functions applicable to different European populations? The PRIME Study. *Eur Heart J* 2003; **24**: 1903–11.

5 Haffner SM, Lehto S, Ronnemaa T, *et al.* Mortality from coronary heart disease in subjects with type 2 diabetes and in non-diabetic subjects with and without prior myocardial infarction. *N Engl J Med* 1998; **339**: 229–34.

6 Kannel WB, McGee DL. Diabetes and cardiovascular disease: the Framingham study. *JAMA* 1979; **241**: 2035–58.

7 Stamler J, Vaccaro O, Neaton JD, *et al.* Diabetes, other risk factors, and 12-yr cardiovascular mortality for men screened in the Multiple Risk Factor Intervention Trial. *Diabetes Care* 1993; **16**: 434–44.

8 National Institute for Health and Clinical Excellence. *Lipid Modification (Clinical Guidelines CG67).* NICE, 2008.

9 National Institute for Health and Clinical Excellence. *Statins for the Prevention of Cardiovascular Events (Technology Appraisal TA94)*. NICE, 2006.

10 Williams B, Poulter NR, Brown MJ, *et al*. Guidelines for management of hypertension: report of the fourth working party of the British Hypertension Society, 2004. *J Human Hypertens* 2004; **18**: 139–85.

11 Srensen HT, Meelemkjaer L, Blot WJ, *et al*. Risk of upper gastrointestinal bleeding associated with the risk of low dose aspirin. *Am J Gastroenterol* 2000; **95**: 2218–24.

12 Antithrombotic Triallists' (ATT) Collaboration. Aspirin in the primary and secondary prevention of vascular disease: collaborative meta-analysis of individual participant data from randomised trials. *Lancet* 2009; **373**: 1849–60.

13 National Institute for Health and Clinical Excellence. *About the Quality and Outcomes Framework*. NICE (http://www.nice.org.uk/aboutnice/qof/qof.jsp).

14 Williams B. Treatment of hypertension in the UK: simple as ABCD? *J R Soc Med* 2003; **96**: 521–2.

15 Calhoun DA, Jones D, Textor S, *et al*. Resistant hypertension: diagnosis, evaluation, and treatment: a scientific statement from the American Heart Association Professional Education Committee of the Council for High Blood Pressure Research. *Hypertension* 2008; **51**: 1403–19.

16 Williams B, Poulter NR, Brown MJ, *et al*. Guidelines for management of hypertension: report of the fourth working party of the British Hypertension Society, 2004 – BHS IV. *J Hum Hypertens* 2004; **18**: 139–85.

17 National Institute for Health and Clinical Excellence. *Hypertension: Clinical Management of Primary Hypertension in Adults* (CG127). NICE, 2011.

18 Royal College of Psychiatrists. *Consensus Statement on High-Dose Antipsychotic Medication (Council Report CR138)*. Royal College of Psychiatrists, 2006.

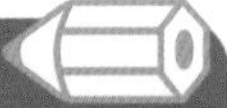

Learning points

- Cardiovascular disease is a common cause of mortality and morbidity.
- Those with a mental disorder are often at increased risk of developing cardiovascular disease because of medication, lifestyle and reduced access to advice on disease prevention.
- The risk of developing coronary heart disease can be estimated using readily available risk calculators.
- All patients should be assessed for reversible health risk factors when first referred for psychiatric assessment and findings should be recorded prominently in the patient record.
- Reducing risk factors such as hypertension, hypercholesterolaemia and smoking reduces risk.
- Patients who report chest pain, breathlessness or 'palpitations' may have cardiovascular disease.
- It can be difficult to determine whether these may be due to life-threatening disease, so referral for further investigation may be needed.
- Patients on medication for psychosis or dementia may develop changes in cardiac rhythm that may present suddenly.
- Interpretation of an ECG is likely to be a skill that most psychiatrists will have long forgotten but ECG machines often provide an interpretation of the ECG; a cardiologist will advise if the ECG is 'abnormal'.
- Psychiatric patients face additional vascular risks compared with the normal population; their care needs to balance effective treatment for both physical and mental disorders.

13 Respiratory disease

Jonathan Corne and Vidya Navaratnum

Respiratory diseases are common in people with mental disorders. This chapter contains information about the management of asthma, chronic obstructive airways disease (COPD), pneumonia, bronchiectasis, tuberculosis, interstitial lung disease and sarcoidosis. Criteria are provided that can be used to assess the severity of respiratory infection.

Introduction

Respiratory disease frequently causes limiting symptoms due to breathlessness and fatigue. Mental health issues may restrict a patient's access to primary care services and so health professionals need to be aware of how to recognise when symptom control is inadequate and how to deal with simple changes to existing treatment before they seek expert help. Respiratory infections which develop in in-patients in mental health units can be treated locally, provided that clinicians can assess disease severity.

Respiratory disease is the third biggest killer in the UK, after cancer and circulatory disorders. There are more than 40 conditions which affect the lungs and/or airways and affect an individual's ability to breathe. They include lung cancer, tuberculosis, asthma, chronic obstructive pulmonary disease (COPD) and respiratory tract infections.

Lung disease is not simply related to smoking. A wide range of other factors affect lung health, including viral lung infections in childhood, passive smoking, genetics, occupational exposure to materials such as asbestos, nutrition and social deprivation. There are clear social class gradients in respiratory disease mortality, with

Mental healthcare professionals need a working knowledge of respiratory illness because:

- those with intellectual difficulties are three times more likely than the general population to die of respiratory disease
- men and women with schizophrenia or bipolar disorder are at greater risk of dying from respiratory disease
- institutional living puts individuals at risk of primary respiratory infection and reinfection
- susceptible patients may not receive 'flu vaccination
- respiratory disease is common in smokers and smoking is more prevalent in people with mental illness
- patients' treatment may be interrupted by respiratory illness
- for each degree of severity of chronic airways disease, those with mental illness have a worse quality of life.

steeper social class gradients for respiratory disease mortality than for mortality in general.

Asthma

Asthma can be defined as chronic airways inflammation that has led to increased responsiveness to various stimuli. Approximately 130 million people worldwide suffer from asthma, with the disease being more prevalent in urban and higher-income societies such as Australia, Europe and America. In the UK alone, up to 7% of the population suffer from asthma.

The aetiology of asthma is multifactorial and is due to a complex interaction of intrinsic and extrinsic factors. The end result is bronchoconstriction due to airways inflammation and hyper-responsiveness. There is strong evidence of a hereditary component to asthma, with increased prevalence in first-degree relatives, although the genetic contribution is complex, involving polygenic inheritance and genetic heterogenicity. The extrinsic component comes from environmental factors such as cigarette smoke, house dust mites and pollen.

Pathophysiologically, asthma may be due to:

- hyper-responsiveness to environmental stimuli
- increased inflammatory cells in bronchi
- hypersecretion of mucus and swelling of mucosa, lead up to oedema
- narrowing of airways
- remodelling of airways.

Diagnosing asthma

The diagnosis of asthma is predominantly clinical, confirmed by a few investigations. Patients present with:

- breathlessness
- wheeze
- chest tightness
- chronic dry cough.

When evaluating a patient with asthma, do not forget to ask about:

- family history of asthma and atopic disease
- home environment
- occupational history
- trigger factors
- responsiveness to treatment.

The key feature is the diurnal or seasonal variation of these symptoms. Examination can be unremarkable, especially if the disease is quiescent. The most common examination findings are diffuse bilateral expiratory wheeze and a prolonged expiratory phase in respiration. There also may be features of associated atopic diseases such as rhinitis and eczema.

Investigation of asthma

The most useful investigation in these patients is peak flow monitoring, which helps to confirm the diagnosis. A peak flow meter is a small portable instrument which measures the maximum speed of expiration, or *peak expiratory flow rate* (PEF). Normal, expected PEF depends on a patient's sex, age and height (Fig. 13.3). In general, peak flow readings are higher when a person is well and lower when the airways are constricted.

Patients are given a peak flow diary to record peak flows over a minimum of 2 weeks. Those with asthma will demonstrate diurnal or seasonal variation of peak flow recordings (usually around 20% variability) as well as morning dipping (prominent symptoms and reduced peak flow recordings first thing in the morning). Formal lung function testing can be useful in older patients with a smoking history, to look for reversibility to bronchodilators.

General management of asthma

Management requires a multidisciplinary team approach. The pivotal aspects of this are patient education, a patient-centred approach to monitoring of the disease and treatment options, and liaison with respiratory nurse specialists.

Pharmacological management of asthma

The pharmacological management of chronic asthma involves a variety of different therapies and a *step-up* regimen. The guidelines produced by the British Thoracic Society and the Scottish Intercollegiate Guidelines Network[1] adopt a stepwise approach to treatment (Figs 13.1 and 13.2), aimed at controlling the disease with minimal side-effects, stepping up or down treatment as necessary.

Drug treatments can be broadly classified as bronchodilators (asthma *relievers*) and anti-inflammatory drugs (asthma *preventers*).

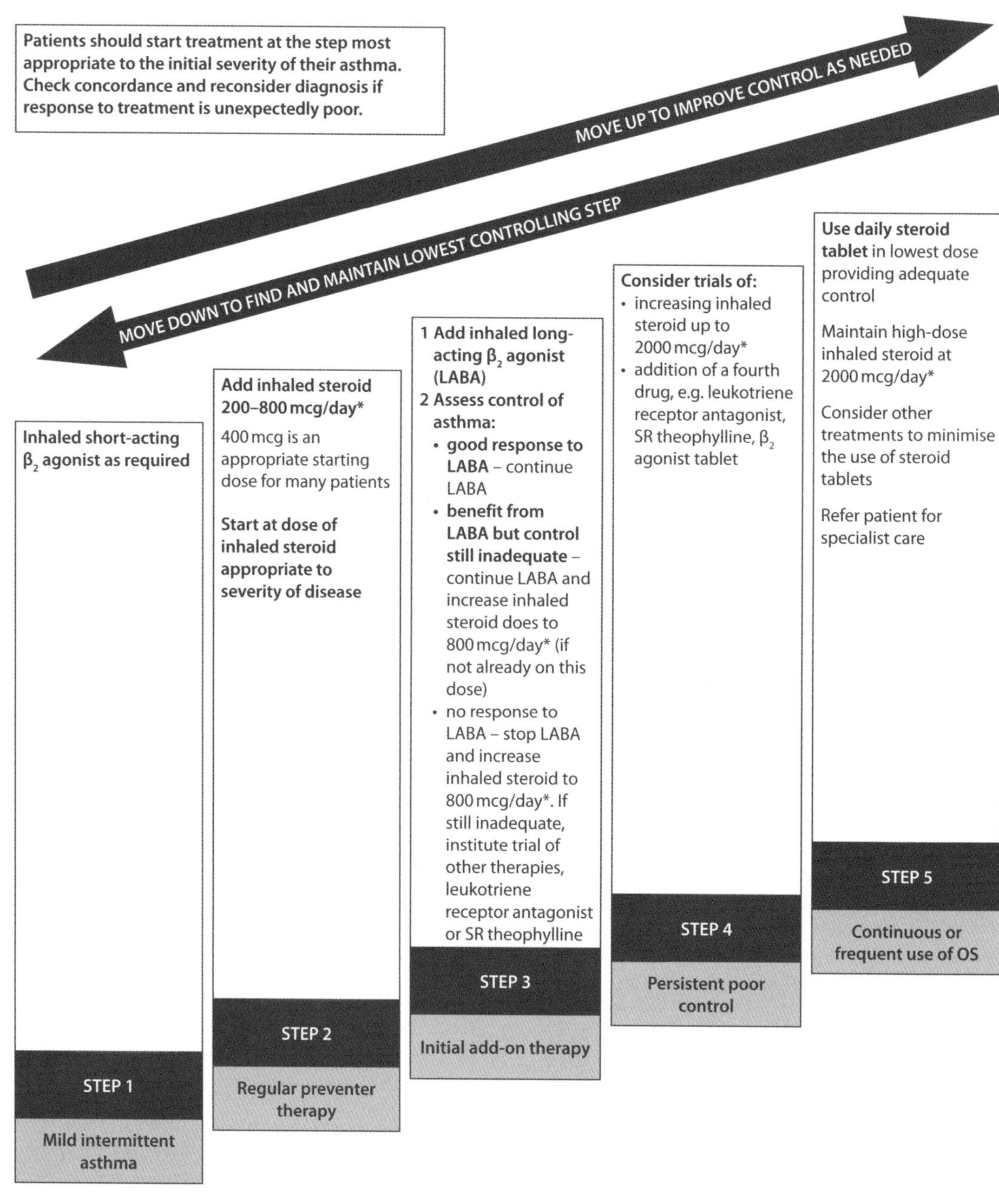

Patients should start treatment at the step most appropriate to the initial severity of their asthma. Check concordance and reconsider diagnosis if response to treatment is unexpectedly poor.
MOVE UP TO IMPROVE CONTROL AS NEEDED
MOVE DOWN TO FIND AND MAINTAIN LOWEST CONTROLLING STEP
Inhaled short-acting β2 agonist as required
STEP 1
Mild intermittent asthma
Add inhaled steroid 200–800 mcg/day*
400 mcg is an appropriate starting dose for many patients
Start at dose of inhaled steroid appropriate to severity of disease
STEP 2
Regular preventer therapy
1 Add inhaled long-acting β2 agonist (LABA)
2 Assess control of asthma:
• good response to LABA – continue LABA
• benefit from LABA but control still inadequate – continue LABA and increase inhaled steroid does to 800 mcg/day* (if not already on this dose)
• no response to LABA – stop LABA and increase inhaled steroid to 800 mcg/day*. If still inadequate, institute trial of other therapies, leukotriene receptor antagonist or SR theophylline
STEP 3
Initial add-on therapy
Consider trials of:
• increasing inhaled steroid up to 2000 mcg/day*
• addition of a fourth drug, e.g. leukotriene receptor antagonist, SR theophylline, β2 agonist tablet
STEP 4
Persistent poor control
Use daily steroid tablet in lowest dose providing adequate control
Maintain high-dose inhaled steroid at 2000 mcg/day*
Consider other treatments to minimise the use of steroid tablets
Refer patient for specialist care
STEP 5
Continuous or frequent use of OS
SYMPTOMS V. TREATMENT

Abbreviations:
OS, oral steroids; SR, sustained release.
*Beclometasone dipropionate or equivalent

Fig. 13.1 Summary of stepwise management of asthma in adults. From British Thoracic Society and Scottish Intercollegiate Guidelines Network guidelines on the treatment of asthma,[1] with permission.

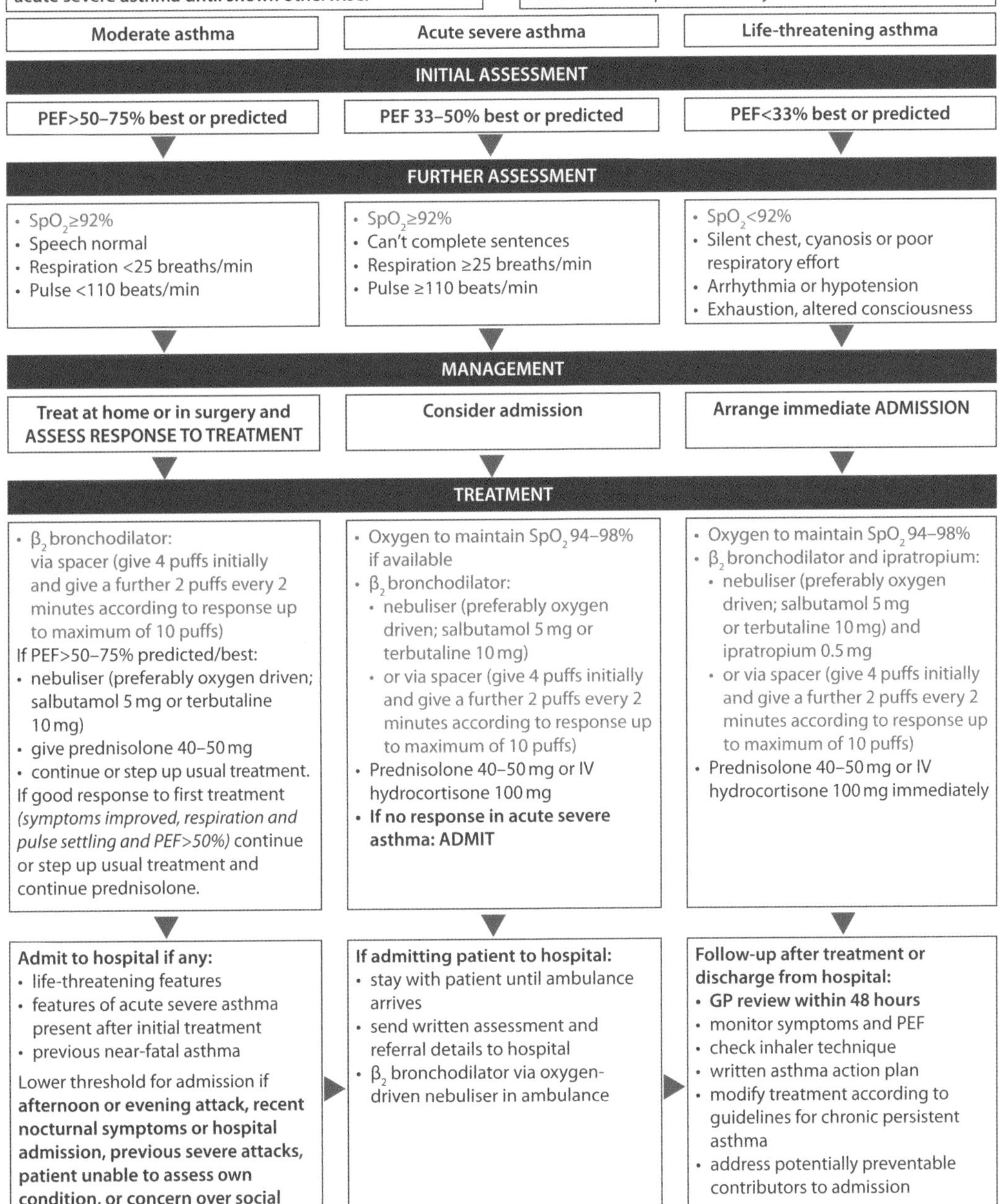

Fig. 13.2 Management of acute severe asthma in adults in general practice. From British Thoracic Society and Scottish Intercollegiate Guidelines Network guidelines on the treatment of asthma,[1] with permission.

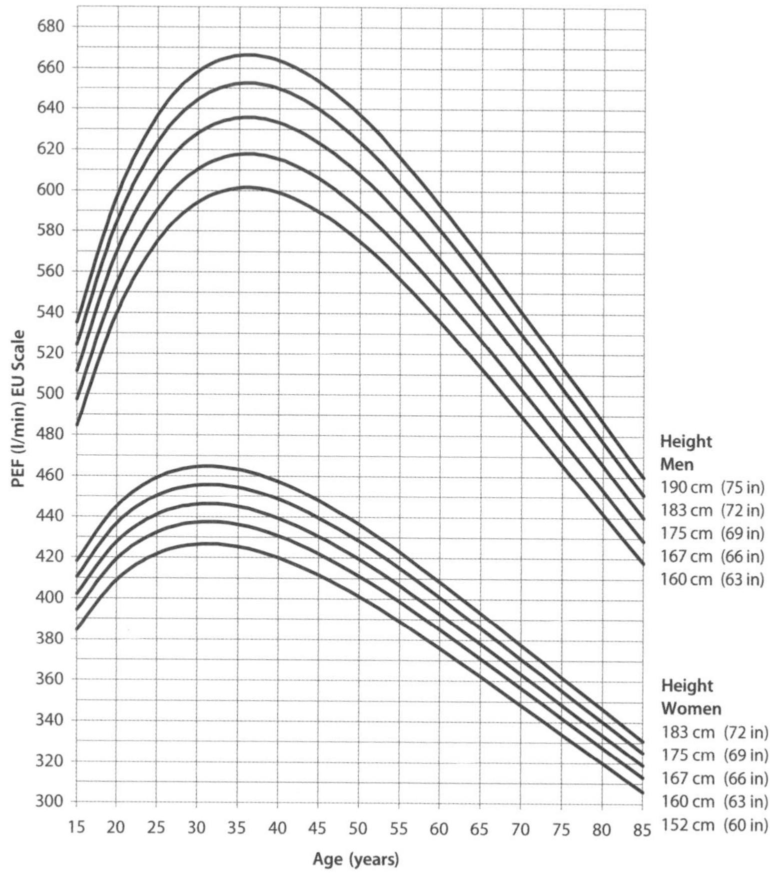

Fig. 13.3 Peak expiratory flow rate, normal values. From British Thoracic Society and Scottish Intercollegiate Guidelines Network guidelines on the treatment of asthma,[1] with permission.

Patients with few symptoms

Very mild disease can sometimes be managed by beta-2 agonists (such as salbutamol) alone, to provide bronchodilation when symptomatic. However, preventive treatment is necessary if bronchodilators are used more than three times a week, symptoms occur more than three times a week or the patient is waking more than once a week with nocturnal symptoms of cough, wheeze or shortness of breath. Inhaled corticosteroids such as fluticasone are the mainstay of preventive asthma treatment since they attenuate the inflammatory process in the airways.

Patients should be made aware that inhaled corticosteroids need to be taken regularly to control symptoms.

Poorly controlled asthma despite inhaled steroids

The next step is the addition of long-acting beta-2 agonists such as salmeterol and formoterol, given *in combination with* an inhaled corticosteroid. Leukotriene receptor antagonists such as montelukast block the pro-inflammatory effects of leukotrienes and can be added if control is not achieved with combinations of long-acting beta-agonist and inhaled corticosteroid. Other drugs used to control asthma, such as theophylline (a phosphodiesterase inhibitor) and omalizumab (a monoclonal anti-IgE administered subcutaneously), are best prescribed by a specialist.

Some prescription medication (see below) can make asthma worse and some over–the-counter

Drugs generally contraindicated in asthma include:
- beta-blockers such as atenolol
- non-steroidal anti-inflammatory drugs such as naproxen
- aspirin
- adenosine.

medication (antihistamines and decongestants), while they may provide some symptomatic relief, can cause nervousness, anxiety, tachycardia and sleep disturbance, so it is important to take a detailed drug history.

When to refer to a respiratory specialist

Most patients with asthma can be managed in the community. Referral to a respiratory physician is recommended when:
- the diagnosis of asthma is in doubt
- the asthma may be 'occupational'
- the asthma is difficult to manage.

Brittle asthma

Brittle asthma is defined as asthma with persistent symptoms or frequent exacerbations despite treatment at steps 4 or 5 of the British Thoracic Society's guidelines (Fig. 13.1). Patients should be assessed carefully to confirm both the diagnosis of asthma and their compliance with therapy.

Brittle asthma is associated with psychological comorbidity and assessment should include psychosocial issues.

Acute severe asthma

Patients with asthma, especially brittle asthma, are prone to *sudden* attacks of *severe* asthma, usually provoked by environmental circumstances such as viral infections, allergen exposure or change in treatment. Underestimation of the severity of the attack is the commonest cause of mortality in these patients.

The occurrence of any of the following indicates a severe asthma exacerbation:
- severe breathlessness – patient unable to complete a sentence in a single breath
- tachypnoea – respiratory rate > 25 breaths/min
- tachycardia – pulse rate > 110 beats/min
- peak flow recording of < 50% predicted.

An arterial blood gas test and a chest X-ray are essential investigations.

It is important that these patients are assessed and treated urgently. The immediate management would include:
- high concentrations of oxygen
- repeated nebulisers – 2.5 mg salbutamol nebulisers every 15–30 minutes *or* multiple doses of salbutamol inhaler via a spacer if a nebuliser is not available
- high-dose systemic corticosteroids – prednisolone 40 mg orally or hydrocortisone 100 mg.

Features of life-threatening asthma

The features of life-threatening asthma can be encapsulated as 'CHEST 92–33':

C – **C**yanosis
H – **H**ypotension
E – **E**xhaustion
S – **S**ilent chest
T – **T**achycardia
92 oxygen saturation < 92%
33 peak expiratory flow rate (PEFR) < 33% predicted.

Chronic obstructive pulmonary disease (COPD)

Chronic obstructive pulmonary disease (COPD) is best described as a slowly progressive disorder that involves alveolar destruction, mucous hypersecretion and non-reversible airways obstruction. In the UK in 2004, over 27 000 men and women died from COPD, most being over the age of 65.

There is a strong and well-established link between tobacco smoking and COPD, and so it is an important comorbidity in patients with other smoking-related diseases such as ischaemic heart disease and lung cancer. There are also certain poorly defined genetic factors that seem to increase an individual's susceptibility to developing the disease. The rare inherited disorder, alpha-1 antitrypsin deficiency, accounts for less than 1% of all COPD.

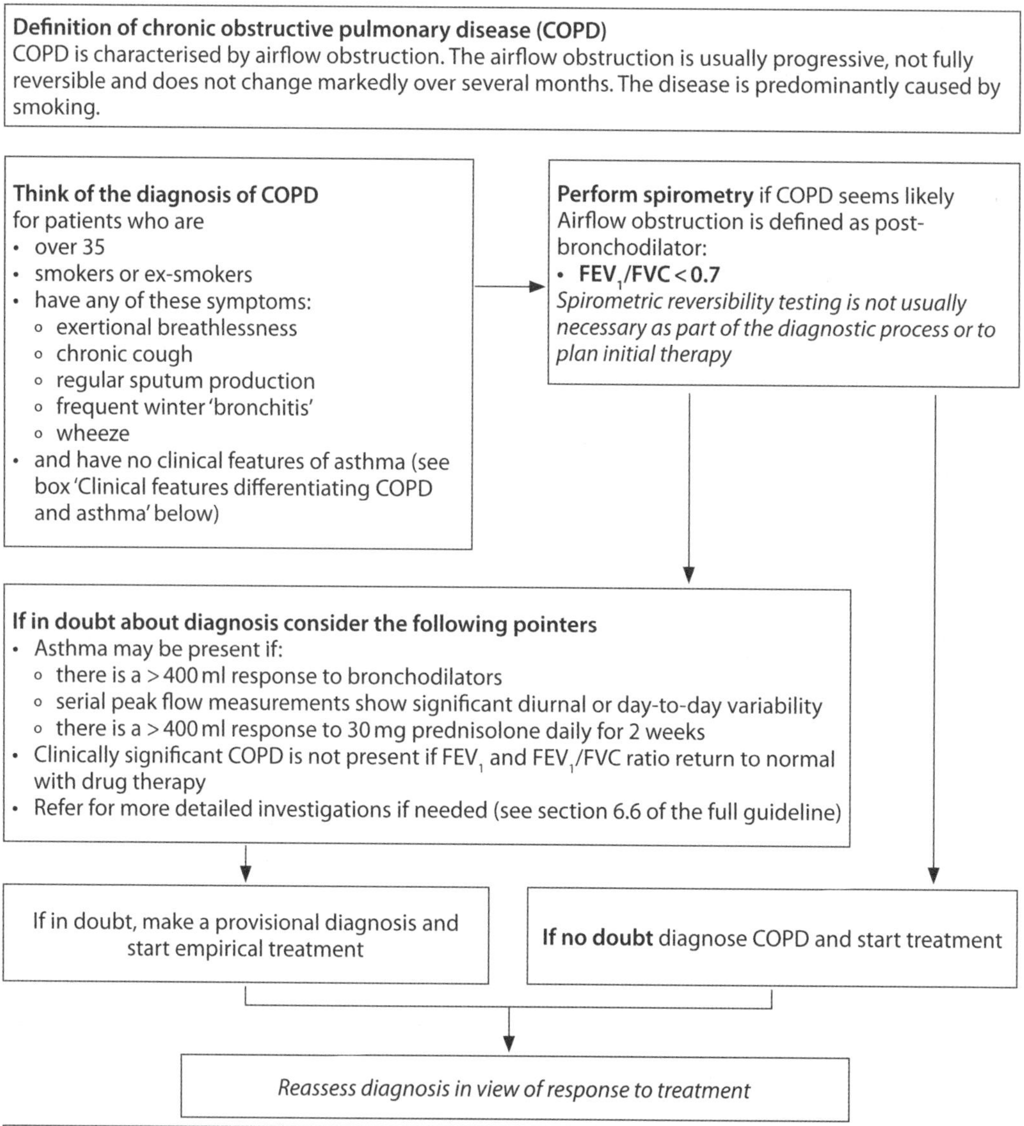

Definition of chronic obstructive pulmonary disease (COPD)
COPD is characterised by airflow obstruction. The airflow obstruction is usually progressive, not fully reversible and does not change markedly over several months. The disease is predominantly caused by smoking.

Think of the diagnosis of COPD
for patients who are
- over 35
- smokers or ex-smokers
- have any of these symptoms:
  - exertional breathlessness
  - chronic cough
  - regular sputum production
  - frequent winter 'bronchitis'
  - wheeze
- and have no clinical features of asthma (see box 'Clinical features differentiating COPD and asthma' below)

→

Perform spirometry if COPD seems likely
Airflow obstruction is defined as post-bronchodilator:
- **FEV_1/FVC < 0.7**

Spirometric reversibility testing is not usually necessary as part of the diagnostic process or to plan initial therapy

If in doubt about diagnosis consider the following pointers
- Asthma may be present if:
  - there is a > 400 ml response to bronchodilators
  - serial peak flow measurements show significant diurnal or day-to-day variability
  - there is a > 400 ml response to 30 mg prednisolone daily for 2 weeks
- Clinically significant COPD is not present if FEV_1 and FEV_1/FVC ratio return to normal with drug therapy
- Refer for more detailed investigations if needed (see section 6.6 of the full guideline)

If in doubt, make a provisional diagnosis and start empirical treatment

If no doubt diagnose COPD and start treatment

Reassess diagnosis in view of response to treatment

Clinical features differentiating COPD and asthma

	COPD	Asthma
Smoker or ex-smoker	Nearly all	Possibly
Symptoms under age 35	Rare	Often
Chronic productive cough	Common	Uncommon
Breathlessness	Persistent and progressive	Variable
Night-time waking with breathlessness and/or wheeze	Uncommon	Common
Significant diurnal or day-to-day variability of sympro ms	Uncommon	Common

Fig. 13.4 An algorithm for the diagnosis of chronic obstructive pulmonary disease (COPD). From NICE clinical guideline CG101,[2] with permission.

Diagnosing COPD

There is a wide spectrum of symptoms and severity in patients with COPD but the predominant symptoms are:

- progressive breathlessness
- wheeze
- productive cough.

A useful classification of COPD is:

- chronic bronchitis – a cough productive of sputum on most days for at least 3 months of the year for 2 successive years (this is often due to smoking-related mucus gland hypertrophy, resulting in mucus hypersecretion)
- airways obstruction – narrowing of the airways along with resistance to airflow produces an obstructive picture on spirometry, namely a reduced FEV1/FVC ratio (< 70%) (see below)
- emphysema – dilation of the terminal airways distal to the terminal bronchioles (destruction of the alveolar wall results in loss of elastic recoil and collapse of the small airways on expiration, with the end result of air trapping and hyperinflation of the chest).

An algorithm for the diagnosis of COPD is presented in Fig. 13.4.

Investigation of COPD

Spirometry is the most common of the pulmonary function tests (PFTs). Spirometry (Table 13.1) measures the volume (FVC – forced vital capacity) and flow (FEV1 – forced expiratory volume in 1 second) of air that a patient can achieve while exhaling. A patient with COPD will have a reduced FEV1 (usually < 80% of predicted) and a reduced FEV1/FVC ratio (< 70%). Most general practitioners have facilities to perform spirometry in their surgeries, but more detailed lung function tests requires referral to a respiratory physician.

A chest X-ray can be undertaken to exclude other diagnoses as well as to identify complications of COPD (see below). A full blood count is also useful as it can sometimes reveal polycythaemia in patients with chronic hypoxaemia, which could predispose them to a stroke. As COPD progresses, it is important to monitor oxygen saturations or arterial blood gases to identify patients who develop hypoxia (low O_2) and/or hypercapnia (high CO_2). Patients with suspected cor pulmonale may also benefit from echocardiography to evaluate pulmonary artery pressures.

Table 13.1 Spirometry

Test	Description
Forced vital capacity (FVC)	Volume of air that can forcibly be blown out after full inspiration. May be normal or marginally reduced in COPD.
Forced expiratory volume in 1 second (FEV1)	Volume of air that can forcibly be blown out in the first second during the FVC manoeuvre. This will be reduced in COPD.
FEV1 % (= FEV1/FVC as a percentage)	This is the ratio of FEV1 to FVC. In healthy adults this should be approximately 75–80%. This ratio will be reduced in COPD

Complications of COPD

Complications of COPD include:

- *Respiratory failure* is characterised by symptoms of progressive breathlessness and hypoxaemia. It worsens with an acute exacerbation.
- *Hypercapnia*, which causes headaches upon waking, general malaise and lethargy.
- *Cor pulmonale* is right heart failure secondary to chronic lung disease. Patients present with peripheral oedema, raised jugular venous pressure, hepatomegaly and tricuspid regurgitation.

General management of COPD

All patients with COPD who are still smoking should be encouraged to stop and should be offered nicotine replacement therapy (unless contraindicated), as well as referral to local support services.

The National Institute for Health and Clinical Excellence (NICE) has produced guidelines on the management of COPD (Fig. 13.5).[2]

Pharmacological management of COPD

The aim is to improve symptoms and activities of daily living, as well as lung function. Management can be difficult.

Patients with mild disease

Beta-2 agonists (either short- or long-acting) can be used to treat breathlessness and exercise limitation.

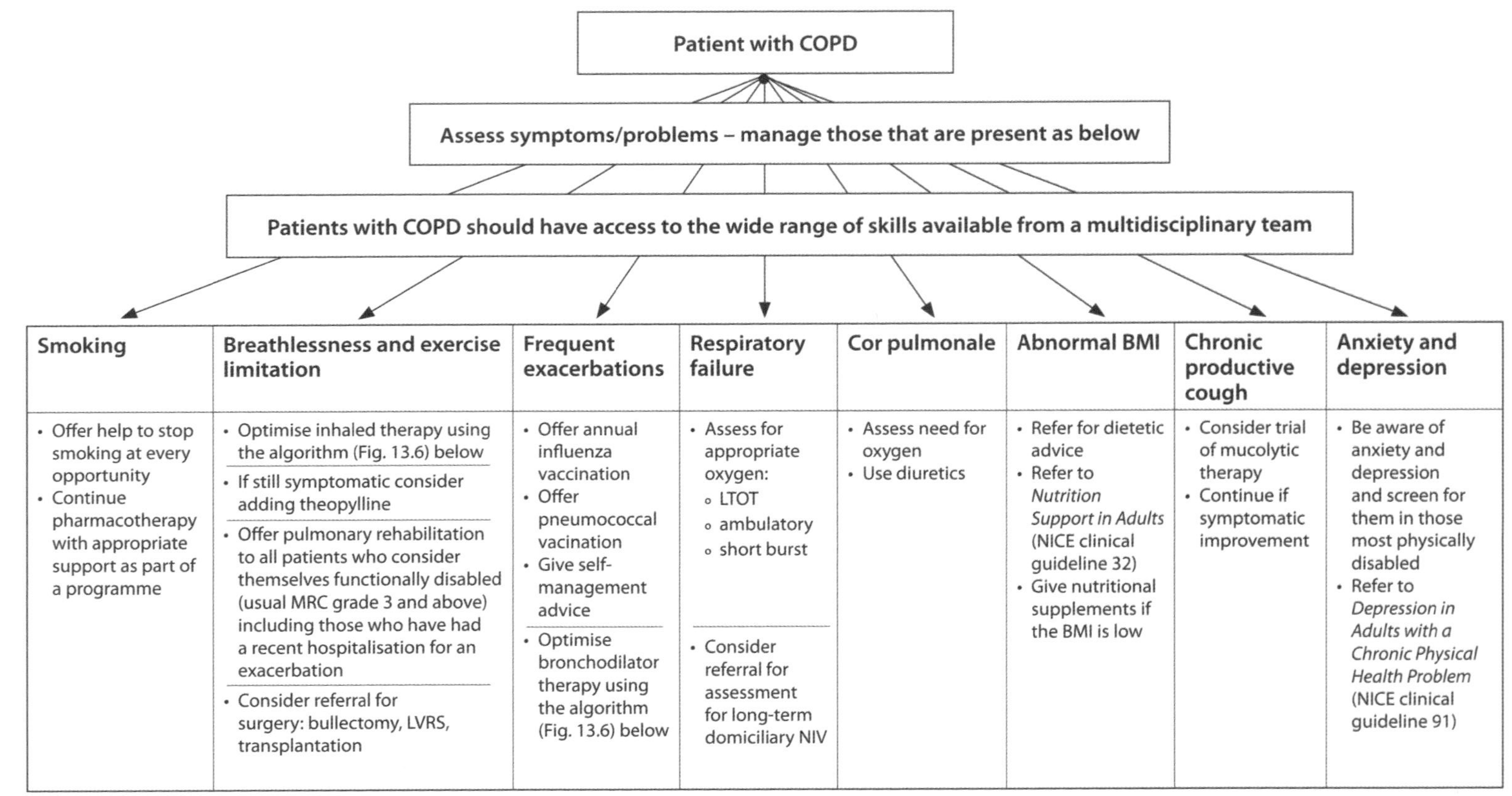

Patient with COPD
Assess symptoms/problems – manage those that are present as below
Patients with COPD should have access to the wide range of skills available from a multidisciplinary team
Smoking
• Offer help to stop smoking at every opportunity
• Continue pharmacotherapy with appropriate support as part of a programme
Breathlessness and exercise limitation
• Optimise inhaled therapy using the algorithm (Fig. 13.6) below
• If still symptomatic consider adding theopylline
• Offer pulmonary rehabilitation to all patients who consider themselves functionally disabled (usual MRC grade 3 and above) including those who have had a recent hospitalisation for an exacerbation
• Consider referral for surgery: bullectomy, LVRS, transplantation
Frequent exacerbations
• Offer annual influenza vaccination
• Offer pneumococcal vacination
• Give self-management advice
• Optimise bronchodilator therapy using the algorithm (Fig. 13.6) below
Respiratory failure
• Assess for appropriate oxygen:
◦ LTOT
◦ ambulatory
◦ short burst
• Consider referral for assessment for long-term domiciliary NIV
Cor pulmonale
• Assess need for oxygen
• Use diuretics
Abnormal BMI
• Refer for dietetic advice
• Refer to *Nutrition Support in Adults* (NICE clinical guideline 32)
• Give nutritional supplements if the BMI is low
Chronic productive cough
• Consider trial of mucolytic therapy
• Continue if symptomatic improvement
Anxiety and depression
• Be aware of anxiety and depression and screen for them in those most physically disabled
• Refer to *Depression in Adults with a Chronic Physical Health Problem* (NICE clinical guideline 91)
Palliative care
Opiates should be used when appropriate for the palliation of breathlessness in patients with end-stage COPD unresponsive to other medical therapy
Use benzodiazepines, tricyclic antidepressants, major tranquillisers and oxygen when appropriate
Involve multidisciplinary palliative care teams

Fig. 13.5 An algorithm for the management of chronic obstructive pulmonary disease (COPD). From National Institute for Health and Clinical Excellence (NICE) clinical guideline CG101.[2] Reproduced with permission. MRC, Medical Research Council; LVRS, lung volume reduction surgery; LTOT, long-term oxygen therapy; NIV, non-invasive ventilation; BMI, body mass index.

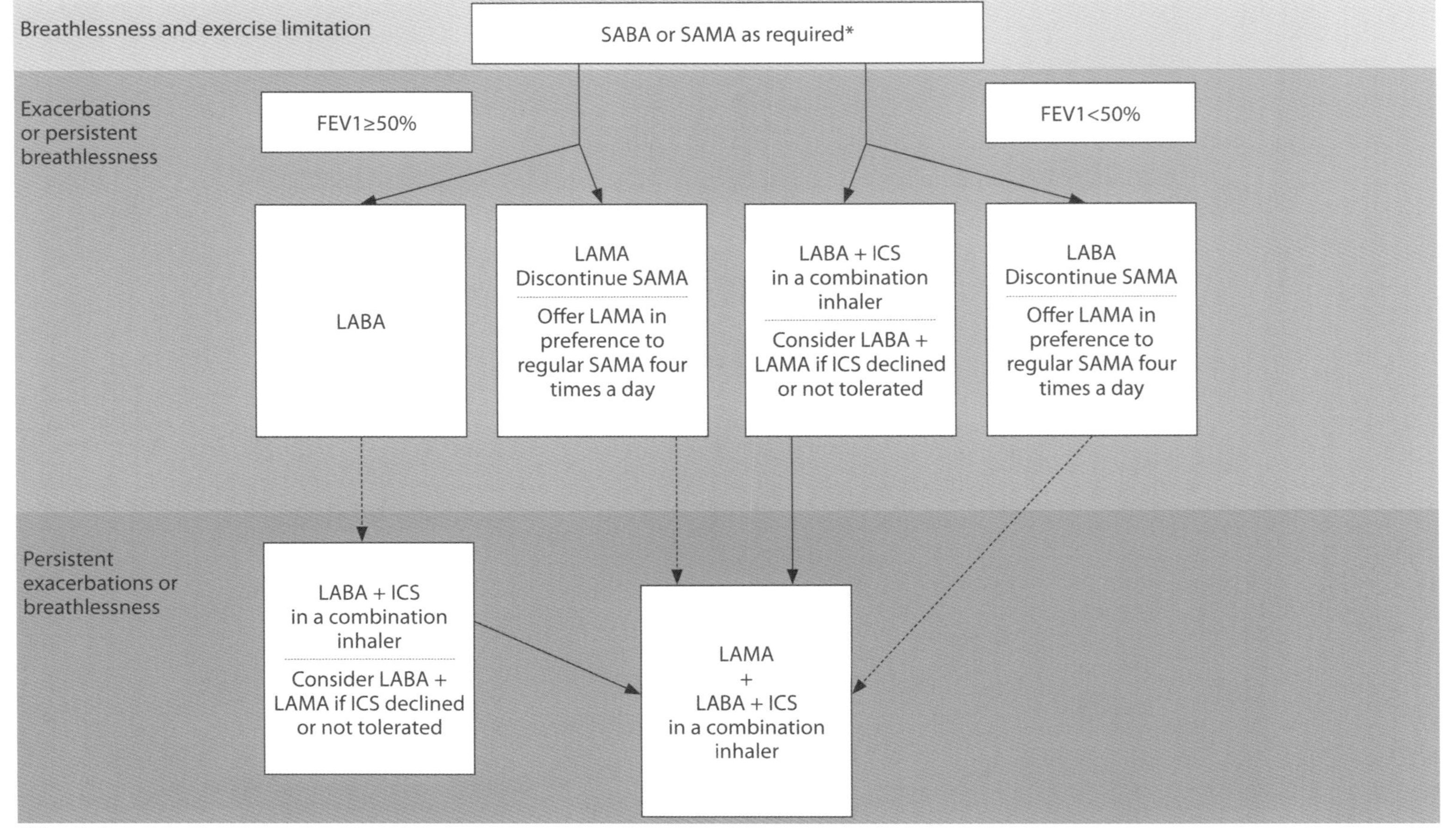

Abbreviations:
SABA, short-acting beta agonist; SAMA, short-acting muscarinic antagonist; LABA, long-acting beta agonist; LAMA, long-acting muscarinic antagonist; ICS, inhaled corticosteroid
*SABA (as required) may continue at all stages
——► Offer therapy (strong evidence) ------► Consider therapy (less strong evidence)

Fig. 13.6 An algorithm for the use of inhaled therapies for chronic obstructive pulmonary disease (COPD). From NICE clinical guideline CG101.[2] Reproduced with permission. This algorithm should be used within the wider context of the management of COPD (see Fig. 13.4, 13.5 and13.7).

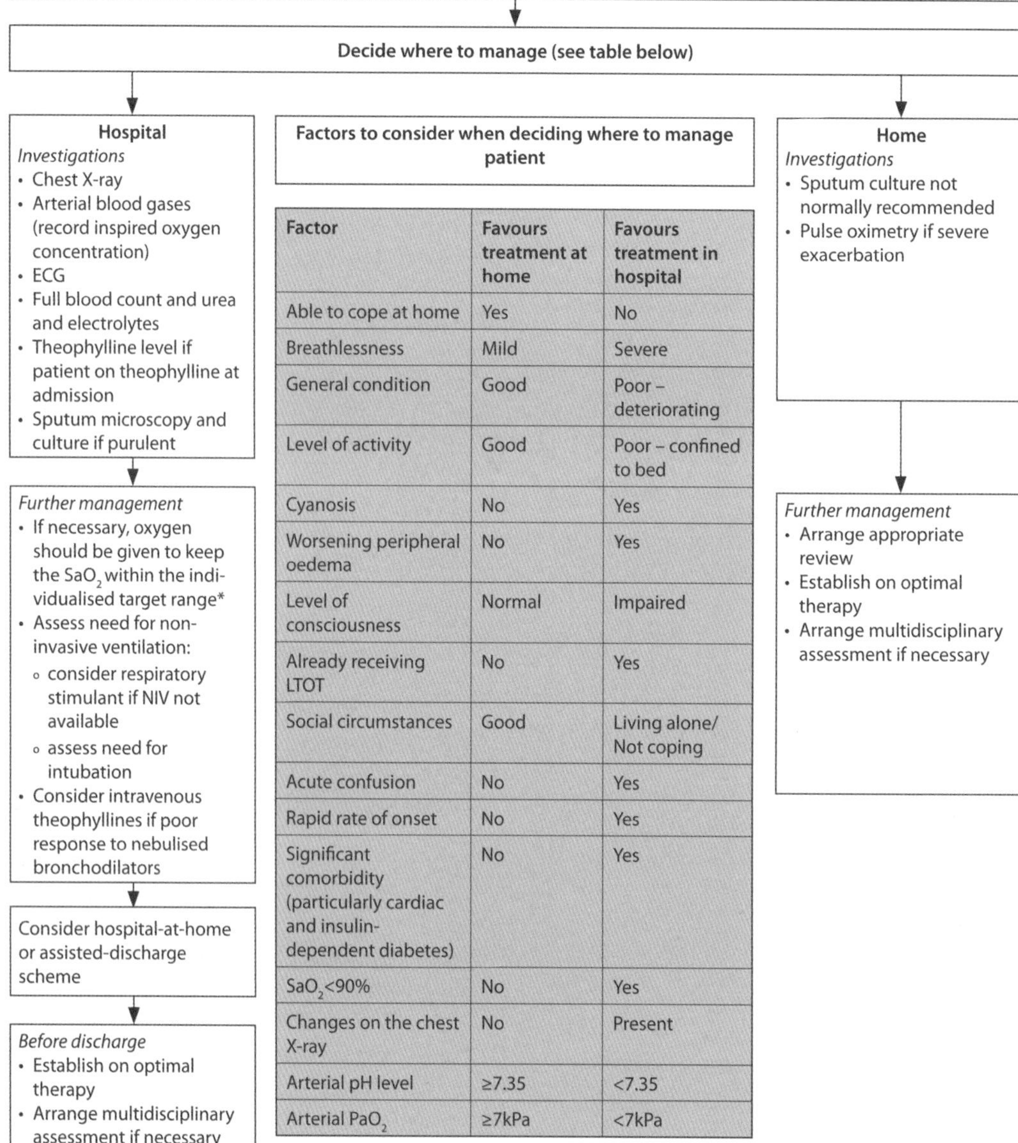

Factor	Favours treatment at home	Favours treatment in hospital
Able to cope at home	Yes	No
Breathlessness	Mild	Severe
General condition	Good	Poor – deteriorating
Level of activity	Good	Poor – confined to bed
Cyanosis	No	Yes
Worsening peripheral oedema	No	Yes
Level of consciousness	Normal	Impaired
Already receiving LTOT	No	Yes
Social circumstances	Good	Living alone/ Not coping
Acute confusion	No	Yes
Rapid rate of onset	No	Yes
Significant comorbidity (particularly cardiac and insulin-dependent diabetes)	No	Yes
SaO_2<90%	No	Yes
Changes on the chest X-ray	No	Present
Arterial pH level	≥7.35	<7.35
Arterial PaO_2	≥7kPa	<7kPa

Abbreviations: ECG, electrocardiogram; NIV, non-invasive ventilation; LTOT, long-term oxygen therapy; SaO_2, oxygen saturation of arterial blood; PaO_2, partial pressure of oxygen in arterial blood
*Readers should refer to local protocols for oxygen therapy

Fig. 13.7 An algorithm for the management of exacerbations of chronic obstructive pulmonary disease (COPD). From NICE clinical guideline CG101,[2] with permission.

Inhaled tiotropium, a long-acting anticholinergic, or one of the long-acting beta-2 agonists, should be given early to provide symptomatic relief in patients with COPD.

An algorithm for the use of inhaled medications is given in Fig. 13.6.

Patients who are still symptomatic

For those who are symptomatic despite tiotropium, or who have recurrent exacerbations (see also below) or whose FEV1 is less than 60% of predicted should be prescribed combinations of inhaled corticosteroids and long-acting beta-agonists; these improve symptoms, reduce exacerbation rates and may attenuate the decline in lung function.

Pulmonary rehabilitation is intended for patients with chronic respiratory problems who consider themselves functionally disabled by COPD, remain symptomatic, or whose pulmonary function has decreased despite medical treatment. It has been shown to be effective in improving exercise tolerance, quality of life and breathlessness, although the impact on mortality is uncertain.

As with asthma, inhaler technique is vital in the delivery of drugs and should be checked regularly.

Management of an acute exacerbation

This is similar to that of an acute asthma attack: the administration of nebulised bronchodilators, steroids and, if appropriate, antibiotics. Some patients with an acute exacerbation will present with type 2 respiratory failure, that is, decreased PaO_2 and elevated $PaCO_2$. Non-invasive ventilation (NIV), that is, the delivery of positive-pressure ventilation using a face or nasal mask rather than an endotracheal tube, may be beneficial in these patients as it avoids complications caused by invasive ventilation, such as infection and airway trauma.

Many hospitals have a coordinated early-discharge scheme for patients who need admission during an exacerbation. Specialist respiratory nurses with an interest in COPD help coordinate such programmes. They review patient inhaler technique, organise the assessment and delivery of home oxygen to appropriate patients and help link patients into the local smoking cessation service. Follow-up in the community can also be arranged with community respiratory nurses.

An algorithm for the management of exacerbations is given in Fig. 13.7, including the factors to consider when deciding where to manage the patient.

When to refer to a respiratory specialist

Like patients with asthma, most patients with COPD can be managed in the community. However, refer any patient if COPD is severe (FEV1 less than 30% of predicted); if functionally disabled by COPD for consideration for pulmonary rehabilitation; if symptoms are disproportionate to lung function; or symptoms are not controlled on 'usual' inhaler therapy.

Pneumonia

Pneumonia, an acute lower respiratory tract illness resulting in inflammation of the lung parenchyma, is an important cause of morbidity and mortality in all age groups. Approximately 1 in 1000 people in the UK are admitted to hospital with pneumonia each year. It is usually classified as 'community acquired' or 'hospital acquired', reflecting the different types of patients and pathogens involved.

- *Community-acquired pneumonia* is usually caused by bacterial infections, most often *Streptococcus pneumoniae* (50–60% of cases), *Haemophilus influenzae*, *Staphylococcus aureus* and atypical organisms such as *Mycoplasma pneumoniae*, *Legionella pneumophila* and *Chlamydia pneumoniae*. It can also be due to viral infection (usually influenza). Guidelines for the treatment of community-acquired pneumonia in adults are available from www.nuh.nhs.uk/antibiotics.
- *Hospital-acquired pneumonia*, that is, pneumonia developing in patients hospitalised for 2 or more days, is usually secondary to other illnesses. It most often involves infection with *Escherichia coli* and *Pseudomonas aeruginosa* following the use of broad-spectrum antibiotics in those with an impaired immune system – the greater the immune system compromise, the more likely is an unusual infection such as *Mycobacterium* and fungal infections.

Symptoms of pneumonia include:

- fever
- shortness of breath
- pleuritic chest pain
- productive cough with purulent sputum
- lethargy, malaise and myalgia.

Infections can also present with urinary, gastro-intestinal symptoms and joint pain in the absence of any respiratory symptoms. A travel history is important as

Box 13.1 Assessing the severity of pneumonia

'CURB-65'

C	Confusion
U	Urea >7 mmol/l
R	Respiratory rate >30/min
B	Blood pressure: systolic <90 mmHg, diastolic <60 mmHg
65	Age 65 years or over

A point is scored for the presence of each factor. If the CURB score is <2 (mild pneumonia) and there are no medical comorbidities, the patient can be treated in the community with oral antibiotics, as long as there are no other signs of severe illness.

Adapted from Lim *et al*, 2003.[3]

some infections have a geographical distribution and the responsible organisms have different profiles of antibiotic resistance.

General assessment gives an overall view of the patient's clinical state. Severe pneumonia warrants urgent hospital admission. Markers include:

- tachycardia – pulse rate > 100 beats per min
- low blood pressure – systolic pressure < 100 mmHg
- tachypnoea – respiratory rate > 20/min
- fever – temperature > 38°C
- reduced perfusion – reduced conscious level, 'dusky' hands or feet or a capillary refill time of greater than 2 seconds indicates that the patient is severely unwell and needs urgent hospital admission.

The 'CURB-65' assessment (see Box 13.1) has been devised to stratify severity specifically in patients with pneumonia.

Examination of the respiratory system of patients with pneumonia may reveal dullness of percussion, bronchial breathing and increased vocal resonance/tactile fremitus, though absence of these signs does not exclude the diagnosis.

Investigation of pneumonia

Investigations include:

- blood tests – full blood count, urea and electrolytes, C-reactive protein and blood cultures
- chest X-ray
- urine for pneumococcal antigen detection
- if an atypical infection is suspected, a serum sample for *Mycoplasma* IgM and/or urine for *Legionella* antigen.

Microbiological investigations are vital so that appropriate antibiotics can be prescribed. If the patient is unwell or hypoxic (Sats<93%), an arterial blood gas is also useful.

When to refer to a respiratory specialist

Patients with a CURB-65 score of 3 or more, or with a comorbidity, should be admitted to hospital.

Treatment of pneumonia

General measures include oxygen at high flow if required; antipyretics and analgesia; and monitoring of fluid balance. Intravenous broad-spectrum antibiotics are administered until the likely pathogen is identified. Amoxicillin, co-amoxiclav and cefuroxime are usually effective in treating pneumonia caused by *Streptococcus pneumoniae* or *Haemophilus influenzae*; erythromycin or clarithromycin may be given to cover atypical organisms such as *Mycoplasma* and *Legionella*. Monitor for complications, which include pleural effusions, empyema, lung abscess, and/or respiratory and/or multi-organ failure.

If these or other complications develop, or the patient fails to respond to treatment (i.e. remains pyrexial), or inflammatory markers such as CRP do not decline by half within 4 days, seek the advice of a respiratory physician.

Patients with pneumonia should be followed up at 6 weeks and those with persistent symptoms or signs or those at higher risk of underlying malignancy (aged over 50 and smokers) should have a follow-up chest X-ray at this time.

Tuberculosis

The World Health Organization estimates that tuberculosis affects 10 million people a year worldwide and up to a third of the world's population have a latent infection with *Mycobacterium tuberculosis*. The clinical presentation stems from a complex interaction between the organism and the patient's immune response. For this reason, tuberculosis can be divided in primary and post-primary tuberculosis.

In the UK there is a statutory requirement for the doctor to notify the public health authorities about any patient who has been diagnosed with tuberculosis.[4]

Primary tuberculosis can affect anyone who has no specific immunity to it. The inhaled organism settles in the lung and causes a reactive lymphadenopathy or Ghon focus, which is asymptomatic – the only telltale sign is calcified nodules on chest X-ray. Occasionally, active progression of the disease can occur at this stage, resulting in a cavitating lesion.

Post-primary tuberculosis results from either reactivation of the infection, usually in the lungs in elderly and immunocompromised patients; or reinfection from another individual. Patients usually present with symptoms such as:

- malaise, lethargy, weight loss and night sweats
- productive cough and haemoptysis.

Tuberculosis can affect any organ in the body and should always be considered in the differential diagnosis of patients with pyrexia of unknown origin. A chest X-ray should be requested, where a cavitating lesion is characteristic. Sputum samples should also be sent to test for acid-alcohol fast bacilli (AAFB).

When to refer to a respiratory specialist

Individuals with suspected (or confirmed) tuberculosis should be referred to a respiratory physician for further investigation and management. Most patients will undergo a 6-month course of quadruple therapy (2 months of rifampicin, isoniazid, pyrazinamide and ethambutol, followed by 4 months of rifampicin and isoniazid). Regular reviews are required, to monitor the toxic side-effects of many of the anti-tuberculous agents and to detect the emergence of drug resistance.

Directly observed therapy (DOT) is not usually needed in most with active tuberculosis but is useful to ensure patient compliance with medication, indirectly helping also to reduce the rates of multidrug-resistant tuberculosis secondary to non-adherence to quadruple therapy. Each patient should have a risk assessment for compliance to therapy and DOT should be considered for those with adverse risk factors such as no fixed abode or a history of non-adherence to treatment.

Miliary tuberculosis

This refers to widespread haematogenous dissemination of tuberculosis, usually characterised by multiple small nodules evident throughout the lung fields on chest X-ray. Symptoms are non-specific – pyrexia, persistent cough or lymphadenopathy. The most important risk factor for developing miliary tuberculosis is immunosuppression, particularly from HIV infection.

Untreated, the mortality approaches 100%. Up to 25% of patients with miliary tuberculosis will also have tuberculous meningitis. They should be referred to either a respiratory physician with an interest in tuberculosis or to a specialist in infectious diseases for further assessment and treatment.

Lung cancer

Lung cancer is the most common cancer worldwide, with 1.3 million new cases diagnosed globally every year, most caused by cigarette smoking. In the UK, about one in four men and one in five women smoke, in total about 12 million. Smoking rates are especially high in the psychiatric community (up to 74% in some studies).

The lifetime risk of developing lung cancer is 1 in 14 for men and 1 in 21 for women, the risk increasing with the number of cigarettes smoked daily. Passive smoking increases risk by up to 1.5%.

Occupational exposure to asbestos and ionising radiation accounts for some lung cancer in non-smokers, and asbestos exposure acts synergistically with tobacco smoke. Genetic predisposition in certain individuals is also acknowledged.

Lung cancer can be classified as small-cell carcinoma (20–30% of cases) or non-small-cell carcinoma (70–80%), based on the histology. Small-cell carcinoma is an aggressive malignancy that has usually metastasised by the time of presentation. At diagnosis, one-third of patients have disease limited to the lungs and their 2-year mortality rate is 25%. When spread is extensive, that is, outside the lungs, the prognosis is extremely poor, with a 5-year survival of less than 5%. Non-small-cell carcinoma usually presents earlier, has a better prognosis and is potentially curable by surgery.

Symptoms to look out for

- Cough/haemoptysis (even if the chest X-ray is normal)
- Chest pain

- Breathlessness/wheeze
- Change in voice, especially new-onset hoarseness
- Weight loss/anorexia
- Malaise/lethargy
- Anaemia.

Patients commonly have no physical signs, but always look out for signs of:

- systemic illness – cachexia, pallor and jaundice
- cervical lymphadenopathy
- clubbed finger nails
- hoarse voice
- localised lung collapse – deviated trachea, dullness to percussion, decreased vocal fremitus
- airways obstruction – fixed monophonic wheeze
- pleural effusions
- Horner's syndrome
- superior vena cava (SVC) obstruction.

Patients with small-cell lung cancer commonly present with symptoms secondary to metastases such as bone pain, jaundice (spread to liver), new-onset seizures, hemiparesis or change in personality (after there is spread to the frontal lobe). There are a host of neuroendocrine syndromes associated with small-cell lung cancer and these can present with psychiatric symptoms, due to the metabolic imbalance caused by, for example, hyponatraemia in the syndrome of inappropriate antidiuretic hormone secretion (SIADH) and hypercalcaemia, either from metastatic spread to bone or parathyroid-like hormone secretion.

Investigating, diagnosing and treating lung cancer

Arrange a chest X-ray for anyone suspected of having lung cancer. However, patients who are smokers or who have been exposed to asbestos who present with symptoms should be referred to a respiratory physician even if their chest X-ray is normal.

Investigations include baseline blood investigations and a staging computerised tomography (CT) scan of the chest, abdomen and pelvis. Tissue diagnosis of the lesion is vital in determining treatment options and prognosis. Patients with central/hilar lesions usually undergo a bronchoscopy and biopsy and those with a peripheral lesion need a CT-guided biopsy.

For small-cell carcinoma, the main treatment is chemotherapy, which may prolong life and reduce symptoms. For non-small-cell tumours, surgery can be curative if the patient is fit enough and the tumour is found at an early stage. For early-staged tumours, if surgery is not possible, intensive radiotherapy can be offered, which can improve the prognosis and quality of life. For more advanced non-small-cell lung cancers, where cure is not possible, chemotherapy is often given to improve both symptoms and quality of life; there may also be some benefit on survival. Palliative radiotherapy can be offered to relieve specific symptoms such as haemoptosis, superior vena cava obstruction, breathlessness due to lung collapse and pain or complications due to bony metastases. Input from palliative care physicians is often appropriate.

All patients with lung cancer should be discussed at a multidisciplinary team meeting, involving respiratory physicians, oncologists, thoracic surgeons, palliative care physicians and radiologists to determine the optimal treatment. In most hospitals, there are respiratory nurse specialists with an interest in lung cancer who help with breaking diagnoses to patients and follow-up with appropriate information and support once treatment options have been given.

> If you suspect lung cancer, refer the patient immediately for assessment. In the UK, patients should be referred to a respiratory physician under the '2-week wait' cancer pathway.

Bronchiectasis

Bronchiectasis is a chronic suppurative lung disease characterised by irreversible dilation of the proximal bronchi. Damage to the bronchial wall is secondary to chronic infection and inflammation.

The pathogenesis includes:

- an accumulation of secretions (usually secondary to defects in mucociliary clearance)
- persistent infection with an accompanying inflammatory response
- tissue damage secondary to the above
- persistent dilation of the bronchi.

Bronchiectasis may be congenital, most commonly due to cystic fibrosis, or acquired, from many causes, including hypogammaglobulinaemia, tumour, foreign body, fibrotic lung disease, autoimmune conditions (especially rheumatoid arthritis) and measles or pertussis infection in childhood. Around a third of cases are idiopathic.

The main symptom is a chronic productive cough with purulent sputum. In the case of intercurrent infection, the sputum is increased in volume and its colour is changed. Haemoptysis can be life-threatening. With chronic infection, systemic symptoms occur – lethargy, malaise, anorexia, weight loss and halitosis.

Clinical examination reveals coarse inspiratory crackles on auscultation of the chest. Patients with chronic severe disease may also appear malnourished (cachexia, short stature) and have digital clubbing.

Investigating, diagnosing and treating bronchiectasis

Patients are usually investigated and managed in secondary care by respiratory physicians. Routine investigations include full blood count and inflammatory markers. Spirometry can be useful in determining whether patients have reversible airflow obstruction. A sputum sample should be sent to microbiology to determine which organisms have colonised the lung secretions and are likely to cause infective exacerbations later. Bronchoscopy is indicated if an endobronchial lesion is the underlying cause.

Diagnosis is usually made with high-resolution CT (HRCT), which can sometimes also reveal an underlying cause. A common finding on the HRCT is the 'signet ring' sign, where the dilated bronchus is more prominent than the vasculature running alongside it.

Like most chronic respiratory conditions, bronchiectasis is best managed with a multidisciplinary team approach. Chest physiotherapy and postural drainage are the mainstay of management. This involves a physiotherapist lightly tapping the patient's chest, back and area under the arms. Breathing is improved by the indirect removal of mucus from the breathing passages.

Antibiotics play an important role in reducing chronic infections and the complications of infective exacerbations. Patients with established airflow reversibility benefit from bronchodilators, either inhaled or nebulised. Surgical options such as a lobectomy may occasionally be appropriate for areas of localised bronchiectasis, especially if complicated by episodes of recurrent or life-threatening haemoptysis.

Interstitial lung disease

This is an umbrella term used to describe a variety of acute and chronic disorders of inflammation and fibrosis of the lung parenchyma. A more accurate description is 'diffuse parenchymal lung disease' (DPLD).

Common causes of DPLD are:

- autoimmune and collagen vascular diseases such as rheumatoid arthritis, systemic sclerosis and sarcoidosis
- drugs such as amiodarone and methotrexate
- occupational and environmental exposure, such as asbestos or birds
- primary respiratory disease, for example idiopathic pulmonary fibrosis (IPF).

Key points in the history are:

- detailed occupational history
- pets, especially birds
- treatment history, including chemotherapy and radiotherapy
- symptoms of vasculitis and connective tissue disease.

Patients report symptoms that are indolent in nature, with progressive breathlessness on exertion being prominent; some will also present with a dry cough. Clinical examination reveals digital clubbing, cyanosis (in advanced disease) and fine end-inspiratory crepitations on auscultation. Patients with aggressive or advanced disease can present with symptoms and signs of right ventricular failure due to cor pulmonale. If due to a connective tissue disorder, signs of this may be present, such as joint deformities in rheumatoid arthritis, sclerodactyly and skin ulceration in systemic sclerosis.

Investigation, diagnosis and treatment

Investigations include blood for an autoimmune screen and a chest X-ray. Most patients will have reticulonodular changes on their chest X-ray, although a normal X-ray does not exclude the diagnosis. Tests of lung function will reveal a restrictive lung defect (reduced FEV and FVC, normal FEV1/FVC ratio, reduced transfer factor).

Diagnosis is based on HRCT, which can show a combination of 'ground glass' shadowing and fibrotic changes; if the diagnosis remains unclear, the patient should be referred for a lung biopsy.

Treatment is targeted at the underlying cause of the DPLD, for example removal of any causative exposure or implementation of immunosuppression for connective tissue disease.

In primary respiratory DPLD (usually IPF), no single pharmacological intervention is particularly effective.

The various forms of primary respiratory DPLD vary in their response to treatment; if treatment is given, it is usually a combination of oral corticosteroids, azathioprine and N-acetyl-cysteine. Patients are given supplemental oxygen for hypoxaemia and are monitored for progression of their disease. Unfortunately, the prognosis of IPF is extremely poor, with a median survival of approximately 3 years.

Sarcoidosis

This multi-system disease is defined by the presence of non-caseating granulomas in affected organs. The aetiology is unknown but involvement of the immune system, resulting in inflammation has been postulated. Clinical presentation is varied but a transient acute illness is followed by a chronic persistent form.

Acute sarcoidosis usually affects young adults; it is characterised by sudden onset of erythema nodosum, arthritis and uveitis. Bilateral hilar lymphadenopathy can be found incidentally on chest X-ray. It is usually a self-limiting illness that resolves spontaneously without treatment.

Chronic sarcoidosis is more indolent and more often found in older patients. It is characterised by non-specific symptoms, such as malaise, lethargy, weight loss, anorexia and night sweats. If the lung parenchyma is involved, the chest X-ray shows peri-hilar reticulonodular shadowing, which may progress to diffuse lung fibrosis and loss of lung function. If the central nervous system is involved, a host of neurological complaints and psychiatric symptoms, such as change in personality, hallucinations and even psychoses, may be evident.

Investigating, diagnosing and treating sarcoidosis

Serum immunoglobulins are raised, as are levels of both calcium and serum angiotensin converting enzyme (ACE), which are useful markers of disease activity but very non-specific. Diagnosis is clinical and radiological, but a transbronchial biopsy of lung tissue (if involved) or the biopsy of an involved lymph node can be extremely useful. Most patients with chronic sarcoidosis are treated with corticosteroids or steroid-sparing agents to suppress inflammation. Patients requiring long-term steroid use also need prophylaxis for complications such as osteoporosis and peptic ulceration.

Suspect sarcoidosis if:

- in a young adult, an unusual rash is associated with joint and eye problems – acute sarcoidosis is generally self-limiting
- in an older patient, malaise, lethargy and night sweats are associated with respiratory symptoms.

In chronic sarcoidosis, psychiatric symptoms may be evident.

Day-to-day issues that commonly present problems for psychiatrists

Acute onset of breathlessness – what to do

Establish the cause (if possible) and treat accordingly. Breathlessness which occurs over *minutes* may be due to any of the following.

- *Pulmonary embolus.* This is often associated with chest pain. It is potentially life-threatening, so give high-flow oxygen and transfer the patient to hospital as an emergency. Treatment may require thrombolysis and anticoagulation.
- *Pneumothorax*, which may be spontaneous or may occur with trauma such as a fall. Give high-flow oxygen and arrange transfer to hospital, where a chest drain may be inserted.
- *Acute asthma* usually occurs in patients already known to have the disease. See guidance above. If the patient does not respond quickly to treatment, or if there are any features of acute severe asthma or life-threatening signs (see above), admit to hospital immediately.
- *Inhaled foreign body.* If severe airway compromise or total obstruction occurs, apply back blows, abdominal thrusts or the Heimlich manoeuvre.
- *Acute heart failure.* This may occur in a patient who has previously had a heart attack. Usually patients present as cold, sweaty and anxious, with tachycardia and creps heard at the lung bases. Give high-flow oxygen, insert a venous cannula (if available), give intravenous furosemide and admit to hospital.

Diagnosing and treating infections of the upper respiratory tract

Acute infections of the upper respiratory tract include pharyngitis/tonsillitis and laryngitis ('common cold'). Symptoms may include a cough, sneezing, sore throat, runny or congested nose, headache and low-grade fever, and may last 7 days or so.

A streptococcal sore throat can cause pain on swallowing.

Treatment is generally to suppress symptoms – analgesics ease headache, sore throat and muscle aches but none shortens the duration of infection.

Antibiotics are not generally recommended as drug resistance may emerge. However, in those at high risk because of an underlying lung disease such as COPD, antibiotics may decrease the period of infection.

How to treat bronchospasm in a patient with asthma who is already taking salbutamol inhalers

Follow the stepwise guidance provided by the British Thoracic Society guidelines (see above) or get advice from a respiratory physician.

If a patient has tuberculosis, who should be contacted to assess the patient and what precautions should staff take?

The World Health Organization advises the following.[5]

- Identify suspected cases of tuberculosis promptly, to limit spread of the disease
- Do three smears on all patients with cough of 3 weeks or more, or who may otherwise be at risk from tuberculosis.
- Strictly follow the standard protocol for management of suspected tuberculosis and know how to treat tuberculosis effectively and promptly.
- Follow the isolation and hospital infection control guidelines.
- Use personal protection equipment appropriately.
- Ensure that diagnosed patients have a realistic plan to continue and complete the treatment after their discharge from hospital.
- Always give proper therapy to control the patient's cough.
- Implement universal precautions and nosocomial infection surveillance programmes.

In the event of identifying a patient with tuberculosis, inform the local Public Health Department immediately.

Managing a patient with COPD

Treatment comprises:

- short-acting bronchodilators (salbutamol inhaler used as required and ipratropium inhaler – these can be used alone or in combination to dilate airways for up to 6 hours)
- long-acting bronchodilators (such as salmeterol or tiotropium) for persistent symptoms or exacerbations
- combination long-acting inhaler plus inhaled steroid.
- oral treatment with theophyllines (best used on the advice of a respiratory specialist) and oral corticosteroids during exacerbations
- mucolytics (carbocisteine), which may aid expectoration
- pulmonary rehabilitation.

It is essential for the patient to stop smoking.

When to refer to a respiratory physician

Refer to a respiratory physician when:

- there is doubt or concern about the diagnosis, investigation or treatment of a patient with breathlessness
- a known respiratory problem is not controlled by existing therapy
- symptoms suggest a malignancy or tuberculosis – persistent cough, blood-stained sputum, weight loss; refer without delay
- there are abnormal findings on a chest X-ray.

Safe doses of oxygen

Oxygen is generally safe. In an emergency treat with the maximum concentration you have available. A nasal cannula can provide up to 40% oxygen, but a face mask can deliver between 40% and 70%.

In any illness where hypoxaemia may occur, put a pulse oximeter on the patient's finger and give oxygen through a nasal cannula or face mask to achieve a target oxygen saturation level of 94–98%, slightly lower in COPD patients (the aim is usually 88–92%).

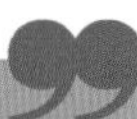

Summary

Respiratory disease is common. Most patients with chronic respiratory disorders such as asthma, chronic bronchitis and emphysema can be managed simply and successfully in the community, but it is important that professionals in contact with patients with mental health problems know when symptom control is inadequate or even life-threatening; and when specialist help is needed. Smoking prevalence is high in those with mental health problems, which makes the recognition of the symptoms and signs of lung cancer especially important.

References

1 British Thoracic Society. *British Guideline on the Management of Asthma: A National Clinical Guideline.* Scottish Intercollegiate Guidelines Network, 2009 (revised 2012).

2 National Institute for Health and Clinical Excellence. *Chronic Obstructive Pulmonary Disease (COPD) – Management of COPD in Adults in Primary and Secondary Care (CG101).* NICE, 2010.

3 Lim WS, van der Eerden MM, Laing R, *et al.* Defining community acquired pneumonia severity on presentation to hospital: an international derivation and validation study. *Thorax* 2003; **58**: 377–82.

4 National Institute for Health and Clinical Excellence. *Clinical Diagnosis and Management of Tuberculosis, and Measures for Its Prevention and Control (CG117).* NICE, 2011.

5 World Health Organization. *The Stop TB Strategy: Building on and Enhancing DOTS to Meet the TB-Related Millennium Development Goals.* WHO, 2006.

Recommended reading

British Thoracic Society Standards of Care Committee. BTS statement on criteria for specialist referral, admission, discharge and follow-up for adults with respiratory disease . *Thorax* 2008; **63** (suppl. 1): i1-16

Lim WS, Baudouin SV, George RC, *et al.* Guidelines for the management of community acquired pneumonia in adults: update 2009. *Thorax* 2009; **64**: 1–61.

National Institute for Health and Clinical Excellence. *Lung Cancer: Diagnosis and Treatment (CG121).* NICE, 2011.

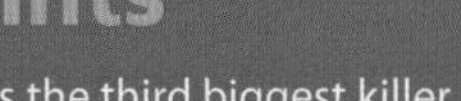

Learning points

- Respiratory disease is the third biggest killer in the UK.
- There are more than 40 conditions which affect the lungs and/or airways and impact on an individual's ability to breathe.
- Usual presenting symptoms of respiratory disease are breathlessness, cough and wheeze; haemoptysis, development of a hoarse voice, weight loss, lethargy and anaemia may indicate lung cancer – arrange urgent referral using the cancer 2-week wait pathway.
- Patients with asthma present with breathlessness, wheeze, chest tightness and a chronic dry cough which varies during the day and with the seasons.
- For patients with asthma, follow the guidelines from the British Thoracic Society, which recommend a stepwise approach using bronchodilators (asthma relievers) and anti-inflammatory drugs (asthma preventers).
- Most patients with asthma can be managed in the community but refer if the diagnosis is in doubt, if the asthma is difficult to manage or if the cause may be 'occupational'.
- In COPD, the main symptoms are progressive breathlessness, wheeze and productive cough; guidelines are available on when to refer to a respiratory physician.
- Short-acting beta-agonists and tiotropium provide symptomatic relief; inhaled corticosteroids and long-acting beta-agonists may be given if symptoms persist despite these, or if exacerbations are recurrent, or FEV1 is less than 60% predicted.
- Patients who develop pneumonia may be treated in the community provided they have a low CURB-65 score. Otherwise, admission to hospital is essential.

14

Neurological disorders

Julie Phukan and James S. Rakshi

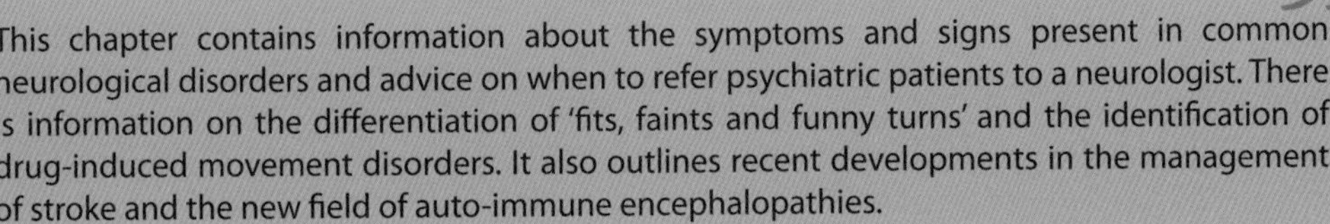

This chapter contains information about the symptoms and signs present in common neurological disorders and advice on when to refer psychiatric patients to a neurologist. There is information on the differentiation of 'fits, faints and funny turns' and the identification of drug-induced movement disorders. It also outlines recent developments in the management of stroke and the new field of auto-immune encephalopathies.

Introduction

The discipline of neurology is highly relevant to the practising psychiatrist. Psychiatrists frequently encounter the coexistence of a neurological disorder in patients with a psychiatric diagnosis (and vice versa). In addition, there is a great deal of overlap of drugs used in the two specialties (e.g. tricyclic antidepressants are used to treat headache and neuropathic pain as well as depression). Moreover, the side-effects of psychiatric medications can mimic those of primary neurological diseases (e.g. Parkinson's disease). It is important to differentiate psychogenic disorders from organic neurological disorders – a feat that can be challenging and only achieved with clinical knowledge of the latter.

Epilepsy

Clinical seizures represent abnormal, excessive excitation and synchronisation of neurons. Epilepsy is defined by two or more unprovoked seizures. Thus provoked seizures (i.e. secondary to exogenous factors, such as alcohol or drug withdrawal) do not constitute epilepsy even if they are repeated.

Seizures are classified as: generalised (myoclonic, atonic, tonic, tonic–clonic, absence); or partial/focal (simple or complex). During simple partial seizures, consciousness is preserved; the patient remains alert and remembers what happened during the seizure. In complex partial seizures, consciousness is impaired. Complex partial seizures usually last up to 3 minutes but may evolve into secondary generalised seizures.[1]

The risk factors for epilepsy include:

- family history
- head trauma
- meningitis
- encephalitis.

It is also worth asking patients if they had a normal gestation and delivery, reached developmental milestones appropriately, had childhood febrile convulsions, were thought of as a daydreamer (perhaps representing absences), or if they have 'clumsy breakfast' syndrome (always dropping things in the morning, as seen in juvenile myoclonic epilepsy). Limb jerks while falling asleep (hypnic) are common in normal individuals.

As for the event itself, take the 'before, during and after' approach.

Before

- Vasovagal precipitants of a seizure can include the patient standing for some time in a hot stuffy room.
- The seizure can be preceded by a sense of derealisation or depersonalisation, nausea, diaphoresis, blurred vision or spots in front of the eyes.

Seizure

- Flashing nightclub lights, sleep deprivation and alcohol may precipitate some seizure types.
- An aura before a seizure can manifest as olfactory disturbances, rising sensation in the abdomen, *déjà vu*, or *jamais vu*.
- Derealisation and depersonalisation can occur in temporal lobe seizures but also in vasovagal events.

Note that cardiac events often occur without warning.

Box 14.1 A scoring system that can be used to differentiate between fainting episodes (syncope) and fits (seizures)

- Feelings of being 'light-headed'
- Sweating before episodes
- Sitting or standing for a long period before the episode

Each of the above characteristics can be given a score of –2.

- Tongue being bitten during an episode
- A sensation of *déjà vu* or *jamais vu* before the episode
- Psychological stress was associated with the loss of consciousness
- If an observer noticed that the person's head turned during an episode
- If someone saw that the person was not responding during an episode, had strange postures, had jerking of the arms or legs, or could not recall the episode
- If anyone noticed that the person was confused after the episode

Each of the above characteristics scores +1, with the exception of tongue biting, which has a score of +2.

Now add up the minus and plus points. If the total score is 1 or more, then the episodes are more likely to be fits. If the total score is less than 1, fainting is the more likely diagnosis.

Adapted from Sheldon *et al*, 2002.[2]

During

Obtain a collateral history and establish the following (see Box 14.1).

- Was the patient completely unaware of the seizure?
- Did the patient bite the tongue?
- Was there any incontinence?
- Were there any jerking movements? Brief myoclonic twitches, usually for less than a minute, and flaccidity are seen in syncope; more prolonged jerks with rigidity occur in seizures.
- Were there automatisms (e.g. lip smacking, chewing, fumbling, grunting, phrase repetitions). More dramatic automatisms occasionally occur, such as screaming, running, disrobing, pelvic thrusting.
- Was there a head turn to either side?
- Did anyone check the patient's pulse?
- Was the patient very pale or blue?
- How long did the event last? (This is notoriously difficult for others to recall.)

Syncope can be associated with limb jerking, incontinence but rarely tongue biting. Up to 20% of events diagnosed as seizures instead represent syncopal or cardiac events. A simple scoring system helps distinguish between syncope and seizures (Box 14.1), and symptoms/signs are included in Fig. 14.1.

After

- Does the patient recall the event or anything before it?
- How long did it take to return to baseline? Unlike after most seizures, recovery in syncope occurs in less than 1 minute.
- Neurological examination should be accompanied by a search for evidence of head trauma (a cause or consequence of seizures) and lateralising features such as post-ictal weakness or aphasia.
- Look out for neurocutaneous features of tuberous sclerosis and neurofibromatosis.
- Cardiovascular examination identifies arrhythmias and valvular disease.

Investigation

Blood tests for infection, metabolic or electrolyte disturbances and a toxicology screen should be performed. Record an electrocardiogram (ECG) and check lying and standing blood pressure.

Elevated serum prolactin levels, when measured 10–20 minutes after a suspected event, are a useful

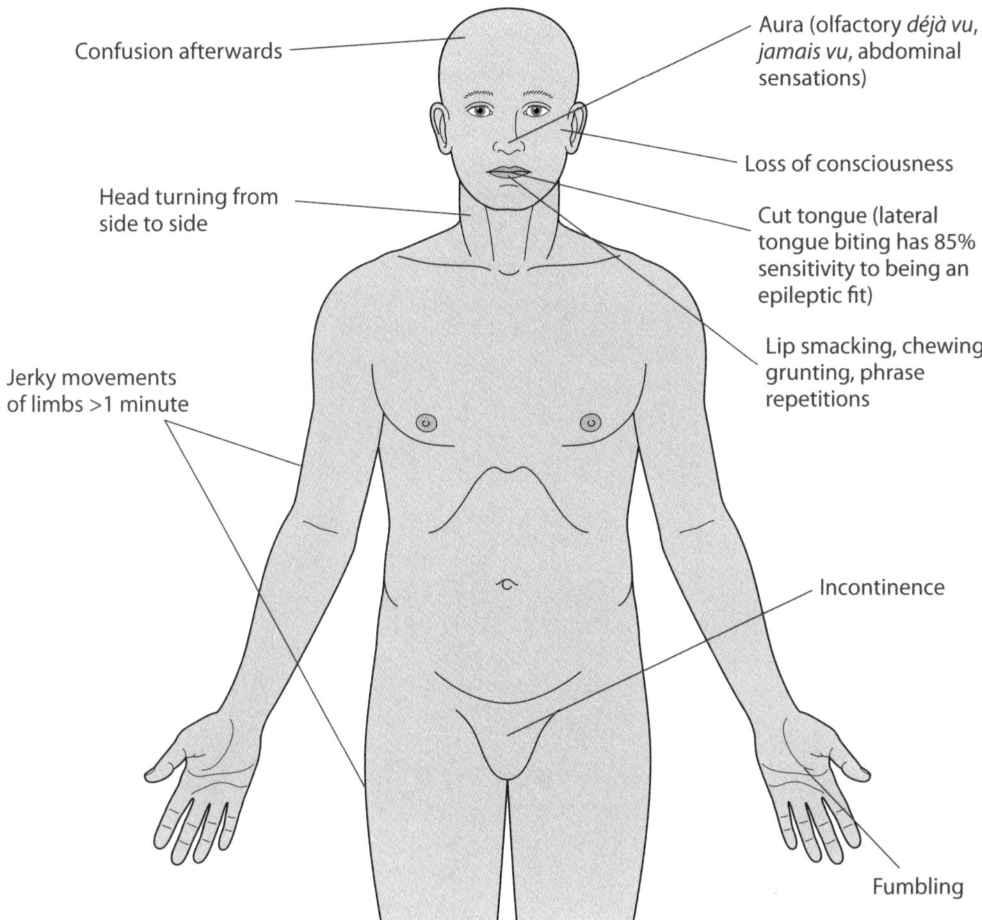

Fig. 14.1 Symptoms and signs of epilepsy.

adjunct for the differentiation of generalised tonic–clonic or complex partial seizure from psychogenic non-epileptic seizures among adults and older children. It is not helpful in distinguishing seizure from syncope.[3]

Lumbar puncture is indicated only if meningitis or encephalitis is suspected and if the potential for brain herniation is excluded.

An electroencephalogram (EEG) can support the diagnosis and identify the specific syndrome if there is clinical suspicion of seizure or epilepsy. In approximately 50% of patients who have epilepsy, a single EEG shows no abnormalities. An EEG obtained from a sleep-deprived patient or video-EEG may then be helpful but, even still, clinical history remains the key for diagnosis.

Emergency computerised tomography (CT) or magnetic resonance imaging (MRI) is indicated if there are seizures and the patient has:[4–6]

- a new focal neurological deficit
- a persistent altered mental status (with or without intoxication)
- a new seizure pattern or new seizure type
- a fever
- head trauma
- persistent headache
- a history of anticoagulant therapy or cancer
- a history or suspicion of immunosuppression, including AIDS.

Magnetic resonance imaging is the high-resolution structural imaging modality of choice for the investigation of epilepsy, although non-contrast CT is acceptable in the first instance if MRI is not readily available or cannot be done for technical reasons (e.g. the patient has a pacemaker, is respirator-dependent) or if access to the patient may be needed during scanning.[5]

Psychiatrists would not normally be expected to perform a lumbar puncture, and anyway EEG cannot exclude epilepsy.

Specific rules regarding epilepsy and driving in the UK are detailed on the website www.direct.gov.uk/en/Motoring/DriverLicensing/MedicalRulesForDrivers/index.htm

Management

Patients may be reassured on two counts:

- epilepsy is common, with about 50 million people affected globally, accounting for 20% of neurology consultations
- epilepsy is manageable – within 5 years of the onset of seizures, up to 60% of patients will have entered long-term remission and only 20% have epilepsy that is refractory to treatment.

Precautions that people with epilepsy may need to take include avoidance of the following:

- heights
- swimming and bathing alone
- precipitants such as excess alcohol use and sleep deprivation.

When to refer to neurology

Psychiatric patients who experience seizures should be referred to a neurology department if:

- diagnosis is required
- seizure control is sub-optimal
- a patient is planning pregnancy or becomes pregnant
- there is a change in seizure type or duration
- there is prolonged agitation or disorientation after a seizure (urgently, as the patient may be in non-convulsive or complex partial status epilepticus).

Treatment

Not all patients with epilepsy need medication. The decision rests upon several factors, including patient preference, risk of further events, ramifications of further seizures and consequences of anti-epileptic drugs.[7]

Epilepsy medications have come a long way since the days of bromide and phenobarbitone. A wealth of new drugs exist – levetiracetam, lamotrigine, topiramate and felbamate – as well as tried and tested carbamazepine and sodium valproate. Decisions should be individualised, based upon the evidence for efficacy and effectiveness of each drug in a given syndrome, potential adverse effect profile, tolerability, formulation and cost. It is not always necessary to monitor the levels of anti-epileptic drugs (Box 14.2).

Lamotrigine is regarded as the drug of choice in young women; it has a good side-effect profile and lower teratogenic potential. Some anti-epileptic drugs interact with the oral contraceptive pill; doses of these may need to be modified. In pregnancies in mothers with epilepsy, 96% produce normal children. Women with epilepsy who might become pregnant should receive pre-conceptual supplementation with folic acid to decrease the risk of neural tube defects. Pregnancy planning is vital, as is optimal seizure control at the lowest dose and least number of anti-epileptic drugs possible before and during pregnancy.

Surgical therapy is considered if seizures and/or medication side-effects significantly impair quality of life. Surgery may be appropriate if seizures arise from an area that can be removed without causing unacceptable neurological deficits.

Box 14.2 Anti-epileptic drug levels

Drug levels are used to assess adherence or toxicity, and are applicable only to a few drugs, e.g. phenytoin, carbamazepine and, to a lesser extent, phenobarbitone.

Clinical response is far more important than the drug level ('treat the patient, not the drug level'). Some patients may be entirely seizure-free despite 'sub-therapeutic' anti-epileptic drug levels; others develop toxicity within or below the range. Clinical judgement is imperative to avoid unnecessary or harmful changes in medication and is best managed by a neurology specialist.

Source: Walters *et al*, 2004.[8]

Aim for monotherapy, but if a second drug has to be added the dosage of the first drug should be optimised beforehand.

Status epilepticus

This refers to a seizure that persists long enough or is repeated frequently enough for recovery not to occur between attacks (International League Against Epilepsy 1981).[1] Status epilepticus requires intensive in-hospital treatment.

Its definition is contentious. Traditionally, generalised convulsive status epilepticus is defined as lasting over 30 minutes. However, neuronal injury may occur and self-termination is unlikely after this period of time, so it has been suggested that 5 minutes is sufficient for diagnosis.[9] A consensus exists that treatments should be initiated *as early as possible*, to avoid the sequelae of prolonged seizure activity.[10] Step-by-step guidelines for acute management of a fit in adults are laid out in Box 14.3.

In an out-of-hospital setting, rectal diazepam or buccal midazolam may be appropriate. (*We strongly encourage doctors to read the National Institute for Health and Clinical Excellence (NICE) guideline on epilepsy, see Recommended reading.*)

An individual who has prolonged convulsive seizures (lasting 5 minutes or more) or serial seizures (three or more seizures in an hour) in the community should receive urgent care and treatment. Rectal diazepam is a safe and effective first-line treatment of prolonged seizures and is recommended in the majority of cases.

Buccal midazolam is currently unlicensed for the treatment of prolonged or repeated seizures. However, for many individuals and in many circumstances it is more acceptable than rectal diazepam and is easier to administer. It should be used according to an agreed protocol drawn up by the specialist and only used following training.

- Healthcare professionals should inform individuals, and their families and/or carers that buccal midazolam is currently unlicensed.
- Treatment should be administered by trained clinical personnel or, if specified within an individually agreed protocol drawn up with the specialist, by family or carers with appropriate training.
- Care must be taken to secure the individual's airway and assess his or her respiratory and cardiac function.

Box 14.3 Acute management of fits in adults

1 Shout for help, call the 'crash team', or dial 999. State 'patient is fitting'.

2 Follow ABCDE resuscitation protocol. Give oxygen by mask. Monitor pulse, blood pressure and oxygen saturation levels and do an ECG, if possible.

3 Gain i.v. access, but if not readily available, consider rectal or buccal administration of medication.[a]

4 First-line drugs: onset of fit

- Lorazepam 4 mg i.v., at rate of 2 mg/min. Repeat same dose if fits not terminated after 5 min
- If lorazepam unavailable, give diazepam 5 mg i.v./min. If fits continue after 5 min, give further diazepam 5 mg i.v.

5 Second-line drugs: fits not controlled by first-line drugs

If the fit does not end after 10 min of the fit starting, and after repeating the dose (as above) of whichever drug was used (lorazepam, diazepam, midazolam), start a phenytoin infusion. Calculate the dose based on the patient's weight (18 mg/kg at 50 mg/min). Use a solution of 10 mg/per ml of phenytoin (i.e. 1000 mg of phenytoin in 100 ml of normal saline). Give the phenytoin i.v. over 20–30 min.

6 Third-line drugs: status epilepticus

- Patient who continues to fit after 15–30 min despite first- and second-line drugs is in practice in status epilepticus
- Contact medical team, if not already done, ITU team, and the on-call anaesthetist
- If available, administer phenobarbitone 700 mg over 7 min in a syringe (10 mg/kg at a rate of 100 mg/min) while awaiting anaesthetist

7 Consider secondary causes of fits: bloods (U&Es, FBC, blood glucose, LFTs, CRP, calcium/phosphate), arterial blood gases, toxicology screen, prolactin level.

8 Consider NES: patient will have normal oxygen saturation and prolactin levels (post event).

9 If 'first fit', patients will need an urgent CT or MRI brain scan to exclude structural lesion. If known epilepsy, check adherence and epilepsy drug levels. Consider secondary causes of fit, e.g. infection.

CRP, c-reactive protein; CT, computed tomography; ECG, electrocardiogram; FBC, full blood count; ITU, intensive treatment unit; IV, intravenous; LFT, liver function tests; MRI, magnetic resonance imaging; NES, non-epileptic seizure; U&Es, urea and electrolytes.

a. If no i.v. access, rectal diazepam 5 mg can be administered. If still fitting after 5 min of the fit starting, second dose of rectal diazepam 5 mg can be given; alternatively, give buccal midazolam (buccolam) 10 mg between lower gums and cheek (repeat 10 min of the fit starting).

Epilepsy and non-epileptic seizures

Of those presenting with non-epileptic seizures (NES), at least 20% *have* epilepsy. NES is important to recognise to allow appropriate psychological and psychiatric intervention and to avoid unnecessary administration

Patients with NES can be misdiagnosed and treated for epilepsy, even to the extent of being intubated and ventilated. If NES is suspected, observe whether the patient resists eye opening and 'screws up' their eyes during the 'fit-like' episode, as this does not occur in an unconscious person. Check whether patient's movements show active resistance or if they appear voluntary or directed. Patients with NES may respond to calm reassurance that their 'fits' will settle. Normal oxygen saturation levels in patients with prolonged generalised movements lasting ≥30 min are more likely to be found in those with NES.

Low oxygen saturations during a fit and raised serum prolactin levels after a fit are more likely to be found in epilepsy than in NES.

of anti-epileptic drugs, and associated risks of toxicity and teratogenicity. It is frequently diagnosed after video-EEG; however, the clinical features listed in Table 14.1 may be supportive of the diagnosis, if not absolute.

Movement disorders

Movement disorders are classified as:

- too little movement – akinetic, hypokinetic or bradykinetic syndromes (used synonymously)
- too much movement (hyperkinesias) – tremor, chorea (dyskinesias), dystonia, myoclonus, tics.

The main akinetic syndrome is idiopathic Parkinson's disease (IDP), which is described in detail in the next section. The main hyperkinesias are briefly described here.

Chorea

Chorea presents with arrhythmic involuntary movements that 'flow' randomly and can look like restlessness and fidgeting, but may at the extreme be disabling, violent movements. Causes include:

- drugs (e.g. L-dopa, neuroleptics, anti-epileptic drugs, digoxin, contraceptive pill, tricyclic antidepressants, and many others)
- Huntington's disease (Box 14.4)
- thyrotoxicosis
- pregnancy
- Wilson's disease
- lupus erythematosus
- polycythaemia
- HIV
- new-variant Creutzfeldt–Jakob disease (nvCJD)
- basal ganglia stroke.

Tetrabenazine, a dopamine-depleting drug, is used for chorea and, compared with neuroleptics, interferes less with cognition and does not cause tardive dyskinesia. However it may cause suicidal ideation, akathisia and Parkinsonism.

Table 14.1 Clinical features that help to distinguish non-epileptic from epileptic seizures

	Non-epileptic seizures	Epilepsy-related seizures
Gradual onset	Common	Rare
Waxing and waning motor activity	Common (stop–start)	Very rare
Biting	Usually tip of tongue, lip	Lateral edge of tongue
Eyes	Closed (even against resistance)	Open
Skin colour	No change	Cyanosis
Movements	Stiffness, shaking	Tonic–clonic
	Crying and thrashing; pelvic thrusting*	
	Lying motionless for over 5 minutes	
Disorientation	Slow, can seem surprised	Prolonged (can be short in some frontal lobe seizures)
Respiration post-event	Tachypnoea, irregular, with brief pauses*	Snoring; regular, and loud

*Occasionally seen in frontal lobe seizures.

Box 14.4 Huntington's disease

Huntington's disease is an autosomal dominant progressive neurodegenerative disorder of the basal ganglia, characterised by chorea, dystonia, cognitive decline and behavioural changes. The mean age of onset is 40; with death typically after 15–20 years. It demonstrates genetic anticipation (i.e. earlier onset and greater severity with each generation). Diagnostic and predictive genetic testing are available but not all patients or family members wish to pursue these. There is no cure – symptomatic treatment forms the mainstay of management.

Dystonia

Dystonia presents with sustained abnormal postures and movements.

In primary dystonia there is no underlying neurodegeneration. Examples include spasmodic torticollis, writer's cramp, oromandibular dystonia, and blepharospasm. Patients may demonstrate a *geste antagoniste* – a sensory trick to ameliorate dystonia (e.g. touching the cheek to correct torticollis).[11]

Secondary dystonia occurs as a component of other basal ganglia disorders, including stroke, Parkinsonian syndromes, Huntington's disease, Wilson's disease and conditions produced by toxins. Investigations and treatments are tailored to the presentation. Botulinum toxin can improve symptoms in up to 80% of focal dystonia patients (e.g. blepharospasm, spasmodic torticollis).

Myoclonus

These brief shock-like movements may be physiological (e.g. sleep/hypnic jerks), essential (idiopathic or hereditary), epileptic or secondary (to metabolic disorders, infections, drugs, brain hypoxia and dementias). Treatment depends upon the underlying cause.

Tics

These brief intermittent stereotyped purposeless movements (motor tics) and sounds (phonic tics) can be suppressed with conscious effort but with rising inner tension and more tics afterwards. They can be simple (e.g. blinking, grimacing, throat clearing, sniffing, grunting) or complex (e.g. jumping, echolalia, coprolalia). Tic disorders can be primary (transient or chronic, the latter including Tourette's syndrome) or secondary to neurodegenerative conditions, infections, head trauma, and exposure to toxins, which usually have other signs and symptoms. Secondary tic disorders usually have other signs and symptoms.

Myoclonic jerks may be caused by clozapine toxicity.

Psychogenic movement disorders

Psychogenic movement disorders account for up to 3% of referrals to movement disorder clinics. Coexisting psychiatric conditions are common. Signs that can help to distinguish them include:[12–14]

- *abrupt onset* (patients frequently report a recent minor injury or precipitating event)
- *quick progression* to maximum severity and disability
- incongruent with recognised organic disease
- *multiple abnormal movements* (although some organic conditions can present in this way)
- *excessively slow* and effortful movements (which may be absent when the patient is not aware of being observed)
- breath-holding
- sudden knee buckling.
- Entrainment: ask the patients to rapidly tap their fingers in the contralateral limb. A psychogenic tremor will assume the frequency of the voluntary movement.
- Distractibility can result in suppression of the movement. For example, during the 'serial 7s' test, the movement attenuates in psychogenic movement disorder, while in organic disease the amplitude often increases.
- Psychogenic disorders tend to respond to suggestion. Tell the patient that vibration can trigger the tremor in some and then apply a tuning fork to the affected part of the body. Converse suggestion also could work: suggesting that the tuning fork will reduce the tremor.

Idiopathic Parkinson's disease

Idiopathic Parkinson's disease (IPD, Fig. 14.2), the main akinetic syndrome, is a progressive neurodegenerative movement disorder caused by the loss of dopaminergic nigrostriatal neurons.

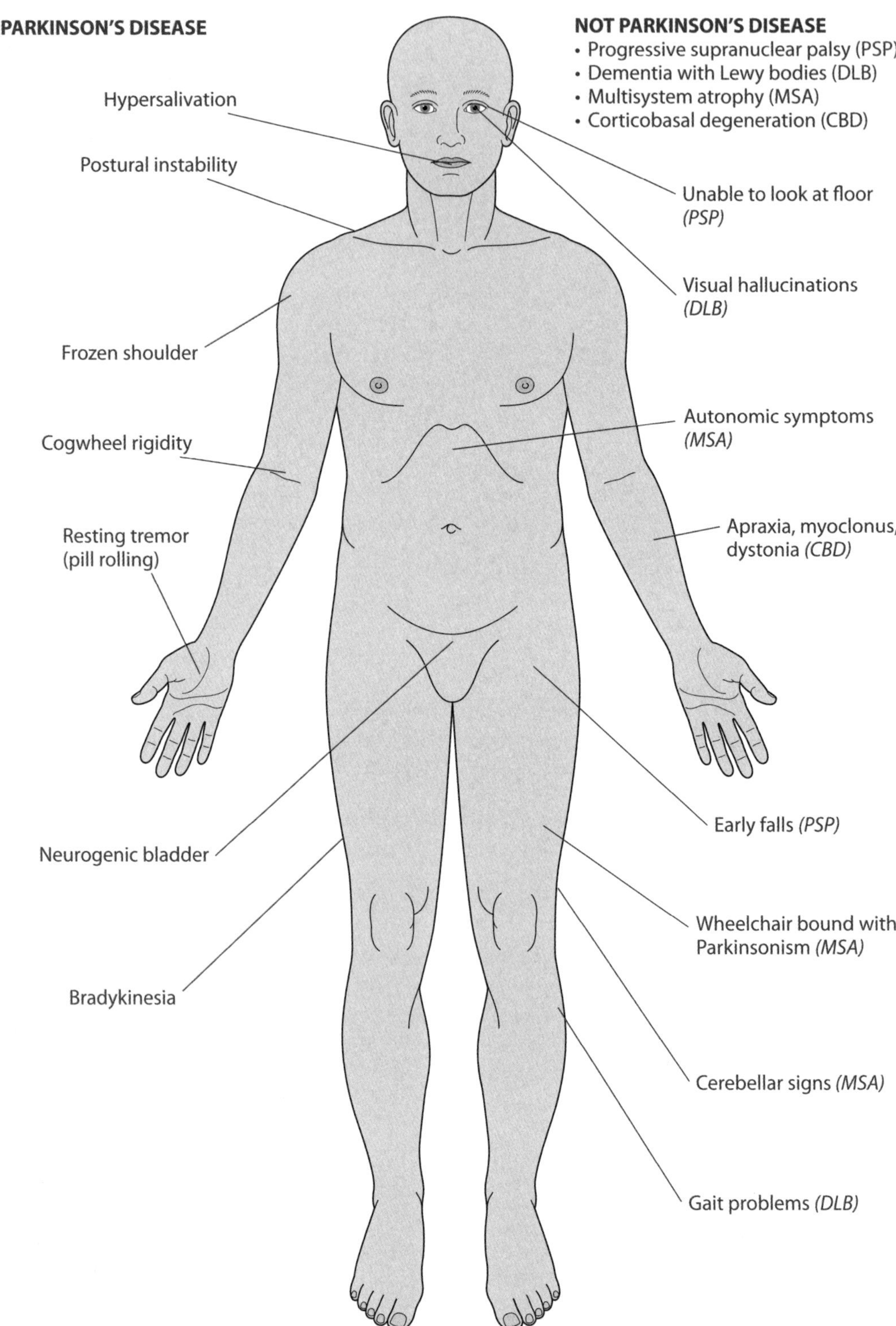

Fig. 14.1 Idiopathic Parkinson's disease and 'Parkinson plus' syndromes (p. 183).

Clinical signs of IPD

- *Bradykinesia* – slowness of initiation of movement, its speed and amplitude. It is best demonstrated by finger tapping (note that the amplitude of movement gets progressively smaller), hand opening and closing, and wrist pronation/supination. Hand weakness (upper or lower motor neuron) may mimic bradykinesia but there is no weakness with IPD. Facial expression is lost (hypomimia), handwriting gets smaller (micrographia) and gait is altered, with asymmetrical reduced arm swing, stooped posture, slow short steps and unsteadiness on turning. In advanced IPD, shuffling is more obvious, gait is festinant (forward propulsion with rapid short steps); there is movement en bloc and the patient may freeze in narrow spaces such as door frames and corridors.
- *Cogwheel rigidity* – increased tone throughout the range of passive movement (when the doctor moves the limb rather than the patient actively moving the limb) about a joint superimposed on a resting tremor. This is best demonstrated with wrist flexion/extension. It may be exaggerated if the patient raises the other arm up and down (synkinesis). If there is no tremor, then rigidity is uniformly increased muscle tone throughout the range of passive movement.
- *Resting tremor* – 'pill-rolling tremor' between thumb and index finger when hands are on lap. It is slower and has more variable amplitude than an essential tremor. It reduces or disappears on action such as picking up a cup or eating, but may reappear on sustained posture (outstretched hands) – the so-called re-emergent tremor.
- *Postural instability* – impairment of reflexes that maintain an upright posture, with a tendency to fall backwards on standing/turning. It is best demonstrated by standing behind the patient and pulling them from behind by the shoulders towards you; it is impaired if more than two steps are taken back or a fall is likely.
- *Non-motor features*. These include autonomic dysfunction (hypersalivation, postural hypotension, bladder and bowel symptoms), sleep disturbance, psychiatric/behavioural problems, cognitive impairment and visual hallucinations.

'Parkinson plus' syndromes

It is important to distinguish IPD from the 'Parkinson plus' syndromes (progressive supranuclear palsy (PSP), dementia with Lewy bodies (DLB), corticobasal degeneration (CBD) and multisystem atrophy (MSA)). 'Plus' refers to involvement of other components of the nervous system (Table 14.2). Treatment tailored to IPD is less effective and can cause adverse events in these other syndromes; for example, neuroleptics are contraindicated in dementia with Lewy bodies since they can cause severe Parkinsonism, neuroleptic malignant syndrome and cognitive decline. Clinical diagnostic criteria to distinguish Parkinson's disease from 'Parkinson plus' syndromes can be found online (www.ncbi.nlm.nih.gov/projects/gap/cgi-bin/GetPdf.cgi?id=phd000042).

Investigations

There is no specific diagnostic test for IPD. Suspect Wilson's disease if onset is early (patient aged under 40 years) and if the Parkinsonism is atypical; copper studies and slit lamp examination are then indicated. MRI is

Table 14.2 'Red flags' suggesting movement disorder, not Idiopathic Parkinson's disease

Sign	Likely syndrome
Little or no response to L-dopa (patient may not notice improvement but partner does)	'Parkinson plus' syndrome
Early falls	Progressive supranuclear palsy (IPD does not usually result in falls in the first 18 months)
Vertical gaze palsy – unable to look down at floor	Progressive supranuclear palsy
Early visual hallucinations and cognitive impairment	Dementia of the Lewy-body type
Wheelchair-bound with Parkinsonism	Multi-system atrophy
Prominent autonomic symptoms	Multi-system atrophy
Cerebellar signs	Multi-system atrophy
Apraxia, myoclonus, dystonia	Corticobasal degeneration
Pyramidal signs	Parkinson's disease with cervical cord compression; multi-system atrophy; corticobasal degeneration; progressive supranuclear palsy

normal in IPD and indicated only if the presentation is or becomes atypical. Single-photon emission computerised tomography (SPECT) scanning, in particular, dopamine transporter (DAT) imaging, is useful where a diagnosis of Parkinsonism is uncertain. The imaging should be abnormal with 'true' IPD, but it cannot usually distinguish between the neurodegenerative Parkinsonian syndromes (IPD, multi-system atrophy, progressive supranuclear palsy, corticobasal degeneration, Lewy-body dementia). It can help to distinguish between these and other 'Parkinson's disease mimics' that do not have *striatal* dopamine loss, such as dystonic, psychogenic or essential tremor, drug-induced Parkinsonism and L-dopa-responsive dystonia (see Table 14.3).[15]

Drug treatment of IPD

Multidisciplinary input and patient education are crucial. Recent studies highlight the importance of most types of regular exercise (e.g walking, swimming, pilates, tai chi) in maintaining and improving gait, balance and mobility.

All patients with suspected IPD should be referred to a specialist before treatment is begun, as recommended by NICE guidelines (see Recommended reading, NICE 2006). More than 16% will have other causes of Parkinsonism.

The choice of drug treatment depends on the predominant symptom (e.g. tremor or bradykinesia), severity, whether the condition is interfering with activities of daily living (ADLs) or work, the patient's wishes and the specialist's recommendation. In general, however, functional disability is an indication for dopaminergic therapy.

What to start?

There is no general agreement on which drug should be used first and what to add next when a patient deteriorates or develops motor complications. L-dopa therapy (in preparations such as sinemet or madopar) is a good start for symptom relief in most patients.

If the IPD is of new onset, mild and, in patients in their 40s to 60s, is interfering with ADLs/work, it is reasonable to start treatment with either a dopamine agonist or a monoamine oxidase (MAO) inhibitor (e.g. rasagiline). However L-dopa is often the first-line treatment in patients over 60 with more severe symptoms (e.g. bradykinesia or rigidity).

In young-onset patients, IPD tends to progress more rapidly due to motor complications, making the condition harder to manage, and more advanced treatments may be required. These patients should be referred to a specialist.

Older patients (over 70) with symptoms that are mild but are interfering with ADLs can start treatment with L-dopa, which is usually well tolerated in the elderly.

Therapies used to treat the motor symptoms of IPD are shown in Table 14.4. No drug has conclusively been shown to be neuroprotective or disease-modifying.

Table 14.3 Causes of secondary Parkinsonism – 'Parkinson's disease mimics'

Diagnosis	Signs
Drug-induced Parkinsonism	Mild symmetrical rigidity/slowness and/or tremor
Essential tremor	On sustained posture and action (see text)
Dystonic hand tremor	Asymmetrical/unilateral hand tremor which may look identical to resting tremor of idiopathic Parkinson's disease (but dopamine transporter (DAT) scan normal)
Vascular Parkinsonism	'Lower-half Parkinsonism' in patients with cerebrovascular disease. Wide-based, small stepping upright gait but good spontaneous movements of the arm, and good facial expression. Gait initiation may be a problem
Normal-pressure hydrocephalus	Slow, shuffling upright gait as in Parkinson's disease but broad-based rather than narrow (gait apraxia). Urinary incontinence and cognitive impairment/dementia
Wilson's disease	Inherited copper overload disorder. Presents in first two decades of life. Bradykinesia and rigidity but also dysarthria, ataxia, 'wing-beating' tremor, psychiatric disturbances, liver failure, cardiomyopathy. Most sensitive test is Kayser–Fleischer rings present in all patients with neurological presentations. Therefore refer to opthalmologist for slit lamp examination. Check serum ceruloplasmin and if low, measure 24-hour urinary copper levels (high)

Therapeutic issues

Motor complications in IPD include dyskinesias, initially in predictable but later unpredictable 'on' and 'off' periods, and dystonia, especially in the morning (e.g. foot inversion). These are due to a combination of dopaminergic therapy and disease progression.

The duration of effect of L-dopa can shorten and motor complications develop, so the drug may need to be taken more frequently (even 1–2 hourly) at lower dosages to maintain efficacy and minimise motor complications.

Nausea and vomiting can occur with all dopaminergic treatments but is more common with dopamine agonists, especially in the elderly. Domperidone (10 mg three times daily) is effective and can be started 48 hours before the patient starts the dopaminergic treatment and continued for several weeks or so thereafter. Elderly patients are more likely to have other side-effects, including confusion and behavioural and psychotic symptoms, and so need to be more closely monitored. Use dopamine agonists with caution in patients with ischaemic heart disease as they can worsen angina.

Excessive tiredness, sleepiness and new or worsening abnormal behaviour including pathological gambling, hypomania/mania, drug hoarding, paranoia and occasionally aggression and hypersexuality can occur with all dopaminergic therapies. Dopamine agonists have been associated with 'punding' (stereotypical motor behaviour and fascination with repetitive mechanical handling, like taking apart and putting back together objects such as a watch or electrical item) and hoarding of objects.

Treatment of advanced and severe IPD

Rasagiline is a new MAO-B inhibitor which does not produce amphetamine metabolites and therefore has a better side-effect profile than selegiline. It has a mild symptomatic effect and is well tolerated.

Combinations of dopaminergic drugs in single-tablet form are available, e.g. L-dopa + carbidopa + catechol-O-methyl transferase (COMT) inhibitor. However, no clear benefit other than reducing the total number of tablets taken has been demonstrated. It has not been shown to increase the time to the development of motor complications.

There are now skin patches and extended-release formulations of dopamine agonists. These are being evaluated as to whether they confer definite clinical benefits over and above what we already have available, at least initially.

In very advanced Parkinson's disease (not all patients reach this stage), patients suddenly and unpredictably 'switch off' and/or have very severe 'off' periods sometimes unresponsive to treatment. They usually also have severe dyskinesias and dystonia. At this stage, the options are:

Table 14.4 Dopaminergic and non-dopaminergic therapies used to treat motor symptoms of idiopathic Parkinson's disease

Drug	Indication
Dopaminergic therapies	
L-dopa	Most effective treatment, thus usually used in all patients aged under 70
Dopamine agonists	Mild, early, or relatively young-onset Parkinson's disease and as add-on treatment
Monoamine oxidase-B inhibitors	Mild, early, young-onset Parkinson's disease and as add-on treatment
Catechol-O-methyltransferase (COMT) inhibitors	An add-on therapy when the effect of L-dopa dose reduces
Amantidine	May reduce dyskinesias
Non-dopaminergic therapies	
Anticholinergics	Mild early tremor in young patients. Avoid use with elderly patients as may cause confusion
Propanolol	Parkinson's patients with mixed tremor: postural/kinetic component

- apomorphine infusion pump – can be as effective as deep-brain stimulation (see below) in reducing 'off' periods and dyskinesias
- deep-brain stimulation (DBS) – contraindicated if there are significant psychiatric or cognitive problems
- continuous duodenal L-dopa infusion ('DuoDopa pump') – works but is expensive and is not widely available
- stem-cell transplantation – trials are underway.

Some patients with 'Parkinson plus' syndromes may respond at least initially to high dose L-dopa.

The non-motor symptoms of IPD

Non-motor symptoms also have a major impact on patients' lives.[16–18]

Depression

Depression is more common in IPD than in age-matched controls. There is no evidence that one class of antidepressant – selective serotonin reuptake inhibitors (SSRIs) or serotonin noradrenalin reuptake inhibitors (SNRIs) – is better than another.

Dementia

The prevalence of dementia among people with IPD is at least double the rate in the general population.[19,20] Clues are periods of confusion unrelated to changes in or timing of medication, and visual hallucinations. Rivastigmine (an acetylcholinesterase inhibitor) is an effective treatment for cognitive impairment and for visual hallucinations.[5]

Dementia with Lewy bodies

This usually similarly presents with cognitive impairment and visual hallucinations (people or animals), and with mild limb Parkinsonism. Gait problems occur earlier. Neuroleptics are contraindicated in patients with Lewy-body dementia since they can cause severe Parkinsonism, neuroleptic malignant syndrome and cognitive decline.

Psychosis

Psychosis arising in IPD is usually a consequence of a change in drug treatment. Dose reduction or withdrawal may resolve the situation. If the psychosis is severe or unrelated to drug treatment, or fails to improve after dose adjustment, clozapine and quetiapine are the drugs of choice. Review non-Parkinson's medication and consider general medical contributory factors.

Sleep disturbance

Sleep may be disturbed in IPD by: difficulty turning in bed, waking up 'off' and rigid, restless legs, pain and depression. Insomnia may respond to L-dopa but not dopamine agonists. Sinemet® CR (L-dopa controlled release) can be very effective. Patients who are drowsy on dopamine agonists during the day can try taking them at night. Restless legs may be related to iron deficiency. Otherwise, simply try to cover the patient at night with their normal dopaminergic therapy or add an alternative dopaminergic drug just at night. Treat pain and depression if present.

Orthostatic/postural hypotension

Hypotension can be difficult to treat. Review medication and exclude general medical contributory factors (e.g. anaemia). Elevating the head of bed 12–15 cm can reduce morning worsening of symptoms. Fludrocortisone 100 μg daily may help and can be increased over months if necessary to 200 μg twice daily. Monitoring of blood pressure can be helpful in assessing drops in blood pressure due to meals and medication.

Bladder and bowel symptoms

Dysautonomia causes a neurogenic bladder with symptoms of an overactive bladder, namely urinary urgency, frequency and urge incontinence. The usual anticholinergics (oxybutynin, tolterodine) cross the blood–brain barrier and may worsen cognition. Treatment with tolterodine could initially be tried or trospium.

Pain

Pain in IPD is under-recognised and multifactorial, arising, for example, from rigidity, predisposition to frozen shoulders (may in fact be an early presentation) and dystonia (responds to L-dopa – dispersible madopar tablets are fast acting). Cervical spondylosis and osteoarthritis may be more problematic because of the greater strain on joints from the surrounding rigid muscles. Sensory pain/disturbance is well recognised but poorly understood in IPD.

Other non-motor symptoms

Difficulties with swallowing partially respond to dopaminergic medications but need to be formally assessed by a speech and language therapist and advice given.

Drooling is a major problem. It is not due to excessive salivation but to reduced swallowing. It may partially respond to increased dopaminergic therapy. Anticholinergics can help, but cause gastrointestinal symptoms and cognitive problems. Glycopyrrolate does not cross the blood–brain barrier and can be effective (up to 2 mg, two or three times daily). Atropine eye drops 0.5 or 1% applied orally one drop each side of mouth can be very effective in controlling drooling without associated side-effects. Treatment-refractory drooling can respond to botulinum toxin injections into the parotid and submandibular glands.

Constipation is very common and can be managed by avoiding anticholinergics, and using stool softeners as well as taking adequate fluids, a high-fibre diet and regular exercise. Osmotic laxatives (e.g. lactulose, or milk of magnesia) are preferred over stimulant laxatives (e.g. senna, bisacodyl). If there is a new history of constipation and an altered bowel habit, particularly if associated with other symptoms, such as bleeding, then a referral for a gastroenterology opinion should be sought to exclude other possible, more serious causes.

Tremor

There are three main types of tremor: resting, intention and postural. Resting tremor occurs with the limb supported against gravity and usually disappears with voluntary movement. It occurs in IPD.

Intention tremor progressively increases in amplitude towards the intended target. It is seen in cerebellar disease – look for other signs of cerebellar disease such as nystagmus and ataxia.

Postural tremor occurs with maintained posture against gravity, such as arms outstretched, and includes physiological tremor and essential tremor (ET). Essential tremor, which also occurs with voluntary action, is usually symmetrical (unlike the asymmetrical pill-rolling rest tremor of IPD) and improves with alcohol. There may be associated head tremor. Writing is of normal size, in contrast to the micrographia seen in IPD. Treatments include primidone and propanolol.

Features of drug-induced tremor

The following may indicate that a patient's tremor has been induced by drugs:[22]

- history of tremorgenic medications – SSRIs, amitriptyline, lithium, valproic acid, neuroleptics, metoclopramide, amiodarone, some respiratory drugs (e.g. salbutamol), which most commonly result in a resting tremor, although SSRIs and lithium also cause action tremor
- temporal relation to commencement of drug or increase in dose
- dose response (in some cases) – drug-induced Parkinsonism is reversible upon cessation within 3 months, although it can be up to 15 months
- subacute symmetric presentation (can be unilateral in drug-induced Parkinsonism, where it is most frequently caused by neuroleptics)
- exclusion of other causes, including metabolic disturbances, Parkinsonian tremor and essential tremor
- lack of progression.

Distinguish between essential tremor and Parkinsonian tremor with the 're-emergence test'.[21] Observe the tremor at rest. Now ask the patient to assume the 'wings of a bird' position: shoulders abducted, fingers of the right hand touching fingers of the left hand in front of the nose. Essential tremor emerges immediately. In IPD, there is a latency of up to 10 seconds between assuming this position and re-emergence of the tremor.

Drugs, particularly neuroleptics, can cause movement disorders (e.g. oculogyria and jaw and neck dystonias) within hours that resolve spontaneously; or tardive disorders that manifest weeks or years later (e.g. torticollis, axial dystonia, opisthotonus trunk movements, akathisia), which have a poor response to treatment.[23]

A DAT-SPECT scan can differentiate between IPD and drug-induced tremor in cases of uncertainty.[24] Management involves checking the drug concentration (e.g. lithium) and dose reduction, or switching/stopping the drug if possible, and sometimes initiating treatment, for example with L-dopa or anticholinergic agents.

Multiple sclerosis

Multiple sclerosis is a demyelinating autoimmune inflammatory disorder of the central nervous system which is possibly caused by environmental and genetic factors. Multiple sclerosis presents in young adults, especially women. First-degree relatives have a 10- to 20-fold increased risk of developing multiple sclerosis.

Some 85% of patients present with relapsing–remitting multiple sclerosis (RRMS), with complete or near-complete recovery of weeks or months after an episode, but 60–70% of patients with RRMS progress to secondary progressive multiple sclerosis within 25 years. However, 10–15% of patients have primary progressive multiple sclerosis with progressive deterioration from the outset – half will be unable to walk unaided within 15 years.

The sites of involvement and the consequent symptoms and signs are set out in Table 14.5.

Cognitive and psychiatric presentations are uncommon. Patients frequently report fatigue.

Uhthoff's phenomenon describes the worsening of symptoms with heat (e.g. a hot bath) or vigorous physical activity.

Table 14.5 Sites of involvement in multiple sclerosis

Site	Sign/symptom
Optic nerve	Acute or subacute visual loss, painful especially with bright light and eye movements. Intravenous steroids hasten recovery but have no effect on long-term prognosis. Ten-year follow-up: 38% of patients with a single episode of optic neuritis will develop multiple sclerosis (22% if the MRI is normal and 56% if at least one lesion is evident on MRI)[25]
Spinal cord	Transverse myelitis presents as asymmetric motor and sensory deficits evolving over hours to days with or without bladder or bowel dysfunction. Lhermitte's sign is the sense of an electric shock going down the spine with neck flexion but occurs in other conditions such as cervical spondylosis
Brain-stem	Ataxia, vertigo, dysarthria, intention tremor

Diagnosis

The diagnosis of RRMS is based upon the confirmation of episodes that occur in different parts of the central nervous system at least 3 months apart; MRI brain and spine scans typically show white-matter plaques of demyelination.

Analysis of the cerebrospinal fluid (CSF) shows oligoclonal bands and an elevated immunoglobulin G (IgG) index, although these findings are not specific to multiple sclerosis. Lumbar puncture and CSF analysis are indicated for suspected multiple sclerosis if the diagnosis of multiple sclerosis is unclear (psychiatrists would not be expected to perform a lumbar puncture). Oligoclonal bands are positive in 95% of patients with a clinical diagnosis of RRMS. Visual evoked potentials can confirm an optic nerve lesion. Key factors to check in the differential diagnosis are in Box 14.5.

Management

Acute treatment with corticosteroid therapy shortens relapse duration but oral steroids are avoided in optic neuritis as the risk of recurrent optic neuritis is increased.

Beta interferons and glatiramer acetate are disease-modifying therapies (DMT) used in patients with relapsing remitting multiple sclerosis with two or more acute relapses within 24 months or in patients with a single relapse (clinically isolated syndrome) at high risk of further relapses. These decrease relapses by about a third. Common adverse effects are inflammation at injection sites, headache, flu-like symptoms and fatigue.

Interferons are contraindicated in patients with current severe depression and/or suicidal ideation. They should be used with caution in patients with previous or current depressive disorders and in those with antecedents of suicidal ideation. It is imperative to monitor for mood changes even in those without a history of mood disorders.

Box 14.5 'Red flags' that suggest a diagnosis other than multiple sclerosis

- Onset age at the extremes (< 10 or > 59 years)
- Hearing loss, especially bilateral
- Headache
- Progressive course (characterises only up to 15% of cases of multiple sclerosis)
- Coexisting systemic or autoimmune disorders
- Significant psychiatric history
- Prominent peripheral nervous system (PNS) signs, lower motor neuron (LMN) signs, bulbar palsy and chorea

Source: Miller *et al*, 2008.[26]

The first oral disease-modifying drugs (fingolimod) for multiple sclerosis have just been licensed and will be on the market this year. However, they need to be reviewed and assessed by NICE before they can be prescribed in the NHS. They are indicated for rapidly evolving severe RRMS, and as a second-line treatment for people whose multiple sclerosis remains active despite treatment with one of the beta-interferon drugs or glatiramer acetate.

Natalizumab, a humanised monoclonal antibody, is recommended in the event of inadequate response to, or intolerance of, other multiple sclerosis therapies. It reduces relapses by 67%.

Mitoxantrone may be considered for selected patients with worsening RRMS or secondary progressive multiple sclerosis (SPMS).

Symptomatic therapies encompass multidisciplinary and medical management of spasticity, fatigue, pain, bladder dysfunction and depression.

Headaches

The cause of headache may be elusive. Headaches can be primary (e.g. migraine, tension-type, cluster) or secondary to other conditions (e.g. intracranial neoplasm, meningitis or subarachnoid haemorrhage). A useful classification has been produced by the International Headache Society.[27]

Migraine

Characteristically, attacks of migraine, with or without aura, last 4–72 hours, are unilateral, pulsating or throbbing, and are worse with routine physical activity (e.g. climbing stairs). Headaches may be accompanied by nausea, vomiting and photophobia, phonophobia and sometimes osmophobia (sensitivity to smell). Box 14.6 outlines key factors about headaches.

Management

Manage by avoiding triggers such as foods (often red wine, cheese), sleep deprivation, stress and dehydration; also avoid codeine due to risk of medication-overuse headache (see below). Start with paracetamol or non-steroidal anti-inflammatory drugs (NSAIDs) for mild to moderate attacks. If the attacks become more severe, contact a neurologist. An anti-emetic is recommended (e.g. domperidone) since peristalsis is often affected even if there is no vomiting.

Investigation

Urgent referral and CT or MRI are indicated if there are new-onset severe headaches, if there is a change in frequency, character or severity of previous headaches, altered consciousness or behaviour, or focal neurological deficit or seizures .

Lumbar puncture is needed if there is suspicion of meningitis, subarachnoid haemorrhage or idiopathic intracranial hypertension.

Box 14.6 Figuring out headaches

- Was there a prodrome? Depression, irritability, euphoria, anorexia, fatigue and food cravings can precede migraine.
- Auras occur in some cases of migraine. They develop over 5 minutes or more, usually last less than an hour, and are *fully reversible*. They may include visual phenomena (spots, flashing lights, zigzag lights), sensory phenomena (paraesthesias, numbness) and speech change (dysphasia).
- The headache itself should be evaluated using the usual 'pain' questions: site, character, radiation, onset, pattern, duration, aggravating and relieving factors. Coughing, sneezing and bending (Valsalva manoeuvre) can worsen migraine but can also precipitate aneurysmal rupture and subarachnoid haemorrhage or the pain produced by a space-occupying lesion. Stress, diet, alcohol and menstruation can precipitate migraine. Ask about the autonomic features of cluster headache (e.g. nasal congestion, conjuctival injection and lacrimation, ptosis). Headache of very sudden onset raises suspicion for subarachnoid haemorrhage, cerebral venous thrombosis and arterial dissection. Migraine evolves over minutes to hours.
- What happened after the headache? For example in migraine, there are sometimes mood and concentration changes.
- Take a family history to cover migraine and aneurysms; also take a drug history, including illicit drugs.
- In the examination pay particular attention to nuchal rigidity and Kernig's sign of meningeal irritation, petechial rash of meningitis, lymphadenopathy of cancer and infection, and temporal artery tenderness/ loss of temporal artery pulsation in giant-cell arteritis.

Preventive treatment for migraine

For frequent disabling migraine, consider preventive treatment such as beta-blockers, serotonin antagonists, tricyclic antidepressants, calcium-channel blockers and anticonvulsants. They should be taken for at least 2 months before trying another agent.

Tension-type headache

Tension-type headaches are the most common type of primary headache. Typically they are bilateral, experienced as pressing/tightening (non-pulsating), of mild or moderate intensity, and not aggravated by routine physical activity such as walking or climbing stairs (unlike migraine). They are featureless, that is, there is no associated nausea (although anorexia may occur) or vomiting, although there may be photophobia or phonophobia (not both). Patients frequently have scalp tenderness. These headaches may become chronic.

Non-pharmacological interventions include patient education, biofeedback, cognitive-based therapy and daily exercise. Mild to moderate acute episodes may respond to acetaminophen, aspirin or NSAIDs. Amitriptyline may be prophylactic. Other preventive medications are as for migraine (see above). It is essential to avoid medication-overuse headache (see below).

Medication-overuse headache ('rebound headache')

These are chronic headaches occurring in the context of overuse of triptans, ergotamines, opioids or combination analgesics for 3 months or more. Advise patients not to take these more than twice a week. The diagnosis is supported if the headache: developed or markedly worsened during medication overuse; and resolves or reverts to its previous pattern within 2 months after discontinuation of the overused medication. It is an important syndrome to identify, given that patients rarely respond to preventive medications while overusing acute medications.

Cluster headaches

These are characterised by severe unilateral orbital, supraorbital and/or temporal pain lasting 15–180 minutes if untreated. Attacks occur up to eight times a day. Other features include: ipsilateral conjunctival injection and/or lacrimation, nasal congestion and/or rhinorrhoea, eyelid oedema, forehead and facial sweating, ipsilateral miosis and/or ptosis and a sense of restlessness or agitation. Importantly, patients with cluster headaches often pace around, unlike migraine patients, who avoid exertion and instead go and lie down in a dark room. Episodes may cluster (i.e. repeat over weeks or months) with remission in between.

Give oxygen, sumatriptan (ideally subcutaneously) and possibly preventive treatment with off-label medications such as verapamil and lithium.

Syndromes related to cluster headache include short-lasting unilateral neuralgiform headache attacks with conjunctival injection and tearing, and chronic paroxysmal headache, both of which manifest as unilateral severe headache and have autonomic features, but are uncommon in general practice.

Idiopathic intracranial hypertension

Idiopathic intracranial hypertension was formerly called 'benign intracranial hypertension'. There may be headache, transient greying out of vision, diplopia due to sixth-nerve palsy and papilloedema. It is particularly common in young overweight females (or those who have recently gained weight). Management aims to lower intracranial pressure and this requires hospitalisation.

Giant-cell arteritis

In patients over 50, suspect giant-cell arteritis (GCA) with headache associated with scalp tenderness (e.g. when brushing hair), jaw claudication, and constitutional symptoms (weight loss, myalgia, anorexia, night sweats and low-grade fever). The major concern is potential visual loss. Examine for temporal artery tenderness and non-pulsatile temporal arteries. Most sufferers have a raised erythrocyte sedimentation rate (ESR). Biopsy of the temporal artery is required to secure the diagnosis (although even this can be negative if there are skip lesions).

Steroids should be given in suspected temporal arteritis after the erythrocyte sedimentation rate is evaluated, to prevent visual loss. Do not wait until after the biopsy.

Stroke

Stroke is an acute focal neurological defect resulting from vascular disease. It is the leading cause of disability worldwide and the third leading cause of death after ischaemic heart disease and cancer. Risk factors include age, smoking, hypertension, ischaemic heart disease, atrial fibrillation, valvular disease, diabetes mellitus, hypercholesterolaemia, alcohol excess, obesity and of course previous strokes and transient ischaemic attacks. Around 85% of strokes are ischaemic (due to thrombus or embolus); the remainder are haemorrhagic. Resulting deficits depend on the arterial territory affected (Table 14.6) and include abrupt onset of hemiparesis, neglect, sensory loss, visual field defects, aphasia, dysarthria and ataxia. See ABCD2 score, p. 446.

Assessment

Once the diagnosis is suspected, seek hospital admission, as a CT brain scan is required urgently to rule out a haemorrhage – there is a 3-hour 'window' to provide clot-busting thrombolysis, although an infarct may not be evident on CT for at least 6 hours. Once haemorrhage is excluded, patients may receive thrombolysis (if they present within 3 hours) and aspirin (unless contraindicated), as these are proven to reduce rates of death and major disability requiring carer dependence.[28,29] Clopidogrel is now the first-line recommendation for people who have had an ischaemic stroke.

A combination of aspirin and dipyridamole is appropriate for people who have had an ischaemic stroke only if clopidogrel is contraindicated or not tolerated (see 2010 NICE guidelines in Recommended reading).

Subsequent management incorporates multidisciplinary input at a stroke unit, investigations to identify stroke aetiology (e.g. ultrasound Doppler scans of the carotid, echocardiography) and addressing vascular risk factors for secondary stroke prevention.

A transient ischaemic attack (TIA) is an episode of neurological dysfunction caused by focal brain, spinal cord or retinal ischaemia, without acute infarction. Subsequent very early risk of stroke is much higher than was previously thought: about 10% at 1 week, 14% at 1 month and 18% at 3 months; hence the need for urgent referral for investigations and secondary prevention.[30–32]

Motor neuron disease

Amyotrophic lateral sclerosis (ALS) is the most common form of motor neuron disease. It is a neurodegenerative disease with a life expectancy of 3–5 years. It is characterised by a combination of:

- upper motor neuron signs (brisk reflexes, clonus)
- lower motor neuron signs (wasting, fasciculations).

Table 14.6 Selected stroke syndromes

Arterial territory affected	Sign/symptoms
Anterior cerebral artery	Contralateral limb weakness greater in legs than arms, contralateral sensory loss, frontal lobe signs (e.g. disinhibition), primitive reflexes, gait apraxia, urinary incontinence
Middle cerebral artery	Contralateral hemiparesis, contralateral sensory loss, Broca's or Wernicke's aphasia if dominant hemisphere, contralateral neglect if non-dominant hemisphere, homonymous hemianopia, gaze preference towards side of lesion
Posterior cerebral artery	Contralateral homonymous hemianopia, alexia without agraphia (i.e. impaired reading with intact writing), memory loss, cortical blindness, visual agnosia, altered mental status
Lacunar stroke[a]	Pure motor hemiparesis, ataxia hemiparesis or pure sensory stroke
Vertebrobasilar artery (posterior circulation)	Vertigo, nystagmus, diplopia, visual field deficits, dysphagia, dysarthria, facial sensory loss, syncope, ataxia. Unlike anterior circulation strokes, which produce findings only on one side of the body, posterior circulation strokes result in crossed findings: ipsilateral cranial nerve deficits and contralateral motor deficits

[a]Lacunar strokes account from up to one-fifth of all strokes. They are especially seen in patients with small-vessel disease (e.g. hypertension and diabetes). They result from occlusion of the small, perforating arteries of the deep subcortical areas of the brain.

Patients with ALS do not have:

- sphincter disturbance (at least in the early stages)
- ocular involvement or ptosis
- prominent sensory symptoms
- involuntary movements.

Patients present with muscle cramping, gait problems (e.g. dragging one leg, tripping), difficulties with fine movements or bulbar symptoms (e.g. sialorrhoea, drooling), dysarthria and dysphagia. Up to 15% of patients develop frontotemporal dementia.

Riluzole is the only licensed drug for ALS and extends survival by about 2 months. Symptomatic management is key (for muscle spasms, malnutrition, emotional lability) with gastrostomy and non-invasive ventilation where indicated. Psychiatric and psychological inputs are called upon to address cognitive, behavioural and mood issues.[33]

Guillain–Barré syndrome

This is characterised by:

- progressive ascending weakness
- ascending flaccid paralysis
- autonomic involvement (arrhythmias, labile blood pressure, urinary retention and paralytic ileus).

It progresses over days to 4 weeks. Cranial nerve and respiratory involvement may follow and about 20% of severely affected patients remain unable to walk after 6 months. Hospital admission is essential. It often follows a prodromal illness or sepsis and 5–8% of patients will die. Patient may initially complain of backache and acute sensory disturbance in hands and feet before or while concurrently developing weakness. There is an increased risk of deep vein thrombosis/pulmonary embolism. The need for ventilation and intensive treatment unit support is assessed by vital capacity (VC) on spirometry. If VC is less than 1.6 l, discuss with anaesthetic ITU team to make them aware of the patient before further possible deterioration.[34]

Myasthenia gravis

This is an autoimmune condition that affects neuromuscular transmission, with antibodies directed against receptors at the neuromuscular junction, causing fatiguable weakness (Box 14.7) or fluctuating weakness affecting the ocular nerve (in 85% of cases) or cranial nerves, or limb or truncal musculature. Bulbar weakness causes dysarthria and dysphagia, and difficulty chewing. Relapses can be precipitated by infection and new medications (e.g. aminoglycosides, steroids, phenytoin, quinine, beta-blockers, anaesthetic agents).

Management

Symptomatic relief is provided by anticholinesterase agents such as pyridostigmine. Some drugs are disease-modifying (prednisolone, azathioprine, cyclosporine). Thymectomy may help some. Hospitalisation is required if dyspnoea, dysphagia, weight loss or rapidly progressive or severe weakness occurs.

Disturbed consciousness

Most patients with a lowered level consciousness will be hospitalised. Two conditions may be encountered in psychiatric practice: akinetic mutism and catatonia.

Akinetic mutism

This presents as wakefulness and awareness with an absence or paucity of speech and spontaneous

Box 14.7 Bedside tests to identify fatiguability in myasthenia gravis

The ice test

In patients with ptosis, place a cube of ice over the eyelid for about 2 minutes which results in an improvement of ptosis (89% sensitivity)[35]

Other tests

Ask the patient:

- to look up for several minutes (examining for ptosis or extra-ocular weakness)
- to close their eyes for 2 minutes – the 'peek' sign refers to widening of the palpebral fissure due to orbicularis oculi fatigue[36]
- to count aloud to 100 (listen for nasal or slurred speech as time goes on)
- to abduct the arms/elevate the legs for 2 minutes – patient with myasthenia gravis unable to maintain posture, arm and/or leg drop down

movement (e.g. facial expression, gestures). There is usually some evidence of conscious behaviour/alertness. Akinetic mutism generally involves bilateral frontal or mesencephalic damage.

Catatonia

Catatonia occurs in up to 40% of psychiatric patients, most commonly associated with mood disorders but also schizophrenia, schizoaffectve disorder, drug intoxication and withdrawal states and extrapyramidal disorders.[37] The DSM-IV criteria are set out in Box 14.8.

Autoimmune encephalopathies

Autoimmune encephalopathies (AiE) are a newly recognised but rare cause of 'new-onset' psychiatric symptoms, for example psychoses, anxiety disorders, mutism, changes in behaviour and personality. Patients may also develop seizures, subacute cerebellar ataxia, symptoms of viral encephalitis, cognitive impairment and confusion. AiEs are associated with various forms of cancer. They are mediated by antibodies to cell surface antigens in the central nervous system involving potassium or calcium channels or receptors. The prognosis is good with immunosuppressive treatments. If you suspect AiE, request an urgent neurological opinion (see p. 336).

Box 14.8 Catatonic schizophrenia: clinical features

Schizophrenia can present with catatonia, although this is rarely seen in the UK nowadays. The clinical presentation includes some of the features outlined below:

- Excitement, agitation or excess, purposeless activity; this can lead to exhaustion
- Stupor: the patient does not respond to their surroundings or become mute
- Immobility: holding the same posture for prolonged periods of time
- 'Waxy flexibility': staying in the same posture that someone else has placed them in
- Stereotypical movements: these can include facial movements and repetition of phrases

For DSM-IV diagnostic criteria, see American Psychiatric Association, 1994.[38]

Thorough history and examination are key to neurological diagnosis. CT and MRI scans are useful only if used in the right context and only if you know what you are looking for! Pattern recognition (e.g. tremor plus rigidity plus bradykinesia = Parkinsonism; headaches plus scalp tenderness plus jaw claudication plus constitutional symptoms = temporal arteritis) is the most important clinical skill to develop.

When to refer to a neurologist

- Epilepsy
  - New onset fit or seizures/focal seizures: urgent referral for MRI brain scan
  - Known epilepsy with poor or worsening control despite increasing or adding medication – refer; may require continuous ambulatory EEG monitoring
  - Known epilepsy and develops new neurological signs: urgent referral
  - Known epilepsy and planning pregnancy or already pregnant
- Parkinson's disease
  - Newly diagnosed: refer to specialist neurologist
  - Possible drug-induced Parkinsonism or other movement disorder: refer to specialist neurologist
- Movement disorders
  - Tremor (functionally disabling and/or 'essential'), chorea, dystonia and myoclonus: refer to neurologist specialising in movement disorder
  - Suspected psychogenic movement disorder: refer for full investigation
- Focal neurological signs
  - Upper motor neuron signs (pyramidal weakness, spasticity/ankle clonus, very brisk reflexes and extensor plantar response)
  - Signs develop acutely (minutes) and Stroke FAST (face, arm, speech test) assessment positive: urgent call 999, stating 'possible stroke'
  - Signs develop sub-acutely or progressively (weeks to months): urgent referral
  - Relapsing remitting course with sensory symptoms: refer
  - Additional lower motor neuron signs (muscle wasting with fasciculations, absent reflexes): refer

    - Sudden loss of neurological function lasting less than 24 hours (unilateral visual loss, motor and/or sensory function): apply the ABCD2 scoring system[39] (see Chapter 31) – refer urgently to TIA clinic
- New-onset motor, sensory or visual symptoms
    - If progressive: urgent referral to neurology clinic
    - If fatigable weakness and/or ptosis: urgent referral, and speech/swallowing refer to accident and emergency (A&E)
    - If visual disturbance (visual failure, diplopia or visual field defect): refer to opthalmologist
- Vertigo
    - If accompanying earache, discharge, tinnitus or hearing loss: refer to ear, nose and throat specialist
    - If other neurological symptoms or signs: urgent referral to neurologist
- Headache
    - Temporal tenderness (on touching, brushing or washing hair) or jaw claudication with raised ESR and over 50 years old: urgent referral to neurologist and start prednisolone enteric coated 60 mg daily immediately before referral
    - Thunderclap headache: urgent referral to A&E for CT head ± lumbar puncture
    - Exertional/coital headaches: refer to neurologist
    - Pyrexia: refer to A&E
- Acute/subacute cognitive impairment
    - With or without behavioural/personality changes ± reduced level of consciousness or seizures: refer to A&E.

References

1 Commission on Classification and Terminology of the International League Against Epilepsy. Proposal for revised clinical and electroencephalographic classification of epileptic seizures. *Epilepsia* 1981; **22**: 489–501.

2 Sheldon R, Rose S, Ritchie D, *et al.* Historical criteria that distinguish syncope from seizures. *J Am Coll Cardiol* 2002; **40**: 142–8.

3 Chen D, So Y, Fisher R. The use of serum prolactin level in diagnosing epileptic seizures: Report of the Therapeutics and Technology Assessment Subcommittee of the American Academy of Neurology. *Neurology* 2005; **65**: 668–75.

4 Krumholz A, Wiebe S, Gronseth G, *et al.* Practice Parameter: evaluating an apparent unprovoked first seizure in adults (an evidence-based review): report of the Quality Standards Subcommittee of the American Academy of Neurology and the American Epilepsy Society. *Neurology* 2007; **69**: 1996–2007.

5 Greenberg MK, Barsan WG, Starkman S. Neuroimaging in the emergency patient presenting with seizure. *Neurology* 1996; **47**: 26–32.

6 Harden CL, Huff JS, Schwartz TH, *et al.* Reassessment: neuroimaging in the emergency patient presenting with seizure (an evidence-based review): report of the Therapeutics and Technology Assessment Subcommittee of the American Academy of Neurology. *Neurology* 2007; **69**: 1772–80.

7 Scottish Intercollegiate Guidelines Network. *Diagnosis and Management of Epilepsy in Adults: A National Clinical Guideline (70).* SIGN, 2003.

8 Walters RJ, Hutchings AD, Smith DF, *et al.* Inappropriate requests for serum anti-epileptic drug levels in hospital practice. *QJM* 2004; **97**: 337–41.

9 Lowenstein DH, Bleck T, Macdonald RL. It's time to revise the definition of status epilepticus. *Epilepsia* 1999; **40**: 120–2.

10 Meierkord H, Boon P, Engelsen B, *et al.* EFNS guideline on the management of status epilepticus in adults. *Eur J Neurol* 2010; **17**: 348–55.

11 Abdo WF, van de Warrenburg BP, Burn DJ, *et al.* The clinical approach to movement disorders. *Nat Rev Neurol* 2010 Jan; **6**: 29–37.

12 Factor SA, Podskalny GD, Molho ES. Psychogenic movement disorders: frequency, clinical profile, and characteristics. *J Neurol Neurosurg Psychiatry* 1995; **59**: 406–12.

13 Fahn S, Williams DT. Psychogenic dystonia. *Adv Neurol* 1988; **50**: 431–55.

14 Hinson VK, Haren WB. Psychogenic movement disorders. *Lancet Neurol* 2006; **5**: 695–700.

15 Suchowersky O, Reich S, Perlmutter J, *et al.* Practice parameter: diagnosis and prognosis of new onset Parkinson disease. *Neurology* 2006; **66**: 968–75.

16 Chaudhuri KR, Healy DG, Schapira AH. Non-motor symptoms of Parkinson's disease: diagnosis and management. *Lancet Neurol* 2006; **5**: 235–45.

17 Miyasaki JM, Shannon K, Voon V, *et al.* Practice Parameter: evaluation and treatment of depression, psychosis, and dementia in Parkinson disease (an evidence-based review): report of the Quality Standards Subcommittee of the American Academy of Neurology. *Neurology* 2006; **66**: 996–1002.

18 Zesiewicz TA, Sullivan KL, Arnulf I, *et al.* Practice Parameter: treatment of nonmotor symptoms of Parkinson disease: report of the Quality Standards Subcommittee of the American Academy of Neurology. *Neurology* 2010; **74**: 924–31.

19 Aarsland D, Anderson K, Larsen JP, *et al.* Risk of dementia in Parkinson's disease – a community-based, prospective study. *Neurology* 2001; **56**: 730–6.

20 Caballol N, Martí MJ, Tolosa E. Cognitive dysfunction and dementia in Parkinson disease. *Mov Disord* 2007; **Sep**: S358–66.

21 Jankovic J, Schwartz KS, Ondo W. Re-emergent tremor of Parkinson's disease. *J Neurol Neurosurg Psychiatry* 1999; **67**: 646–50.

22 Alvarez MV, Evidente VG. Understanding drug-induced parkinsonism: separating pearls from oysters. *Neurology* 2008; **70**: e32–4.

23 Morgan JC, Sethi KD. Drug-induced tremors. *Lancet Neurol* 2005; **4**: 866–76.

24 Kägi G, Bhatia KP, Tolosa E. The role of DAT-SPECT in movement disorders. *J Neurol Neurosurg Psychiatry* 2010; **81**: 5–12.

25 Beck RW, Trobe JD, Moke PS, *et al.* High- and low-risk profiles for the development of multiple sclerosis within 10 years after optic neuritis: experience of the optic neuritis treatment trial. *Arch Ophthalmol* 2003; **121**: 944–9.

26 Miller DH, Weinshenker BG, Filippi M, *et al.* Differential diagnosis of suspected multiple sclerosis: a consensus approach. *Mult Scler* 2008; **14**: 1157–74.

27 Headache Classification Subcommittee of the International Headache Society. *The International Classification of Headache Disorders (2nd edn): Cephalagia.* Blackwell Publishing, 2004.

28 Adams HP, del Zoppo G, Alberts MJ, *et al.* Guidelines for the early management of adults with ischemic stroke. *Stroke* 2007; **38**: 1655–711.

29 National Institute of Neurological Disorders and Stroke rt-PA Stroke Study Group. Tissue plasminogen activator for acute ischemic stroke. *N Engl J Med* 1995; **333**: 1581–7.

30 Coull AJ, Lovett JK, Rothwell PM. Population based study of early risk of stroke after transient ischaemic attack or minor stroke: implications for public education and organisation of services. *BMJ* 2004; **328**: 326.

31 Easton JD, Saver JL, Albers GW, *et al.* Definition and evaluation of transient ischemic attack: a scientific statement for healthcare professionals from the American Heart Association/American Stroke Association Stroke Council *et al. Stroke* 2009; **40**: 2276–93.

32 Rothwell PM, Giles MF, Chandratheva A, *et al.* Effect of urgent treatment of transient ischaemic attack and minor stroke on early recurrent stroke (EXPRESS study): a prospective population-based sequential comparison. *Lancet* 2007; **370**: 1432–42.

33 Andersen PM, Borasio GD, Dengler R, *et al.* EFNS task force on management of amyotrophic lateral sclerosis: guidelines for diagnosing and clinical care of patients and relatives. *Eur J Neurol* 2005; **12**: 921–38.

34 van Doorn PA, Ruts L, Jacobs BC. Clinical features, pathogenesis, and treatment of Guillain–Barré syndrome. *Lancet Neurol* 2008; **7**: 939–50.

35 Sethi KD, Rivner MH, Swift TR. Ice pack test for myasthenia gravis. *Neurology* 1987; **37**: 1383–5.

36 Osher RH, Griggs RC. Orbicularis fatigue: the 'peek' sign of myasthenia gravis. *Arch Ophthalmol* 1979; **97**: 677–9.

37 Taylor MA, Fink M. Catatonia in psychiatric classification: a home of its own. *Am J Psychiatry* 2003; **160**: 1233–41.

38 American Psychiatric Association. *Diagnostic and Statistical Manual of Mental Disorders (4th edn).* APA, 1994.

39 Johnston SC, Rothwell PM, Nguyen-Huynh MN, *et al.* Validation and refinement of scores to predict very early stroke risk after transient ischaemic attack. *Lancet* 2007; **369**: 283–92.

Recommended reading

ACEP Clinical Policies Committee, Clinical Policies Subcommittee on Seizures. Critical issues in the evaluation and management of adult patients presenting to the emergency department with seizures. *Ann Emerg Med* 2004; **43**: 605–25.

Bateman DE. Neurological assessment of coma. *J Neurol Neurosurg Psychiatry* 2001; **71** (suppl 1): i13–7.

Bates D. The management of medical coma. *J Neurol Neurosurg Psychiatry* 1993; **56**: 589–98.

International Headache Society. *The International Classification of Headache Disorders* (2nd edn). Blackwell, 2004.

Miyasaki JM, Shannon K, Voon V, *et al. Practice Parameter: Evaluation and Treatment of Depression, Psychosis and Dementia in Parkinson Disease.* American Academy of Neurology, 2006 (http://www.aan.com/professionals/practice/guidelines/pda/Eval_Dementia_PD.pdf).

National Institute for Health and Clinical Excellence. *Parkinson's Disease: Diagnosis and Management in Primary and Secondary Care* (CG35). NICE, 2006.

National Institute for Health and Clinical Excellence. *Clopidogrel and Modified-Release Dipyridamole for the Prevention of Occlusive Vascular Events* (review of technology appraisal guidance 90) (TA210). NICE, 2010.

National Institute for Health and Clinical Excellence. *The Epilepsies: The Diagnosis and Management of the Epilepsies in Adults and Children in Primary and Secondary Care* (CG137). NICE, 2012.

Phukan J, Hardiman O. The management of amyotrophic lateral sclerosis. *J Neurol* 2009; **256**: 176–86.

Sheldon R, Rose S, Ritchie D, *et al.* Diagnostic questions to determine whether loss of consciousness is due to seizures or syncope: historical criteria that distinguish syncope from seizures. *J Am Coll Cardiol* 2002; **40**: 142–8.

Summary

The key to making a neurological diagnosis is to take a thorough history and make a thorough physical examination. Investigations such as CT scans and MRI scans are only helpful if used in the right context, and only if you know what you are looking for in the first place. Pattern recognition is the most important clinical skill to develop.

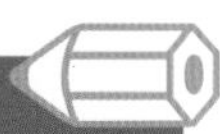

Learning points

- When evaluating an episode of lost consciousness, use the 'before, during, after' approach of questioning. A simple scoring system can be used to distinguish between seizure and syncope.
- An EEG cannot exclude epilepsy. It is best to consult an neurologist before ordering one.
- Epilepsy and non-epilepsy (psychogenic) seizures coexist in at least 20% of patients presenting with seizures. Things suggestive of non-epileptic seizures include gradual onset of the seizure, stop–start motor activity, eyes closed (even against resistance), biting of the tip of the tongue (as opposed to its lateral edges) and lying motionless for over 5 minutes.
- Parkinson's disease is marked by bradykinesia, cogwheel rigidity, resting tremor and postural instability but also by non-motor features such as insomnia, behavioural and cognitive impairment, and bladder and bowel symptoms.
- It is important to identify the 'Parkinson plus' syndromes (e.g. Lewy-body dementia, progressive supranuclear palsy, multisystem atrophy) by noting the 'red flags'. Treatment used in idiopathic Parkinson's disease may be ineffective in the syndromes or may even cause deterioration.
- All patients with suspected idiopathic Parkinson's disease should be referred to a specialist before treatment is commenced.
- Drug-induced tremor is suggested by a temporal relation to the commencement or increase in the dosage of a drug, subacute symmetric presentation and lack of progression.
- Psychogenic movement disorders account for up to 3% of referrals to movement disorder clinics. Look out for features such as abrupt onset, quick progression, excessively slow and effortful movements, suppression with distraction, entrainment and response to suggestion.
- Oral steroids for optic neuritis are not recommended due to the risk of subsequent recurrent optic neuritis. Disease-modifying treatment with beta-interferons or glatiramer acetate should be considered as soon as possible following a definite diagnosis of multiple sclerosis with active, relapsing disease and may also be considered for selected patients with a first attack, who are at high risk of multiple sclerosis.
- Urgent referral and CT or MRI are indicated if there are new-onset severe headaches, change in frequency, character or severity of previous headaches, altered consciousness or behaviour, focal neurological deficit or seizures.
- Patients who present with 3 hours of stroke (and sometimes 4.5 hours according to more recent guidelines) may be eligible for thrombolysis. Refer instantly if a stroke is suspected.

15

Endocrinology

Theingi Aung, Charles N. Antonypillai, Josephine Tuthill, Niki Karavitaki and John A. H. Wass

Endocrine disorders may present with psychiatric symptoms. In addition, endocrine conditions can be caused by psychotropic medication. This chapter describes the clinical presentations and investigations of key endocrine disorders, along with tips on when to refer to an endocrinologist.

Introduction

Endocrine disorders can masquerade as psychiatric disorders and vice versa. Psychiatrists need the knowledge and skills to be able to tell the difference.

Endocrine diseases can present with mild or serious psychiatric symptoms. It has been reported that a mother murdered her child before the psychosis caused by her Cushing's syndrome was recognised.

Many patients see psychiatrists for symptoms of anxiety before the underlying adrenaline release from a phaeochromocytoma or in response to hypoglycaemia is recognised. Many psychotropic drugs raise prolactin levels and cause hypogonadism.

This chapter outlines the psychological aspects of endocrine disorders as well as endocrine conditions caused by medications used for psychiatric conditions. It also gives guidance on diagnosis and when to refer to an endocrinologist.

Diabetes mellitus is covered in Chapter 16.

Psychiatric conditions that may be caused by endocrine disorders are included on p. 360.

Endocrine conditions presenting with psychiatric symptoms

The psychiatric manifestations of endocrine disorders are outlined in Table 15.1. The sections below discuss these disorders by organ system.

Pituitary/hypothalamus

Cushing's syndrome

The syndrome actually covers all cases – Cushing's disease is pituitary-dependent Cushing's syndrome.

Mood disturbances (depression, concentration difficulties, insomnia, memory disturbances and irritability, psychosis and anxiety) are some of the commonest presentations of Cushing's syndrome and occur with all of its causes. In one study, 83% of patients with Cushing's syndrome were diagnosed with an affective disorder, 67% with endogenous depression,

Table 15.1 Psychiatric manifestations of endocrine disorders

Endocrine disorder	Psychiatric symptoms
Cushing's syndrome	Depression, psychosis, insomnia, anxiety
Acromegaly	Affective disorders (depression, dysthymia)
Hyperprolactinaemia	Irritability, depression
Growth hormone deficiency	Depression, anxiety, impaired self-esteem
Gonadotrophin deficiency	Depression, anxiety, irritability, insomnia, poor memory
Hypothalamic syndrome	Behavioural change, somnolence, eating disorder
Hyperthyroidism	Emotional lability, anxiety, restlessness, rarely psychosis
Hypothyroidism	Depression, paranoia, cognitive impairment, slowing of intellectual function
Hypercalcaemia	Depression, tiredness, confusion, coma if extreme
Hypocalcaemia	Seizures
Addison's disease	Mild disturbance in mood, motivation and behaviour. Psychosis and delirium more rarely
Phaeochromocytoma	Panic attacks, anxiety
Insulinoma	Irritability, confusion, aggression, coma, anxiety
Polycystic ovary syndrome	Affective disorder

and 27% with mania or hypomania.[1] Furthermore, there is a more than 50% increased rate of psychotic symptoms in patients with the syndrome.[2]

Cushing's syndrome can either be adrenocorticotrophic hormone (ACTH) dependent (pituitary adenoma or ectopic ACTH secretion) or ACTH independent (mainly adrenal).

The clinical features include a round plethoric facial appearance, weight gain (mainly truncal obesity), buffalo hump, supraclavicular fat pads, skin manifestations (thin and easily bruising skin, purple striae), proximal myopathy (manifested as an inability to stand up from a sitting position without support), menstrual irregularity, low libido and impotence. Hypertension, diabetes mellitus or impaired glucose tolerance, osteopenia or osteoporosis can also be associated with the syndrome.

The symptoms of Cushing's syndrome may precede the diagnosis by many years. Clinical suspicion of the condition should lead to appropriate investigations and referral. Screening tests include a 24-hour urinary collection of free cortisol (UFC) on two occasions and an overnight dexamethasone suppression test (ONDST) (administer 1 mg of dexamethasone at midnight and check serum cortisol levels at 9 a.m. the next day – the normal level is < 50 nmol/l).[3] False positives (lack of normal suppression) occur in gross obesity, primary depressive disorders, anorexia nervosa and other illnesses which upset circadian rhythm, such as heart failure and malignancy.

Correctly diagnosing the cause of Cushing's syndrome and managing the complex nature of the disease can be challenging. Treatment depends on aetiology, and definitive management should be given at an endocrine unit with a multidisciplinary approach. After successful treatment, symptoms will reverse with time, including psychiatric symptoms.[4]

When making a diagnosis of Cushing's syndrome, check if the patient has a round face, thin skin and if their leg muscle size is disproportionate to their weight, indicating presence of a myopathy.

Functioning and non-functioning pituitary tumours

Psychiatric manifestations of pituitary tumours are much less common than with Cushing's syndrome. Prolactinomas occur most commonly, followed by

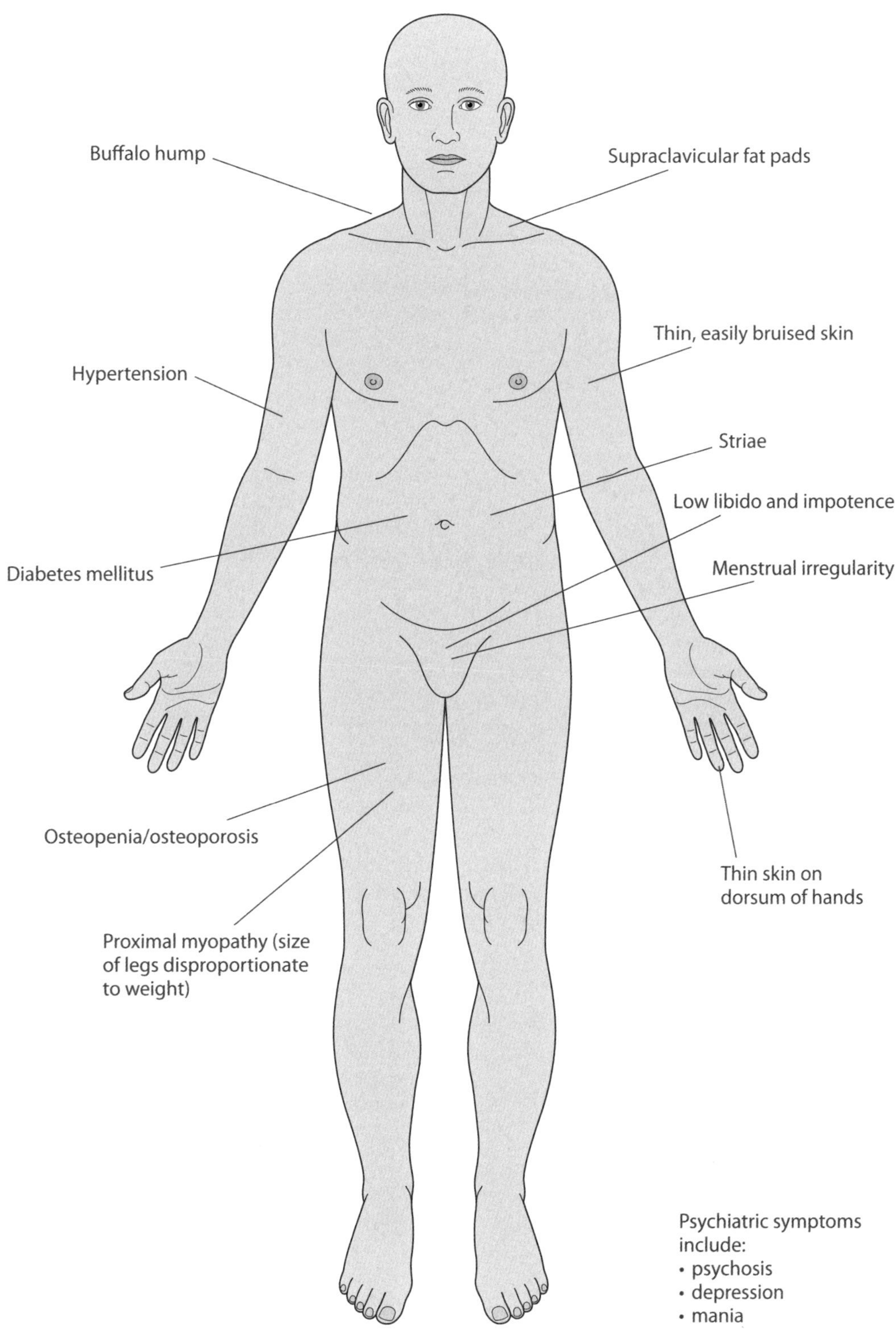
Buffalo hump
Supraclavicular fat pads
Thin, easily bruised skin
Hypertension
Striae
Low libido and impotence
Diabetes mellitus
Menstrual irregularity
Osteopenia/osteoporosis
Thin skin on dorsum of hands
Proximal myopathy (size of legs disproportionate to weight)
Psychiatric symptoms include:
• psychosis
• depression
• mania

Fig. 15.1 Cushing's syndrome.

non-functioning pituitary adenomas, acromegaly and Cushing's syndrome.

Symptomatic pituitary tumours occur in around 1 in 10 000, but pituitary magnetic resonance imaging (MRI) reveals an abnormal 'incidentaloma' in 10% of the population.[5] Headaches may occur, usually with larger tumours but occasionally with microadenomas (< 1 cm) of the pituitary. Hypopituitarism (growth hormone deficiency, secondary hypogonadism, hypothyroidism or hypoadrenalism) can cause fatigue, with clinical features depending on the type and degree of hormonal insufficiency.

Prolactinoma

Prolactinomas are the commonest functioning pituitary tumour; there is a female preponderance.[3] Clinical symptoms and signs of hyperprolactinaemia in women include oligoamenorrhoea, infertility and galactorrhoea. In men, hypogonadism, decreased libido, erectile dysfunction, infertility, gynaecomastia and, in rare instances, galactorrhoea can be seen. Irritability and depression can also be presenting symptoms.

Although rare, prolactinomas may occur in children, typically with mass effect, pubertal delay or both. Macroprolactinomas (tumours > 1 cm) can cause mass effects (headache, bitemporal visual field defect and cranial nerve palsies due to invasion of the cavernous sinus). Aggressive tumours can occasionally erode bone, leading to leakage of cerebrospinal fluid (CSF) and secondary meningitis.

People with prolactinomas have prolactin levels above 3000 mU/l. Other causes of high prolactin (raised, but usually < 3000 mU/l) should be excluded, including physiological causes such as pregnancy and lactation, medications such as antidepressants and antipsychotics, chronic renal disease, severe liver disease and hypothyroidism. Pituitary imaging for tumour localisation is needed after biochemical confirmation. Endocrine referral and advice are necessary.

In patients with pituitary adenomas, there is a predictable sequence of onset of hormone deficiency, with growth hormone going first, then gonadotrophins, prolactin and lastly thyroid-stimulating hormone (TSH) and ACTH.

Non-functioning pituitary adenomas and hypopituitarism

These present with headaches and hypogonadism due to hypopituitarism. Clearly, no excessive levels of pituitary hormones are found. Diagnosis is often delayed, particularly in men in whom sexual dysfunction goes unrecognised or is falsely attributed to ageing.

Growth hormone deficiency

Growth hormone deficiency affects psychological and physical well-being. It can be secondary to a pituitary tumour or can follow surgery or radiotherapy, and occurs in both adults and children.

Symptoms include depression, anxiety and reduced muscle mass with central obesity. Growth hormone deficiency is also related to increased cardiovascular risk and fracture risk from osteoporosis. Impaired self-esteem and social withdrawal are also early symptoms.

Although insulin-like growth factor (IGF-1) may be used as a measure of the growth hormone axis, it may still be in the reference range in 50% of patients who are growth hormone deficient. Hence definitive dynamic testing (insulin tolerance test/glucagon test) should be performed in a specialist endocrine unit.

Gonadotrophin deficiency

Gonadotrophin deficiency can be primary (testicular or ovarian failure), secondary (pituitary or hypothalamic) or have non-endocrine causes (physical and psychological stress, systemic illness, anabolic steroid and recreational drug usage). It can manifest with psychiatric symptoms (depression, anxiety, irritability, insomnia and poor memory), diminished libido, impotence, reduced muscle and bone mass, and diminished body hair. Anaemia can be found in the chronic hypogonadal state because testosterone stimulates erythropoietin.

An early-morning (9 a.m.) testosterone level should be checked with measurements of leuteinising hormone (LH) and follicle stimulating hormone (FSH) to differentiate between primary and secondary causes of hypogonadism. An inappropriately low or normal FSH and LH with a low testosterone or oestrogen (hypogonadotrophic hypogonadism) suggests a pituitary or hypothalamic aetiology needing an MRI scan of the pituitary and should engender a referral to endocrinology for further evaluation and assessment for hormone replacement. A low testosterone or oestrogen level with high compensatory FSH and LH (hypergonadotrophic hypogonadism) indicates a local

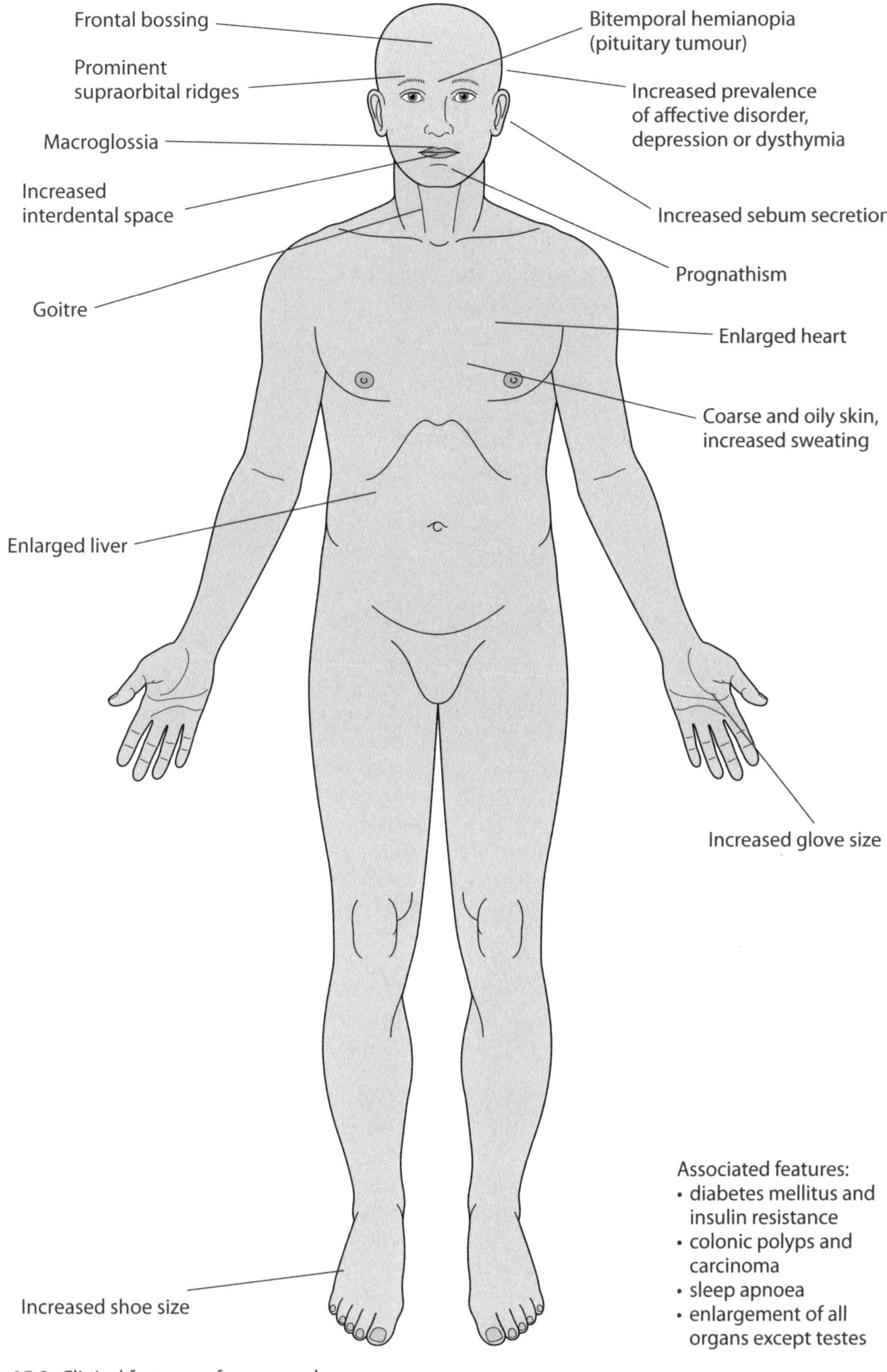
Frontal bossing
Prominent supraorbital ridges
Macroglossia
Increased interdental space
Goitre
Bitemporal hemianopia (pituitary tumour)
Increased prevalence of affective disorder, depression or dysthymia
Increased sebum secretion
Prognathism
Enlarged heart
Coarse and oily skin, increased sweating
Enlarged liver
Increased glove size
Associated features:
• diabetes mellitus and insulin resistance
• colonic polyps and carcinoma
• sleep apnoea
• enlargement of all organs except testes
Increased shoe size

Fig. 15.2 Clinical features of acromegaly.

gonadal defect and also needs appropriate referral and investigations.

Acromegaly

Acromegaly is associated with an increased prevalence of affective disorder, major depression and dysthymia.[6]

It is a rare endocrine condition with a prevalence of 40–50 cases per million population, and mainly presents between the ages of 30 and 50 years. The disease is secondary to hypersecretion of growth hormone, the commonest cause of which is a pituitary adenoma – macroadenoma (80% of cases) more often than microadenoma.

Prolonged excessive production of growth hormone causes well-recognised clinical signs: changed facial features (frontal bossing, prognathism, increased interdental space, macroglossia, coarse and oily skin), increased sweating, occasional headache, an increase in ring or shoe size, deep voice, organomegaly (macrosomia, goitre, heart, liver and kidneys), joint pains (back, knees and hips) and tiredness. The pressure effects of a pituitary macroadenoma on the optic chiasm can cause visual field defects, classically a bitemporal hemianopia. Other associated features include hypertension, sleep apnoea, insulin resistance and diabetes mellitus, colonic polyps and carcinoma, and heart valve regurgitation.

As disease progress is insidious, diagnosis can be considerably delayed (up to 15 years) and comparison with old photographs is often helpful to recognise the changes. Single IGF-1 and basal growth hormone measurements can be useful for the diagnosis if elevated. The definitive test is an oral glucose tolerance test (OGTT), which should be performed. Failure of suppression of growth hormone to less than 0.5 ng/ml after a glucose load is diagnostic of acromegaly.

Endocrine referral should be sought for diagnostic confirmation, tumour localisation, and for definitive treatment and follow-up.

Hypothalamic syndrome

This is uncommon and is mainly due to large tumours (e.g. craniopharyngioma) or various infiltrative disorders, (e.g. sarcoidosis). Clinical features include hyperphagia, obesity, loss of thirst sensation and behavioural change, including disinhibition and somnolence. Disturbances of temperature regulation can give rise to hypothermia or hyperthermia. Management can be challenging and needs a multidisciplinary team approach.

Thyroid

Hyperthyroidism

Thyrotoxicosis can be associated with various psychiatric symptoms, such as emotional lability, anxiety, restlessness and, rarely, frank psychosis. Psychotic symptoms in the context of hyperthyroidism typically present as an affective psychosis and up to 50% of adult men with hyperthyroidism have sexual dysfunction.[7]

Thyrotoxicosis can be due to autoimmune stimulation of the thyroid (Graves' disease), a toxic nodule (single or multinodular) and, rarely, thyroid inflammation (thyroiditis). Other rare causes include thyroid-stimulating hormone (TSH) secreting pituitary tumours (< 1% of all pituitary tumours), pituitary thyroid resistance syndrome or struma ovarii (an ovarian tumour containing functional thyroid tissue). Over-replacement of thyroid hormone should also be considered if a patient is taking thyroxine.

Symptoms include heat intolerance, weight loss with increased appetite, palpitations, sweating, menstrual disturbances, insomnia, fatigue and diarrhoea. In severe cases, there may be signs of congestive cardiac failure. Graves' ophthalmopathy (due to swelling of extraocular muscles and inflammation of the orbital contents) and ophthalmoplegia can also be present in addition to above features.

Clinical signs such as fine tremor, sinus tachycardia or atrial fibrillation, goitre or thyroid nodule(s), thyroid eye disease (exophthalmos, especially in Graves' disease) and hair loss should be looked for in clinical examination. Localised dermopathy (pretibial myxoedema) and thyroid acropachy of the nails can also be found, though rarely. Thyroiditis can be associated with tenderness of the gland and flu-like symptoms, including sore throat.

The diagnosis is mainly clinical but is confirmed biochemically by blood tests showing low TSH and high free thyroxine (fT4) and free triiodothyronine (fT3). Thyroid receptor antibodies are positive in Graves' disease. Ultrasound of the thyroid or thyroid uptake scans can differentiate Graves' disease from multinodular goitre.

Referral to an endocrine team is advised, and if there is severe Graves' ophthalmopathy, referral to an ophthalmologist is also needed. Medical treatment can be started with thionamides (carbimazole is widely used in the UK) after warning the patient about the side-effects. Agranulocytosis is a potentially fatal but rare side-effect (0.1–0.5%)[3] and it is necessary to report any sign of infection (e.g. sore throat) and urgently

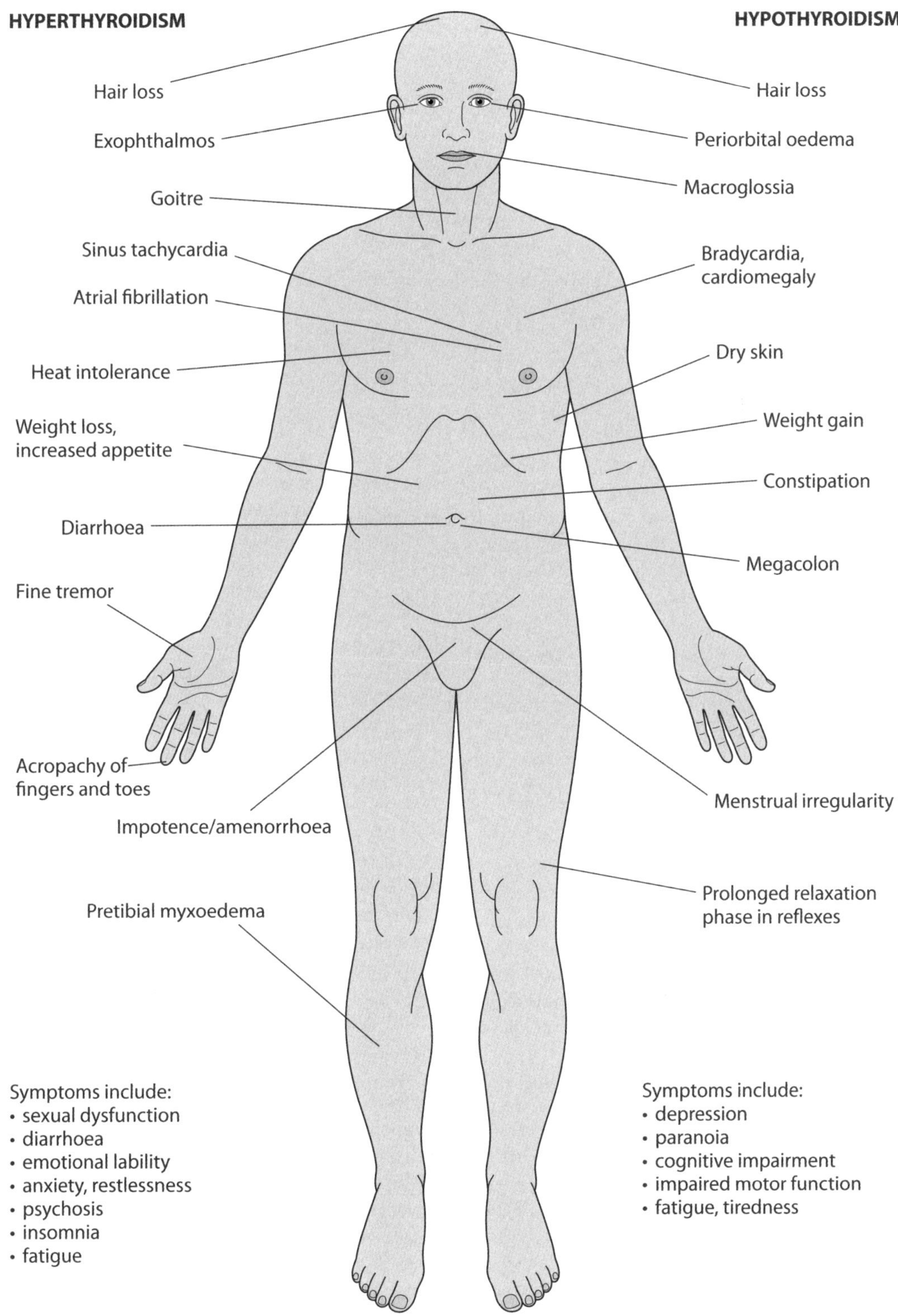
HYPERTHYROIDISM
HYPOTHYROIDISM
Hair loss
Exophthalmos
Goitre
Sinus tachycardia
Atrial fibrillation
Heat intolerance
Weight loss, increased appetite
Diarrhoea
Fine tremor
Acropachy of fingers and toes
Impotence/amenorrhoea
Pretibial myxoedema
Hair loss
Periorbital oedema
Macroglossia
Bradycardia, cardiomegaly
Dry skin
Weight gain
Constipation
Megacolon
Menstrual irregularity
Prolonged relaxation phase in reflexes
Symptoms include:
• sexual dysfunction
• diarrhoea
• emotional lability
• anxiety, restlessness
• psychosis
• insomnia
• fatigue
Symptoms include:
• depression
• paranoia
• cognitive impairment
• impaired motor function
• fatigue, tiredness

Fig. 15.3 Signs and symptoms of hyperthyroidism and hypothyroidism.

check the white-cell count. Other side-effects include a skin rash (4%) and peripheral polyarthropathy. Until the carbimazole works, symptomatic tachycardia can be controlled by beta-adrenergic antagonists such as propranolol (unless contraindicated).

Hypothyroidism

Psychological manifestations of hypothyroidism consist of depression, paranoid feelings, severe cognitive impairment, and slowing of mental intellectual and motor function.

Hypothyroidism is a common disorder, arising more often in women than men and increasing in incidence with age. In a community survey in the UK,[8] an abnormally high serum TSH concentration was recorded in 7.5% of women and 2.8% of men. Of individuals aged 65 years or more, 1.7% had overt hypothyroidism and 13.7% had mild hypothyroidism.

The commonest cause of hypothyroidism is autoimmune disease. Other causes include previous thyroid surgery, radiation and radio-iodine treatment or drugs (e.g. amiodarone, which contains iodine). Central causes include pan-hypopituitarism (e.g. following pituitary surgery), isolated TSH deficiency or hypothalamic disorders (e.g. neoplasm or infiltrative disorders).

Symptoms of hypothyroidism can be insidious in onset and non-specific, which can delay the diagnosis. The severity spectrum of symptoms varies from asymptomatic to myxoedemic coma. Fatigue, tiredness, dry skin, hair loss, constipation, difficulty in losing weight and menstrual irregularity occur. Sometimes, obstructive sleep apnoea may be present. There may be a goitre. In long-standing and severe cases, the clinical signs include pale, coarse skin, periorbital puffiness, a prolonged relaxation phase of deep-tendon reflexes, and organomegaly (macroglossia, cardiomegaly, megacolon). Myxoedemic coma is the extreme severe clinical presentation of hypothyroidism; it can be precipitated by cold exposure or infection.

The diagnosis is clinical but is confirmed biochemically with thyroid function tests. A high TSH with low fT4 and fT3 is diagnostic of primary hypothyroidism. A low TSH with a low fT4 and fT3 suggests central hypothyroidism (secondary to pituitary or hypothalamic disease).

Thyroxine replacement is an easy and effective treatment for hypothyroidism. The starting dose depends on each individual. A low starting dose (0.25–0.5 mg) followed by a gradual incremental dose increase, alongside regular (6-weekly) TSH monitoring, is recommended, especially for older people or those with heart disease. If in doubt, an endocrinologist should be consulted.

> If an elevated TSH is found after thyroxine replacement (median dose 1.25 mg daily), this is likely to be due to poor adherence, after malabsorption (e.g. due to coeliac disease) has been excluded.

Parathyroid (and calcium) disorders

Hypercalcaemia

Hypercalcaemia may cause depression and fatigue. The most common endocrine cause is primary hyperparathyroidism, which occurs more commonly in women over the age of 65 years.[3] It can sometimes be associated with multiple endocrine neoplasia (MEN) types I and II. Type I is the association of hyperparathyroidism with pancreatic and pituitary disease. Type II is hyperparathyroidism with phaeochromocytoma (see below) and medullary carcinoma of the thyroid. Other causes of hypercalcaemia include vitamin D intoxication and familial hypocalciuric hypercalcaemia (FHH), caused by a mutation in the calcium-sensing receptor. Malignancy-related hypercalcaemia must be excluded. Drugs (e.g. lithium) can also cause hypercalcaemia.

Hypercalcaemia can be, and often is, asymptomatic until the calcium level is very high (> 3 mmol/l). Symptoms can be non-specific and include polyuria, polydypsia, headache, constipation, vomiting and abdominal pain. Renal stones, nephrocalcinosis, osteoporotic fractures or bone pain can also occur. A careful family history is important to exclude the autosomal dominant disorder of FHH and the MEN syndromes. There are rarely clinical signs of hypercalcaemia.

In hyperparathyroidism, the serum calcium level is high with a low phosphate level and elevated level of parathyroid hormone. Vitamin D, renal and liver function tests must be requested as baseline measurements. The 24-hour urinary calcium is high, except in hypocalciuric hypercalcaemia, when it is low. Renal ultrasound and sometimes an evaluation of bone mineral density should be requested to exclude end-organ damage from chronic hypercalcaemia.

A patient with acute symptomatic hypercalcaemia (> 3 mg/dl) may need hospital admission for urgent rehydration and for appropriate investigations as to the cause. Patients with primary hyperparathyroidism should be referred to endocrinology for further work-up and for the consideration of definitive treatment, including parathyroid surgery.

Hypocalcaemia

Hypocalcaemia is rare but may cause seizures. The important endocrine causes include destruction of the parathyroid glands secondary to radiation, infiltration, autoimmune processes or surgery. Other causes include vitamin D deficiency. Symptoms depend on the rate of onset and the severity of hypocalcaemia. Acute hypocalcaemia presents with tingling and numbness, muscle spasm and seizures. Blood tests including calcium and phosphate, parathyroid hormone and vitamin D should be done and replacement carried out with calcium and vitamin D after endocrine referral.

The endocrine and other disorders that can lead to secondary osteoporosis are listed in Box 15.1.

Box 15.1 Bone health: endocrine and other disorders that can lead to secondary osteoporosis

- Coeliac disease
- Hypogonadism
- In men, Klinefelter's syndrome; in women, Turner's syndrome and early menopause (<45 years)
- Hyperthyroidism
- Hyperparathyroidism
- Hypovitaminosis
- Myeloma
- Mastocytoma (tumour of mast cells)
- Anorexia nervosa
- Cushing's syndrome
- Exogenous steroids

Adrenal gland

Addison's disease

Conditions causing damage to both adrenal glands result in primary adrenal failure (Addison's disease), and consequently glucocortocoid (cortisol) and mineralocorticoid (aldosterone) deficiency. Around 80% of cases in the UK are due to an autoimmune adrenalitis.

Psychiatric symptoms are seen in 65% of those with Addison's disease.[9] These are mainly mild disturbances in mood, motivation and behaviour. Psychosis and delirium occur more rarely, but are associated with severe disease and can be the presenting feature of Addisonian crisis. Very rarely catatonia and self-mutilation are seen in Addison's disease.[9]

The common physical signs and symptoms of adrenal insufficiency are fatigue, loss of energy, weight loss, reduced muscle strength, anorexia, nausea, syncope, postural hypotension and hyperpigmentation due to raised levels of ACTH.[10] These patients may also have severe hypotension or hypovolaemic shock and hypoglycaemia. This can be a life-threatening condition and should be managed with intravenous steroids if diagnosed early.

Adrenoleukodystrophy (ALD) is a rare condition and should be considered in any young man presenting with adrenal insufficiency, particularly when there are associated neuropsychiatric symptoms. ALD is X-linked and is characterised by the accumulation of very-long-chain fatty acids (VLCFA) as a result of defective beta-oxidation.[9]

Routine biochemistry may reveal hyponatraemia, hyperkalaemia and raised blood urea levels. The diagnosis should be confirmed by a short synacthen test, where 250 μg of synacthen is injected either intravenously or intramuscularly and cortisol is measured just before and 30 and 60 minutes after the injection. Failure of cortisol to rise to >580 nmol/l confirms adrenal insufficiency.[3] The ACTH will be high in these patients. The patient should be referred to a specialist at this stage. If acute adrenal insufficiency is suspected, the patient should be treated empirically with steroids, preferably hydrocortisone, after a blood test has been taken for cortisol and until the diagnosis can be confirmed. Long-term steroids should never be stopped

Long-term steroids should never be stopped abruptly as this can lead to acute adrenal insufficiency. Doses of long-term steroids may need to be increased in febrile illnesses, stress or injury.

Consider Addison's disease as a possible diagnosis if a patient is losing weight and skin pigmentation is increasing. Loss of appetite is an almost invariable feature of Addison's disease.

abruptly as this can result in acute adrenal insufficiency and doses may need to be increased in febrile illnesses, stress or injury.

Phaeochromocytoma

Many patients have seen a psychiatrist with symptoms before the correct diagnosis is made. The most important symptoms from the mental health point of view are panic attacks and anxiety disorder. There are also case reports where patients with phaeochromocytoma have presented initially with paranoid illness and depression and the above symptoms have settled following removal of the tumour.[11]

Phaeochromocytomas are adrenal tumours that secrete catecholamines. In healthy individuals catecholamines are secreted during times of stress and result in adrenergic symptoms such as tachycardia, sweating, tremulousness and a feeling of apprehension. Similar symptoms are seen in phaeochromocytoma and are usually associated with hypertension and headache. Characteristically, but not always, these symptoms appear in paroxysms.

A history of hypertension, sweating, palpitations or headache may indicate a phaeochromocytoma. One of these symptoms is present in 80% of patients with phaeochromocytoma.[12]

If a phaeochromocytoma is suspected the recommended initial screening test is a 24-hour urinary catecholamines test on two occasions. If the levels are raised the patient should be referred to a specialist. Several drugs can interfere with this test, however. The important ones are antihypertensives such as alpha- and beta-blockers, monoamine oxidase inhibitors, tricyclic antidepressants and phenothiazines.[3] If a phaeochromocytoma is suspected, beta-blockers should not be used as the first drug to control the hypertension. Beta-blockade without adequate alpha-blockade can precipitate a catecholamine crisis.

Tricyclic antidepressants and phenothiazines can precipitate a crisis in a patient with a pheochromocytoma.

Pancreas

Insulinoma

Insulinomas are rare tumours of the pancreatic islet cells that secrete insulin, leading to frequent episodes of hypoglycaemia. Insulinoma patients are frequently seen with anxiety symptoms caused by adrenaline release in response to hypoglycaemia before the correct diagnosis is made.

The clinical manifestations of hypoglycaemia can be classified into adrenergic features, which are the result of activation of the sympathetic system, and neuroglycopenic features, which are due to glucose deficiency in the brain. The adrenergic features are sweating, pallor, tachycardia and tremor. The neuroglycopenic features are irritability, confusion, aggression and coma.[3] Sometimes the neuroglycopenic features are mistaken for psychiatric disorders or behavioural disturbances and are managed accordingly. For this reason, the diagnosis of insulinomas has taken up to 20 years in some patients[13] and there may be sufferers in whom it is never diagnosed. Patients with an insulinoma tend to gain weight.

If an insulinoma is suspected, capillary blood glucose (CBG) should be measured at the time of symptoms. If the CBG demonstrates hypoglycaemia (< 2.2 mmol/l) it is useful to take immediate blood samples for plasma assessment of glucose, insulin and C peptide before the management of hypoglycaemia (a high insulin level and low C peptide level is seen with exogenous insulin administration). This will help the specialist in making the diagnosis. Overnight 15-hour fasting with blood glucose and insulin monitoring will pick up 80% of insulinoma patients. If hypoglycaemia is not demonstrated despite a strong suspicion of an insulinoma, the patient can be referred to a specialist to arrange an in-patient supervised 72-hour fast, which is the gold standard for the diagnosis.[3]

Ovary/testis

Polycystic ovary syndrome

Polycystic ovary syndrome (PCOS) is a common condition, affecting one in 15 women worldwide.[14] This clinical syndrome is characterised by irregular periods, androgen excess and insulin resistance. The patients may also have polycystic ovaries on imaging.[3] Psychiatric disorders, especially affective disorders, have been described in patients with PCOS.[15] On the other hand,

Insulinoma may cause anxiety, irritability, sweating, pallor, tachycardia and tremor. Episodes of confusion and aggression may occur before meals and be relieved by eating.

sodium valproate, which is used in the treatment of bipolar disorder, epilepsy and migraine, can cause PCOS in 7% of the patients treated with the drug.[16] Epilepsy, bipolar disorders and migraines are common conditions that are also often associated with disturbances in menstrual function in adolescent girls.[16]

Endocrine conditions caused by psychiatric medications

Drug-induced hyperprolactinaemia

Drug-induced hyperprolactinaemia is common with antipsychotics and some antidepressant medications. Hyperprolactinaemia can induce hypogonadism, which has adverse consequences on bone as well as other organs. Drugs that inhibit the dopamine (D_2) receptors in the hypothalamic–pituitary axis result in raised prolactin levels. Many drugs used in psychiatry have this potential (Table 15.2). There are now newer antipsychotics and antidepressants that have minimal or no effect on the prolactin levels.[17]

If a patient is found to have a raised prolactin level (raised, but usually < 3000 mU/l) and is on medication that is known to cause hyperprolactinaemia it is important to establish whether medication is indeed the underlying cause. The other differential diagnoses are primary hypothyroidism, prolactinomas (prolactin usually > 3000 mU/l), hypothalamic–pituitary tumours causing stalk compression, and renal failure. To make the diagnosis, the suspected drug can be either withdrawn or substituted with another drug that does not cause hyperprolactinaemia, and the prolactin test repeated to see whether it has normalised.[17] The above drug changes should clearly be made under the close supervision of a psychiatrist. If this is not possible, an MRI scan of the hypothalamic–pituitary region can be performed to exclude a sinister cause, such as a pituitary tumour.[17]

If the drug-induced hyperprolactinaemia is mild with normal menstrual periods and no galactorrhoea the patient can be reassured. If hyperprolactinaemia is symptomatic with galactorrhoea and menstrual irregularities in a female or erectile dysfunction in a male an alternative drug should be considered. If switching medication is not possible, and if the major concern is decreased oestrogen or testosterone levels, then simple substitution with oestrogen or testosterone is possible. If the concern is osteoporosis after measurement of bone mineral density, a bisphosphonate can be used if the fracture risk is elevated in patients of the right age group (usually over 65 years).[17]

Thyroid disorders

Lithium is the main culprit here. It can cause a goitre and hypothyroidism in a significant number of patients.

Table 15.2 Psychiatric medications causing endocrine problems

Endocrine condition	Psychiatric medication causing endocrine manifestation
Drug-induced hyper-prolactinaemia	Chlorpromazine Trifluoperazine Fluphenazine Perphenazine Monoamine oxidase inhibitors Selective serotonin reuptake inhibitors Tricyclic and tetracyclic antidepressants Thioxanthenes, butyrophenones
Thyroid disorder	Lithium
Sodium disturbances (including SIADH)	Typical and atypical antipsychotic agents Tricyclic antidepressants Non-selective serotonin reuptake inhibitors Selective serotonin reuptake inhibitors Anticonvulsants

SIADH, syndrome of inappropriate antidiuretic hormone

The annual incidence of hypothyroidism in patients on lithium is 1.5%. Therefore it is recommended that thyroid function should be monitored annually in those who are on lithium. Those with pre-existing autoimmune thyroid disease have a higher chance of developing hypothyroidism. It will be advisable to measure the thyroid peroxidase antibodies prior to treatment and, if positive, to check thyroid function more frequently than yearly. The hypothyroidism can be treated with thyroxine in order to render TSH into the normal range. Furthermore, it is not necessary to discontinue lithium.[18]

The goitre induced by lithium is usually smooth. It is worth investigating further if there is an irregularly shaped thyroid gland or if there are signs of nodular enlargement, so that malignancies are not missed.[18]

Lithium is also associated with thyrotoxicosis but this is extremely rare. The aetiologies are Graves' disease, toxic multinodular goitre and silent thyroiditis. The management options are antithyroid medications and radio-iodine treatment.[19]

Sodium disturbances

Hyponatraemia

Hyponatraemia represents an excess of body water relative to body sodium content and is frequently defined as a serum sodium concentration of less than 135 mEq/l. Hyponatraemia is the most common electrolyte disorder, occurring in up to 6% of hospitalised patients,[20] and can result in severe morbidity and even mortality if left untreated.

Psychiatric disorders are among the clinical conditions associated with an increased risk of hyponatraemia. The potential risk factors for the development of hyponatraemia in psychiatric patients are related to the conditions that increase water consumption (psychogenic polydipsia), including delusional states, obsessive–compulsive behaviour and a dry mouth associated with the anticholinergic adverse effects of many psychotropic drugs. The risk of hyponatraemia is increased with the use of the many types of psychotropic drugs that are associated with the syndrome of inappropriate antidiuretic hormone (SIADH) (Table 15.2). Desmopressin (DDAVP), a synthetic arginine vasopressin (AVP) agonist, is frequently used to treat nocturnal enuresis in psychiatric patients[21] and over-dosage can cause excessive water retention and hyponatraemia.

The clinical presentation depends on the rate of decline of the serum sodium and the severity of hyponatraemia. Symptoms include nausea and malaise as the earliest findings, followed by headache, lethargy and obtundation, and eventually seizures, coma and respiratory arrest if the plasma sodium concentration falls below 115–120 mEq/l. Acute-onset hyponatraemia may induce delirium and behavioural changes, which may resemble psychomotor agitation or retardation.[20] In chronic hyponatraemia, symptoms are relatively non-specific, including fatigue, nausea, dizziness, gait disturbances, forgetfulness, confusion, lethargy and muscle cramps. An accurate diagnosis of hyponatraemia secondary to SIADH may be delayed in psychiatric patients, as the symptoms may resemble primary psychiatric disorders or the adverse effects of many psychotropic drugs.[21]

Determination of plasma and urine osmolality, along with urine and serum sodium levels, will help in the identification of the aetiology. Hyponatraemia associated with psychogenic polydipsia and drug-induced SIADH are associated with euvolemic hyponatraemia. In psychogenic polydipsia there will be a low plasma osmolality (< 280 mOsm/kg) and low urine osmolality (< 100 mOsm/kg), whereas in SIADH there will be a low plasma osmolality (< 280 mOsm/kg) with a relatively high urine osmolality (> 100 mOsm/kg).[21]

Chronic hyponatraemia is managed with fluid restriction (500–700 ml per day) and removal of any underlying cause such as drug-induced SIADH. Demeclocycline can be added to fluid restriction. Newer agents such as the AVP-receptor antagonists look very promising.[21] Correction of hyponatraemia should be limited to no more than 10–12 mEq/l on the first day of treatment and less than 6 mEq/l per day thereafter in these patients.[20]

Nephrogenic diabetes insipidus

The commonest side-effect of lithium is nephrogenic diabetes insipidus (NDI), which affects 40% of patients.[22] These patients present with polyuria and polydipsia but it is important to differentiate this from psychogenic polydipsia. In NDI, as opposed to psychogenic polydipsia, the patient will have hyponatraemia, with a high plasma osmolality and low urine osmolality. If NDI is suspected it is worth referring the patient to a specialist

> Careful monitoring of serum sodium is critical because of an increased risk of irreversible osmotic demyelination in patients with chronic hyponatraemia that is corrected too quickly.

endocrinologist as the diagnostic test is an 8-hour water deprivation test. If lithium can be discontinued it should be, although the NDI may not reverse completely in those on long-term treatment.[23] If the treatment cannot be discontinued amiloride can be added, but this needs specialist supervision.[22]

When to refer to an endocrinologist

Psychiatrists may need access to expert help from an endocrinologist to investigate patients with symptoms that may have an endocrine cause and to provide advice on what is a typical (or unexpected) response, or *rate* of response, to endocrine manipulation for patients with a pre-existing endocrine problem who are admitted to a psychiatric unit; in addition, patients may develop symptoms *de novo* that require investigation.

A psychiatrist should consider referral on symptomatic or clinical grounds or if 'routine' investigations raise suspicion of an endocrine disorder in the following contexts:

- unexplained hypercalcaemia – to investigate for parathyroid disease or other cause
- abnormal thyroid test result –
  - if suggestive of an overactive thyroid – to determine most appropriate treatment
  - if suggestive of an underactive thyroid – to stabilise on thyroid replacement therapy
  - if thyroid nodule – to establish if lesion is benign or malignant
- abnormal glucose level –
  - to confirm diagnosis and type of diabetes mellitus
  - determine most appropriate treatment
  - for advice on monitoring for complications
- blood pressure consistently elevated above 140/90 mmHg or symptomatic hypotension –
  - to screen for underlying cause
  - for advice on drugs to prescribe and to avoid
- irregular periods or amenorrhoea –
  - to investigate cause, including genetic testing if appropriate
  - for advice on treatment, including hormone replacement
- unexplained milk production, irregular periods, infertility or impaired sexual function suggestive of hyperprolactinaemia, with hypothyroidism, pregnancy and drug cause excluded
  - to investigate for pituitary tumour
- obesity
  - to exclude secondary cause where appropriate
  - to assess comorbidity, including sleep apnoea
  - to advise on management, including suitability for bariatric surgery.

Summary

Many endocrine conditions may present with psychiatric symptoms and indeed may sometimes be missed for years. Particularly in women over the age of 65, hypothyroidism and hypercalcaemia are comparatively common. Very severe psychiatric morbidity can accompany Cushing's syndrome. In the patient with new-onset anxiety, phaeochromocytoma and hypoglycaemia should be considered.

Many psychiatric drugs cause endocrine disturbances. For the most part, these are easily managed, but the optimum management of hypogonadism and potential bone morbidity in patients with psychiatric disorders who are hyperprolactinaemic remain unclear.

References

1 Haskett RF. Diagnostic categorization of psychiatric disturbance in Cushing's syndrome. *Am J Psychiatry* 1985;**142**: 911–16.

2 Starkman MN, Schteingart DE, Schork MA. Depressed mood and other psychiatric manifestations of Cushing's syndrome: relationship to hormone levels. *Psychosom Med* 1981; **43**: 3–18.

3 Turner HE, Wass JAH. *Oxford Handbook of Endocrinology and Diabetes*. Oxford University Press, 2009.

4. Starkman MN, Schteingart DE, Schork MA. Cushing's syndrome after treatment: changes in cortisol and ACTH levels, and amelioration of the depressive syndrome. *Psychiatry Res* 1986; **19**: 177–88.

5 Fernandez A, Karavitaki N, Wass JA. Prevalence of pituitary adenomas: a community-based, cross-sectional study in Banbury (Oxfordshire, UK). *Clin Endocrinol (Oxf)* 2010; **72**: 377–82.

6 Sievers C, Dimopoulou C, Pfister H, *et al*. Prevalence of mental disorders in acromegaly: a cross-sectional study in 81 acromegalic patients. *Clin Endocrinol (Oxf)* 2009; **71**: 691–701.

7 Carani C, Isidori AM, Granata A, *et al*. Multicenter study on the prevalence of sexual symptoms in male hypo- and hyperthyroid patients. *J Clin Endocrinol Metab* 2005; **90**: 6472–9.

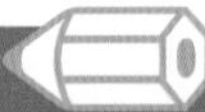

Learning points

- Psychiatric manifestations may precede the onset of physical symptoms in endocrine disorders.
- In new-onset anxiety, phaeochromocytoma and hypoglycaemia should be considered.
- Mood disturbances are some of the commonest presentations of Cushing's syndrome.
- If an elevated TSH is found after thyroxine replacement for hypothyroidism, suspect poor compliance.
- If acute adrenal insufficiency is suspected, the patient should be treated empirically with steroids, preferably hydrocortisone, after a blood test has been taken for cortisol.
- Long-term steroids should never be stopped abruptly as this can result in acute adrenal insufficiency. Steroid doses may need to be increased in febrile illnesses, stress or injury.
- In patients with a phaeochromocytoma, beta blockade without adequate alpha blockade can precipitate a catecholamine crisis.
- To diagnose drug-induced hyperprolactinaemia, the suspected drug can be either withdrawn or substituted with another drug that does not cause hyperprolactinaemia, and the prolactin test repeated to see whether it has normalised.
- The goitre induced by lithium is usually smooth. If there is an irregularly shaped thyroid gland or signs of nodular enlargement, further investigation is required so that malignancies are not missed.
- Correction of hyponatraemia must be limited to no more than 10–12 mEq/l on the first day of treatment, and less than 6mEq/l per day thereafter.

8 Tunbridge WM, Evered DC, Hall R, *et al.* The spectrum of thyroid disease in a community: the Whickham survey. *Clin Endocrinol (Oxf)* 1977; **7**: 481–93.

9 Anglin RE, Rosebush PI, Mazurek MF. The neuropsychiatric profile of Addison's disease: revisiting a forgotten phenomenon. *J Neuropsychiatry Clin Neurosci* 2006; **18**: 450–9.

10 Arlt W, Allolio B. Adrenal insufficiency. *Lancet* 2003; **361**: 1881–93.

11 Medvei VC, Cattell WR. Mental symptoms presenting in phaeochromocytoma: a case report and review. *J R Soc Med* 1988; **81**: 550–1.

12 Lenders JW, Eisenhofer G, Mannelli M, *et al.* Phaeochromocytoma. *Lancet* 2005; **366**: 665–75.

13 Piccillo GA, Musco A, Manfrini S, *et al.* Two clinical cases of insulinoma misdiagnosed as psychiatric conditions. *Acta Biomed* 2005; **76**: 118–22.

14 Norman RJ, Dewailly D, Legro RS, *et al.* Polycystic ovary syndrome. *Lancet* 2007; **370**: 685–97.

15 Bruce-Jones W, Zolese G, White P. Polycystic ovary syndrome and psychiatric morbidity. *J Psychosom Obstet Gynaecol* 1993; **14**: 111–16.

16 Joffe H, Hayes FJ. Menstrual cycle dysfunction associated with neurologic and psychiatric disorders: their treatment in adolescents. *Ann N Y Acad Sci* 2008; **1135**: 219–29.

17 Molitch ME. Drugs and prolactin. *Pituitary* 2008; **11**: 209–18.

18 Lazarus JH. Lithium and thyroid. *Best Pract Res Clin Endocrinol Metab* 2009; **23**: 723–33.

19 Barclay ML, Brownlie BE, Turner JG, *et al.* Lithium associated thyrotoxicosis: a report of 14 cases, with statistical analysis of incidence. *Clin Endocrinol (Oxf)* 1994; **40**: 759–64.

20 Douglas I. Hyponatremia: why it matters, how it presents, how we can manage it. *Cleve Clin J Med* 2006; **73** suppl 3: S4–12.

21 Siegel AJ. Hyponatremia in psychiatric patients: update on evaluation and management. *Harv Rev Psychiatry* 2008; **16**: 13–24.

22 Grunfeld JP, Rossier BC. Lithium nephrotoxicity revisited. *Nat Rev Nephrol* 2009; **5**: 270–6.

23 de Angelis L. Lithium treatment and the geriatric population. *Int J Clin Pharmacol Ther Toxicol* 1990; **28**: 394–8.

16

Diabetes

Muhammad Ali Karamat and Stephen C. L. Gough

Diabetes is a major health risk in the general population and is even more prevalent in people with mental disorders. This chapter describes the clinical presentation, screening tests and treatment of diabetes, including when to refer to a specialist diabetic clinic.

Diabetes is a disease which often shows itself in families in which insanity prevails. (Sir Henry Maudsley, *The Pathology of Mind*, 1897)

Introduction

Type 2 diabetes mellitus is an extremely common, lifelong health condition. According to latest figures from Diabetes UK, 2.9 million people are known to suffer from diabetes in the UK while another 850 000 remain undiagnosed. By 2025 there will be more than 4 million people with diabetes in the UK. In England the current prevalence of diabetes is estimated at around 5.5%.[1] Type 2 diabetes is a global epidemic with an estimated worldwide prevalence of 8.3% (366 million) in 2011 that is forecast to rise to 9.9% (552 million) in 2030.[2] In addition, 280 million people have impaired glucose tolerance that is forecast to increase to 398 million by 2030.[2]

While the above numbers are of concern, even more worrying is the fact that the proportion of people with diabetes among patients with severe mental illness is much higher. The prevalence of diabetes in schizophrenia has been found to be about 20%[3] and depression is associated with a 60% increase in rates of type 2 diabetes.[4] In addition, diabetes is considered to be one of the most psychologically demanding of the chronic medical illnesses and is often associated with several psychiatric disorders, including depression. According to a large meta-analysis, the prevalence of depression in diabetes was found to be 17.6% *v.* 9.8% in the general population.[5] The prevalence of depression in diabetes was also reported to be higher in women (23.8%) than in men (12.8%).[5]

Physical symptoms and signs

The symptoms of type 1 and type 2 diabetes are similar. The main difference, which may not always be apparent, is that type 1 diabetes usually develops over weeks or even days, whereas type 2 diabetes may go undiagnosed for many years, because early symptoms

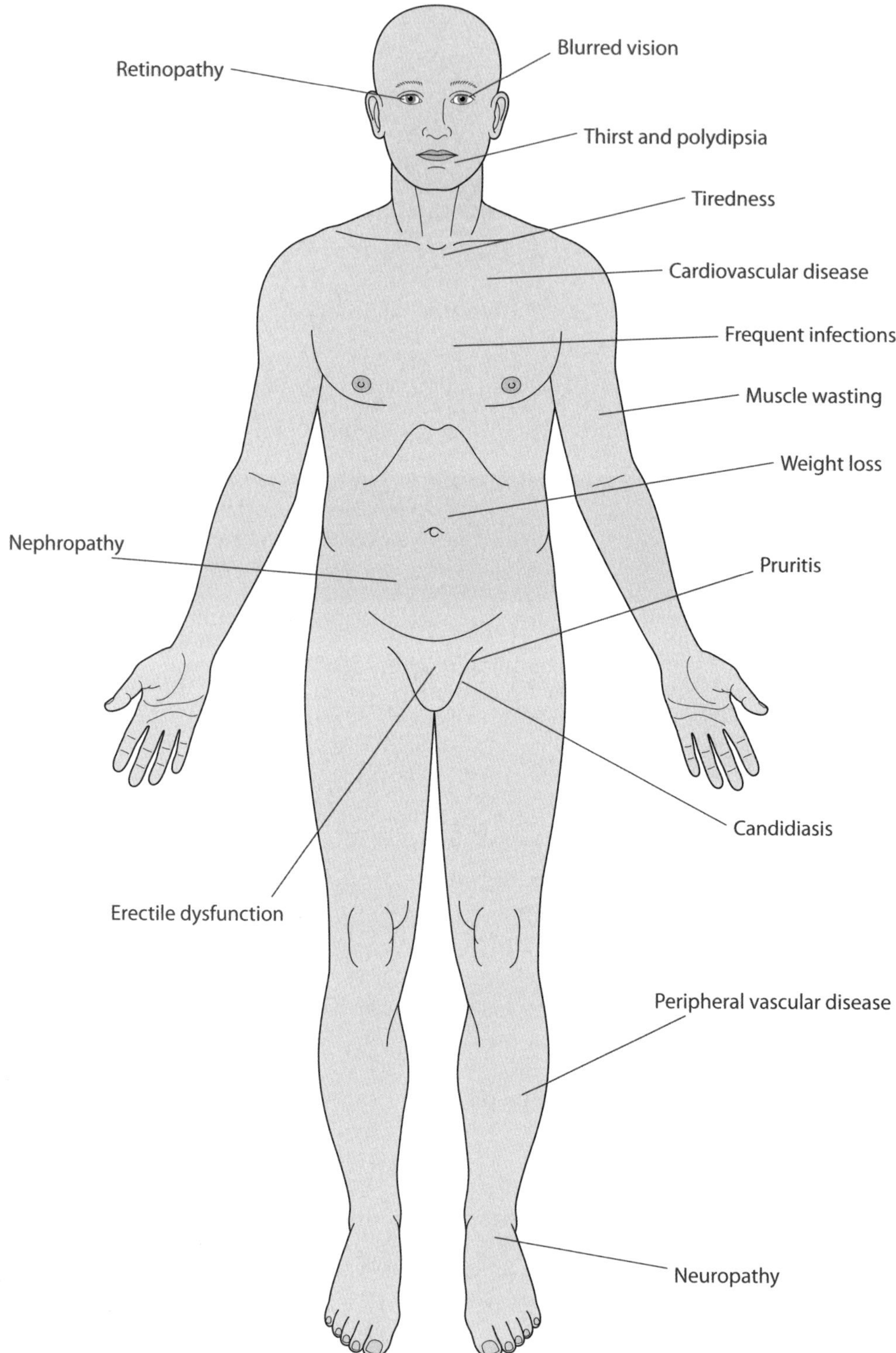

Fig. 16.1 Symptoms and signs of diabetes mellitus.

- Type 1 diabetes: onset is usually sudden, with weight loss and muscle wasting as well as the more usual symptoms of diabetes. Diabetic ketoacidosis is classically seen with type 1 diabetes.
- Type 2 diabetes: onset is slower, often undiagnosed for years, as early symptoms may be non-specific or even absent. A hyperosmolar hyperglycaemic state may occur in elderly patients.

may be non-specific or even absent. The symptoms of diabetes can include:

- polydipsia (increased thirst)
- polyuria (increased frequency of micturition)
- tiredness
- weight loss (classically associated with type 1 diabetes)
- muscle wasting
- frequent infections
- pruritis
- frequent episodes of thrush (candidiasis)
- blurred vision.

In addition to the short-term metabolic disturbances that produce the above symptoms, people with diabetes are at an increased risk of diabetes-related complications over a more prolonged period. These include both *macrovascular* (cardiovascular disease) and *microvascular* complications, and are present in up to 50% of patients with type 2 diabetes at the time of diagnosis. The microvascular complications include diabetic eye disease (retinopathy), diabetic kidney disease (nephropathy) and diabetic neuropathy, including, for example, peripheral neuropathy and autonomic dysfunction such as erectile dysfunction.[6]

Patients with type 1 diabetes can present with diabetic ketoacidosis, which is defined as a triad of:

- hyperglycaemia (blood sugar > 15 mmol/l)
- ketonuria
- metabolic acidosis (serum bicarbonate < 15 mmol/l).

Diabetic ketoacidosis has a mortality rate of 5–10%,[7] although improved awareness and more prompt medical action have probably reduced this figure. Nevertheless, it should still be considered as a medical emergency – patients need to be transferred to an acute hospital for urgent treatment with intravenous fluids, insulin and potassium. It can also occur in patients with type 2 diabetes but is much less common.

A rarer diabetic emergency, seen in more elderly patients with type 2 diabetes, is hyperosmolar hyperglycaemic state (HHS), previously known as hyperosmolar non-ketotic state (HONK). This is associated with severe hyperglycaemia (blood sugar > 30 mmol/l) and dehydration, but no ketonuria or acidosis. These patients need to be treated urgently but cautiously with intravenous fluids and insulin.

People with diabetes have a higher risk of myocardial infarction (MI) than non-diabetic individuals. People *with* type 2 diabetes who have *never* had an MI have as high a risk of having a first heart attack as people *without* type 2 diabetes but *with* a history of MI have of having another MI.[8] This is of great importance in clinical practice.

In terms of cardiovascular risk, consider each person with type 2 diabetes as if they have already had a myocardial infarction.

Screening tests

These include tests of random blood glucose levels and fasting blood glucose levels, the 75 g oral glucose tolerance test (OGTT) and tests of glycosylated haemoglobin ($HbA1_c$) levels. If the symptoms described above are present, the diagnosis of diabetes is confirmed with any of the following:

- random glucose ≥ 11.1 mmol/l
- fasting glucose ≥ 7 mmol/l
- OGTT with a fasting glucose level of ≥ 7 mmol/l or a 2-hour value of ≥ 11.1 mmol/l.

In asymptomatic individuals, two positive tests are needed.

During recent years World Health Organization and Diabetes UK have reviewed HbA1c as a diagnostic tool for diabetes and agreed that a cut-off of 6.5% (48 mmol/mol) can be used as a diagnostic test for diabetes providing that stringent quality assurance tests are in place. Diabetes UK link to recommendations for diagnostic criteria for diabetes (www.diabetes.org.uk/About_us/Our_Views/Care_recommendations/New_diagnostic_criteria_for_diabetes_/).

'Pre-diabetes' is a separate entity and helps define people who are at high risk of developing diabetes. This includes people with impaired fasting glycaemia (fasting glucose 6.1–7.0 mmol/l) and impaired glucose tolerance (2-hour glucose 7.8–11.0 mmol/l).

Monitoring

Restoring blood sugar levels to as near normal as possible will reduce diabetes-related complications. Monitoring of treatment effects can be performed using both home blood glucose readings and laboratory determinations of $HbA1_c$, a measure of longer-term control which provides an average glucose reading over a 6- to 8-week period. Reducing $HbA1_c$ is the key to addressing complications. Data from the UK Prospective Diabetes Study[9] demonstrated the association of good blood glucose control with a reduced burden of microvascular and macrovascular complications. Each 1% reduction in mean $HbA1_c$ is associated with:

- a 21% reduction in the risk of developing any end-point related to diabetes (including death)
- 14% reduction in the risk of developing a myocardial infarction
- 37% reduction in the risk of developing microvascular complications

Glycaemic control is, however, only one risk factor for complications; others, including blood pressure[10] and lipid levels, are important, particularly in preventing cardiovascular complications.[11] The audit standards of the UK General Medical Services (GMS) contract recognise the importance of control of blood glucose, blood pressure and cholesterol, independent of clinical targets, in the management of diabetes.[12]

Good diabetes care can be difficult to implement; it can be quite complex and time-consuming, drawing on many areas of healthcare management. The necessary lifestyle changes, the complexities of management and the side-effects of therapy make self-monitoring and education for people with diabetes central parts of diabetes management.

What to expect from primary care?

Primary care should initially offer screening, followed by structured diabetes education to every person and/or their carer at and around the time of diagnosis, with annual reinforcement and review. All patients should be provided with individualised and ongoing nutritional advice from a healthcare professional with specific expertise and competencies in nutrition, for example a dietitian. Many guidelines recommend a general $HbA1_c$ target for most newly diagnosed patients with type 2 diabetes of < 6.5%, although individual targets may be above this, depending upon the clinical circumstances, including, for example, the presence of comorbidities.

> For most people with type 2 diabetes, treatment with aspirin, statin and ACE inhibitor is recommended to reduce vascular risk, unless there are specific contraindications.

Thereafter, $HbA1_c$ should be checked every 2–6 months unless the patient is stable on therapy.

Self-monitoring of blood glucose should be offered to all those on insulin or any other agent that has the propensity to cause hypoglycaemia. In most cases the first oral antidiabetic agent of choice is metformin. The role of the new incretin-based therapies is less clear; these are gastrointestinal hormones that cause an increase in insulin release from islet cells, such as dipeptidyl peptidase-4 (DPP4) inhibitors and glucagon-like peptide-1 (GLP-1) receptor agonists. If a second agent is required, options include sulfonylureas, thiazolidinediones or for some patients newer agents like DPP4 inhibitors and GLP-1 receptor agonists as well as insulin injections can be used.

Comprehensive treatment requires:

- statins – to achieve a total cholesterol level < 4.0 mmol/l
- aspirin – for patients aged over 50
- angiotensin-converting enzyme (ACE) inhibitor – the agent of choice in most patients with a blood pressure > 145/90 mmHg, or below the age of 50 years with multiple cardiovascular risk factors
- thiazide diuretic or calcium-channel blocker – consider using in patients of African-Caribbean origin as they may not respond to ACE inhibitors
- calcium-channel blocker, if there is a possibility of the patient becoming pregnant.

The blood pressure target in most patients is < 140/80 mmHg. For those with retinopathy or nephropathy the target is < 130/80 mmHg. Patients with diabetes should be offered annual retinopathy, neuropathy and nephropathy screening, which includes a check of urinary albumin/creatinine ratio (ACR), as part of their annual review.

When to refer

While many primary healthcare professionals with an interest in diabetes can provide the general care for

A weight gain of 7–11 kg by a patient aged over 18 years, which is common in people with severe mental illness, is associated with a twofold increase in the risk of diabetes.

people with diabetes, there will be times, depending upon their level of expertise, when referral to a specialist is needed. Those referred will include:

- patients with newly diagnosed type 2 diabetes
- patients with poorly controlled type 2 diabetes
- patients who require more expert podiatry input
- patients with newly diagnosed type 1 diabetes
- patients with poorly controlled type 1 diabetes
- patients with complex problems with lipid, blood pressure and cardiovascular disease
- patients with renal complications
- all patients who have developed retinopathy and require tight diabetic control.

What to expect from secondary care

In general terms, secondary care should be able to provide more complex specialist support and care. While it may also provide many of the services available in primary care – including, for example, structured education – secondary care should be able to manage more complex treatment regimens and manage diabetes-related complications. Insulin initiation, although moving more and more into the community, is still often performed in hospital diabetes out-patient departments. In addition, the initiation of novel therapies, including, for example, incretin-based therapies, in most instances takes place in secondary care.

It is beyond the scope of this chapter to provide detailed information on the management of the complications of diabetes. However, many centres now have subspecialty multidisciplinary clinics, including, for example, diabetic eye clinics, diabetic renal clinics, diabetic foot clinics and diabetic pregnancy clinics.

In very basic terms, once diabetic nephropathy is confirmed, patients should be offered ACE inhibitors with dose titration aiming for a blood pressure of under 130/80 mmHg. Angiotensin-2 receptor blocking agents (AIIRB) can be used as a substitute for ACE inhibitors if the latter are not well tolerated. Patients should be referred to ophthalmologists if there is any evidence of maculopathy or pre-proliferative retinopathy. Urgent review should be arranged if there is any evidence of neovascularisation and emergency review for sudden loss in vision, rubeosis iridis, vitreous haemorrhage or retinal detachment. Patients should be assessed annually for neuropathic symptoms and, when clinically indicated, autonomic neuropathy. If there is any suggestion of foot problems, appropriate assessment should be arranged via podiatry.

Why diabetes is associated with severe mental illness

A number of common or shared factors are believed to contribute to the higher incidence of type 2 diabetes among patients with severe mental illness (SMI). These include obesity, sedentary lifestyles and the use of psychotropic medications. Low birth weight and genetic pre-determinants may also be involved.

Important lifestyle factors associated with SMI and predisposing to diabetes include reduced dietary fibre, reduced fruit and vegetable intake, and increased intake of saturated fat. Physical inactivity and smoking are also risk factors. A weight gain of 7–11 kg by someone over 18 years, which may not be uncommon in people with SMI, is associated with a twofold increase in the risk of diabetes.[13] Studies have suggested that lower birth weight is related to the occurrence of type 2 diabetes mellitus, hypertension and hyperlipidaemia. Prenatal nutritional deficiency may also play a role in the origin of some cases of schizophrenia.[14] Schizophrenia, bipolar affective disorder and type 2 diabetes are common diseases with complex modes of inheritance, which include both genetic factors and environmental determinants. As 'susceptibility genes' are beginning to be identified, there is increasing interest in the possibility of shared susceptibility loci between the conditions.[15] Finally, studies have also examined the effect of acute psychotic stress on glucose homeostasis in non-diabetic people. Results indicate that beta-cell function and insulin sensitivity are inversely correlated with acute psychotic stress.[16] At present, however, it remains unclear whether this link is causal, as hormones released at the time of stress, including during an acute psychotic episode, are known to cause abnormalities of glucose homeostasis.

Antipsychotic medications and diabetes

> The risk of significant weight gain is great with clozapine and olanzapine, moderate with risperidone, quetiapine, amisulpride and zotepine and least with aripiprazole.

The possible role of antipsychotic medication in the development of abnormal glucose tolerance and diabetes has generated enormous interest in recent years. Antipsychotic drugs, both the 'typical' and the 'atypical', are known to induce weight gain and may also produce abnormalities in glucose and lipid metabolism. These modifications, in addition to risk factors intrinsic to the psychiatric illness (physical inactivity, smoking, diabetes – see above), are likely to increase the risk of cardiovascular complications.

Before prescribing medication, all risk factors must be taken into account. Good practice would also suggest that a clinical and metabolic assessment should be made at the time of starting treatment and at regular intervals thereafter. It should be remembered that most cases of emergent diabetes occur within 3 months, which would, therefore, seem like a sensible time for a first metabolic follow-up. Depending on the results, follow-up every 6–12 months may be appropriate.

A basic assessment should include:

- clinical history
- examination of blood pressure
- blood tests for glucose (random or fasting)
- glycosylated haemoglobin ($HbA1_c$)
- lipid profile.

In case of similar antipsychotic efficacy, when considering antipsychotic drugs, the clinician should consider the risk of inducing further metabolic disorder alongside the intrinsic risk factors of the patient. Nonetheless, the key consideration should always be the control of the mental illness (Box 16.1). Without this, it is very difficult to manage diabetes and increased cardiovascular risk, as patient empowerment is crucial. Diabetes induced by antipsychotic medication can be managed with standard diabetes treatments.

Some antipsychotic drugs have been reported to be more likely associated with a higher risk of metabolic disorders than others.[17] Clear guidance is now being provided in pharmacological formularies and is also available in *The Maudsley Prescribing Guidelines*.[18] The risk of iatrogenic diabetes seems to be more marked with clozapine, olanzapine, risperidone and quietapine than with amisulpride and aripiprazole. Nevertheless, the risk/benefit ratio often remains largely in favour of treatment.[19]

Obesity and overweight are not only risk factors for the development of diabetes but are also associated with other morbidities. Avoidance of weight gain is, therefore, an important health issue. With respect to antipsychotic drugs, clozapine and olanzapine appear to be associated with the greatest risk of clinically significant weight gain. Risperidone, quetiapine and amisulpride generally show low to moderate levels of weight gain and a modest risk of clinically significant increases in weight. Aripiprazole is generally associated with minimal mean weight gain.

Box 16.1 Steps to take for a patient starting an antipsychotic drug

When starting an antipsychotic drug:

- select antipsychotic based upon efficacy
- provide lifestyle advice
- conduct a baseline metabolic assessment: blood pressure, random or fasting blood glucose, $HbA1_c$ and lipid profile
- repeat 3–4 monthly
- inform general practitioner/diabetologist.

The Maudsley Prescribing Guidelines are recommended for more information about routine monitoring.

Box 16.2 Steps to take for a patient already on antipsychotic drug

For patients already prescribed an antipsychotic drug:

- provide lifestyle advice
- educate and advise about symptoms of diabetes
- perform the metabolic/Joint British Societies (JBS2) assessment annually
- perform tests of random plasma glucose, $HbA1_c$ and lipid profile.

JBS2: Joint British Societies' guidelines on prevention of cardiovascular disease in clinical practice.[20]

Refer to Chapter 12 for cardiovascular risk factors.

Although observational studies, large retrospective database analyses and controlled experimental studies, including randomised clinical trials, indicate that the second-generation 'atypical' antipsychotics are associated with differing effects on glucose and lipid metabolism, those with the greatest effect in terms of weight gain are not always associated with the greatest effect on glucose and lipid metabolism. Lack of data makes it difficult to draw conclusions concerning weight gain and diabetes risk with amisulpride, although amisulpride appears to have less risk of treatment-emergent dyslipidaemia than does olanzapine. Similar comments can be made for aripiprazole. Clozapine and olanzapine may have a direct effect on glucose regulation, independent of adiposity.

As type 2 diabetes is increased in patients with SMI and with the current degree of uncertainty around drug effects, it would therefore be advisable to consider all antipsychotic drugs as having the potential to cause weight gain, diabetes and increased cardiovascular risk; therefore appropriate risk screening and management of all patients are required (Box 16.2).

- Always obtain a personal and family history of obesity, diabetes, dyslipidaemia, hypertension and cardiovascular disease and ask women about a history of gestational diabetes.
- Record baseline height, weight and umbilical circumference and calculate body mass index.
- Record baseline blood pressure, fasting plasma glucose and lipid levels and repeat at 12 weeks and then annually.
- Record patients' weight at each visit.

In-patient management of diabetes

Suboptimal glycaemic control in hospitalised psychiatric patients with type 2 diabetes mellitus can have adverse consequences, including:

- increased neurological ischaemia
- delayed wound healing
- an increased infection rate
- poorer outcome of the primary illness.

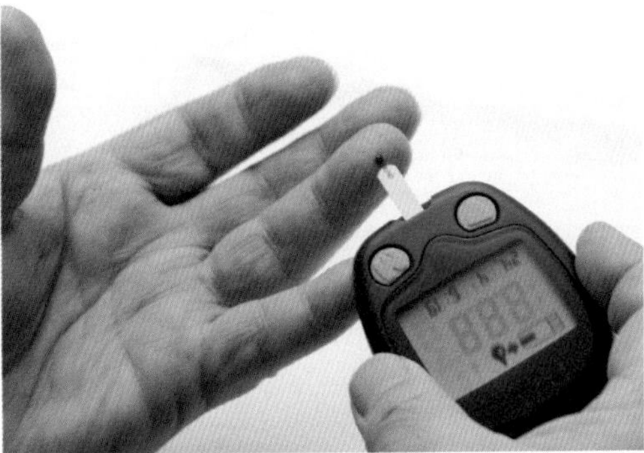

Fig. 16.2 A person with diabetes using a glucose meter.

If possible, hospitalised patients with diabetes should continue their existing anti-hyperglycaemic treatment. Poor long-term glycaemic control, as evidenced by clinical findings and elevated glycosylated haemoglobin levels, is common in psychiatric patients who are admitted to hospital. During the hospital stay, it may be possible to thoroughly investigate the problems that have led to poor control and to develop a therapeutic regimen that can be maintained after discharge. The patient and family members can also be educated about diabetes self-management, and both the management and the prevention of long-term complications can be addressed.[21]

The medical issues encountered by patients with SMI are usually complex. A team approach is vital and allows input from staff representing the various disciplines involved in treating the patient.[22–24] Multidisciplinary rounds allow the psychiatrists, medical physicians, caseworkers, pharmacists, nurses and nutritionists to provide a comprehensive and holistic package of patient care.[25,26] There is a need for hospital policies and training to focus on the treatment of diabetes for psychiatric in-patients.

Interface between community and hospital

A 2004 consensus conference of the American Diabetes Association, American Psychiatric Association, American Association of Clinical Endocrinologists and

North American Association for the Study of Obesity recommended several baseline evaluations at the initiation of medication use.[27] Clinicians should obtain from patients a personal and family history of obesity, diabetes, dyslipidaemia, hypertension and cardiovascular disease. Women should be asked about a history of gestational diabetes. Baseline height, weight and umbilical circumference should be measured and body mass index calculated. Baseline blood pressure, fasting plasma glucose and lipid levels should be checked. Ideally, patients' weight should be monitored at each visit. Blood pressure, glucose and lipid levels should be rechecked at 12 weeks and annually thereafter. In addition, nutrition and wellness classes for patients and their families can be helpful, and, increasingly, exercise groups need to be incorporated into mental health programmes to promote healthy lifestyles.[28]

When to refer a patient with diabetes to a specialist clinic

- Most patients with diabetes can have the diagnosis of diabetes confirmed and be managed by their own general practitioner, without the need for referral to a specialist clinic.
- Any patient in whom there are additional concerns over management of glycaemia control or other diabetes-related complications can be referred to a specialist clinic. Concerns may include:
  - unstable glycaemia control, including, suboptimal $HbA1_c$, hypo- and hyperglycaemia
  - the use of injectable therapies, including insulin and GLP-1 analogues
  - the development of diabetes-related complications.

Summary

Psychiatric disorders can be a risk factor for, as well as a complication of, diabetes. The use of antipsychotic medications, while associated with an increased risk of type 2 diabetes, cannot completely explain the association between these two chronic disease states. There is undoubedtly a complex interaction between multiple genetic and environmental factors that predispose the patient with SMI to type 2 diabetes. Screening for cardiovascular and metabolic risk factors is important in all psychiatric patients, as they are at high risk of diabetes and cardiovascular disease. Baseline screening should include questions about personal and family history of diabetes risk factors and measurement of blood pressure, blood glucose and serum lipids. Diabetes risk reduction, including counselling about diet, control of blood pressure, lowering of lipid levels, weight loss and increased physical activity, can have a positive impact on both diabetes and the psychiatric illness, and requires widespread implementation.

References

1 Diabetes UK. Reports and Statistics: Diabetes Prevalence 2011 (Oct 2011). Diabetes UK (http://www.diabetes.org.uk/Professionals/Publications-reports-and-resources/Reports-statistics-and-case-studies/Reports/Diabetes-prevalence-2011-Oct-2011).

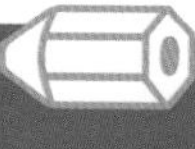

Learning points

- Diabetes in the UK population is rising
- Intensive glycaemic control and control of lipids and blood pressure reduce the microvascular and macrovascular complications associated with diabetes
- Patients with SMI are at an increased risk of diabetes
- Antipsychotic agents also increase the risk of type 2 diabetes
- All psychiatric patients should be regularly screened for diabetes and cardiovascular disease
- A multidisciplinary team approach is the key to good management

2 International Diabetes Federation. IDF Diabetes Atlas (Fifth Edition). IDF, 2011 (http://www.idf.org/diabetesatlas/5e/the-global-burden).

3 Bushe C, Leonard B. Association between atypical antipsychotic agents and type 2 diabetes: review of prospective clinical data. *Br J Psychiatry* 2004; **184** (suppl 47): s87–93.

4 Mezuk B, Eaton WW, Albrecht S, *et al.* Depression and type 2 diabetes over the lifespan, a meta-analysis. *Diabetes Care* 2008; **31**: 2383–90.

5 Ali S, Stone MA, Peters JL, *et al.* The prevalence of co-morbid depression in adults with type 2 diabetes: a systematic review and meta-analysis. *Diabet Med* 2006; **23**: 1165–73.

6 UKPDS Group. UK Prospective Diabetes Study 6. Complications in newly diagnosed type 2 diabetic patients and their association with different clinical and biochemical risk factors. *Diabetes Res* 1990; **13**: 1–11.

7 Park C. Diabetic ketoacidosis. *J R Coll Physicians Edinb* 2006; **36**: 40–3.

8 Haffner SM, Lehto S, Rönnemaa T, *et al.* Mortality from coronary heart disease in subjects with type 2 diabetes and in nondiabetic subjects with and without prior myocardial infarction. *N Engl J Med* 1998; **339**: 229–34.

9 Stratton IM, Adler AI, Neil HA, *et al.* Association of glycaemia with macrovascular and microvascular complications of type 2 diabetes (UKPDS 35): prospective observational study. *BMJ* 2000; **321**: 405–12.

10 UK Prospective Diabetes Study Group. Tight blood pressure control and risk of macrovascular and microvascular complications in type 2 diabetes: UKPDS 38. *BMJ* 1998; **317**: 703–13.

11 Colhoun HM, Betteridge DJ, Durrington PN, *et al.* Primary prevention of cardiovascular disease with atorvastatin in type 2 diabetes in the Collaborative Atorvastatin Diabetes Study (CARDS): multicentre randomised placebo-controlled trial. *Lancet* 2004; **364**: 685–96.

12 British Medical Association. *Revisions to the GMS Contract 2006/07: Delivering Investment in General Practice.* BMA, 2006.

13 Colditz GA, Willett WC, Rotnitzky A, *et al.* Weight gain as a risk factor for clinical diabetes mellitus in women. *Ann Intern Med* 1995; **122**: 481–6.

14 Susser E, Neugebauer R, Hoek HW, *et al.* Schizophrenia after prenatal famine. Further evidence. *Arch Gen Psychiatry* 1996; **53**: 25–31.

15 Gough SC, O'Donovan MC. Clustering of metabolic comorbidity in schizophrenia: a genetic contribution? *J Psychopharmacol* 2005; **19** (6 suppl): 47–55.

16 Shiloah E, Witz S, Abramovitch Y, *et al.* Effect of acute psychotic stress in nondiabetic subjects on beta-cell function and insulin sensitivity. *Diabetes Care* 2003; **26**: 1462–7.

17 Newcomer JW. Second-generation (atypical) antipsychotics and metabolic effects: a comprehensive literature review. *CNS Drugs* 2005; **19** (suppl 1): 1–93.

18 Taylor D, Paton C, Kapur S. *The Maudsley Prescribing Guidelines in Psychiatry.* Informa Healthcare, 2012.

19 Chabroux S, Haffen E, Penfornis A. Diabetes and second-generation (atypical) anti-psychotics. [In French.] *Ann Endocrinol (Paris)* 2009; **70**: 202–10.

20 Joint British Societies' guidelines on prevention of cardiovascular disease in clinical practice. *Heart* 2005; **91** (suppl V).

21 Lilley SH, Levine GI. Management of hospitalized patients with type 2 diabetes mellitus. *Am Fam Physician* 1998; **57**: 1079–88.

22 Samet JH, Friedmann P, Saitz R. Benefits of linking primary medical care and substance abuse services: patient, provider, and societal perspectives. *Arch Intern Med* 2001; **161**: 85–91.

23 Schwarz M, Landis SE, Rowe JE. A team approach to quality improvement. *Fam Pract Manag* 1999; **6**: 25–30.

24 Keawe'aimoku Kaholokula J, Schirmer TN, Elting D. Identifying and prioritizing diabetes care issues among mental health professionals of a multi-ethnic, state psychiatric hospital. *Diabetes Spectrum* 2004; **17**: 123–8.

25 Lambert TJ, Velakoulis D, Pantelis C. Medical comorbidity in schizophrenia. *Med J Aust* 2003; **178** Suppl: S67–70.

26 Meiklejohn C, Sanders K, Butler S. Physical health care in medium secure services. *Nurs Stand* 2003; **17**: 33–7.

27 American Diabetes Association, American Psychiatric Association, American Association of Clinical Endocrinologists, North American Association for the Study of Obesity. Consensus Development Conference on Antipsychotic Drugs and Obesity and Diabetes. *J Clin Psychiatry* 2004; **65**: 596–601.

28 Llorente MD, Urrutia V. Diabetes, psychiatric disorders, and the metabolic effects of antipsychotic medications. *Clin Diabetes* 2006; **24**: 18–24.

17 Hepatology

Vidyasagar Ramappa and Guruprasad P. Aithal

Members of the mental health team need to be aware of liver disease because it can be caused by alcohol, commonly prescribed antipsychotic medication and infection, and can result in encephalopathy and dementia. This chapter describes the risk factors for liver disease, symptoms and signs, tests of liver function, and disease management.

Introduction

The liver is one of the largest organs in the body at a weight of around 1–1.5 kg, and is critical to a number of physiological processes. It receives a dual blood supply: approximately 20% from the oxygen-rich hepatic artery (from the systemic circulation) and 80% from the portal vein, which delivers nutrient-rich blood from the stomach, intestines, pancreas and spleen (from the portal circulation).[1]

The liver has numerous functions to maintain homeostasis and health; therefore, diseases of the liver affect other organ systems. Such diseases lead to:

- a tendency to 'clot' readily
- a tendency to bruise and bleed due to a low platelet count (thrombocytopenia)
- muscle wasting
- renal dysfunction
- cognitive decline
- encephalopathy
- neuropsychiatric manifestations such as mood disturbances, personality change and memory loss.

While the last may be the presenting symptoms in some *without* known liver disease, they may precede specific symptoms or signs of hepatic decompensation.

The high prevalence of alcohol and substance misuse (see Chapters 22 and 23) in patients with chronic liver disease necessitates close collaboration between specialists from both psychiatry and hepatology in the joint management of both risk behaviour as well as the consequences of liver disease.

This chapter focuses on the neuropsychiatric manifestations of liver disease, the interface of psychiatry with hepatology, the use of medication in patients with liver disease and hepatotoxicity.

Liver disease

The liver has sufficient reserves to compensate for even advanced structural and architectural change resulting from disease processes. Therefore, liver disease is often suspected on the basis of the presence of risk factors in the context of non-specific symptoms. In most instances, the diagnosis can be deduced from the presence of supportive physical signs, a few laboratory tests and an ultrasound scan of the liver as well as the biliary tree. In some instances more detailed imaging and liver biopsy may be necessary for confirmation of the diagnosis.

History

Patients use a variety of expressions to describe their often non-specific complaints, commonly:

- fatigue and malaise – described variously as lethargy, weakness, increased sleepiness, lack of stamina or poor energy
- nausea (with or without vomiting) – if this follows a meal, gallstone disease may be associated
- a continuous dull ache in the right upper abdominal quadrant – this is due to an acute swelling of the liver in acute hepatitis
- intense but intermittent pain – this can be due to intermittent distension of the gallbladder or biliary tree secondary to biliary obstruction (sometimes referred to as 'biliary colic')
- jaundice – in the presence of known liver disease is generally a reasonable indicator of its severity
  - jaundice associated with tea-coloured urine is the hallmark of liver and biliary disease
  - in the absence of dark urine, jaundice is an indicator of unconjugated hyperbilirubinaemia, which is typical of haemolytic anaemias
- itching – indicates bile flow obstruction (or sluggish flow; cholestasis), usually accompanied by pale stools
- easy bruising – due to a low platelet count or abnormal blood coagulation.

The symptoms commonly experienced by patients with liver disease are listed in Box 17.1.

Chronic liver disease may remain asymptomatic until signs of decompensation of cirrhosis and so suspicion of liver disease should be based on risk factors (Table 17.2).

Physical examination

The physical examination of people with chronic liver disease is often unremarkable, unless signs of decompensation have developed. However, a thorough examination is desirable to seek signs suggesting potential risk factors:

- needle tracks in intravenous drug users
- Dupuytren's contracture with chronic alcohol misuse
- spider angiomas, gynaecomastia and oedema suggestive of chronic liver disease or cirrhosis
- palpable spleen and ascites suggestive of portal hypertension
- jaundice, bruising and encephalopathy suggestive of decompensation.

Laboratory investigations

There are some important considerations when blood tests are performed for people suspected to have liver disease. First of all, tests commonly called 'liver function

Box 17.1 Symptoms of liver and biliary disease

Non-specific symptoms:

- fatigue
- malaise
- poor appetite
- nausea
- vomiting

Specific symptoms:

- tea-coloured urine
- yellow discoloration of skin (jaundice)
- itching
- pale stools
- easy bruising
- abdominal distension (ascites)
- pain/discomfort in the right upper quadrant

Box 17.2 Risk factors for liver disease

- Alcohol misuse/dependency
- Metabolic syndrome (obesity, diabetes mellitus, hypertension, dyslipidaemia)
- Intravenous drug misuse
- Previous surgery/blood transfusions
- Tattoos, piercings
- Medications – herbal remedies, over-the-counter drugs, oral contraception, antibiotics
- Occupational exposure to toxins
- Travel to areas where hepatotropic viruses are endemic
- Promiscuous sexual behaviour
- Family history of liver disease

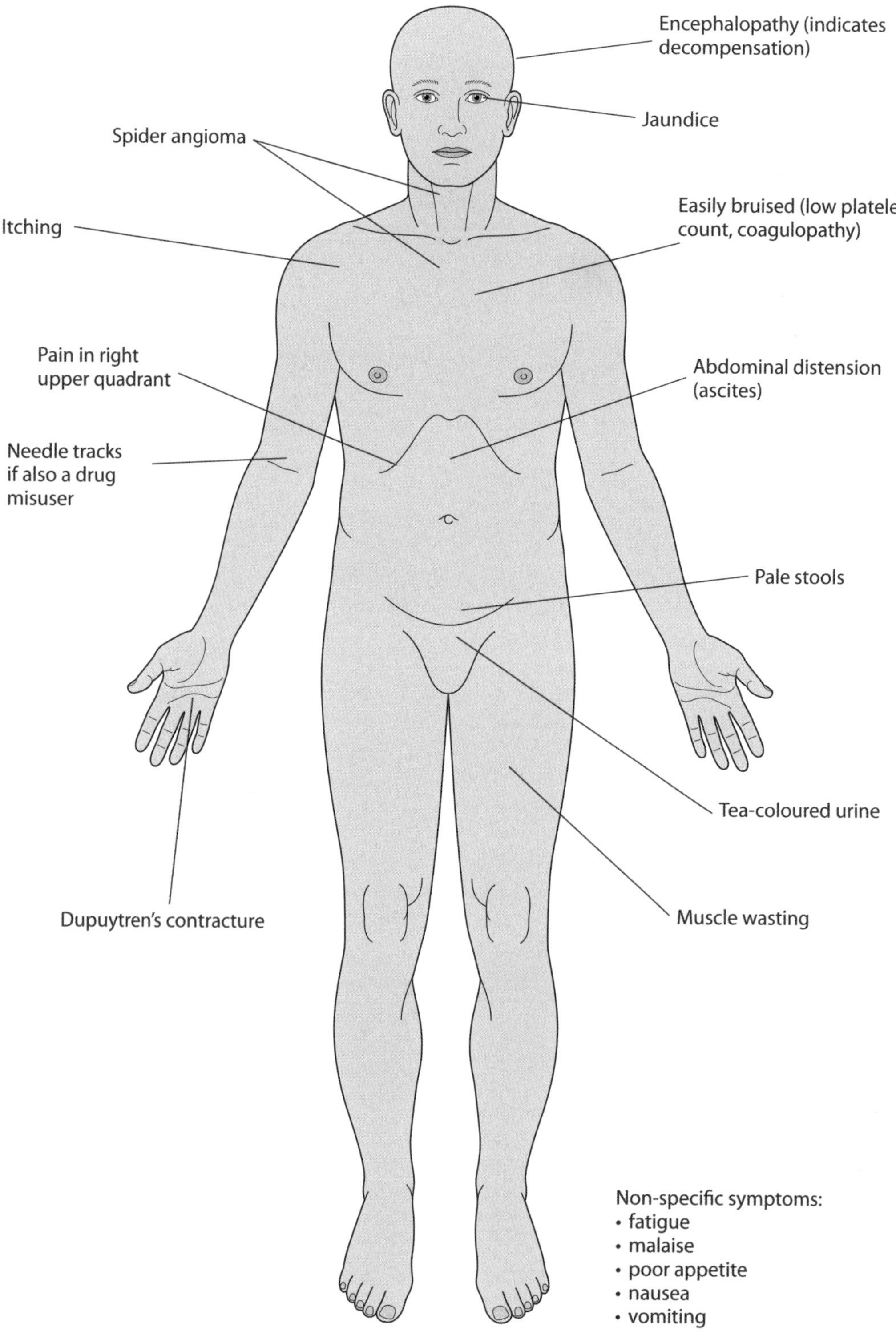

Fig. 17.1 Symptoms and signs of liver disease.

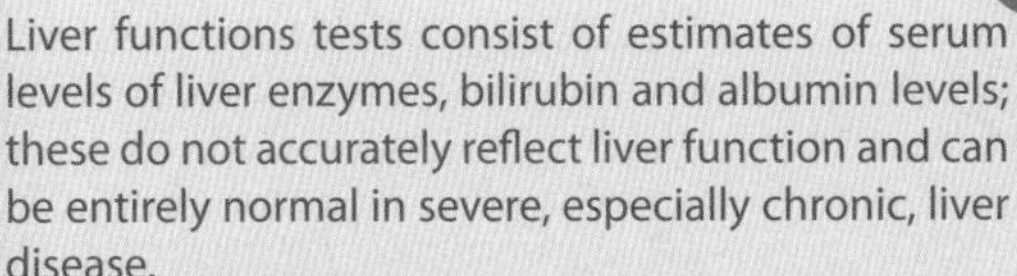
Liver functions tests consist of estimates of serum levels of liver enzymes, bilirubin and albumin levels; these do not accurately reflect liver function and can be entirely normal in severe, especially chronic, liver disease.

tests' consist of estimates of serum levels of liver enzymes, bilirubin and albumin levels. However, liver enzymes:

- do not accurately reflect function of the liver or the extent of liver injury or the presence of liver disease and they can be entirely normal, especially in chronic liver diseases (a 'false negative' test)
- can be raised in systemic disease unrelated to the liver pathology (a 'false positive' test)
- can occasionally be useful in assessing the response to treatment and to monitor progress in specific circumstances such as autoimmune hepatitis.

For the sake of simplicity, liver tests can be grouped as tests differentiating hepatocellular from cholestatic disease, which help direct the clinician to investigate appropriately, and tests that reflect liver function (Box 17.3).

Box 17.3 Tests for liver disease

Tests differentiating hepatocellular from cholestatic disease, which help direct the clinician to investigate appropriately.

- *Liver cell injury*. Alanine transaminase (ALT) and aspartate transaminase (AST) are sensitive indicators of liver cell injury. Modest elevation (ALT up to 200 IU/l; normal is < 40) occurs in any liver disease but ALT > 400 IU/l is often associated with acute conditions such as acute viral hepatitis, ischaemic hepatitis (resulting from circulatory shock or heart failure) and drug- or toxin-induced hepatitis (e.g. paracetamol overdose, adverse hepatic reactions to drugs).[2] Alcoholic liver disease causes a disproportionate rise in AST compared with ALT, unlike in other hepatocellular diseases.[3]
- *Cholestasis*. Alkaline phosphatase (ALP) and gamma glutamyl transpeptidase (GGT) *individually* are non-specific. Alone, a raised ALP level (< 1.5 times the upper limit of normal) is common in the sixth decade of life but if doubled and accompanied by a rise in GGT level, suspect cholestatic or infiltrative liver disease. Alone, an elevated GGT level suggests enzyme induction from chronic excess alcohol[4] or from a medication such as an anti-epileptic.[5]

Tests that reflect liver function:

- *Serum bilirubin*. Alone, a raised bilirubin level may be *unconjugated* – suggesting haemolysis or Gilbert's syndrome (hereditary, benign) – or *conjugated* – suggesting liver or biliary disease.
- *Serum albumin*. A low albumin level with raised polyclonal immunoglobulin (Ig) levels suggests liver decompensation. Elevated IgA is seen commonly in alcoholic liver disease, IgG in auto-immune hepatitis and IgM in primary biliary cirrhosis.
- *Coagulation screen*. Apart from factor VIII, clotting factors are synthesised exclusively in the liver. Measurement of clotting using prothrombin time or the international normalised ratio (INR) is a good indicator of synthetic liver function. Chronic cholestasis can lead to vitamin K malabsorption and a prolonged prothrombin time due to deficiency of vitamin K-dependent clotting factors II, VII, IX and X. A prolonged prothrombin time despite parenteral vitamin K is usually a marker of poor synthetic reserve.[6,7]
- *Imaging*. Where liver tests suggest cholestasis, ultrasound can be used to look for evidence of biliary obstruction.
- *Liver biopsy*. Biopsy is needed where a diagnostic dilemma exists after initial investigations.

Clinical approach to liver disease

Identify the pattern of liver disease

This may be acute or chronic.

- In hepatocellular disease (viral hepatitis, auto-immune disease, alcoholic liver disease), the clinical presentation is dominated by liver cell injury, inflammation and necrosis.
- In cholestatic disease, biliary excretion is slowed due to drugs, gallstones or tumour.
- With a mixed pattern, the above two coexist, as in viral hepatitis or drug-induced liver injury.

Assess the severity of disease

In acute liver failure, encephalopathy, prothrombin time, creatinine levels and the degree of metabolic acidosis determine the need for liver transplantation.

In chronic liver disease, 'grading' of necro-inflammation and 'staging' of the amount of scarring are usually based on liver histology.[8] New techniques, such as transient elastography ('fibroscan'), are being increasingly used in place of histology. Once cirrhosis is established, the Child–Pugh score may be useful (see below); in those with liver failure, more subtle scoring

Table 17.1 Stages of hepatic encephalopathy

Clinical stage	Mental status	Asterixis (flapping tremor)	Neuromuscular function	Findings on electro-encephalography (EEG)
Minimal	Normal	–	Subtle changes on psychomotor test	–
Stage 1	Euphoria/depression; reversed sleep pattern; mild confusion	±	Tremor, incoordination, apraxia	Normal/slowing
Stage 2	Drowsy	+	Ataxia, slurred speech	Triphasic
Stage 3	Increased somnolence but arousable	+	Hypoactive reflexes, myoclonus, rigidity	Triphasic
Stage 4	Coma	–	Dilated pupils, decerebrate posturing, absent doll's eye reflex	Delta

systems such as Mayo End-Stage Liver Disease (MELD)[9] and UK End Stage Liver Disease (UKELD) are useful in estimating prognosis.[10]

Hepatic encephalopathy

Hepatic encephalopathy is a potentially reversible neuropsychiatric syndrome ranging from subtle abnormalities only detectable on psychometric testing to an altered sensorium associated with either acute or chronic liver failure, wherein neuropsychiatric signs are more noticeable. Numerical clinical staging (Table 17.1) is useful for clinical assessment and to assess response to treatment. The classification of hepatic encephalopathy is set out in Table 17.2.[11]

Minimal hepatic encephalopathy

This condition occurs in the context of chronic liver disease; patients may appear normal on clinical and neurological examination, but there is impairment on psychometric tests such as the trail-making or digit symbol test, and subtle changes in cognition, behaviour and intellect and measurement of evoked potentials. These tests are sensitive and quite specific for the diagnosis of minimal hepatic encephalopathy in the context of chronic liver disease.[12]

Pathogenesis

Ammonia plays a major role in the pathogenesis of hepatic encephalopathy (Fig. 17.2). Hyperammonaemia has been thought to be an end-result of breakdown of urea by colonic bacteria. Recently, the focus has changed to the role of glutaminase in the small intestine and kidneys, which catalyses glutamine to yield glutamate and ammonia. In cirrhosis, an inability to detoxify ammonia by urea synthesis and porto-systemic shunting increases ammonia in the systemic circulation. Hyperammonaemia leads to accumulation of glutamine within astrocytes, generating an osmotic stress causing astrocytes to take in water and swell. In addition, hyperammonaemia increases oxidative stress

Table 17.2 Classification of hepatic encephalopathy

Type	Presentation, manifestation, symptoms
Type A (acute)	In acute liver failure, hepatic encephalopathy is an essential clinical component, with 25% of patients developing significant brain swelling and increased intracranial pressure
Type B (bypass)	Under rare circumstances, ammonia from the gut bypasses the liver via porto-systemic shunts in the absence of cirrhosis to cause encephalopathy
Type C (cirrhosis)	In cirrhosis, hepatic encephalopathy is a consequence of portal hypertension and is observed in up to 70% of the patients with existing porto-systemic shunting

Adapted from Ferenci *et al*, 1998.[11]

and GABA-ergic neural activity, leading to inhibition of the central nervous system.[13–19]

Most cases of hepatic encephalopathy have some precipitating factors; common precipitants are listed in Table 17.3.

Other problems that may resemble or coexist with hepatic encephalopathy are listed in Table 17.4.

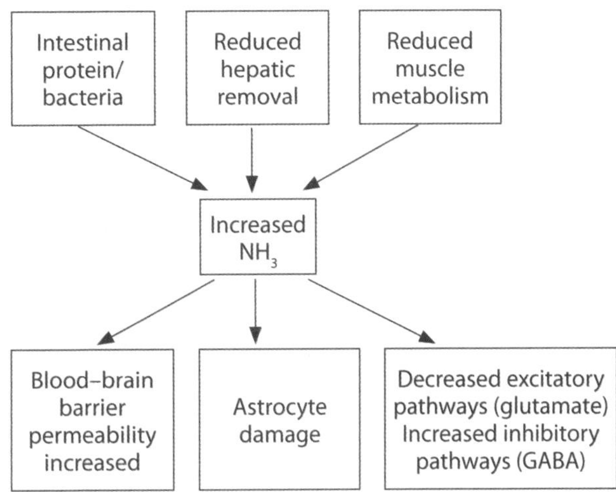

Fig. 17.2 Role of ammonia in hepatic encephalopathy.

Treatment of hepatic encephalopathy

Diets and supplements. Very large protein loads (such as blood rich in protein, from gastrointestinal bleeding) can precipitate encephalopathy.[20] However, protein energy malnutrition is frequent in advanced liver disease; dietary protein restriction may adversely affect the outcome and is not recommended.

Branched-chain amino acids are beneficial in hepatic encephalopathy, but their use is limited by patient compliance and high costs.[21,22]

Thiamine deficiency may have a synergistic effect, with hyperammonaemia accounting for some of the manifestations of hepatic encephalopathy, so prompt and adequate *thiamine supplementation*, either orally or intravenously depending on specialist advice, should be considered in all patients with chronic liver failure. Concomitant hypokalaemia should be corrected as it

able 17.3 Factors that precipitate hepatic ncephalopathy

ctor	Putative causes
uid and ectrolyte nbalance	Over-diuresis, hyponatraemia, hypokalaemia; large-volume paracentesis; vomiting, diarrhoea
eeding	Varices; gastroduodenal ulcers
fections/ epsis	Spontaneous bacterial peritonitis, chest/urinary sepsis
arge protein ad	Gastrointestinal bleed; high-protein diet
rugs	Opiates, sedatives and hypnotics
iscellaneous	Constipation

able 17.4 Differential diagnosis for hepatic encephalopathy

ifferential diagnosis	Background	Manifestations
yponatraemia (serum odium usually < 125 mmol/l; common aggravating factor)	Ascites, diuretic therapy, recurrent paracentesis	Apathy, drowsiness, nausea, hypotension
lcohol withdrawal	Abrupt cessation of alcohol intake	Motor and autonomic over-activity, hallucinations, tremors, agitation
ernicke's encephalopathy	Chronic alcohol excess, malnutrition	Ophthalmoparesis, ataxia, sensory neuropathy, confusion
orsakoff's psychosis	Chronic alcohol excess, malnutrition	Confabulation
ubdural haematoma	History of head trauma	Localising signs, seizures
ilson's disease	Chronic liver disease in the young (< 40 years of age at presentation), family history of liver disease	Extrapyramidal signs, especially dystonia, tremors, cerebellar features, haemolysis and renal impairment

increases renal ammonia production and may promote conversion of ammonium into ammonia, which can cross the blood–brain barrier.

Lactulose works by causing an osmotic diarrhoea, reducing the time for intestinal bacteria to metabolise protein into ammonia; and by acidifying the bowel lumen, so promoting the conversion of ammonia (NH_3) to ammonium (NH_4^+) and reducing its absorption.[23,24] The dose is increased until there are two or three soft bowel motions every day.

Antibiotics decrease the bacterial conversion of protein to ammonia. It is now clear that non-absorbable rifaximin is an effective treatment either on it's own or as an adjunct to lactulose in hepatic encephalopathy.[25]

Flumazenil, a benzodiazepine receptor antagonist, has theoretical benefits, but is too short-acting to be of clinical value.[26]

L-ornithine stimulates the urea cycle and initial results from randomised controlled trials are encouraging.[22,27]

Hyponatraemia in chronic liver disease[28–30]

In cirrhosis, splanchnic vasodilation leads to arterial under-filling and hypovolaemia, causing baroreceptors to stimulate hypersecretion of the antidiuretic hormone arginine vasopressin. This leads to hyponatraemia, which may be aggravated by diuretic-induced sodium loss.

More than half of hospitalised patients with cirrhosis have hyponatraemia, which usually develops over several days or weeks. Patients may develop symptoms which are indistinguishable from hepatic encephalopathy:

- progressive fatigue
- apathy
- nausea.

It is important to measure the serum sodium concentration, as it is an independent and a major determinant of quality of life in patients with cirrhosis.[31] In patients with hyponatraemia, there is an inverse relationship between serum sodium levels and the frequency of hepatic encephalopathy as well as other complications of cirrhosis such as spontaneous bacterial peritonitis and hepato-renal syndrome.

Hyponatraemia may worsen with hypotonic fluids such as 5% dextrose and hypertonic saline aggravates oedema in patients with cirrhosis.

Prevention and management

Fluid management and dilutional hyponatraemia

The aim of therapy is to increase solute-free water excretion. Hypotonic fluids such as 5% dextrose worsen hyponatraemia; hypertonic saline solution worsens oedema and ascites. Fluid restriction to no more than 1.5 litres per day is often used, but is of limited success. Plasma expansion with albumin may transiently correct hyponatraemia and prevent short-term complications.

Vaptans are vasopressin receptor antagonists acting specifically on the distal collecting tubule; these induce clearance of solute-free water only (aquaretics) and are effective in correcting hyponatraemia in advanced cirrhosis.[32]

Diuretic resistance and renal dysfunction are indicators of a poor prognosis in hyponatraemia secondary to advanced liver disease.

Interface of psychiatry and hepatology

Mortality from cirrhosis in the UK has increased threefold in the past few decades and ninefold among those aged 25–44 years. Alcohol consumption rose 120% between 1950 and 2000, so that the average consumption of alcohol is now 22 units per adult per week, with 25% drinking at hazardous or harmful levels. Hospital admissions for alcohol-related conditions are increasing by 80 000 per year.[33] Three common chronic liver diseases, all of which are more prevalent, are alcoholic liver disease, non-alcoholic fatty liver disease and hepatitis C infection. Unsurprisingly, alcohol-related problems and hepatitis C infections are two common conditions where optimal management relies upon collaboration between hepatology and liaison psychiatry teams.

Alcohol-related liver disease

Quantity, duration and pattern of alcohol consumption are important risk factors in the development of liver disease. The current guidance from the Royal College of Physicians suggests an upper limit for safe drinking of 21 units for men and 14 units for women a week (Table 17.5)[34] (see Chapter 22).

Table 17.5 Terminology related to problem drinking

Description	Pattern
Sensible	< 21 units a week for men; < 14 units a week for women
Heavy	> 50 units a week for men; > 35 units a week for women
Binge	Regularly drinking in a single session: > 10 units for men; > 7 units for women
Hazardous	Heavy and binge drinkers whose drinking patterns pose considerable risk to own and others' health
Harmful	Heavy and binge drinkers whose drinking is causing physical and psychological harm to self and causing harm to the physical, mental or social well-being of others

The pathology of alcohol-related liver disease comprises the following, although there is significant overlap and these rarely exist in the pure form:[35]

- *Fatty liver* (Fig. 17.3). This may be identified on routine blood tests, with an AST:ALT ratio of 3 or more a useful indication of an alcohol aetiology. It occurs in 90% of heavy and binge drinkers, who usually have no liver-related symptoms and in whom the only abnormal sign is a smooth non-tender liver.
- *Alcoholic hepatitis* (Fig. 17.4). This occurs in 10–20% of patients with alcohol liver disease, where fatty infiltration is associated with inflammatory infiltrates and fibrosis or coexisting cirrhosis. It may present with systemic symptoms such as low-grade fever, malaise, jaundice and abdominal pain with a recent history of excess drinking. Signs of chronic liver disease may be evident and the liver tender and enlarged. When coagulopathy and encephalopathy are present, mortality is about 50% within 3 months.
- *Cirrhosis* (Fig. 17.5). This is usually apparent with episodes of hepatitis. Abdominal ultrasound may show evidence of portal hypertension (splenomegaly and collateral vessels), hence implying cirrhosis. Ascites, variceal bleeding, jaundice and encephalopathy indicate decompensated cirrhosis.

Treatment

Abstinence from alcohol is the cornerstone of treatment as it is the critical determinant of the prognosis, even

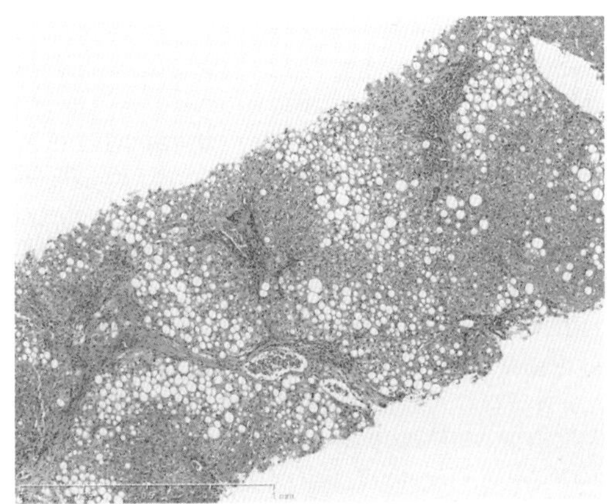

Fig. 17.3 Fatty changes in liver.

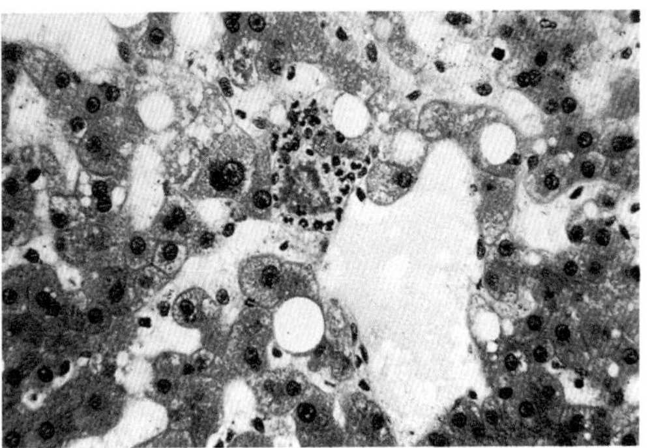

Fig. 17.4 Liver biopsy in alcoholic hepatitis. © SpringerImages (www.springerimages.com). With kind permission from Springer Science and Business Media B.V.

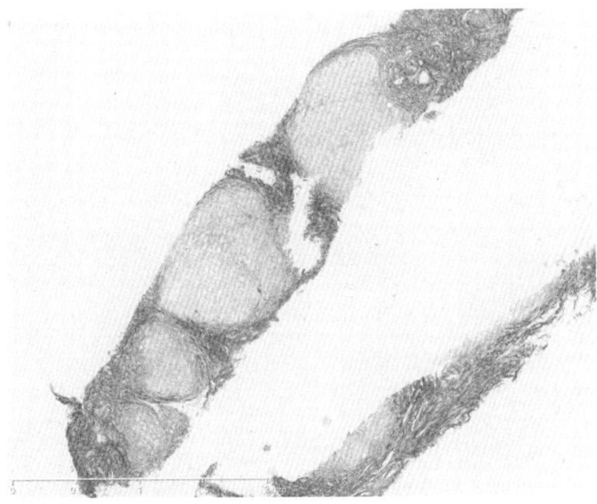

Fig. 17.5 Cirrhosis of the liver.

in patients with established cirrhosis.[36] Hence, alcohol counsellors and alcohol liaison services should be routinely involved in the management of these patients.

Glucocorticoids to suppress inflammation may improve the short-term outcome in selected patients with acute severe alcoholic hepatitis.[37–39]

Pentoxiphylline (an anti-tumour necrosis factor-alpha agent) is an alternative to glucocorticoids, as tumour necrosis factor is the key cytokine accounting for the liver injury and systemic inflammatory response.[40,41]

Diuretics and therapeutic paracentesis afford symptom control by reducing ascites in decompensated cirrhosis.

Antibiotics are warranted in spontaneous bacterial peritonitis.

Non-selective beta-blockers and/or *transjugular porto-systemic shunt* (TJPSS) may reduce portal pressures and varices.

Liver transplantation may be offered in advanced liver disease only to patients who have achieved significant sobriety.

Alcohol withdrawal syndrome

This occurs in individuals who abruptly stop alcohol consumption following prolonged heavy drinking. Symptoms, described in Table 17.6, depend upon the amount of alcohol consumption, the pattern of drinking and the time since withdrawal.

Patients with minor symptoms and hallucinations usually have a clear sensorium, but in delirium tremens there is an acute confusional state with clouding of consciousness. Delirium tremens has a mortality rate of 1–5%. Risk factors for delirium tremens include concomitant acute medical illness, a history of delirium tremens or withdrawal seizures, heavy alcohol use, older age and more severe symptoms at presentation.

The Clinical Institute Withdrawal Assessment for Alcohol (CIWA-Ar) scale is a validated-10 item assessment tool which stratifies patients based on the scoring as mild, moderate, severe or at risk of delirium tremens.[42]

Treatment

The goal is to provide a safe withdrawal in a dignified manner and prepare patients for ongoing therapy for dependence.

Benzodiazepines are the most commonly used class of drugs to treat withdrawal symptoms. Long-acting benzodiazepines (chlordiazepoxide or diazepam) give a smoother onset of therapy.[43] Intramuscular absorption of lorazepam is reliable when a parenteral route of administration is needed. Treatment may be given based on the CIWA-Ar score, using a fixed-schedule or symptom-triggered regimen. It is important to review the response frequently and if necessary to modify the prescription to ensure that the patient receives an adequate dose, but avoid precipitating hepatic encephalopathy in those with a decompensated liver. Additionally, nutritional deficiencies may need to be corrected.

In Wernicke's encephalopathy (see below), withdrawal can be managed in an out-patient setting or an in-patient setting for those with cirrhosis or at risk of developing delirium tremens. In severe cases, *haloperidol* may need to be used to treat agitation and hallucinations. *Clonidine* has been shown to improve the autonomic symptoms of withdrawal.

Long-term management

Follow-up is essential to address the underlying problem of addiction, aiming towards low-risk drinking or abstinence, especially for those with advanced fibrosis. Management is likely to include:

- counselling
- brief interventions
- cognitive–behavioural therapy
- family therapy
- pharmacotherapy.

Table 17.6 Evolution of the clinical manifestations of alcohol withdrawal syndrome

Symptoms/syndrome	Time to emergence
Insomnia, tremors, anxiety, hypervigilance, loose stools, diaphoresis, tachycardia, nausea, anorexia	6–12 hours
Hallucinations: auditory, visual, tactile	12–24 hours
Seizures	24–48 hours
Delirium tremens: visual hallucinations, disorientation, agitation, autonomic overactivity	48–72 hours

A range of ion channels, neurotransmitter receptors and enzymes are involved in the different components of alcohol dependence. *Disulfiram*, *acamprosate*, *baclofen*, *naltrexone* and *gabapentin* have been investigated as anti-craving medications but their role in the management of alcohol dependence has yet to be established.

Wernicke's encephalopathy

This metabolic encephalopathy results from thiamine deficiency. It is characterised by:

- ophthalmoplegia – with treatment, this usually recovers in days to weeks, although some patients may be left with nystagmus
- ataxia – this usually improves in the first week but takes 1 –2 months to resolve and some may be left with ataxia
- confusion – this usually resolves within 1– 2 days, but the global psychomotor retardation noted will take weeks to months to resolve
- memory loss.

Wernicke's encephalopathy is seen in 12–14% of heavy drinkers.[44] It is a medical emergency with an estimated mortality of up to 20% in untreated cases. Only 20% are clinically diagnosed in life, with the majority identified on autopsy or in retrospect.[45] Of those who survive, 85% have long-term neurological damage, with 25% needing long-term institutionalisation.[46]

Prevention and treatment

Inadvertent high carbohydrate feeds or dextrose infusion prior to replenishing thiamine reserves may hasten the accumulation of lactate and precipitate Wernicke's encephalopathy, therefore prompt and adequate thiamine supplementation is critical in those at risk.

Korsakoff's psychosis

Wernicke's encephalopathy and Korsakoff's psychosis are considered to be the *acute* and *chronic* phases, respectively, of the same disease process. Korsakoff's is characterised by neuronal loss and micro-haemorrhages in the periventricular region and periaqueductal grey matter, causing:

- memory disturbance in the setting of a clear level of consciousness (patients have severe impairment of current/recent memory and to a lesser extent remote memory)
- false recollection of events or 'confabulations', are considered the hallmark of Korsakoff's syndrome.

In dementia thought to be caused by alcohol consumption, computerised tomography is required only if there are atypical features, such as localising neurological signs or a history of head trauma.

Treatment

Once established, Korsakoff's syndrome is considered irreversible. Adequate *thiamine* supplementation is often tried at the time of first presentation, but the mainstay of management involves a multidisciplinary approach including physiotherapy and occupational therapy, with continued care in specialised Korsakoff's units or residential homes.

Alcohol-related dementia

Up to 29% of individuals with dementia have a history of heavy drinking and up to 23% of elderly patients treated for problem drinking also have dementia.[47–49] Diagnosing alcohol-related dementia can be difficult and is based on clinical patterns and the exclusion of other disorders, especially those that are potentially reversible. Patients presenting with a history of alcohol excess and cognitive impairment can be assumed to have alcohol-related dementia if the following criteria are met:[50]

- alcohol withdrawal has been treated
- no sedatives have been given for 48 hours
- serum sodium levels are normal or stable at above 120 mmol/l
- serum ammonia levels are normal, or hepatic encephalopathy has been clinically excluded
- thyroid function is normal.

Computerised tomography is required only if there are atypical features, such as localising neurological signs or a history of head trauma. Thiamine should be given to all patients with confusion and alcohol excess (ideally as 2–3 days of intravenous therapy), as in-patients if necessary.

Hepatitis C infection

Worldwide, more than 170 million people are infected with hepatitis C virus (HCV), one of the leading causes of progressive liver disease in the Western world and a common indication for liver transplantation.[51,52] Around

85% of those exposed to HCV develop chronic hepatitis, of whom 10–20% progress to cirrhosis and 1–5% develop hepatocellular carcinoma (HCC).[53,54]

There are several known risk factors:

- a history of intravenous drug use, via the sharing of needles or other drug paraphernalia, including cookers, cotton, spoons and water – the prevalence of HCV is high (30–90%) in this group[55]
- transfusion of blood or blood products prior to implementation of HCV screening – the prevalence is about 10% in this group
- iatrogenic medical or dental exposure
- prior haemodialysis[56]
- tattoos and piercings
- sexual transmission – prevalence in sexual partners of HCV-infected persons is 1–5%[57,58]
- mother–infant transmission – though this is rare.

There is a high prevalence of substance misuse and alcohol dependency in patients with severe mental health illness that contributes to the 10–20% prevalence in this group.[59,60] Conversely, 85% of HCV-infected individuals have a psychiatric illness, the commonest being depression, anxiety and personality disorders.[61] Thus screening this high-risk population may be justified to help prevent the spread of HCV infection.

Screening and diagnosis

It is important to identify HCV infection because of the implications for the future health of the individuals concerned and for the control of further spread of infection. However, uptake of HCV testing is low in individuals with substance misuse and alcohol dependency, complicated by difficulty with venous access in people who inject drugs. However, the development of 'dried blood spot testing' has increased the uptake of HCV testing in specialist drug clinics.

Prevention

Individuals infected with HCV should be counselled:

- to stop using illicit drugs
- to avoid, if drug misuse is to continue, reusing or sharing syringes, needles, water, or cotton (injection sites should be swabbed with a new alcohol swab and syringes and needles should be disposed of after a single use into a safe, puncture-proof container)
- to avoid sharing tooth brushes and dental or shaving equipment
- to cover any bleeding wound to prevent contact of their blood with others (see p. 240).

Treatment of HCV infection

Ribavarin and *pegylated interferon* may be given for 24–48 weeks based on genotype and other parameters related to the pathology as well as viral kinetics.[62] Prior to starting interferon, depressive or anxiety symptoms should be stabilised. Regular screening and evaluation should be available for those at risk of neuropsychiatric problems. Various neuropsychiatric side-effects may occur with interferon, ranging from mild symptoms of anxiety and depression, psychomotor retardation, cognitive impairment and fatigue, to severe side-effects such as suicidal ideation and psychosis. Psychotic, manic or hypomanic symptoms are rare and usually warrant stopping treatment. Antipsychotics should be given if symptoms of mania and psychosis do not respond.[63]

'Needs adapted' approach

A strategy to reduce the burden of HCV infections in intravenous drug users should include:

- treatment of chronic HCV – intravenous drug users are less likely to adhere to treatment, largely because of the side-effects
- prevention of new infections – active intravenous drug users are prone to reinfection
- Creating specialist hepatitis services (in a 'needs adapted' setting) to facilitate the link with community addiction services, which will allow HCV treatment to be delivered within the community, with an acceptable level of compliance and effectiveness.

Medications and the liver

Patients with liver disease with a coexisting primary or secondary psychiatric disorder need effective treatment. An understanding of pharmacokinetics in liver disease will provide a logical basis to the choice of psychotropic medication and its dose, and alert the clinician to the potential adverse effects.

Through the portal circulation, the liver is highly exposed to drugs and other substances absorbed from the gastrointestinal tract. Most drugs are readily taken up by the liver but the lipophilic nature of most drugs prevents their excretion in the bile or the urine. However, the liver is sufficiently adaptable and induces metabolic pathways that include alteration of the drug molecule by a variety of processes.

Psychotropic medication and other drugs can be metabolised by one or more metabolic pathways

Table 17.7 Examples of drugs grouped according to the key aspects influencing their bioavailability

Extensive first-pass metabolism	Phase I metabolism	Phase II metabolism
Amitriptyline	Diazepam	Temazepam
Bupropion	Chlordiazepoxide	Lorazepam
Chlorpromazine	Amitriptyline	Oxazepam
Desipramine	Imipramine	
Dextropropoxyphene	Chlorpromazine	
Doxepin	Thioridazine	
Imipramine	Risperidone	
Nortriptyline	Meperidine	
Olanzapine	Propoxyphene	
Quetiapine		
Sertraline		
Venlafaxine		

affecting bioavailability. In liver disease, choosing a drug not needing phase I or needing only phase II metabolism may be advantageous (see Table 17.7).[64,65]

Liver disease may affect the pharmacokinetics, from absorption, metabolism and distribution through to elimination of the drug.

Absorption

In liver cirrhosis, portal hypertension and the resulting splanchnic congestion leads to *delayed* absorption of medications via the gut. Using osmotic laxatives like lactulose to treat or prevent encephalopathy further *reduces* absorption by reducing small-bowel transit time.

Distribution

The volume of distribution of drugs varies greatly in direct proportion to the degree of portal hypertension. Hypoalbuminaemia, ascites and oedema increase the volume of distribution. The presence of a porto-systemic shunt bypasses some metabolism in the liver and so less drug is available for liver metabolism.[66,67]

Protein binding

Most psychotropic drugs are highly protein bound; exceptions include venlafaxine, lithium, gabapentin, topiramate and methylphenidate. In liver cirrhosis, low albumin and altered protein binding to the drug leads to *increased availability* of pharmacologically active, unbound drug in the plasma; and for some drugs, such as benzodiazepines, a very low serum albumin increases dose-related side-effects, so consider a dose reduction when prescribing them.[65,67,68]

Considerations during prescription

The changes in pharmacokinetics and dynamics cannot be explained by a single mechanism. Thus a clinician prescribing psychotropic medications for patients with underlying liver disease has to bear in mind the following:

- the severity of liver disease, including the presence or absence of encephalopathy
- the therapeutic window of the psychotropic drug and drug monitoring
- the major metabolic mechanism of the drug
- the possible drug–drug interactions.

There are several validated clinical scoring systems to rate the severity or prognosis of liver disease. The Child–Pugh score (Table 17.8) is a semi-quantitative tool used most widely because of its simplicity. Indeed, it may oversimplify the complexities of drug biotransformation but is nevertheless a useful guideline[69] for dosing psychotropic medications (in addition to the guidance issued by the *British National Formulary*). However, in the context of hepatic encephalopathy, psychotropic medications, especially those with anticholinergic side-effects, can significantly worsen the symptoms of delirium in hepatic encephalopathy. As a general

Table 17.8 Child–Pugh score and recommendations for dose modification

Parameter	Score 1	Score 2	Score 3
Ascites	None	Slight, medically controlled	Moderate/severe, poorly controlled
Encephalopathy	None	Stage 1–2	Stage 3–4
Bilirubin (μmol/l)	<34	34–51	>51
Albumin (g/l)	>35	28 – 35	<28
Prothrombin time prolongation (s)	1–3	4–6	>6
Total score	5–6	7–9	10–15
Child–Pugh score (class of liver disease – see text)	A	B	C
Initiation dose as % of normal dose (refer to drug information/*British National Formulary*)	75–100%	50–75%	25–50%

measure, psychotropic dosing can be titrated according to the Child–Pugh score. Patients with:

- class A liver disease can usually tolerate 75–100% of a standard initial dose without any major side-effects
- class B liver disease should be dosed with more caution, owing to the prolonged half-life and delay in the distribution phase of the drugs – the initial dose should be 50% of the standard initial dose
- class C liver disease requires even more caution – use a low dosing schedule combined with frequent therapeutic monitoring wherever feasible, and use drugs which are lipophilic.

These strategies reduce the risk of cumulative toxicity.[70–72]

Drugs such as lithium can be problematic in patients with advanced cirrhosis who are overloaded with fluid as a result of complex changes in body fluids due to renal dysfunction, variable diuretic therapy and therapeutic drainage of ascites or diarrhoea from lactulose usage. As total body water decreases, intra- and extracellular fluid equilibrates slowly, causing previous therapeutic drug levels to become toxic. A coordinated approach involving the psychiatrist, hepatologist and other medical carers is absolutely essential.

Adverse hepatic reactions

As the liver plays a central role in the biotransformation of most drugs, hepatotoxicity is a potential complication of many medications. Idiosyncratic adverse hepatic reactions by their very nature are not predictable from the pharmacological effect of the drug and, hence, are not often detected until the medication has been used by large numbers after marketing. Although these are rare events, with a frequency varying from 1 in 1000 (e.g. chlorpromazine) to 1 in 10 000 users (e.g. tricyclic antidepressants), they can have serious consequences, including acute liver failure and death. Therefore, clinicians should be aware of the potential hepatotoxicity, be able to recognise the adverse effects and be ready to withdraw medication promptly to prevent serious outcomes (see Table 17.9).[73]

Clinically and pathologically, drug-induced liver injury mimics a wide variety of hepatobiliary diseases, and hence is prone to be missed or incorrectly diagnosed; this may be due to the difficulty of proving causality in the absence of a definitive test, the apparent lack of a temporal relationship of drug intake with clinical manifestation of disease, or an alternative explanation for the clinical syndrome.[74] When the diagnosis is not certain, early involvement of hepatologists is important, as prompt withdrawal of the causative agent is the critical step in management.

When to refer to a gastroenterologist or hepatologist

Refer urgently for hospital admission any patient with:

- jaundice
- clinical signs of chronic liver disease

Table 17.9 Examples of idiosyncratic hepatotoxicity secondary to medications used in neuropsychiatric conditions

Hepatocellular pattern	Cholestatic pattern	Mixed pattern
Fluoxetine Paroxetine Sertraline Risperidone Valproic acid Bupropion Trazodone Nefazodone	Chlorpromazine Haloperidol Mirtazapine	Tricyclic antidepressants (amitriptyline, imipramine, desipramine) Carbamazepine Phenobarbital Trazodone Phenytoin

- suspected hepatic encephalopathy
- suspected focal lesion within the liver
- alanine transaminase levels over five times the upper limit of normal.

Refer to the hepatology out-patient department any patient with:

- persistent unexplained elevation of liver biochemistry results
- raised bilirubin levels in association with raised liver enzyme levels (an isolated rise in bilirubin levels is almost always Gilbert's disease, which is benign)
- evidence of a dilated biliary system on imaging.

Note that an isolated rise in gamma-glutamyl transpeptidase (GGT) may be due to:

- alcohol abuse
- fatty liver or non-alcoholic steatohepatosis (NASH) if associated with risk factors such as diabetes mellitus, dyslipidaemia and obesity
- enzyme-inducing drugs such as phenytoin, carbamazepine and barbiturates.

An isolated rise in AST is uncommon in liver disease and is usually of skeletal or cardiac origin. Check skeletal muscle and cardiac enzymes and refer to a liver specialist only if no other cause is found.

An isolated rise in alkaline phosphatase is not usually due to liver disease, but more likely of bone origin, either Paget's disease or malignancy.

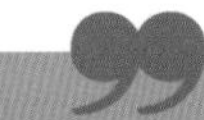

Summary

Within the National Health Service, liver disease does not have the same high profile as, for example, vascular disease. This is likely to change, for two reasons. First, the number of alcohol-precipitated admissions to hospital increases yearly, so chronic liver disease and alcohol-related dementia may become more prevalent. Second, intravenous drug dependency exposes individuals to hepatitis C infection, and such individuals may not readily seek medical help when symptoms of liver disease become apparent. Mental health specialists need to be aware of the potential harm that psychotropic medication can pose, not only because these medications can cause liver disease but also because liver disease can alter the pharmacokinetics of many commonly prescribed medications, leading to unpredictable changes in drug absorption and metabolism.

References

1 Ghany M, Hoofingale JH. Approach to the patient with liver disease. In *Harrison's Principles of Internal Medicine* (16th edn) (ed DL Kasper *et al*): 1808–13. McGraw-Hill, 2005.

2 Kew MC. Serum aminotransferase concentration as evidence of hepatocellular damage. *Lancet* 2000; **355**: 591–2.

3 Cohen JA, Kaplan MM. The SGOT/SGPT ratio – an indicator of alcoholic liver disease. *Dig Dis Sci* 1979; **24**: 835–8.

4 Perrillo RP, Griffin R, De Schryver-Kecskemeti K, *et al*. Alcoholic liver disease presenting with marked elevation of serum alkaline phosphatase. A combined clinical and pathological study. *Am J Dig Dis* 1978; **23**: 1061–6.

Learning points

- Incidence of and mortality from cirrhosis has increased in the UK in the past three decades in parallel with increased hospital admissions for alcohol-related conditions.
- Chronic liver diseases remain asymptomatic even in the presence of advanced structural and architectural changes; therefore liver disease should be suspected in those with risk factors.
- Laboratory tests performed routinely as 'liver function tests' do not accurately reflect function of the liver nor can estimate the degree of liver injury especially in chronic liver diseases.
- Hepatic encephalopathy is a potentially reversible neuropsychiatric syndrome ranging from subtle abnormalities only detectable on psychometric testing as in minimal hepatic encephalopathy to altered sensorium associated with either acute or chronic liver failure.
- Abstinence from alcohol is the cornerstone of treatment in all stages of alcoholic liver disease as it is the critical determinant of the prognosis; hence, alcohol liaison services should be routinely involved in the management of these patients.
- Clinically and pathologically, drug-induced liver injury mimics a wide variety of hepatobiliary diseases; therefore, clinicians should be aware of the potential and be prepared to withdraw medication promptly to prevent serious outcomes.

5 Lee WM. Drug-induced hepatotoxicity. *N Engl J Med* 2003; **349**: 474–85.

6 Mammen EF. Coagulation defects in liver disease. *Med Clin North Am* 1994; **78**: 545–54.

7 Denson KW, Reed SV, Haddon ME. Validity of the INR system for patients with liver impairment. *Thromb Haemost* 1995; **73**: 162.

8 Ishak K, Baptista A, Bianchi L, *et al.* Histological grading and staging of chronic hepatitis. *J Hepatol* 1995; **22**: 696–9.

9 Kamath PS, Wiesner RH, Malinchoc M, *et al.* A model to predict survival in patients with end-stage liver disease. *Hepatology* 2001; **33**: 464–70.

10 Neuberger J, Gimson A, Davies M, *et al.* Selection of patients for liver transplantation and allocation of donated livers in the UK. *Gut* 2008; **57**: 252–7.

11 Ferenci P, Lockwood A, Mullen K, *et al.* Hepatic encephalopathy – definition, nomenclature, diagnosis, and quantification: final report of the working party at the 11th World Congresses of Gastroenterology, Vienna, 1998. *Hepatology* 2002; **35**: 716–21.

12 Dhiman RK, Chawla YK. Minimal hepatic encephalopathy. *Indian J Gastroenterol* 2009; **28**: 5–16.

13 Felipo V, Butterworth RF. Neurobiology of ammonia. *Prog Neurobiol* 2002; **67**: 259–79.

14 Hazell AS, Butterworth RF. Hepatic encephalopathy: an update of pathophysiologic mechanisms. *Proc Soc Exp Biol Med* 1999; **222**: 99–112.

15 Jalan R, Shawcross D, Davies N. The molecular pathogenesis of hepatic encephalopathy. *Int J Biochem Cell Biol* 2003; **35**: 1175–81.

16 Jalan R. Pathophysiological basis of therapy of raised intracranial pressure in acute liver failure. *Neurochem Int* 2005; **47**: 78–83.

17 Shawcross DL, Wright G, Olde Damink SW, *et al.* Role of ammonia and inflammation in minimal hepatic encephalopathy. *Metab Brain Dis* 2007; **22**: 125–38.

18 Shawcross DL, Wright GA, Stadlbauer V, *et al.* Ammonia impairs neutrophil phagocytic function in liver disease. *Hepatology* 2008; **48**: 1202–12.

19 Wright G, Jalan R. Ammonia and inflammation in the pathogenesis of hepatic encephalopathy: Pandora's box? *Hepatology* 2007; **46**: 291–4.

20 Conn HO. Animal versus vegetable protein diet in hepatic encephalopathy. *J Intern Med* 1993; **233**: 369–71.

21 Als-Nielsen B, Koretz RL, Kjaergard LL, *et al.* Branched-chain amino acids for hepatic encephalopathy. *Cochrane Database Syst Rev* 2003; CD001939.

22 Morgan MY. Branched chain amino acids in the management of chronic liver disease. Facts and fantasies. *J Hepatol* 1990; **11**: 133–41.

23 Mortensen PB. The effect of oral-administered lactulose on colonic nitrogen metabolism and excretion. *Hepatology* 1992; **16**: 1350–6.

24 Conn HO, Leevy CM, Vlahcevic ZR, *et al.* Comparison of lactulose and neomycin in the treatment of chronic portal-systemic encephalopathy. A double blind controlled trial. *Gastroenterology* 1977; **72**: 573–83.

25 Bass NM, Mullen KD, Sanyal A, *et al.* Rifaximin treatment in hepatic encephalopathy. *N Engl J Med* 2010; **362**: 1071–81.

26 Pomier-Layrargues G, Giguere JF, Lavoie J, *et al.* Flumazenil in cirrhotic patients in hepatic coma: a randomized double-blind placebo-controlled cross-over trial. *Hepatology* 1994; **19**: 32–7.

27 Morgan MY, Blei A, Grungreiff K, *et al.* The treatment of hepatic encephalopathy. *Metab Brain Dis* 2007; **22**: 389–405.

28 Bekheirnia MR, Schrier RW. Pathophysiology of water and sodium retention: edematous states with normal kidney function. *Curr Opin Pharmacol* 2006; **6**: 202–7.

29 Gerbes AL, Gulberg V, Gines P, *et al.* Therapy of hyponatremia in cirrhosis with a vasopressin receptor antagonist: a randomized double-blind multicenter trial. *Gastroenterology* 2003; **124**: 933–9.

30 Schrier RW. Water and sodium retention in edematous disorders: role of vasopressin and aldosterone. *Am J Med* 2006; **119**: S47–53.

31 De LL, Klein L, Udelson JE, *et al.* Hyponatremia in patients with heart failure. *Am J Cardiol* 2005; **96**: 19–23L.

32 Schrier RW, Gross P, Gheorghiade M, *et al.* Tolvaptan, a selective oral vasopressin V2-receptor antagonist, for hyponatremia. *N Engl J Med* 2006; **355**: 2099–112.

33 NHS Information Centre. *Statistics on Alcohol: England 2009*. Department of Health, 2009.

34 Royal College of Physicians. *Alcohol – Can the NHS Afford It?* Royal College of Physicians, 2001.

35 Lieber CS. Alcoholic liver injury: pathogenesis and therapy in 2001. *Pathol Biol (Paris)* 2001; **49**: 738–52.

36 Powell WJ, Jr, Klatskin G. Duration of survival in patients with Laennec's cirrhosis. Influence of alcohol withdrawal, and possible effects of recent changes in general management of the disease. *Am J Med* 1968; **44**: 406–20.

37 Carithers RL, Jr, Herlong HF, Diehl AM, *et al.* Methylprednisolone therapy in patients with severe alcoholic hepatitis. A randomized multicenter trial. *Ann Intern Med* 1989; **110**: 685–90.

38 Maddrey WC, Boitnott JK, Bedine MS, *et al.* Corticosteroid therapy of alcoholic hepatitis. *Gastroenterology* 1978; **75**: 193–9.

39 Ramond MJ, Poynard T, Rueff B, *et al.* A randomized trial of prednisolone in patients with severe alcoholic hepatitis. *N Engl J Med* 1992; **326**: 507–12.

40 Akriviadis E, Botla R, Briggs W, *et al.* Pentoxifylline improves short-term survival in severe acute alcoholic hepatitis: a double-blind, placebo-controlled trial. *Gastroenterology* 2000; **119**: 1637–48.

41 Strieter RM, Remick DG, Ward PA, *et al.* Cellular and molecular regulation of tumor necrosis factor-alpha production by pentoxifylline. *Biochem Biophys Res Commun* 1988; **155**: 1230–6.

42 Sullivan JT, Sykora K, Schneiderman J, *et al.* Assessment of alcohol withdrawal: the revised clinical institute withdrawal assessment for alcohol scale (CIWA-Ar). *Br J Addict* 1989; **84**: 1353–7.

43 Mayo-Smith MF. Pharmacological management of alcohol withdrawal. A meta-analysis and evidence-based practice guideline. American Society of Addiction Medicine Working Group on Pharmacological Management of Alcohol Withdrawal. *JAMA* 1997; **278**: 144–51.

44 Torvik A, Lindboe CF, Rogde S. Brain lesions in alcoholics. A neuropathological study with clinical correlations. *J Neurol Sci* 1982; **56**: 233–48.

45 Blansjaar BA, Vielvoye GJ, Van Dijk JG, *et al.* Similar brain lesions in alcoholics and Korsakoff patients: MRI, psychometric and clinical findings. *Clin Neurol Neurosurg* 1992; **94**: 197–203.

46 Cook CC, Hallwood PM, Thomson AD. B vitamin deficiency and neuropsychiatric syndromes in alcohol misuse. *Alcohol Alcohol* 1998; **33**: 317–36.

47 Pierucci-Lagha A, Derouesne C. Alcoholism and aging. 2. Alcoholic dementia or alcoholic cognitive impairment? [In French.] *Psychol Neuropsychiatr Vieil* 2003; **1**: 237–49.

48 Gupta S, Warner J. Alcohol-related dementia: a 21st-century silent epidemic? *Br J Psychiatry* 2008; **193**: 351–3.

49 Ritchie K, Villebrun D. Epidemiology of alcohol-related dementia. *Handb Clin Neurol* 2008; **89**: 845–50.

50 Oslin DW, Cary MS. Alcohol-related dementia: validation of diagnostic criteria. *Am J Geriatr Psychiatry* 2003; **11**: 441–7.

51 Davis GL, Albright JE, Cook SF, *et al.* Projecting future complications of chronic hepatitis C in the United States. *Liver Transpl* 2003; **9**: 331–8.

52 Wasley A, Alter MJ. Epidemiology of hepatitis C: geographic differences and temporal trends. *Semin Liver Dis* 2000; **20**: 1–16.

53 Liang TJ, Rehermann B, Seeff LB, *et al.* Pathogenesis, natural history, treatment, and prevention of hepatitis C. *Ann Intern Med* 2000; **132**: 296–305.

54 Takahashi M, Yamada G, Miyamoto R, *et al.* Natural course of chronic hepatitis C. *Am J Gastroenterol* 1993; **88**: 240–3.

55 Sweeting MJ, Hope VD, Hickman M, *et al.* Hepatitis C infection among injecting drug users in England and Wales (1992–2006): there and back again? *Am J Epidemiol* 2009; **170**: 352–60.

56 Fabrizi F, Martin P, Dixit V, *et al.* Quantitative assessment of HCV load in chronic hemodialysis patients: a cross-sectional survey. *Nephron* 1998; **80**: 428–33.

57 Haley RW, Fischer RP. Commercial tattooing as a potentially important source of hepatitis C infection. Clinical epidemiology of 626 consecutive patients unaware of their hepatitis C serologic status. *Medicine (Baltimore)* 2001; **80**: 134–51.

58 Lauer GM, Walker BD. Hepatitis C virus infection. *N Engl J Med* 2001; **345**: 41–52.

59 Dinwiddie SH, Shicker L, Newman T. Prevalence of hepatitis C among psychiatric patients in the public sector. *Am J Psychiatry* 2003; **160**: 172–4.

60 Rosenberg SD, Goodman LA, Osher FC, *et al.* Prevalence of HIV, hepatitis B, and hepatitis C in people with severe mental illness. *Am J Public Health* 2001; **91**: 31–7.

61 El-Serag HB, Kunik M, Richardson P, *et al.* Psychiatric disorders among veterans with hepatitis C infection. *Gastroenterology* 2002; **123**: 476–82.

62 Booth JC, O'Grady J, Neuberger J. Clinical guidelines on the management of hepatitis C. *Gut* 2001; **49** (suppl 1): 11–21.

63 Crone CC, Gabriel GM, DiMartini A. An overview of psychiatric issues in liver disease for the consultation–liaison psychiatrist. *Psychosomatics* 2006; **47**: 188–205.

64 Pond SM, Tozer TN. First-pass elimination. Basic concepts and clinical consequences. *Clin Pharmacokinet* 1984; **9**: 1–25.

65 Howden CW, Birnie GG, Brodie MJ. Drug metabolism in liver disease. *Pharmacol Ther* 1989; **40**: 439–74.

66 Klotz U. Pathophysiological and disease-induced changes in drug distribution volume: pharmacokinetic implications. *Clin Pharmacokinet* 1976; **1**: 204–18.

67 Leipzig RM. Psychopharmacology in patients with hepatic and gastrointestinal disease. *Int J Psychiatry Med* 1990; **20**: 109–39.

68 Blaschke TF. Protein binding and kinetics of drugs in liver diseases. *Clin Pharmacokinet* 1977; **2**: 32–44.

69 Albers I, Hartmann H, Bircher J, *et al.* Superiority of the Child–Pugh classification to quantitative liver function tests for assessing prognosis of liver cirrhosis. *Scand J Gastroenterol* 1989; **24**: 269–76.

70 Schlatter C, Egger SS, Tchambaz L, *et al.* Pharmacokinetic changes of psychotropic drugs in patients with liver disease: implications for dose adaptation. *Drug Saf* 2009; **32**: 561–78.

71 Huet PM, Villeneuve JP. Determinants of drug disposition in patients with cirrhosis. *Hepatology* 1983; **3**: 913–18.

72 Bass NM, Williams RL. Guide to drug dosage in hepatic disease. *Clin Pharmacokinet* 1988; **15**: 396–420.

73 Hussaini SH, Farrington EA. Idiosyncratic drug-induced liver injury: an overview. *Expert Opin Drug Saf* 2007; **6**: 673–84.

74 Chalasani N, Fontana RJ, Bonkovsky HL, *et al.* Causes, clinical features, and outcomes from a prospective study of drug-induced liver injury in the United States. *Gastroenterology* 2008; **135**: 1924–34.

18

Blood-borne viruses

Yusri Taha and Will Irving

Infection with blood-borne viruses can have potentially serious consequences both for patients and for the staff caring for them. This chapter presents information about infection with hepatitis B, hepatitis C and the human immunodeficiency virus (HIV): the methods of transmission of these viruses, treatment and disease prevention.

What are blood-borne viruses?

Many viruses may be found within the bloodstream of an infected host. The term 'blood-borne viruses' (BBV) refers specifically to those viruses whose natural history involves the presence of mature and infectious viral particles over prolonged periods in the bloodstream of a host. Many viruses fulfil these criteria but the 'big three' are:

- hepatitis B virus (HBV)
- hepatitis C virus (HCV)
- human immunodeficiency virus (HIV).

Individuals attending psychiatric clinics, or resident in psychiatric wards, may have particular risk factors which increase their chances of being infected with a BBV (e.g. injecting drugs or a history of having done so, sexual promiscuity, body piercing, tattooing). This chapter covers the salient features of BBV infections, including consideration of risks to healthcare staff looking after patients infected with a BBV. Although HBV, HCV and HIV are all blood-borne, there are many differences between them, including basic virology, routes of spread, approaches to diagnosis, consequences of infection, treatment options and prevention strategies.

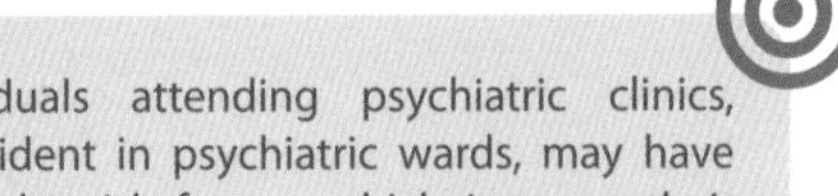

Individuals attending psychiatric clinics, or resident in psychiatric wards, may have particular risk factors which increase their chances of being infected with a blood-borne virus. These include injecting drugs (or history of having done so), sexual promiscuity, body piercing and tattooing.

Hepatitis B

Basic virology

Replication of HBV requires a reverse transcription step in which RNA is copied. Reverse transcriptase inhibitor (RTI) drugs, many of which were developed against HIV infection, can be used to treat HBV infection.

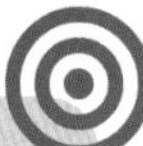

In relation to HBV, the UK is a low-prevalence country, with a carriage rate of 0.1–0.5%. The most important routes of transmission of HBV infection in the UK are through injecting drug use and sexual contact.

Epidemiology and routes of spread

The prevalence of chronic HBV infection varies considerably between countries, from over 10% in China to < 1% in northern Europe. This reflects differences in the predominant routes of transmission. The spread of HBV is through:

- vertical transmission – mother-to-baby transmission
- horizontal transmission – for example inapparent transmission between children through exposure to blood via cuts, abrasions
- sexual transmission
- other parenteral exposure.

On a global scale, vertical and horizontal transmission are by far the most important; in countries where these predominate, very high HBV carriage rates (over 10%) result. The UK is a low-prevalence country, with a carriage rate of 0.1–0.5%, and the most important routes of transmission of HBV infection are through injecting drug use and sexual contact.

'Other parenteral exposure' encompasses a wide range of possible risk behaviours, including being a recipient of a blood or blood product transfusion, sharing of contaminated needles and syringes for recreational drug use, use of contaminated needles in tattooing or body-piercing parlours and acupuncture clinics, needle-stick exposure of healthcare workers, sharing of contaminated razors or toothbrushes, and reuse of inappropriately sterilised needles for medical purposes.

A working knowledge of the routes of HBV spread allows identification of population subgroups who might be at increased risk of HBV infection (Box 18.1).

Box 18.1 Assessments of patients who may have hepatitis B

History

- Country of origin (is it high-, medium- or low-prevalence for HBV?)
- Injecting drug use (past or present)
- Blood or blood product transfusion (especially if abroad)
- Men who have sex with men
- Sexual promiscuity
- Family history of chronic liver disease or hepatocellular carcinoma
- Sexual partner/household contact of patient with acute or chronic hepatitis
- Occupational exposure to blood/body fluids (healthcare, morticians, embalmers, police and emergency services)

Examination

- Signs of venous damage resulting from needle access
- Tattoos (especially if 'do it yourself')
- Body piercing
- Signs of chronic liver disease/cirrhosis

Investigation

- Send serum for hepatitis B surface antigen testing

Diagnosis

There are several laboratory markers of infection. Viral antigens include:

- hepatitis B core antigen – HBcAg – which forms a protective coat around the viral genome
- hepatitis B surface antigen – HBsAg – the outer protein shell of the virus, which is helpful in diagnosis, as a positive HBsAg indicates acute or chronic HBV infection
- hepatitis B e antigen – HBeAg – which is a surrogate marker of virus replication.

Immunocompetent hosts should therefore generate anti-HBc, anti-HBs and anti-HBe antibodies in response to infection. In addition, there are now sensitive assays for quantifying the viral load (HBV DNA).

Acute and chronic infection and infectivity can be determined for any individual:

- if HBsAg and immunoglobulin M (IgM) anti-HBc are positive, the infection is acute
- HBeAg is a marker of intense viral replication, so positivity correlates with very high HBV DNA levels and a high degree of infectivity
- Anti-HBe positive carriers have much reduced levels of HBV DNA and so are much less infectious.

The presence of hepatitis B surface antigen, HBsAg, in the blood is the hallmark of hepatitis B virus infection.

These, though, are generalisations and it is always best to seek advice from a local microbiology department.

The significance of the various diagnostic markers for HBV infection is summarised in Table 18.1.

Patients with chronic HBV infection are at potential risk of developing serious liver disease. Only 1% of acute infections cause sufficient damage to the liver to result in liver failure, but the mortality rate is then 70%.

Consequences of infection

The possible outcomes of HBV infection are illustrated in Fig. 18.1 and have been reviewed by Liaw & Chu.[1]

In adults, about half of acute infections are asymptomatic. Acute icteric hepatitis B is clinically indistinguishable from many other forms of acute icteric hepatitis. About 1% of acute infections cause sufficient damage to the liver to result in liver failure (fulminant hepatitis), with 70% mortality.

About 5–10% of adults with acute HBV infection fail to clear virus from the liver and become chronically infected. They may be asymptomatic or have non-specific symptoms of lethargy and tiredness; they may be unaware of their infected status. Chronic inflammatory hepatitis leads to cirrhosis, with considerably increased risk of developing hepatocellular carcinoma.

The risk of chronicity is age-dependent – around 90% of neonates who acquire infection from their carrier mothers will become chronically infected, while for children under the age of 5, this risk is of the order of 30%.

Help and support are available for patients from the British Liver Trust (www.britishlivertrust.org.uk, email: info@britishlivertrust.org.uk, free helpline: 0800 652 7330).

Treatment options

There is no specific treatment for acute HBV infection.

Chronic HBV infection can be treated with either:

- immunomodulatory drugs – interferon injections for 1 year
- reverse transcriptase inhibitors (lamivudine, entecavir, telbivudine, adefovir, tenofovir), which differ in cost, side-effect profiles, potency, anti-HIV activity, and propensity for inducing resistance mutations.

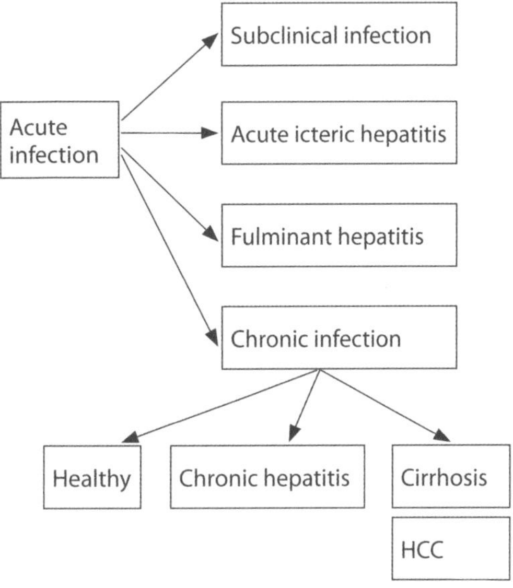

Fig. 18.1 Outcomes of infection with the hepatitis B virus. HCC, hepatocellular carcinoma.

All HBV carriers require specialist assessment and long-term follow-up by a hepatologist, infectious diseases physician or gastroenterologist with an interest in liver disease.

Table 18.1 Diagnostic markers for hepatitis B virus infection

	HBsAg	IgM anti-HBc	IgG anti-HBc	HBeAg	Anti-HBe	Anti-HBs	HBV DNA
Acute HBV infection	+	+	+	+	–	–	+++
Cleared HBV infection	–	–	+	–	+	+	–
Chronic HBV, low risk	+	–	+	–	+	–	±
Chronic HBV, high risk	+	–	+	+	–	–	+++
Responder to HBV vaccine	–	–	–	–	–	+	–

Box 18.2 When to refer patients with hepatitis B

Most cases of chronic HBV infection in the UK are *not* diagnosed. There should be a low threshold for considering testing a psychiatric patient for HBV infection, as many such individuals will have identifiable risk factors for HBV infection.

Ask your laboratory to test a blood sample for hepatitis B surface antigen. *All* HBsAg-positive patients should be referred to an appropriate specialist for further assessment and management, irrespective of their current state of health or liver function tests.

First-line therapy should be either tenofovir or entecavir, as these are high-potency drugs with high genetic barriers to resistance. They suppress virus replication but without leading to viral elimination. A number of detailed guidelines from expert advisory groups are available.[2]

Prevention

Hepatitis B (Fig. 18.2) is spread by chronic carriers of the virus. Those individuals therefore need to be educated as to the precautions they should take to avoid onward transmission, for example by not sharing toothbrushes, razors, appropriate mopping up of blood spills and ensuring vaccination of sexual partners and household contacts.

HBV infection can be prevented by both passive and active immunisation. Passive immunisation is with intramuscular hepatitis B immunoglobulin (HBIg). Active immunisation is with vaccines containing purified HBsAg. Multiple doses are required to achieve satisfactory immune responses. The standard course is three injections at 0, 1 and 6 months, and a booster dose 5 years after the initial course. Protection is directly proportional to the amount of anti-HBs synthesised in response to the vaccine. Around 5–10% of adults fail to respond by generating anti-HBs and so are not protected. Such individuals need to be aware of their non-responder status, so that appropriate passive immunisation can be given should they be exposed to HBV.

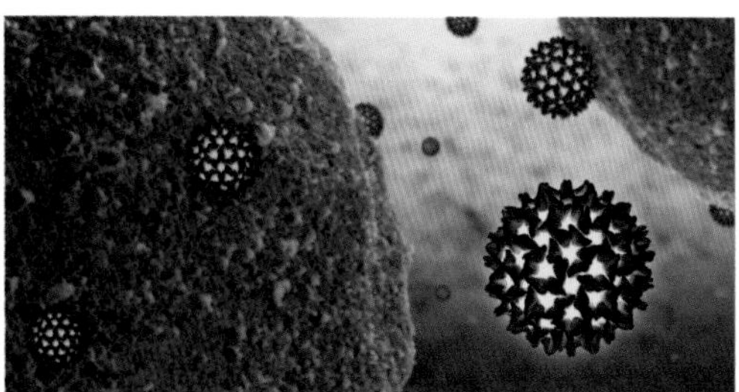

Fig. 18.2 The hepatitis B virus.

> Individuals need to be educated to prevent infecting others – they should avoid sharing a toothbrush or razor, advise sexual partners to be vaccinated, and be careful about cleaning up any blood spills.

The World Health Organization and the European Union recommend that HBV vaccine be offered universally. However, the UK is one of a few countries which persist with a selective vaccination policy, targeting the vaccine at those deemed to be at increased risk of infection, as listed in the Department of Health's 'Green Book', *Immunisation Against Infectious Disease*.[3] Most vaccine in the UK is administered to those occupationally at risk. It is much more difficult to vaccinate those at risk through their lifestyle (e.g. injecting drug users, sex workers, men who have sex with men), and therefore rates of acute HBV infection in the UK have not declined significantly in the past few years. See Box 18.2 for guidance on when to refer to a specialist.

> Individuals who fail to respond to hepatitis B immunisation need to be aware of their status so that passive immunisation can be given if they are exposed to potentially infected material.

Hepatitis C

Basic virology

Hepatitis C virus is an RNA virus and is a distant relative of yellow fever virus. There are many genotypes, requiring different treatments.

Epidemiology and routes of spread

As with HBV, the prevalence of HCV infection varies considerably across different parts of the world. The greatest risk factor for hepatitis C is exposure to contaminated needles or other medical instruments (some countries reuse non-sterilised needles). In contrast to HBV, HCV is not efficiently spread sexually, and mother-to-baby rates of transmission are low. In the UK, infection is driven by recreational drug use, via sharing of contaminated needles and syringes.

The groups at increased risk of HCV infection in the UK are listed in Box 18.3.

Diagnosis

Anti-HCV antibodies in serum are diagnostic. If absent, HCV infection is effectively ruled out unless:

- the exposure/infection occurred within the past 12 weeks, or
- the patient is immunosuppressed and may therefore not generate an effective humoral immune response.

Anti-HCV positivity indicates past infection – the virus may have been cleared or the infection could be chronic. A further test for HCV RNA is therefore essential.

Consequences of infection

Acute HCV infection presents with clinical hepatitis in just 15% of cases but only 25% of acutely infected individuals clear the virus spontaneously, so most become chronically infected. This inflammatory hepatitis results in cirrhosis and an increased risk of hepatocellular carcinoma.

The symptoms in chronic HCV infection are non-specific, such as fatigue and difficulty concentrating; most patients are asymptomatic until end-stage liver disease becomes apparent. The risk of serious liver disease is greater in men, those infected at an older age, and those who drink alcohol, which acts synergistically with HCV in inducing liver damage.

Patients with chronic HCV infection need long-term monitoring and follow-up by a specialist in hepatology, gastroenterology or infectious diseases. Liver biopsy remains the gold standard for the assessment of disease severity.

HCV RNA test result:

- Anti-HCV positive, HCV RNA *negative* = infection is cleared, so not infectious and not at risk of chronic liver disease.
- Anti-HCV positive, HCV RNA *positive* = currently infected, so infectious and at risk of (and may already have) serious liver disease. ARRANGE SPECIALIST REFERRAL.

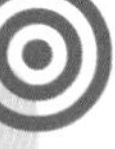

Family and household members, and sexual partners, of a patient with HCV infection are at much lower risk of acquiring infection than is the case with HBV.

Box 18.3 Assessments of patients who may have hepatitis C

History

- Injecting drug use (past or present)
- Country of origin (high risk = Egypt, Pakistan, Eastern Europe, Mediterranean)
- Blood or blood product transfusion (especially if abroad)
- Family history of chronic liver disease/hepatocellular carcinoma
- Sexual partner/household contact of patient with hepatitis
- Occupational exposure to blood/body fluids (healthcare, morticians, embalmers, police and emergency services)

Examination

- Signs of venous damage resulting from needle access
- Tattoos (especially if 'do it yourself')
- Body piercing
- Signs of chronic liver disease/cirrhosis

Investigation

- Send serum for anti-HCV testing (any positive samples should be automatically tested for HCV RNA)

Help and support are available for patients from the Hepatitis C Trust (www.hepctrust.org.uk, email: admin@hepctrust.org.uk, free helpline: 0845 223 4424).

Treatment options

Treatment regimens vary according to genotype but the National Institute for Health and Clinical Excellence (NICE) recommends[4] 6–12 months of:

- a combination of pegylated interferon once weekly via subcutaneous injection and
- ribavirin orally.

Both are associated with significant side-effects: with interferon, flu-like symptoms, fatigue, depression,

Full psychiatric assessment, treatment and support may be necessary before therapy is given for HCV infection, as psychiatric comorbidity is an important potential contraindication to the use of pegylated interferon.

Box 18.4 When to refer patients with hepatitis C

Many cases of chronic HCV infection in the UK are *not* diagnosed. There should be a low threshold for considering testing a psychiatric patient for HCV infection, as many such individuals will have identifiable risk factors for HCV infection.

Ask your laboratory to test a blood sample for antibodies to HCV. *All* patients with chronic HCV infection should be referred to an appropriate specialist for further assessment and management, irrespective of their current state of health or liver function tests.

Alcohol is a potent co-factor for progression of HCV-related liver disease. HCV-infected patients should therefore be given harm-reduction advice, including limitation of alcohol intake.

bone marrow suppression and induction of autoimmune diseases; with ribavirin, haemolytic anaemia. New directly acting antiviral agents acting against HCV have recently (2012) been licensed and approved for use in the UK. Information on when to refer to a specialist is outlined in Box 18.4.

Prevention

Standard infection control procedures such as screening of blood, organ and tissue donors, and provision of adequate supplies of clean needles and syringes, both for medicinal and for recreational drug use, are the mainstays of prevention of HCV transmission. There is no form of passive or active protection.

Human immunodeficiency virus (HIV)

Major advances in HIV diagnostics and the introduction of new and novel classes of drugs active against this virus have helped to transform HIV in high-income countries from a deadly infection into a treatable chronic condition, with long-term management goals centred on quality of life and monitoring for metabolic disturbances related to treatment.

Basic virology

The HIV-1 and HIV-2 viruses cause the acquired immunodeficiency syndrome (AIDS). HIV predominantly infects CD4+ T-lymphocytes but macrophages are infected as well. Understanding the viral replication cycle has allowed for the design and development of specific anti-HIV drugs.

Epidemiology and routes of spread

Over 33 milllion people live with HIV but this is increasing, as new HIV infections continue to occur in numbers that exceed the number of deaths due to AIDS (2.6 million *v.* 1.8 million, respectively, in 2009). Anti-HIV therapy has extended the lives of those infected. About 68% of all HIV-infected people reside in sub-Saharan Africa, where heterosexual transmission is responsible for the vast majority of cases. Elsewhere, HIV disproportionately affects men who have sex with men (MSM), intravenous injecting drug users (IVDUs) and sex workers.

In North America and Europe, MSM remain the most important risk group for HIV, while IVDUs are less commonly affected, particularly in Europe.[5] Young people (aged 15–24) account for approximately 45% of new HIV infections worldwide.

Diagnosis

Infection with HIV is now a treatable condition and most people living with it remain fit and well on treatment. Diagnosing HIV infection late in the disease significantly increases morbidity and mortality risk, so healthcare professionals should dispel myths about testing and encourage testing by patients with appropriate risk factors (Box 18.5). The HIV test remains confidential and optional within any healthcare setting.

Infection with HIV is diagnosed by demonstrating anti-HIV antibodies in the blood. A negative test

HIV infection has been transformed from a deadly infection into a treatable chronic condition by an understanding of the virus and advances in treatment.

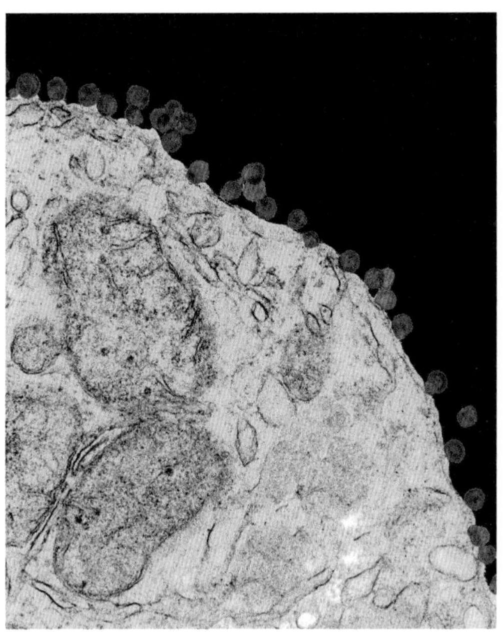

Fig. 18.3 HIV particles budding from a lymphocyte.

Box 18.5 Testing for HIV infection

All doctors and nurses should be able to obtain informed consent for an HIV test in the same way that they do for other medical investigations.

The test should be offered to all injecting drug users (past and present) and all individuals infected with another blood-borne virus.

Other risk factors include country of origin (high-risk is sub-Saharan Africa), sexual promiscuity, men who have sex with men, and being the sexual partner or child of an HIV-positive individual

Clinical indicator diseases, either non-specific or *AIDS-defining* (see Table 18.2), should trigger a test for HIV infection.

For HIV-negative injecting drug users, the test should be repeated annually or whenever symptoms suggestive of seroconversion illness develop.

generally excludes HIV infection, unless the exposure was within the preceding 12 weeks. In the 'window period' between exposure to the virus and a positive anti-HIV test, the HIV viral load is high and the patient is likely to be very infectious. Demonstrating HIV p24 antigen may help to detect infection earlier during this period. The standard diagnostic test is an HIV p24/antibody combined test.

A simple point-of-care test (POCT), similar to a pregnancy test, is now available, which allows patients to receive results of their tests within 15–30 minutes of blood sample collection.

Consequences of infection

Many patients become symptomatic within 10–30 days of initial exposure to the virus, and present with a glandular fever-like illness with high temperature, maculopapular rash, sore throat, headache and cervical lymphadenopathy. Without a high index of suspicion, this illness may be diagnosed as a non-specific viral infection when in reality it is an acute HIV syndrome when seroconversion is occurring.

Patients then enter a largely asymptomatic chronic phase of the infection (clinical latency) that may last as long as 10 years, during which the virus continues to replicate (Fig. 18.3), being detectable at a relatively stable level within the patient's blood. HIV infection causes inexorable damage to the immune system in an untreated patient, as evidenced by a continuous decline in CD4+ T-lymphocytes in peripheral blood. Patients may then present with non-specific symptoms and signs, such as fever, weight loss, night sweats, lymphadenopathy and evidence of declining immune function, such as reactivation of latent herpes virus infections and oral candidiasis. Ultimately, the immune system damage is so overwhelming that the patient's condition is defined as AIDS. There are over 20 AIDS-defining illnesses, including opportunistic infections, malignancies and neurological diseases (Table 18.2). The HIV disease stages over time are depicted in relation to CD4+ T-lymphocyte cell count and HIV RNA load in Fig. 18.4.

Treatment options

In an asymptomatic patient with no clinical or laboratory signs of actual or impending immunodeficiency, close monitoring (of HIV viral load and CD4+ T-cell count) with no specific treatment is adequate. The decision to initiate anti-HIV therapy is dependent on a number of factors, most importantly viral load, CD4 count, and presentation with relevant symptoms and signs. Specific anti-HIV treatment is then offered in the form of combination therapy of at least three drugs. Response is

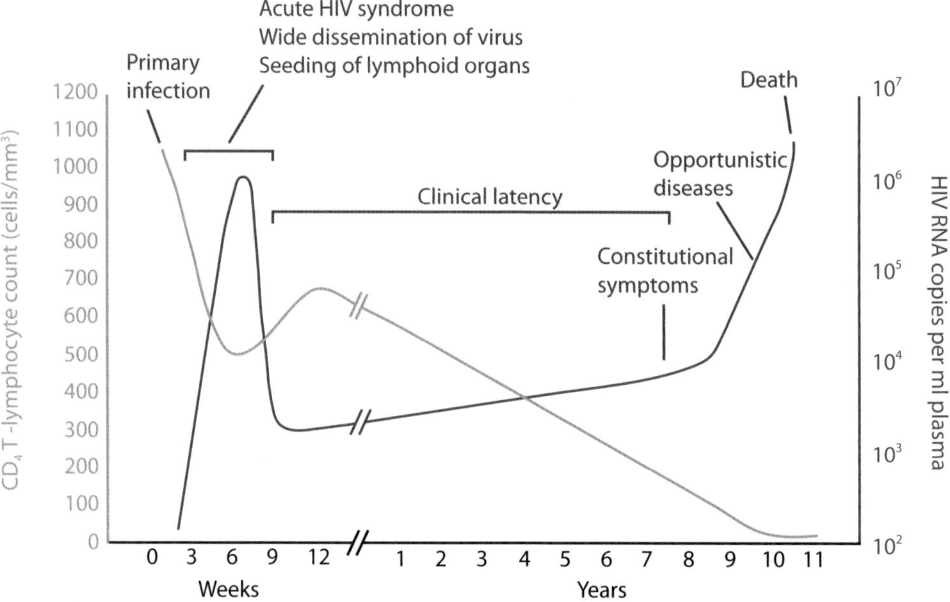

Fig. 18.4 Natural history of HIV infection, from primary infection to development of AIDS. Source: Pantaleo *et al*, 1993 (Fig. 1).[6] Reproduced with permission.

monitored by serial measurements of the HIV RNA viral load. Prophylaxis against and treatment for HIV-related opportunistic infections, particularly *Pneumocystis jiroveci*, are required in at-risk and symptomatic patients, respectively.

Antiretroviral therapy aims to halt immunological damage or possibly reverse it and so avert the associated risks of opportunistic infections and other morbidities, prolonging survival.

Drug toxicity, drug–drug interactions, treatment failure and drug resistance remain significant problems. Key questions in relation to therapy are briefly discussed below.

When to initiate antiretroviral therapy?

Immediate treatment is universally recommended in:

- all symptomatic HIV-infected or AIDS patients
- individuals with a CD4+ cell count of less than 350 cells/mm^3
- coinfection with hepatitis B or hepatitis C viruses, particularly if the CD4+ cell count falls below 500 cells/mm^3.

Special considerations pertain when decisions on initiation of treatment are made in patients with comorbidities such as cardiovascular, renal and psychiatric diseases. The British HIV Association (BHIVA) issues and regularly updates treatment guidelines.[7]

What antiretroviral therapy?

Combination triple therapy is offered as first-line treatment to inhibit specific steps in the virus cycle (Table 18.3).

From where to deliver antiretroviral therapy?

Management is best done by a multidisciplinary team comprising an HIV physician, a pharmacist and specialists in the fields of psychology and Social Services. Close laboratory monitoring of viral load and CD4+ cell count is essential, although access to such tests may not be easily available in resource-limited settings.

How to ensure adherence to therapy?

Treatment, once initiated, will be lifelong. Non-adherence is the single most important risk factor for the development of resistance against anti-HIV medications. Specific assessment with regard to depression, substance misuse and lack of motivation of patients to commence therapy should be undertaken at the outset. Addressing these issues prior to the start of treatment greatly

Table 18.2 Clinical indicator conditions for HIV infection in adults

Clinical area	AIDS-defining conditions	Other conditions that warrant HIV testing
Respiratory	Tuberculosis	Bacterial pneumonia
	Pneumocystis jiroveci infection	Aspergillosis
Neurology	Cerebral toxoplasmosis	Aseptic meningitis/encephalitis
	Primary cerebral lymphoma	Space-occupying lesion of unknown cause
	Cryptococcal meningitis	Guillain–Barré syndrome
	Progressive multifocal leukoencephalopathy	Transverse myelitis
		Peripheral neuropathy
		Dementia
Dermatology	Kaposi's sarcoma	Severe or recalcitrant seborrhoeic dermatitis
		Severe or recalcitrant psoriasis
		Multidermatomal or recurrent herpes zoster
Gastroenterology	Persistent cryptosporidiosis	Oral candidiasis
		Oral hairy leukoplakia
		Chronic diarrhoea of unknown cause
		Weight loss of unknown cause
		Hepatitis B or C infection
Oncology	Non-Hodgkin's lymphoma	Anal cancer or anal intraepithelial dysplasia
		Lung cancer
		Seminoma
		Head and neck cancer
		Hodgkin's lymphoma
Gynaecology	Cervical cancer	Vaginal intraepithelial neoplasia
		Cervical intraepithelial neoplasia, grade 2 or above
Haematology		Any unexplained blood dyscrasia, including: thrombocytopenia, neutropenia, lymphopenia
Ophthalmology	Cytomegalovirus retinitis	Infective retinal diseases, including herpes virus and toxoplasma
Otolaryngology		Lymphadenopathy of unknown cause
		Chronic parotitis
Other		Mononucleosis-like syndrome
		Pyrexia of unknown origin
		Any sexually transmitted infection

Adapted from UK national guidelines for HIV testing.[8]

enhances the chances of success. Chronic depression may adversely affect outcome,[9] lower CD4+ cell count over time,[10] and increase rates of non-adherence and alcohol misuse.[11]

Specific issues that have been shown to adversely affect adherence to treatment among substance misusers include instability of lifestyle, lack of social support, clinician discomfort with treating illicit drug users and medical complications related to addiction. Adherence, viral load suppression and CD4+ T-cell count recovery are significantly worse in illicit drug users than in former and non-users.[12]

Table 18.3 Antiretroviral drug classes and mechanisms of action

Drug class (abbreviation)	Mechanism of action	Examples
Nucleoside/nucleotide analogue reverse transcriptase inhibitors (NRT1)	Prevent conversion of viral RNA into DNA	Zidovudine, abacavir, tenofovir
Non-nucleoside analogue reverse transcriptase inhibitors (NNRTI)	Prevent conversion of viral RNA into DNA	Efavirenz, nevirapine
Protease inhibitors (PI)	Prevent processing of viral proteins into infectious units	Lopinavir, atazanavir, darunavir
Entry inhibitors (EI)	Prevent entry of virus into cells by blocking virus interaction with cell membrane or receptors	Enfuvirtide, maraviroc
Integrase inhibitors (INI)	Prevents insertion of virus DNA into human genome	Raltegravir

Prevention

Prevention of HIV infection remains the ultimate goal despite the great success in controlling the infection through the use of multiple drug therapy. Established and potential preventive measures include the following:

- *Standard infection control procedures.* These include screening of blood, organ and tissue donors and provision of adequate supplies of clean needles and syringes for both medical and recreational drug use
- *Modification of high-risk behaviour.* Efforts made over 25 years to modify high-risk behaviour and advocate the concept of safe sex, mostly through the use of condoms, have met with variable success.
- *Post-exposure prophylaxis (PEP).* Antiretroviral medications may prevent HIV infection in: people exposed through contaminated needle-stick injuries and splash incidents (see below); those who engage in unprotected sexual intercourse with a discordant HIV-positive partner; and babies born to HIV-infected mothers.
- *Male circumcision.* This offers significant protection for men against HIV infection. Modelling indicates that the population-level impact of this intervention will be greater than the individual-level impact if a large proportion of men become circumcised. This may result in a large and sustained fall in prevalence of HIV in endemic areas.
- *Development of a vaccine against HIV.* This offers the best hope for control and containment of the HIV epidemic but remains an elusive goal.

Mother to child transmission is preventable and is almost completely eliminated by use of combination antiretroviral therapy (cART), Caesarean section when required, and avoidance of breastfeeding. See Box 18.6 for information on when to test and refer patients with HIV infection.

Issues for healthcare providers

Risk to health workers

Patients infected with HBV, HCV, or HIV are not only at risk of serious disease themselves, but also pose an infection risk to those around them. Healthcare workers, or other staff present in wards or residential settings, may be exposed to the blood or body fluids of their patients through a number of scenarios, including needle-stick

Box 18.6 When to test and refer patients with HIV infection

Testing patients for HIV infection is straightforward and should be encouraged. There should be a low threshold for considering testing a psychiatric patient for HIV, as many such individuals will have identifiable risk factors for HIV infection. The standard diagnostic test is the HIV p24/antibody combination test.

All patients with HIV infection should be referred to an appropriate specialist for further assessment and management, irrespective of their current state of health.

Treatment of HIV infection is with a potent combination of anti-retroviral drugs. Treatment is monitored by serial viral load testing. Adherence to therapy is vital.

or splash exposures during medical procedures, patients suffering accidental cuts or trauma, or even purposeful acts on the part of the patient, such as biting. Healthcare workers as a group are therefore recognised as being at increased risk of BBV infection.

The risks of transmission via needle-stick injuries, and the possible post-exposure interventions, are summarised in Table 18.4. What to do immediately after such an incident is outlined in Box 18.7.

HBV exposure

All healthcare workers:

- should be vaccinated against HBV and their anti-HBs response should be measured 6–10 weeks after the third vaccine dose
  - at-risk non-responders should have a second course of vaccination
  - suboptimal responders should have a fourth vaccine dose
  - non-responders should be aware of their status so that they can take appropriate action (i.e. obtain passive immunisation with HBIg) following an exposure incident.

Current guidance on occupational exposure to BBVs is available on the Health and Safety Executive website (www.hse.gov.uk/biosafety/blood-borne-viruses/index.htm). Management of an exposure incident requires an urgent risk assessment to establish whether the exposure has the potential to transmit a BBV, and if so, what action should be taken. The risk assessment should be performed by appropriately trained clinical personnel and will consider the following factors:

- *What is known about the source?* If the BBV status of the source is not already known, then a request should be made of that individual for provision of a blood sample for appropriate testing. This approach should be made by another member of the management team, not the needle-stick recipient. Most source patients will not be infected by a BBV and appropriate reassurance can then be provided to the recipient.
- *Which body fluid was the recipient exposed to?* Blood carries the highest risk, but BBV can be transmitted by other body fluids, especially if they are also contaminated by blood.
- *What was the route of exposure?* Intact skin is impervious to BBV; however, transmission may occur through non-intact skin (e.g. with cuts, abrasions, or chronic dermatitis). Splashing of blood/body fluids onto mucous membranes may result in virus transmission, although the risk is considerably lower than for percutaneous exposure.
- *Other considerations* include the nature of the exposure – directly, or indirectly through a needle or other medical device, whether or not the recipient was wearing any protective equipment, and the HBV immune status of the recipient.

Table 18.4 Risk of transmission of blood-borne viruses from patient to healthcare worker, and intervention

Infection	Transmission rate (patient to healthcare worker)	Intervention
Hepatitis B	Up to 30%[a]	Post-exposure prophylaxis with vaccine and/or HBIg
Hepatitis C	1–3%	Monitor recipient. Early therapy if transmission occurs
HIV	0.3%	Post-exposure prophylaxis with antiretroviral drugs

a. There is a wide variability in infectiousness of hepatitis B carriers. The risk stated is that of transmission following needle-stick exposure in unvaccinated individuals.

Management options

Management options for a significant exposure include:

- administration of passive HBIg to a recipient known to be a vaccine non-responder, or not to have been vaccinated
- active immunisation with hepatitis B vaccine, using an accelerated course, according to the HBV status of the donor and the immune status of the recipient.

HCV exposure

In the absence of any form of either passive or active immunisation for HCV, management of an HCV exposure incident is based on monitoring the recipient for evidence of acquisition of infection with HCV. This involves testing the recipient for HCV RNA at 6 weeks and for anti-HCV and HCV RNA at 12 weeks after the incident. If evidence of infection is detected, the recipient should be referred immediately to an appropriate specialist for consideration of antiviral therapy, as treatment at this early stage of HCV infection is very successful (sustained viral response rates approach 100%).

Box 18.7 What to do after someone has been exposed to a blood-borne virus

Undertake immediate first aid. Where the eyes or mouth have been exposed to blood or body fluids, they should be washed copiously with water. Puncture wounds should be encouraged to bleed, but not scrubbed or sucked, and should be washed with soap and water.

Any mucocutaneous or percutaneous exposure to blood or body fluids should be reported to someone with specialist knowledge and expertise, who can advise on the need for further management. Arrangements will differ in different settings, but possible sources of specialist advice include:

- specialist-led occupational health departments
- virology/microbiology departments
- infectious diseases specialists
- genitourinary medicine specialists
- accident and emergency departments
- local health protection units.

Risk assessment will be by the appropriate expert and will involve consideration of a number of factors (see text). Testing of the source patient, with informed consent, for evidence of infection with a BBV is standard practice.

Management options include reassurance, HBV immunisation, hepatitis B immunoglobulin, post-exposure monitoring for evidence of HCV acquisition and post-exposure prophylaxis for HIV infection.

HIV exposure

If there is a significant risk of HIV transmission, the recipient should be offered post-exposure prophylaxis (PEP), that is, a regimen of three anti-HIV drugs taken for 4 weeks. The UK Chief Medical Officers' Expert Advisory Group on AIDS provides details on schedules recommended for HIV PEP, which should be started as soon as possible after the exposure incident – all hospitals should always have an emergency supply of HIV PEP available.

If there is any doubt about whether PEP is necessary, for example because the HIV status of the source is unknown, it is best to start PEP and then review the need for its continuation later, perhaps when laboratory test results become available.

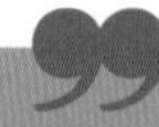

Summary

Blood-borne viruses have important implications not only for those carrying the virus but also for those looking after them. Most professionals, if not all, will be aware that needle-stick injury carries risk of virus transmission, but even simple splash exposure to blood from an infected individual cannot be ignored. Chronic infection with blood-borne viruses has important consequences for affected individuals but staff need to be cognisant of how infectious each patient is, so that appropriate precautions can be taken to protect healthcare workers. Non-specific signs of lethargy and tiredness may suggest chronic infection.

References

1 Liaw Y-F, Chu C-M. Hepatitis B virus infection. *Lancet* 2009; **373**: 582–92.

2 European Association for the Study of the Liver. EASL clinical practice guidelines: management of chronic hepatitis B. *J Hepatol* 2009; **50**: 227–42.

3 Department of Health. Hepatitis B. In *Immunisation Against Infectious Diseases* (ed D Salisbury, M Ramsay, K Noakes): pp. 161–84. TSO (The Stationery Office), 2006.

4 National Institute for Health and Clinical Excellence. *Peginterferon Alfa and Ribavirin for the Treatment of Mild Hepatitis C (Technology appraisals, TA106).* NICE, 2006.

5 UNAIDS. *UNAIDS Report on the Global AIDS Epidemic.* UNAIDS, 2010 (http://www.unaids.org/en/media/unaids/contentassets/documents/unaidspublication/2010/20101123_globalreport_en.pdf).

6 Pantaleo G, Graziosi C, Fauci AS. New concepts in the immunopathogenesis of human immunodeficiency virus infection. *New Engl J Medicine* 1993; **328**: 327–35 (Fig. 1).

7 William I, Churchill D, Anderson J, *et al. British HIV Association Guidelines for the Treatment of HIV-1 Infected Adults with Antiretroviral Therapy.* BHIVA, 2012.

8 Palfreeman A, Fisher M, Ong E, *et al.* Testing for HIV: concise guidance. *Clin Med* 2009; **9**: 471–6.

9 Ickovics JR, Hamburger ME, Vlahov D, *et al.* Mortality, CD4 cell count decline, and depressive symptoms among HIV-seropositive women: longitudinal analysis from the HIV Epidemiology Research Study. *JAMA* 2001; **285**: 1466–74.

10 Ghebremichael M, Paintsil E, Ickovics JR, *et al.* Longitudinal association of alcohol use with HIV disease progression and psychological health of women with HIV. *AIDS Care* 2009; **21**: 834–41.

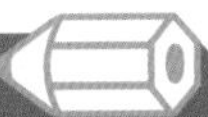

Learning points

- Hepatitis B
  - Testing positive for HBsAg indicates current infection which may be acute or chronic
  - 5–10% of adults infected with hepatitis B become chronic carriers
  - Prevent infection by immunisation with HBsAg vaccine and educate chronic carriers
- Hepatitis C virus
  - Transmission is by 'blood-to-blood' injecting drugs, blood transfusion, needle-stick injury
  - Sexual transmission is inefficient other than in HIV-positive men, who have sex with men
  - 80% infections with hepatitis C are not cleared and are asymptomatic until end-stage liver disease develops
  - Chronic infection leads to chronic hepatitis, cirrhosis and hepatocellular carcinoma
  - No vaccine is available for hepatitis C
- Human immunodeficiency virus (HIV)
  - Transmission is by sexual contact, mother-to-baby and blood exposure
  - Monitor progress by testing for viral load and CD4 counts
  - Clinically may present with HIV seroconversion illness, lasting a few weeks
  - Infection leads to inexorable loss of CD4+ T-cells
  - Infection leads to acquired immunodeficiency syndrome (AIDS)
- Management of HIV-infected individual
  - Dilemmas include when to start treatment and with which drug
  - Treatment is with combination antiretroviral therapy (cART)
  - Adherence to therapy is of utmost importance
  - Resistance arises through mutations in the viral genome
  - No vaccine is available
  - Sexual transmission can be reduced by safe sex practices and male circumcision
  - Mother to child transmission is preventable
- Management of needle-stick exposure to blood-borne viruses
  - Patients should be tested for HBV, HCV, HIV infection
  - Exposure to hepatitis B – depends on vaccine status of recipient, and may vary from nothing through to accelerated course of vaccination and passive immunisation
  - Exposure to hepatitis C – test recipient at 6 weeks for hepatitis C virus RNA, and at 12 weeks for anti-HCV and HCV RNA. If evidence of infection, consider therapy with pegylated interferon alone
  - Exposure to HIV – consider post-exposure prophylaxis, with 4 weeks of triple antiretroviral drugs

11 Yun LW, Maravi M, Kobayashi JS, *et al.* Antidepressant treatment improves adherence to antiretroviral therapy among depressed HIV-infected patients. *J Acquir Immune Defic Syndr* 2005; **38**: 432–8.

12 Lucas GM, Cheever LW, Chaisson RE, *et al.* Detrimental effects of continued illicit drug use on the treatment of HIV-1 infection. *J Acquir Immune Defic Syndr* 2001; **27**: 251–9.

19

Sexual health

Kevan Wylie and David Burton

Sexual health is an important aspect of health that can be easily ignored by mental health professionals. While treatment of sexual disorders may be beyond the remit of most psychiatrists, this chapter describes the interactions between mental disorders, their treatment and sexual function. It also covers key factors about sexually transmitted infections.

Introduction

Good sexual health is important for sexual and general well-being. *Sexual health* means many things to different people. Although in the UK the term is usually used to describe freedom from sexually transmitted infection, a wider definition includes the absence of sexual dysfunction, good sex education and awareness, and the ability to have sexual pleasure within satisfactory relationships (if desired), with ease of access to services where clinicians can advise on matters such as contraception and healthy pregnancy (Chapter 20). While all of this is not necessarily within the remit of a psychiatrist to manage, an awareness of the importance of asking about sexuality and related themes and appropriate signposting may lead to a patient's more satisfactory engagement with any proposed mental health intervention.

The prevalence of sexual dysfunction in the community is difficult to establish, due to problems with sampling and definition. In community epidemiological studies, the prevalence of sexual disorder is estimated to be around 30% of men and over 40% of women.[1,2] Sexual difficulty seems be short-lived however, as the prevalence of disorders persisting for 6 months or longer is substantially less.[3] Comorbidity with mental health disorders is common, as is iatrogenic sexual dysfunction secondary to psychotropic medication.

Sexual dysfunctions

Diagnostic classification

Sexual dysfunctions are described in DSM-IV-TR[4] as being characterised by disturbance in sexual desire and in the psychological and physiological changes that characterise the sexual response. Aetiological factors include organic disease, psychological and psychiatric disturbance, or a combination of these. Common contributory factors to sexual dysfunction include:

- anxiety and depression
- low self-esteem
- disturbed body image
- alcohol and illicit substance misuse
- medication for vascular, neurological and endocrinological disease
- the consequences of surgery
- ageing.

Nine sexual dysfunctions are described in DSM-IV-TR:

- sexual desire disorder or loss of libido
  - hypoactive sexual desire disorder (HSDD) – there is a low interest in sex
  - sexual aversion disorders – there is objection to having the genitalia observed or touched, but this may be situation-specific
- sexual arousal and erectile dysfunction
- orgasmic disorders, including premature ejaculation
- sexual pain disorders
  - vaginismus
  - dyspareunia, or pain during intercourse – this may affect men and women
- other disorders of ejaculation
  - inhibited ejaculation
  - retrograde ejaculation, where the ejaculate passes into the bladder rather than being expelled.

Additionally, the DSM-IV classification covers paraphilias (sexual arousal disorders), but this is controversial as many of these disorders are common within the community and rarely present to clinicians – for example, fetishism, sadomasochism and voyeurism. Some paraphilias are more likely to present to mental health professionals, such as exhibitionism, paedophilia and bestiality.

Management

A comprehensive psychosexual history should be undertaken to obtain a clear description of the extent of the sexual problems or dysfunction. A concurrent medical, surgical, relationship and family history is recommended. Enquiry should be made about iatrogenic factors, including surgery and prescribed medications, as well as major life events such as diagnoses of cancer.

Investigation may involve blood tests to exclude diabetes mellitus, low testosterone levels, dyslipidaemia and raised prolactin levels. Specialist investigations in consultant-led centres are sometimes indicated following primary blood investigations and physical examination; these include assessment of penile rigidity, blood flow and thermal clearance investigations for arousal disorders in men and women, and selective nerve conduction studies for orgasmic disorders in both men and women.

> Drug history should include past and present medication, prescribed or otherwise, and illicit drug use. This should include both enzyme- and non-enzyme-inducing antibiotics.

For the majority of patients, normalisation of an age-related process and reassurance of exclusion of serious underlying disease processes are important. When the patient is in a relationship, it is often prudent to see the patient with the partner, and where appropriate to arrange interventions such as communication training and negotiation skills. Assessment of sexual dysfunction in the partner is also important.

> When the patient is in a relationship, offer to:
>
> - see the patient with the partner
> - assess the partner for sexual dysfunction
> - arrange appropriate interventions, such as communication training and negotiation skills.

Many of the treatment strategies for sexual dysfunction currently involve off-license use of medications, although some conditions do have more licensed treatments; for example, licensed treatments for erectile dysfunction include phosphodiesterase inhibitors such as sildenafil, vardenafil and tadalafil. Dosing regimens vary considerably to suit individual requirements. For males with low testosterone levels, treatment with testosterone therapy is indicated after appropriate investigations.[5] Testosterone is licensed for both surgically menopausal women (as a transdermal patch) and for naturally menopausal women (as an implant). More detailed accounts of treatment options are available elsewhere.[6]

Medication-induced sexual dysfunction

A review of a clinical pharmacological database revealed:[7]

- 736 medications specifically listed as decreasing libido
- 651 that caused erectile dysfunction
- 211 affecting ejaculation
- 57 with effects on orgasmic function.

Psychotropic medications are particularly prone to induce sexual dysfunction (additionally, some dysfunctions feature as part of the primary mental health problem, as with depression or schizophrenia). Antidepressant medications have a marked effect on sexual dysfunction,

Many medications contribute to sexual dysfunction through adverse effects on libido, erectile function, ejaculation and orgasm. Psychotropic medications affect sexual dysfunction in addition to any sexual dysfunction that may occur with the primary mental health problem.

whether they are tricyclics, monoamine oxidase inhibitors (MAOIs) or selective serotonin reuptake inhibitors (SSRIs). Anxiolytics and mood stabilisers (including lithium, carbamazepine and phenytoin) may adversely affect sexual function. It is important to establish the extent of an individual's sexual life and expectations, as the prescription of medication which induces sexual dysfunction may be a major factor in non-compliance in both the short and the medium term.

Several newer atypical medications are less likely to produce sexual dysfunction. Clayton & Balon have reviewed sexual dysfunction within psychiatric illness, its treatment and the need for early identification and incorporation of patient preference for successful management.[8] The SSRIs can have deleterious effects on sexual desire, erectile function and ejaculation. Men using SSRIs may experience discomfort during masturbation.[9]

Individual psychotropic drugs affect sexual function in 25.8–80.3% of patients.[10] In this, they may be ranked worst to least as follows:

- sertraline
- venlafaxine
- citalopram
- paroxetine
- fluoxetine
- imipramine
- phenelzine
- duloxetine
- escitalopram
- fluvoxamine.

A number of reasons for under-reporting of sexual side-effects in patients on antipsychotic mediations have been proposed.[11] They include factors relating to the patient, the health professional, the medication, the mental illness and the environment.

There is no evidence that the antidepressants agomelatine, amineptine, bupropion, moclobemide, mirtazapine and nefazodone adversely affect sexual function.

Sexually transmitted infections

The WHO estimates that, worldwide, over 340 million adults aged 15–49 years are diagnosed with a curable sexually transmitted infection (STI); 17 million are in Western Europe. The incidence of STIs in the UK has been increasing steadily since the mid-1990s, with 397 990 new cases presenting at genitourinary medicine (GUM) clinics in 2007.[12]

Mental disorders such as depression are associated with STIs;[13] this may be attributed to individual risk behaviour.[14] The types of behaviour exhibited include having multiple sex partners and infrequent use of condoms.

The natural sequelae of STI include:

- chronic liver disease
- neurological decompensation
- problems related to reproduction and pregnancy.

Patients with suspected STIs may be embarrassed, distressed or anxious about the consultation. It is important therefore that the clinician be appropriately responsive and respectful in order to convey a sense of privacy and confidentiality. The need for a welcoming environment is paramount in assisting this cause.

History

Identifying the patient's concerns and reason for attendance dictates the direction of the interview. Open and less intrusive starting questions will also help to encourage rapport.

Urogenital symptoms of urethral discharge, vaginal discharge and genital ulceration form the main symptoms of enquiry for a patient with an STI (Box 19.1).

Documentation should include associated abdominal pain, dysuria, dyspareunia, itch, burning, swelling, suspicious odour, urinary frequency, skin rash and eye symptoms. Constitutional symptoms such as fever and vomiting should also be noted.

A detailed approach to the sexual history should include dates of last sexual intercourse, previous partners (regular and casual), previous STIs and use of contraceptive devices (Box 19.2). Hepatitis B and HIV risk assessment is prudent (e.g. previous known exposure,

Box 19.1 Causes of main symptoms of an STI

Urethral discharge
Chlamydia trachomatis
Neisseria gonorrhoeae
Mycoplasma genitalium
Gardnerella vaginalis
Herpes simplex virus
Trichomonas vaginalis
Candida albicans
Papillomavirus

Vaginal discharge
Trichomonas vaginalis
Candida albicans
Gardnerella vaginalis
Herpes simplex virus 1 (HSV1)
Mycoplasma genitalium
Chlamydia trachomatis
Neisseria gonorrhoeae

Genital ulceration
Herpes simplex virus
Treponema pallidum
Haemophilus ducreyi
Klebsiella granulomatis

testing, results, treatments and blood transfusions). Risk assessment is also crucial, not only in identifying those populations at increased exposure, but also in establishing contact tracing.

A full past medical and surgical history assists in identifying associated conditions, which may influence or relate to the presenting condition. A good drug history should include the use of current medication as well as previous therapy, particularly for treated STIs (e.g. use of antibiotics). Current or past drug misuse should be explored and known drug allergies must be noted.

The psychiatric consultation should establish risk factors associated with transmission of STIs. Depressive symptoms are associated with certain HIV risk behaviours (see also below), such as increased number of lifetime sex partners, drug and alcohol misuse and having sex in exchange for money.[14] When symptoms suggest cognitive impairment in patients with HIV, the clinician should screen for depression. Cognitive impairment may lead to poor judgement and unsafe sexual practices.

Box 19.2 Core components of the sexual history

- Symptoms/reason for attendance
- Last sexual intercourse (LSI): date, partner's gender, sites of exposure, condom use
- Previous sexual partner: details as for LSI
- Previous STIs
- For women: last menstrual period (LMP), contraceptive and cytology history
- HIV history
- Hepatitis B and C risk assessment
- Establish mode of giving results
- Establish competency/child protection concerns (if age < 16 years)

Physical examination

Usually in a genitourinary setting, examination of the mouth, throat and skin is warranted in patients presenting with suspected STI. Assessment of the horizontal and vertical group of inguinal lymph nodes forms a crucial part of the physical examination. Closer inspection of external genitalia is necessary to find pubic lice, erythema, swelling, chancres and ulcers. Bimanual palpation should be undertaken to note size, shape and consistency of the uterus and cervix and to elicit adnexal tenderness. See Table 19A (p. 261) for more information on STIs.

Investigations and monitoring

Both the history and examination will guide choice of investigation. For example, asymptomatic heterosexual men require urethral swabs and smear with urine analysis for testing for gonorrhoea and chlamydia. Asymptomatic men who have sex with men (MSM) will require additional rectal and oropharyngeal specimens.[15] Infections may coexist at the time of presentation. Full screening should therefore be considered in symptomatic patients who have come into contact with one STI (Box 19.3).

In deciding upon appropriate pharmacological therapy, the prescriber should be aware of any potential drug interactions (see p. 269, Table 20.3). Additionally, antibiotics have reported psychiatric side-effects.[16] Penicillins can cause symptoms of irritability, anxiety and hallucinations, and cephalosporins may cause

Box 19. 3 Full screening for symptomatic patients with a sexually transmitted infection

Men

- Urethral smear for Gram staining
- Urethral swab for gonococcal culture and chlamydia
- Urine analysis
- Serology for syphilis and HIV (with counselling)
- Rectal and throat swabs for *Gonorrhoea* and *Trichomonas* (if indicated)

Women

- Urethral smear and swab for gonococcal culture placed in Amies medium
- First-pass urine for chlamydia DNA amplification
- Lateral vaginal wall swab for *Candida* and *Trichomonas* culture
- Endocervical smear and swabs for gonococci and chlamydia
- Serology for syphilis and HIV (with counselling)
- Rectal and throat swabs for *Gonorrhoea* and *Trichomonas* (if indicated)
- Cervical cytology

sleep disturbances and hallucinations. Acyclovir in HIV can cause lethargy and psychosis; lower dosing or withdrawal of the responsible drug is advised. Patients may require additional psychotropic medication to control symptoms.

Close collaboration should exist between the psychiatrist, primary care and GUM clinics to coordinate management. Primary care should continue to monitor and recognise those patients who may need referral to the mental health team for further evaluation. Involvement of the psychiatrist, community mental health nurses and social workers may be required where advice and treatment strategies for psychotherapy need to be employed.

Prevention and treatment

Patients with mental health disorders should be counselled on the risks of acquiring and transmitting HIV to a partner and methods to reduce this.[17] Behavioural interventions through counselling on risk reduction are effective in reducing both self-reports of unprotected sex and rates of STIs, and in reducing risk of HIV infection.[18]

Box 19.4 Theories behind preventive models

- *Health belief model.* Perception of risk and anticipation of positive and negative outcomes when demonstrating preventive behaviour
- *Social cognitive theory.* Modelling of behaviours by peers and demonstrating self-efficacy (i.e. controlling one's own behaviour under a variety of circumstances)
- *Theories of reasoned action and planned behaviour.* Attitudes and perceived social norms influence the intention of the individual to perform certain behaviour

Three broad theoretical counselling factors have guided risk-reduction strategies for STIs (Box 19.4). Preventive counselling models all recognise the importance of having achievable goals and reinforcing clients' positive steps in achieving them.[11] One-to-one counselling, with a clear and focused outcome on consistent condom use, for example, can help to change the attitudes and self-efficacy of patients[19] (Box 19.5). Motivational enhancement and behavioural skills training are two of the techniques employed in reducing HIV risk in the psychiatric outpatient setting.[13]

Poorly controlled psychiatric disorders can hinder the success of the treatment of the STI, by impairing the cognition and physical functioning of the individual. Close monitoring of the patient in the community is necessary, as risk behaviour and non-adherence to treatment may disrupt management goals and generate barriers to counselling.[14]

HIV and psychiatric illness

Disproportionate rates of AIDS/HIV are well reported among adults with psychiatric disorders.[20,21] The prevalence is estimated to be as much as eight times higher than that in the general population.[22] Conversely, people with HIV are likely to experience mental health problems and emotional stress, and psychiatric disorders

Antiretroviral drugs, especially the most potent, ritonavir, can have significant interactions with psychopharmacotherapy.

Box 19.5 Principles of HIV/STI prevention counselling

Keep the session focused on HIV/STI risk reduction

- Counselling session should be tailored to the patient and should help to address their personal STI/HIV risk rather than give predetermined information
- Counsellor should not allow session to be distracted by the patient's other problems
- Counselling techniques that may be employed to facilitate focus on risk reduction include open-ended questions, role-play and attentive listening.

Include an in-depth, personalised assessment of risk

- Assist the patient to identify concrete, acceptable measures to reduce personal STI/HIV risk
- Risk assessment should explore prior risk-reduction efforts, identifying patient's success and challenges

Acknowledge and provide support for positive steps patient has already made

- Confirm and encourage belief that change is possible

Clarify critical rather than general misconceptions

- Counsellor should focus on patient's current risk rather than hold a general discussion of the mode of transmission in STI/HIV

Negotiate concrete, achievable behaviour change to reduce STI/HIV risk

- Steps should be acceptable to the patient
- Counsellor should assist in helping the patient achieve steps which pose the most critical risk which the patient wishes to change
- The steps should be small, explicit and achievable, not global
- The counsellor and patient should identify barriers to and support for the achievement of the steps
- Patients with ongoing risk behaviour may benefit from additional support

Seek flexibility in the prevention approach and counselling process

- Counsellor should avoid a generic prevention message (e.g. 'always use condoms')
- The length of the counselling session may vary, depending on client risk and profile

Provide skill-building opportunities

- Counsellor can demonstrate or ask the patient to demonstrate problem-solving activities through role-play (e.g. use of male latex condoms)

Use explicit language when providing test results

- Avoid an in-depth technical discussion, which may diffuse the importance of the prevention message

Ensure patient returns to same counsellor

- A consistent patient–counsellor relationship helps the patient feel secure and increases the likelihood of effective risk reduction

Use a written protocol to help the counsellor conduct an effective session

- A structured protocol will help to keep the counsellor and supervisor on the subject of risk reduction
- The protocol can include examples of open-ended questions and lists of explicit risk-reduction steps

Ensure ongoing support by supervisors and administrators

- Provide training opportunities
- Include staff appraisals and evaluations

Avoid using counselling sessions for data collection

- If possible, paperwork should be completed by the end of the counselling session
- Avoid checklist risk assessments driven by data collection

Avoid the provision of unnecessary information

- Providing too much information/discussion of theoretical risks can detract from prevention and may cause the patient to lose interest.

Adapted from: Rietmeijer, 2007.[24]

Poorly controlled Axis I and Axis II psychiatric disorders can hinder the successful treatment of STIs, by impairing cognition and the physical functioning of the individual.

are highly prevalent in HIV-affected individuals.[23] The psychiatric disorders present in patients with HIV may be the result of contracting the infection or caused by side-effects of treatment.

Antiviral drugs in the form of highly active anti-retroviral therapy (HAART) are an effective method of suppressing HIV and form the mainstay of treatment. Both the presence of and treatment for HIV infection can lead to psychological decompensation of new and pre-existing neuropsychiatric disorders. Psychiatric conditions that can result (as a side-effect) from HIV treatments include depression, insomnia, sleep disturbance and mania (Table 19.1).[16,25] Treatment of mental health problems in patients with HIV is further complicated by the drug interactions of psychotropic medication with HAART (Table 19.2). Most of the medications employed for use in psychiatry are metabolised by enzymes in the cytochrome P450 pathway. Antiretroviral drugs, most notably the protease inhibitors, also act via the enzymes of this pathway, causing significant changes in drug levels. Of the protease inhibitors used in HAART therapy, ritonavir is the most potent, with the greatest reported number of drug interactions with psychopharmacotherapy.[26]

Antidepressants are the psychotropic drugs most frequently prescribed for HIV patients.[23] The choice of antidepressant will depend on the drug's side-effect profile and drug interactions:

- Use of tricyclic antidepressants is limited owing to their anticholinergic adverse effects and interactions with protease inhibitors, leading to increased risk of toxicity.
- Fluoxetine has been shown to be the most effective of the SSRIs in the treatment of major depression in HIV patients.[27]
- Increased plasma levels of fluoxetine have been reported with concurrent use of ritonavir. Close monitoring of patients and a low starting dose are therefore advised.[28]
- The newer-generation antidepressants serotonin and serotonin–noradrenaline reuptake inhibitors (SNRIs) offer an alternative treatment for depression. Venlafaxine has been reported to reduce the plasma

Table 19.1 Psychiatric side-effects of common antiretroviral therapies

Agent	Psychiatric side-effects
Nucleoside reverse transcriptase inhibitors (NRTIs)	
Abacavir	None reported
Didanosine	Insomnia, mood change, nervousness, confusion, seizures, peripheral neuropathy
Emtricitabine	None reported
Lamivudine	Insomnia, mood disorders
Stavudine	Abnormal dreams, drowsiness, depression, anxiety, cognitive dysfunction, mania
Tenofovir	None reported
Zalcitabine	Mood changes, convulsions, sleep disturbances
Zidovudine	Convulsions, dizziness, drowsiness, depression, anxiety, insomnia, loss of mental acuity, unusually vivid dreams, confusion
Non-nucleoside reverse transcriptase inhibitors (NNRTIs)	
Efavirenz	Anxiety, depression, sleep disturbances, impaired concentration, abnormal dreams headaches, dizziness; *less commonly* psychosis, mania, suicidal ideation, amnesia, convulsions
Nevirapine	None reported
Protease inhibitors	
Amprenavir	Sleep disturbances, fatigue, dizziness
Indinavir	Sleep disturbances, fatigue, dizziness
Lopinavir with rotonavir	Confusion, depression, anxiety, agitation, amnesia, abnormal dreams
Nelfinavir	None reported
Ritonavir	Anxiety, drowsiness
Saquinavir	Mood changes

Patients with pre-existing bipolar disorder tend to present either: early (primary mania), with the traditional symptoms; or late (secondary mania), at the onset of AIDS, with marked cognitive impairment, dementia and pronounced irritable mood (as opposed to elation).

Table 19.2 Drug interactions of pharmacological treatments used in the HIV patient (psychotropics with antiretroviral agents)

Psychotropic	Interactions with antiretroviral agents	Recommendations
Antidepressants		
Tricyclics	Imipramine effective. Side-effect profile increased by amprenavir and ritonavir	Reserved for patients who do not respond to SSRI due to side-effect profile of tricyclic
Selective serotonin reuptake inhibitors (SSRIs)	Plasma concentration of SSRI raised by ritonavir Plasma concentration of sertraline reduced by efavirenz Protease inhibitor/non-nucleoside reverse transcriptase inhibitor (NNRTI) may affect activity of CYP450	Low initial dose of SSRI, slow titration, close monitoring for toxic reaction (reported cases of serotonin syndrome)
Serotonin–noradrenaline reuptake inhibitors (SNRIs)	Reported lower plasma concentration of indinavir	No reported ill effects
Antipsychotics		
Olanzapine	Decreased plasma concentration with ritonavir through enhanced activity of liver enzyme CYP1A2	Increase starting dose
Clozapine	Increased plasma concentration in concurrent use with amprenavir and ritonavir	Lower starting dose and slower titration. Close monitoring for toxic effects Note risk of developing dyslipidaemia and hyperglycaemia Avoid concomitant use with ritonavir due to increased risk of toxicity and agranulocytosis
Pimozide	Increased plasma concentration in concurrent use with ritonavir, saquinavir, nelfinavir, lopinavir, indinavir	Avoid concomitant use with protease inhibitors and efavirenz due to increased risk of ventricular arrhythmias
Aripiprazole	Decreased plasma concentration with efavirenz Metabolism inhibited by protease inhibitors	Increase dose of aripiprazole Decrease dose of aripiprazole
Risperidone	Increased serum levels due to inhibition of metabolism by ritonavir	Consideration of dosing level
Anxiolytics		
Benzodiazepines	Increased risk of prolonged sedation and respiratory depression with amprenavir Increased risk when midazolam is given with efavirenz, indinavir, nelfinavir, ritonavir	Avoid concomitant use
Buspirone	Increased plasma concentration when used with ritonavir	Increased risk of toxicity
Mood stabilisers		
Sodium valproate	Increased plasma concentration of zidovudine	Increased risk of toxicity with nephrotoxic and myelosuppressive drugs
Carbamazepine	Reduced plasma concentration of both drugs when used concurrently Reduced plasma concentration of amprenavir, indinavir, lopinavir, saquinavir, nelfinavir, tipranavir Plasma concentration increased by ritonavir	Avoid use of etravirine – manufacturer advice
Lamotrigine	Decreased plasma concentration with lopinavir and ritonavir	Dose adjustments

Source: Brogan & Lux, 2009.[31]

concentration of ritonavir.[29] Caution with the use of duloxetine in patients with impaired liver function is advised as it can cause elevation of liver enzymes.[30]

Bipolar disorder

In bipolar disorder, depressive episodes are typically longer in duration than those of elevated mood.[32] Patients, especially those who also misuse drugs, are at high risk for HIV infection.[33]

Patients with HIV tend to present early (primary mania) with the traditional symptoms or late (secondary mania). Late-presenting mania is associated with the onset of AIDS and often includes marked cognitive impairment, dementia and pronounced irritable mood (as opposed to elation) and is more severe throughout its clinical course.[34] The differences in presentation have been linked to central nervous system involvement during secondary mania. Sodium valproate is recommended for the treatment of mania.[25] Lamotrigine is an alternative, but careful and close monitoring of the blood dyscrasias is required. Use of lithium requires close monitoring, especially in patients with HIV-related neuropathy or in whom renal toxicity is of concern.

Psychotic disorders

Psychotic disorders are broadly classified as primary (e.g. schizophrenia or delusional disorder) or secondary (as a result of medical condition or substance misuse); their onset may pre-date the onset of HIV. Psychotic episodes in HIV patients are characterised by both variable and fluctuating symptoms that occur over hours to days. Presenting symptoms include persecutory, grandiose and somatic delusions with or without auditory and visual delusions and visual hallucinations.[35] Conventional antipsychotic medications carry an increased risk of extrapyramidal side-effects in HIV patients and so, generally, atypical antipsychotic agents should be used.[31] Treatment-related LSD-like psychotic episodes have been reported with efavirenz. Caution and close monitoring of hepatic function are advocated when prescribing antipsychotics in HIV positive patients.[25,31,36]

Anxiety disorders

Anxiety disorders are prevalent among HIV-positive individuals and are associated with HIV-related symptoms of fatigue and physical dysfunction.[37] Potential clinical subtypes of anxiety include:

- post-traumatic stress disorder
- adjustment disorder
- generalised anxiety
- social phobia
- panic disorder.

Both post-traumatic stress disorder and adjustment disorder are associated with pre-HIV episodes brought about by other significant life events.[38] Precipitating factors related to the onset of anxiety disorders include adaptation and living with the diagnosis of HIV infection, failure of antiretroviral therapy, concerns related to the side-effects of therapy and medical set-backs. The psychiatrist should establish the exact cause of concern before initiating any form of therapy.

Benzodiazepines should be avoided with HIV-positive anxious patients as there can be problematic drug interactions.[25] For example, alprazolam, midazolam and triazolam are potent activators of the CYP pathway that can interact with ritonavir. Ritonavir acts to inhibit their metabolism, causing a reduction in clearance, and then oversedation.[39] Short-acting benzodiazepines such as lorazepam can, though, be prescribed.[25] Additionally, SSRIs such as citalopram or sertraline are widely prescribed and are more beneficial, as they do not interfere with antiretrovirals. See Table 19.3 for treatment of psychiatric disorders in HIV.

Severe anxiety is a predictor of poor compliance with HAART therapy. Patients may also benefit from interventions such as counselling to improve adherence and treatment success.[40]

HIV-associated dementia

In some individuals, HIV infection can lead to a syndrome of neurological dysfunction, so-called HIV-associated neurocognitive disorder (HAND). This broad description includes HIV-associated dementia (HAD) (Box 19.6) as

Treatment-related LSD-like psychotic episodes have been reported with efavirenz use. Caution and close monitoring of hepatic function are advocated when prescribing antipsychotics in HIV-positive patients.

In the HIV-positive anxious patient, benzodiazepines may be problematic, as they interact with antiviral agents. Short-acting benzodiazepines such as lorazepam can be prescribed, or SSRIs such as citalopram or sertraline which do not interfere with antivirals.

Table 19.3 Psychiatric disorders in HIV and treatment

Psychiatric disorder	Prevalence	Notes	Consequences in HIV	Treatment
Depressive spectrum disorder	Reported prevalence 2–30% Patients with HIV 2–7 times more likely to meet diagnostic criteria for major depressive disorder than general population	Primary consequence of CNS effect/ reaction to stigma/emotional or coping/ combination	Anorexia, insomnia, fatigue, HAD and suicide Increased sexual activity, multiple partners[5]	Prefer – citalopram, sertraline and mirtazapine with plasma monitoring Avoid – fluoxetine, St John's wort with PIs and NNRTI, venlafaxine with indinavir[13]
Mania	Reported prevalence <10%	Primary or secondary to HIV Two-cluster presentation Early on in the course of HIV or late stage of AIDS	Increased sexual activity, multiple partners,[5] sex trading, injecting drug use Complicated by cognitive impairment through HIV-associated CNS involvement	Prefer – sodium valproate and lamotrigine as mood stabiliser. May need higher doses in concurrent use with PIs/NNRTI Close monitoring of lithium in patients with HIV-related neuropathy or renal toxicity (narrow therapeutic index)
Psychosis	Prevalence rates 0.5–15% Higher risk of HIV infection than general population	Primary (schizophrenia, schizoaffective disorder) or secondary (psychosis caused by medical condition, i.e. HIV)	Increased potential for extrapyramidal side-effects with conventional antipsychotics	Prefer – amisulpride, olanzapine, sulpride and risperidone (use not advocated with ritonavir)[13]
Anxiety	Present in up to 12% of asymptomatic individuals	Potential consequences of HIV diagnosis include PTSD, adjustment disorder, GAD triggered by new diagnosis, antiretroviral failure	Can compromise adherence to HAART therapy	Prefer – promethazine and zopiclone Benzodiazepines for acute management may include short-acting lorazepam. Consider psychotherapy Avoid – midazolam[13]

CNS, central nervous system; GAD, generalised anxiety disorder; HAD, HIV-associated dementia; HAART, highly active antiretroviral therapy; NNRTI, non-nucleoside reverse transcriptase inhibitor; PI, protease inhibitors; PTSD, post-traumatic stress disorder. For references (nos 5 & 13), see list at the end of this chapter.

Source: adapted from Antinori *et al*, 2007.[41]

Box 19.6 HIV-1-asssociated dementia (HAD)

To meet the criteria the patient should show:

- marked impairment of cognitive functioning in at least two domains, determined during neuropsychological testing, and being at least two standard deviations greater than the demographic mean
- marked interference with activities of daily living (work, home and social activities)
- a pattern of criteria not demonstrative of delirium (e.g. clouding of consciousness)
- no evidence of other pre-existing causes of dementia

Close collaboration with coordination of patient management should exist between the psychiatrists, primary care and GUM clinics, especially in those patients in whom drug compliance is an issue.

well as other HIV-associated cognitive impairments. Symptoms related to HAD are a result of subcortical dysfunction and include a triad of features:

- cognitive impairment (subcortical dementia, focal cognitive deficit)
- behavioural abnormalities (depression, apathy, mania, agitation)
- disturbed motor function (tremor, ataxia, bradykinesia, gait and postural abnormalities).

Adherence to HAART therapy is the most promising treatment strategy to overcome HAD; optimal antiretroviral therapy, which may include the use of drugs that can penetrate the central nervous system, such as zidovudine, is therefore better than the primary use of psychotropic medication to control altered behaviour in HAD.[25]

Summary

An understanding of the risk factors, prevention and treatment strategies relating to STI/HIV infection in patients with mental disorder is necessary to deliver an effective and holistic, patient-centred approach for control of both the physical and mental disorder.

Learning points

- When the patient is in a relationship: see the patient with the partner, assess the partner for sexual dysfunction, arrange appropriate interventions such as communication training and negotiation skills.
- Many medications contribute to sexual dysfunction through adverse effects on libido, erectile function, ejaculation and orgasm.
- There is no evidence that the antidepressant medications agomelatine, amineptine, bupropion, moclobemide, mirtazapine and nefazodone adversely affect sexual function.
- Poorly controlled Axis I and Axis II psychiatric disorders can hinder the success of treatment, by impairing cognition and physical functioning of the individual.
- Antiretroviral drugs, especially the most potent, ritonavir, can have significant interactions with psychopharmacotherapy.
- Patients with pre-existing bipolar disorder tend to present early (primary mania), with the traditional symptoms, or late (secondary mania) and at the onset of AIDS, with marked cognitive impairment, dementia and pronounced irritable mood (as opposed to elation).
- Treatment-related LSD-like psychotic episodes have been reported with efavirenz use.
- When prescribing antipsychotic medications in HIV-positive patients caution and close monitoring of hepatic function are advocated.
- In the HIV-positive anxious patient, benzodiazepines may be problematic, interacting with antiviral agents.
- Short-acting benzodiazepines such as lorazepam or SSRIs such as citalopram or sertraline do not interfere with antiviral agents.
- Close collaboration with coordination of patient management should exist between psychiatrists, primary care and GUM clinics, especially in those patients in whom drug compliance is an issue.

Appendix

Table 19A Sexually transmitted diseases

Specific infection	Prevalence and clinical features	Investigation for diagnosis	Management	Complications
Chlamydia trachomatis	Most encountered bacterial STI: up to 5–10% of women <24 years[42] 70% of women: 50% men asymptomatic[42] In women lower abdominal pain, intermenstrual bleeding, dysuria, purulent vaginal discharge In men ascending infection gives epididymitis Rectal infection in MSM	Examination reveals mucopurulent cervicitis/ contact bleeding EIA (40–70% sensitivity)/ NAAT (90% sensitivity) of urethral/endocervical swabs and first-void urine in men[42]	Uncomplicated chlamydia – doxycycline 100 mg × 2 daily for 1 week/ azithromycin 1 g single dose Contraindicated in pregnancy, therefore use erythromycin 500 mg × 2 daily for 14 days Contact tracing Abstain from sexual intercourse	Natural sequelae if untreated include infertility, pelvic inflammatory disease, endometriosis, perihepatitis (Fitz-Hugh–Curtis syndrome), salpingitis, Bartholin's gland abscess, Reiter's syndrome Increased risk of HIV infection × 3–4[43]
Neisseria gonorrhoeae	50% of women: <10% men asymptomatic[44] In men: urethral discharge (>80%), dysuria (>50%) In women: increased vaginal discharge (50%), dysuria, postcoital bleeding, pelvic pain	Swab and culture sensitivity 95%[44] Microscopy sensitivity: 90% in urethral specimens, 50% in endocervical specimens Alternative test includes NAAT – gives sensitivity of 90% for endocervical swabs	Uncomplicated Ceftriaxone 250 mg IM as single dose/cefixime 400 mg oral as a single dose/spectinomycin 2 g IM as a single dose/ ampicillin 3 g plus probenecid 1 g single dose Contact tracing Abstain from sexual intercourse until partner treated Repeat swabs to check infection has cleared	Rectal infection in MSM and ascending infection giving rise to epididymitis Female infertility, ophthalmia neonatorum of the newborn Coexisting *Chlamydia trachomatis*, *Trichomonas vaginalis*, *Candida albicans* and syphilis[44]
Trichomonas vaginalis	Reported increased prevalence in study population 3.1% *v.* 15.7% in women with a psychiatric disorder[43] Infects only the urogenital tract In women: vaginal discharge frothy, offensive, dyspareunia In men: present as asymptomatic partner, urethral discharge, irritation, and urinary frequency	Examination reveals inflamed vaginal mucosa and vulval erythema. Phase-contrast background microscopy sensitive in 70% of female specimens/30% male specimens[45]	Metronidazole 2 g orally single dose/400 mg × 2 7 days Contact tracing Simultaneous treatment Abstain from sex until partner completes treatment 95% cure rate No evidence of teratogenicity from metronidazole use during 1st trimester	Preterm delivery and LBW Increased risk of HIV Coexisting gonorrhoea/ chlamydia

contd

Table 19A contd

Syphilis *Treponema pallidum* (see national guideline[46])	Can be asymptomatic Three stages of symptomatology: • primary syphilis – single painless ulcer (chancre) develops around 3 weeks after exposure; spontaneous resolution • secondary syphilis – constitutional symptoms, fever, sore throat, malaise and skin rashes appear 4–10 weeks after onset of primary chancre • tertiary syphilis (late stage) – presentation of gumma syphilis (bone and skin involvement), cardiovascular syphilis (aortic regurgitation and aortitis), and neurosyphilis	Serological testing includes use of treponemal enzyme immunoassay EIA, *Treponema pallidum* hemagglutination (TPHA) and cardiolipin (non treponemal) test Veneral Disease Research Laboratory (VDRL)	Antibiotic treatment and follow-up employed at specialist genitourinary medicine clinic	Secondary syphilis may involve any organ, causing nephritis, meningitis, arthritis and hepatitis Congenital syphilis Late syphilis can cause cortical neuronal loss; gradual decline in memory and cognitive function, psychosis, dementia and emotional lability
Genital herpes, *Herpes simplex* virus 1/2 (see national guideline[47])	HSV infection gives rise to constitutional symptoms, fever, malaise and headache Primary infection: multiple painful ulcers which may coalesce with tender inguinal lymphadenopathy Recurrence: usually milder than first episode Symptom prodrome of tingling, itching and pain prior to recurrence	Viral culture specificity 100%	Salt-water bathing Analgesia Topical anaesthetic, e.g. 5% lidocaine ointment Aciclovir 200 mg × 5 daily for 5 days Can be used in pregnancy and breastfeeding	Can co-occur in HIV HSV encephalitis
HIV (see national guideline[48])	Asymptomatic in first years of infection May present with mild systemic illness with constitutional symptoms Opportunistic infections may present in unusual ways	Serology for antibodies to HIV	CD4 count and HIV viral load measurements, no treatment if immune function normal Antiretroviral therapy if CD4 count 250–350 × 109/l HAART therapy can be used in pregnant women, but avoid breastfeeding to reduce vertical transmission	Susceptibility to opportunistic infections

CD4, cluster of differentiation 4; EIA, enzyme immunoassay; HAART, highly active antiretroviral therapy; HSV, *Herpes simplex* virus; IM, intramuscular; LBW, low birth weight; MSM, men who have sex with men; NAAT, nucleic acid amplification technique; STI, sexually transmitted infection.

References

1 Dunn KM, Croft PR, Hackett GI. Sexual problems: a study of the prevalence and need for health care in the general population. *Family Practice* 1998;**15**: 519–24.

2 Laumann EO, Michael RT, Gagnon JH. A political history of the national sex survey of adults. *Fam Plann Perspectives* 1994; **26**: 34–8.

3 Mercer CH, Fenton KA, Johnson AM, *et al.* Sexual function problems and help seeking behaviour in Britain: national probability sample survey. *BMJ* 2003; **327**: 426–7.

4 American Psychiatric Association. *Diagnostic and Statistical Manual of Mental Disorders (4th edn, text revision) (DSM-IV-TR).* APA, 2000.

5 Wang C, Nieschlag E, Swerdloff R, *et al.* Investigation, treatment, and monitoring of late-onset hypogonadism in males: ISA, ISSAM, EAU, EAA, and ASA Recommendations. *Eur Urology* 2009; **55**: 121–30.

6 Wylie K, Rees M, Hackett G, et al. Androgens, health and sexuality in women and men. *Maturitas* 2010; **67**: 275–89.

7 Verhulst J, Reynolds JK. Sexual pharmacology: love potions, pills, and poisons. *J Fam Psychother* 2009; **20**: 319–43.

8 Clayton AH, Balon R. The impact of mental illness and psychotropic medications on sexual functioning: the evidence and management (CME). *J Sex Medicine* 2009; **6**: 1200–11.

9 Corona G, Ricca V, Bandini E, *et al.* Selective serotonin reuptake inhibitor-induced sexual dysfunction. *J Sex Medicine* 2009; **6**: 1259–69.

10 Serretti A, Chiesa A. Treatment-emergent sexual dysfunction related to antidepressants: a meta-analysis. *J Clin Psychopharmacol* 2009; **29**: 259–66.

11 Murthy S, Wylie KR. Sexual problems in patients on antipsychotic medication. *Sex Relationship Ther* 2007; **22**: 97–107.

12 The UK collaborative Group for HIV and STI surveillance. *Testing Times: HIV and other Sexually Transmitted Infection in the United Kingdom, 2007.* Helath Protection Agency, Centre for Infection, London, 2007.

13 Chen Y, Wu J, Yi Q, *et al.* Depression associated with sexually transmitted infection in Canada. *Sex Transm Infect* 2008; **84**: 535–40.

14 Hutton H, Lyketsos C, Zenilman J, *et al.* Depression and HIV risk behaviours among patients in a sexually transmitted disease clinic. *Am J Psychiatry* 2004; **161**: 912–4.

15 Ison CA, Lewis DA. Chancroid. In *Sexually Transmitted Infections: UK National Screening and Testing Guidelines* (eds J Ross, C Ison, C Carder, *et al*): 47–51. British Association for Sexual Health and HIV (BASHH), 2006 .

16 Turjanski N, Lloyd GG. Psychiatric side-effects of medications: recent developments. *Adv Psychiatr Treat* 2005; **11**: 58–70.

17 Carey MP, Carey KB, Maisto SA, *et al.* Reducing HIV-risk behavior among adults receiving outpatient psychiatric treatment: results from a randomized controlled trial. *J Consult Clin Psychol* 2004; **72**: 252–68.

18 Crepaz N, Horn AK, Rama SM, *et al* (HIV/AIDS Prevention Research Synthesis Team). The efficacy of behavioral interventions in reducing HIV risk sex behaviors and incident sexually transmitted disease in black and Hispanic sexually transmitted disease clinic patients in the United States: a meta-analytic review. *Sex Transm Dis* 2007; **34**: 319–32.

19 Guillebaud J. *Contraception Today (5th edn).* Informa Healthcare, 2003.

20 Erbelding E, Hutton H, Zenilman J, *et al.* The prevalence of psychiatric disorders in sexually transmitted disease clinic patients and their association with sexually transmitted disease risk. *Am Sex Transm Diseases Assoc* 2004; **31**: 8–12.

21 Meade C, Sikkema K. HIV risk behaviour among adults with severe mental illness: a systematic review. *Clin Psychol Rev* 2005; **25**: 433–57.

22 Rosenberg S, Goodman L, Osher F, *et al.* Prevalence of HIV, Hepatitis B and Hepatitis C in people with severe mental illness. *Am J Public Health* 2001; **91**: 31–7.

23 Thompson A, Silverman B, Dzeng L, *et al.* Psychotropic medications and HIV. *Clin Infectious Diseases* 2006; **42**: 1305–10.

24 Rietmeijer CA. Risk reduction counseling for prevention of sexually transmitted infections: how it works and how to make it work. *Sex Transm Inf* 2007; **83**: 2–9.

25 Royal College of Psychiatrists. *Guidelines for the Prescribing of Medication for Mental Health Disorders for People with HIV Infection (Council Report CR127).* Royal College of Psychiatrists, 2004.

26 Forstein M, Cournos F, Douaihy A, *et al. Guideline Watch: Practice Guideline for the Treatment of Patients with HIV/AIDS.* American Psychiatric Association, 2006.

27 Caballero J, Nahata MC. Use of selective serotonin-reuptake inhibitors in the treatment of depression in adults with HIV. *Ann Pharmacother* 2005; **39**: 141–5.

28 DeSilva KE, Le Flore DB, Marston BJ, *et al.* Serotonin syndrome in HIV-infected individuals receiving antiretroviral therapy and Fluoxetine. *AIDS* 2001; **15**: 1281–5.

29 Levin GM, Nelson LA, DeVane CL, *et al.* A pharmokinetic drug interaction study of venlafaxine and indinavir. *Psychopharmacol Bull* 2001; **35**: 62–71.

30 Westanmo AD, Gayken J, Haight R. Duloxetine: a balanced and sective norepinephrine-and serotonin reuptake inhibitor. *Am J Health System Pharm* 2005; **62**: 2479.

31 Brogan K, Lux J. Management of common psychiatric conditions in the HIV positive population. *Curr HIV/AIDS Rep* 2009; **6**: 108–15.

32 Grant BF, Stinson FS, Hasin DS, *et al.* Prevalence, correlates and co-morbidity of bipolar disorder I and Axis I and II disorders: results from the National Epidemiologic Survey on alcohol and related conditions. *J Clin Psychiatry* 2005; **66**: 1205–15.

33 Meade CS, Graff FS, Griffin ML, *et al.* High-risk behaviour among patients with co-occurring bipolar and substance use disorders: associations with mania and drug abuse. *Drug Alcohol Depen* 2008; **92**: 296–300

34 Cruess DG, Evans DL, Repetto MJ, *et al.* Prevalence, diagnosis and pharmacological treatment of mood disorders in HIV disease. *Soc Biol Psychiatry* 2003; **54**: 307–16.

35 Dolder CR, Patterson TL, Jeste DV. HIV, psychosis and aging: past, present and future. *AIDS* 2004; **18** (suppl I): S35–42.

36 Repetto MJ, Petitto JM. Psychopharmacology in HIV infected patients. *Psychosom Medicine* 2008; **70**: 585–92.

37 Hinkin CH, Castellon SA, Atkinson JH, *et al.* Neuropsychiatric aspects of HIV infection among older adults. *J Clin Epidemiol* 2001; **54**: S44–52.

38 Owe-Larsson B, Sall L, Salamon E, *et al.* HIV infection and psychiatric illness. *Afr J Psychiatry* 2009; **12**: 115–28.

39 Wynn G, Cozza K, Zapor M, *et al.* Antiretrovirals, part III: Antiretrovirals and drugs of abuse. *Psychosomatics* 2005; **46**: 79–87.

40 Campos LN, Guimarães MDC, Remien RH. Anxiety and depression symptoms as risk factors for non-adherence to antiretroviral therapy in Brazil. *AIDS Behav* 2010; **14**: 289–99.

41 Antinori A, Arendt G, Becker JT, *et al.* Updated research nosology for HIV-associated neurocognitive disorders. *Neurology* 2007; **69**: 1789–99.

42 Horner PJ, Boag F. *2006 UK National Guideline for the Management of Genital Tract Infection with Chlamydia trachomatis.* British Association of Sexual Health and HIV, 2006.

43 King C, Feldman J, Waithaka Y, *et al.* Sexual risk behaviors and sexually transmitted infection prevalence in an outpatient psychiatry clinic. *Sex Transm Dis* 2008; **35**: 877–82.

44 British Association for Sexual Health and HIV. *National Guideline on the Diagnosis and Treatment of Gonorrhoea in Adults 2005.* BASHH, 2005.

45 Clinical Effectiveness Group, British Association for Sexual Health and HIV. *United Kingdom National Guideline on the Management of Trichomonas vaginalis.* BASHH, 2007.

46 Kingston M, French P, Goh B, *et al*; Syphilis Guidelines Revision Group 2008, Clinical Effectiveness Group. UK National Guidelines on the Management of Syphilis 2008. *Int J STD AIDS* 2008; **19**: 729–40.

47 Clinical Effectiveness Group. *2007 National Guideline for the Management of Genital Herpes.* British Association for Sexual Health and HIV, 2007.

48 Nandwani R. *2006 United Kingdom National Guideline on the Sexual Health of People with HIV: Sexually Transmitted Infections.* British Association for Sexual Health and HIV, 2006.

20

Contraception, pregnancy, the puerperium and breastfeeding

David Burton and Kevan Wylie

The topics covered include the care of patients with mental health problems during pregnancy and in the puerperium; and the psychiatric treatments which could affect the well-being of the pregnant woman, the fetus and the breastfed baby. Methods of contraception are also described. It is beyond the scope of this chapter to address the physical complications of pregnancy and the puerperium. Close liaison between mental health services and obstetric services is recommended.

Introduction

The arrival of a newborn is often one of the most joyous and eagerly anticipated events of family life. But pregnancy and the puerperium may be a source of stress and anxiety, which can be compounded by physical and mental disorder.[1–4] Carers of expectant mothers must be sensitive to the signs of psychological instability. Pregnant women with a new or pre-existing mental health disorder offer challenging treatment scenarios for clinicians. The potential harm through continued use of psychotropic medication to mother and fetus needs to be balanced against the effects of the mental disorder.[5] This chapter describes methods of contraception, mental disorders occurring in pregnancy and the safety of the most frequently prescribed drugs used in treating mental disorders during the antenatal and postnatal periods.

Contraception.

Data from the World Health Organization (WHO) suggest that, of the 200 million pregnancies that occur each year, 75 million are unwanted. Around 40 million abortions are undertaken worldwide, of which half are performed in unsafe conditions. Contraceptive technology offers a relatively inexpensive method of reducing both unwanted pregnancy and the incidence of sexually transmitted infections (STIs).

The key features of the contraceptive products that may influence the choice of a patient with a mental disorder are discussed. Three useful websites for information on contraception are those of the sexual health charity FPA (www.fpa.org.uk), NHS Direct (www.nhsdirect.nhs.uk) and the Faculty of Sexual and Reproductive Healthcare of the Royal College of Obstetricians and Gynaecologists (www.fsrh.org). In addition, the short book on contraception by Guillebaud is recommended (see Recommended reading).

Of particular note to the psychiatrist are the drug interactions that occur between the hormonal contraceptive devices and liver-enzyme-inducing medication (see below), which includes St John's wort, anti-epileptic medication and barbiturates.

The patient and, when appropriate, her GP, obstetrician or gynaecologist, *must* be consulted if physical conditions in pregnancy or the puerperium are suspected or found.

Table 20.1 Contraceptive methods that depend on the user

	Combined oral contraceptive pill	Progesterone-only pill	Contraceptive patch
Failure rate	< 1/100 if taken as per instruction	< 1/100 if taken as per instruction	< 1/100 if taken as per instruction. Less effective in women > 90 kg
Delivery and method	Oral medication containing progestogen and oestrogen	Oral medication containing progestogen	Patch contains oestrogen and progestogen. Daily dose released into bloodstream via skin
Side-effects/risks	Headaches, nausea, vomiting, breast tenderness, weight changes, depression, 'spotting' in early cycle	Headaches, irregular menses	Headaches, nausea, vomiting, breast tenderness, weight changes, depression, 'spotting' in early cycle
Contraindication	Pregnancy Smokers over 35 years of age History of severe depression Risk factors for venous thromboembolism Migraine Hypertension Diabetes with renal or arterial complications Liver disease	Pregnancy Severe arterial disease Ovarian cysts Ectopic pregnancy Breast cancer Unexplained bleeding from vagina	Pregnancy Smokers over 35 years of age History of severe depression Risk factors for venous thromboembolism Migraine Hypertension Diabetes with renal or arterial complications Liver disease
Benefits	Protects against cancer of uterus, colon, ovary Can reduce period pain and premenstrual symptoms Does not interfere with intercourse	Can be used in women who smoke and are over 35 Does not interfere with intercourse	Weekly application *v.* daily application Not affected by diarrhoea and vomiting Can reduce period pain and premenstrual symptoms Does not interfere with intercourse

Contraception

Contraceptive advice needs to be tailored to the patient. The contraceptive method chosen is dependent on the woman's preference, physical health, pregnancy risk and lifestyle. Discussion should centre on both contraception and disease prevention. Communication with primary carers may help in deciding and monitoring the method of contraception. Contraceptive choice on the part of patients on long-term medication may include discussion with primary care, secondary care and community mental health providers.

Contraceptives are broadly divided into those that depend on the user to take them properly (Table 20.1) and those that do not (Table 20.2).

Pregnancy commonly confers a higher risk to maternal and fetal outcome in women with physical and mental disorders. Contraceptive advice and counselling creates an active period for control of disease processes, during which avoidance of unwanted pregnancy can be achieved. Mood-stabilising drugs such as lithium, tricyclic antidepressants and anxiolytics can alter the normal menstrual cycle. Fertility tests and barrier methods of contraception should be considered in these circumstances.

Hormonal methods

Combined oral contraceptive

These preparations contain the hormones oestrogen, usually synthetic ethinylestradiol, and some form of progestogen, with differing ratios of progestogen to oestrogen to mirror the hormonal changes during normal ovarian cycles.

Table 20.2 Contraceptive methods that do not depend on the user

	Intrauterine system (IUS)	Intrauterine device (IUD)	Implanon	Contraceptive injection
Failure rate	< 1/100 women will be pregnant in 1 year	< 1/100	< 1/1000 women will be pregnant in 3 years	< 1/100 women will be pregnant in 1 year
Delivery and method	T-shaped device with slow-release progestogen is placed into the uterus	Small copper-containing device is placed into the uterus	Implant placed just under the skin of the inner area of the upper arm. Device is the length of a hair-grip	IM injections given every 12 weeks
Side-effects/risks	Headaches Breast tenderness Small increased risk of PID within first 20 days of insertion Perforation of uterus Expulsion or displacement	Irregular bleeding between menses Increased risk of pelvic infection within first 20 days of insertion Perforation of uterus Expulsion or displacement	Acne Breast tenderness Changes in weight, mood and libido Irregular periods or spotting	Weight gain Irregular bleeding between periods Headache Abdominal pain Dizziness Breast tenderness
Contraindications	Pregnancy Previous ectopic pregnancy Uterine or breast neoplasm Immunosuppression Pelvic infection Untreated STIs Severe arterial disease or thrombosis Problems with uterus or cervix	Pregnancy Previous ectopic pregnancy Pelvic infection Untreated STI Problems with uterus or cervix	Pregnancy Active liver disease Current breast cancer or within the past 5 years Migraine Arterial disease Unexplained vaginal bleed	Osteoporosis or risk factors Under 19 years of age
Benefits	Does not interrupt sex Can be used during breast-feeding Can be used as an alternative to COC Works for 5 years	Does not interrupt sex Can be used during breast-feeding Can be used as an alternative to COC Works for 5–10 years	Works for 3 years Does not interrupt sex May protect against pelvic inflammatory disease	Lasts for 12 weeks Does not interrupt sex Can be used during breast-feeding May give protection against PID and uterine neoplasm

COC, combined oral contraceptive; IM, intramuscular; PID, pelvic inflamatory disease; STI, sexually transmitted infection.

If a combined oral contraceptive pill is missed for over 12 hours, patients should be advised to immediately use barrier methods of contraception for the next 7 days.

Once-daily pills are taken for 21 days followed by a 7-day break, during which a light withdrawal bleed takes place. Women are protected from pregnancy from day 1 of taking the pill and during the 7-day break. Forgotten pills are a source of anxiety. If a pill is missed for over 12 hours, patients should be advised to immediately use barrier methods of contraception for the next 7 days.

Contraindications

A history of circulatory disease, pregnancy, oestrogen-dependent neoplasms, active disease of the liver and undiagnosed bleeding of the genital tract are *absolute* contraindications to the use of combined oral contraceptives (COCs) (Box 20.1).

Low-dose COCs do not appear to confer an increased risk of depression in individuals with a history of depression compared with those without a prior history,[1] although their use is associated with increased rates of anxiety and depression for reasons which are unclear[2] and caution is advised in postpartum depression and bipolar disorder owing to lack of data.

Circulating levels of ethinylestradiol may reduce the antidepressant effects of *tricyclic antidepressants* and may lead to unwanted antimuscarinic effects such as dry mouth and constipation.[4] The side-effect profile of COCs

Box 20.1 Contraindications to the combined oral contraceptive

Circulatory diseases
Thrombo-embolic disease
Ischaemic heart disease
Focal migraine
Transient ischaemic attacks or stroke
Hyperlipidaemia
Hypertension
Arteritis
Diabetes
Heavy smoking
Gross obesity
Liver disease/impaired liver function
Breast cancer
Pregnancy
Hyperprolactinaemia
Abnormal genital tract bleeding

Box 20.2 Drugs that induce liver enzymes

Anti-epileptic (enzyme inducers):
- carbamazepine
- felbamate
- lamotrigine
- oxcarbazepine
- phenytoin
- phenobarbital
- primidone
- rufinamide
- topiramate

Antibiotics:
- rifampicin
- rifabutin

Antifungal:
- griseofulvin

Antiretroviral (protease inhibitors):
- amprenavir
- atazanavir
- nelfinavir
- lopinavir
- saquinavir

Antiretroviral (non-nucleoside reverse transcriptase inhibitors):
- efavirenz
- nevirapine

Other:
- St John's wort

Clinicians should consider the possibility of drug interaction when prescribing contraceptives, especially those containing hormonal composites.

Depo-Provera given as a single intramuscular dose of 150 mg should be considered in psychiatric patients with comorbidities, on multiple medications and who misuse drugs and alcohol. Care should be taken if there are significant risks of thromboembolic disease.

should be considered in patients who are most at risk for relapse of depression or other mood deterioration.

Drug interactions

Liver-enzyme-inducing medication, acting via the cytochrome P450 pathway, can reduce the efficacy and clinical effect of hormonal contraceptive devices (Box 20.2) so patients taking medications such as *St John's wort* or *carbamazepine* should use alternative contraceptive measures during, and for 4 weeks after, cessation of the liver-inducing medication.[4]

The serum levels and the anti-seizure effects of the non-enzyme-inducing anticonvulsant *lamotrigine* may be reduced in women starting on a COC.[5] Close monitoring when initiating or discontinuing a COC is recommended with patients on lamotrigine.[6]

Antibiotics can also reduce the effectiveness of COCs by impairing the absorption of oestrogen. An additional form of contraception is recommended for 7 days after a patient finishes a short-term course of antibiotics. Those on long-term antibiotics should use contraceptives that are unaffected by drug interaction (e.g. IUS-Mirena or progestogen-only injections – see Table 20.3).

Progestogen-only pills

The progestogen-only pill (POP, 'mini' or 'everyday' pill) is taken daily without a pill-free interval, at the same time of day to within 3 hours (12 hours for Cerazette®); if it is taken outside this window, it is ineffective. It is less effective if taken concurrently with medication such as *St John's wort* or *anti-epileptic drugs.* POPs are a useful alternative for patients in whom COCs are contraindicated, for example women with migraine or breast cancer and in smokers aged over 35 years. Its own contraindications are listed in Box 20.3.

Broad-spectrum antibiotics do not affect POP efficacy. However, *rifampicin* and *rifabutin* may reduce the effectiveness of POPs,[7] so users on long-term

Table 20.3 Interactions between drugs and contraceptives

	Combined oral contraceptive	Progestogen-only pill	Implanon	Depot injection	Mirena	Intrauterine device
Anticonvulsant therapy						
Phenytoin, carbamazepine, barbituates, primidone, topiramate, oxcarbazepine	3	3	2	1	1	1
Lamotrigine	3	1	1	1	1	1
Antiretroviral therapy						
Nucleoside reverse transcriptase inhibitor	1	1	1	1	2/3	2/3
Non-nucleoside reverse transcriptase inhibitor	2	2	2	1	2	2
Ritonavir	3	3	2	1	2/3	2/3
Antimicrobial therapy						
Broad spectrum	1	1	1	1	1	1
Antifungals	1	1	1	1	1	1
Antiparasitic	1	1	1	1	1	1
Rifampicin or rifabutin	3	3	2	1	1	1

1 = A condition for which there is no restriction for the use of the contraceptive method
2 = A condition where the advantages of using the method generally outweigh the theoretical or proven risk
3 = A condition where the theoretical or proven risks usually outweigh the advantages of using the method

Source: World Health Organization, 2010.[8]

Box 20.3 Contraindications to progestogen-only pills

Known or suspected pregnancy
Known or suspected carcinoma of the breast
Current deep-vein thrombosis/pulmonary embolism without adequate anticoagulation
Less than 6 weeks postpartum
Liver disease

therapy should consider additional barrier methods of contraception.

Contraceptive injection

Progestogen-only injectable preparations such as Depo-Provera are given as a single intramuscular injection which is effective for 2–3 months. Injection cycles of 12 weeks offer protection from pregnancy. Drug levels remain constant, so any side-effects cannot be alleviated immediately; patients should be prepared for these to continue during and for a while after treatment. Depo-Provera should be considered in psychiatric patients with comorbidities, on multiple medications and those who misuse drugs and alcohol.

Contraceptive implant

Implanon is a progestin-only implant that works for 3 years. It gives immediate protection if inserted during the first 5 days of the menstrual period; outside this, alternative contraception should be used. Normal fertility can be resumed as soon as the implant is taken out. It can be used in patients on antiretroviral, anticonvulsant and antimicrobial therapy,[7] when it is essential to avoid pregnancy.

Intrauterine devices

Intrauterine system

The T-shaped intrauterine system (IUS) Mirena releases a low dose of the progestogen levonorgestrel and can last for 5 years. Threads attached to the end of the device allow the user to check that the IUS is not displaced. Mirena is not affected by concurrent use of anti-epileptic medication and is not subject to user failure.[7,9] It should not be used by women with hormone-sensitive tumours such as oestrogen-positive breast cancer.

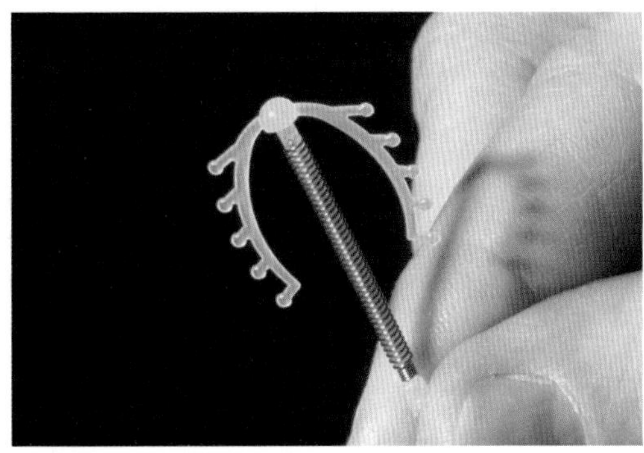

Fig 20.1 An intrauterine contraceptive device.

Intrauterine devices

The intrauterine device (IUD) (Fig. 20.1), unlike the IUS, contains copper, and offers an alternative when progestogen is contraindicated, for example by active liver disease. Menstrual periods tend to be longer and heavier compared with IUS use.

Barrier methods

Condoms, the leading method for protection from STIs, including HIV, are very effective if used correctly. They are, however, prone to user failure due to technique and compliance. Users should be informed of emergency contraception, especially when condoms are the sole method of contraception.

Emergency contraception

Two methods of emergency contraception are available for use after unprotected sexual intercourse or where conventional methods have failed due to user error.

Free emergency contraception and advice can be obtained from National Health Service (NHS) walk-in centres, general practitioners, and contraception, sexual health and genitourinary medicine clinics. Most pharmacies also offer the emergency pill for sale. Patients should be made aware that advice and treatment are given in strictest confidence.

Emergency contraceptive pill

Sometimes erroneously referred to as 'the morning-after pill', this method can be used for up to 72 hours after unprotected intercourse. It is most effective the sooner it is taken. Menses may occur on time or may be a few days early or late.

The copper IUD

The copper device is the most effective emergency contraceptive device. It can be inserted up to 5 days post ovulation. Menses will occur as normal. Patients should be instructed to take a pregnancy test if their normal period has not occurred within 3 weeks of having the IUD fitted. The IUD can be removed during the next menstrual period.

Mental conditions during in pregnancy

Mental health teams should work closely with the patient's obstetric and physical healthcare teams. For medical emergencies, see Chapter 31, for example diagnosis and management of collapse (p. 434), sepsis (p. 441) and fits (p. 437).

Hyperemesis gravidarum

Hyperemesis gravidarum is a rare but potentially fatal condition affecting up to 0.3–2% of expectant mothers.[13] Its hallmark feature is intractable nausea and vomiting sufficient to produce at least 5% loss of body weight, dehydration and sequential electrolyte imbalance.[14,15] The aim of psychiatric consultation is to screen for depressive or anxiety disorders and assess the patients' ability to cope with distress.[14] Following this the psychiatrist can focus on improving coping skills and reassure the patient that her emotional feeling will improve as the symptoms resolve.[14]

Nausea and vomiting occur in 80% of normal pregnancies.[16] Examination should be undertaken to explore other possible causes, as physical symptoms of epigastric pain, abdominal tenderness, fever, headache and dysuria may suggest alternative diagnoses. Hyperemesis gravidarum typically presents at 4–8 weeks' gestation and settles at 14–16 weeks, but may progress throughout pregnancy.[15] Investigations are listed in Box 20.4.

Box 20.4 Investigations for hyperemesis gravidarum

- Full blood count – raised haematocrit
- Urea and electrolytes – hyponatraemia, hypokalaemia and low urea
- Liver function test
- Calcium – to exclude hypercalcaemia
- Thyroid function test
- Arterial blood gas (ABG) – not routinely performed
- Urine analysis – ketonuria, urinary tract infection
- Pelvic ultrasound – confirm gestational age, multiple pregnancy and exclude molar pregnancy

Management

Parenteral fluid such as normal saline intravenously may reduce nausea and correct electrolyte deficits. Dextrose solution should be avoided, as it may increase the body's requirement for thiamine and therefore increase the risk of Wernicke's encephalopathy.[17] Thiamine hydrochloride (25–50 mg three times a day) or Pabrinex® (100 mg diluted in 100 ml normal saline intravenously over 30–60 minutes) should be considered in severe and prolonged cases of hyperemesis.[16,18]

Anti-emetics may also be considered and are effective in reducing the frequency of nausea in early pregnancy.[19] Suggested first-line therapy includes the use of cyclizine 50 mg (three times a day, orally, intramuscularly or intravenously) or promethazine 25 mg orally at night).[16] Two suggested dose regimens are: [17]

- prochlorperazine, 5 mg orally three times a day or 12.5 mg intramuscularly or intravenously three times a day; and/or
- chlorpromazine, 10–25 mg orally three times a day or 25 mg intramuscularly three times a day.

Depression

Depression occurs in up to 15% of all pregnancies in the UK.[6,7] Psychosocial risk factors include:

- a history of depressive disorder
- an unwanted or unplanned pregnancy
- a low level of education
- high neuroticism.[10]

As depression rates are higher during pregnancy than at other points in a woman's life,[9] family-planning options should be discussed with all women who have an affective disorder and are of reproductive age.[2] Women who regularly take medication to treat their depression should not abruptly stop taking it once they conceive and should be made aware of the risk of depressive relapse if they do so.[11] Those with a history of recurring depression or bipolar disorder should be referred to perinatal services or, if those are unavailable, to general psychiatric services for specialist management during pregnancy.[2] Women who have depression and have been symptom-free for over a year can reduce or gradually discontinue their antidepressant therapy before conceiving.[12] Close monitoring for relapse is still recommended during pregnancy and the puerperium.

Postnatal blues ('baby blues')

Postnatal blues is a normal and short-lived presentation following normal delivery, affecting 15–85% of women.[20] Its aetiology is uncertain but it has been associated with history of anxiety, depressed mood during the last trimester and fears of labour.[21] Depressive symptoms occur 3–5 days postnatally and resolve within 2 weeks, without the need for medical intervention.[20] Mothers require reassurance and supportive therapy may be offered.

Postnatal blues is a risk factor for postpartum depression (PPD).[22]

Depression after delivery

This is defined as a major depressive disorder (MDD) with a postpartum onset. Postpartum depression is one of the most common new-onset psychiatric complications of pregnancy,[22] affecting up 15%.[5] The clinical features are akin to those that may occur at any stage in the woman's life.[23] To fulfil the criteria of MDD the mother should display depressed mood or loss of interest in the pleasure of daily activities for at least 2 weeks. Risk factors include: a history of depression; a history of other psychiatric disorder; a recent stressful life event; and poor social support.[24] Useful screening tools in the early detection and identification of postnatal depression include the Edinburgh Postnatal Depression Scale[23,25] and the Postpartum Depression Predictors Inventory – Revised.[24] It is important to note that the psychiatric interview is the only acceptable method for definitive diagnosis of PPD.[1] See Table 20.4 for the stepped care approach to management.

Clinical features

For confirmation of the diagnosis, anhedonia and depressed mood should be present for at least 2 weeks. Diagnosis is complicated as a disrupted sleep pattern, upset appetite and fatigue are likely soon after a birth. More suggestive diagnostic features worth exploring include early-morning waking before the baby and feelings of worthlessness and hopelessness.[25]

Table 20.4 Stepped-care approach to postpartum depression

Step	Who is responsible	What is the focus	What they do
1	General practitioner, practice nurse, midwife, obstetrician, health visitor	Recognition	Assessment
2	Primary care team, primary care mental health worker, therapist	Mild disorder	Watchful waiting, guided self-help, e.g. computerised cognitive–behavioural therapy, exercise, brief psychological intervention
3	Primary care team, primary care mental health worker, clinical psychologists/ therapists	Moderate or severe disorder	Medication, psychological interventions, social support
4	Mental health specialists, including perinatal and crisis teams	Psychosis, severe disorder	Medication, complex assessment and complex psychological interventions, combined treatments
5	In-patient care	Risk to life, severe self-neglect	Medication, combined treatment, electroconvulsive therapy

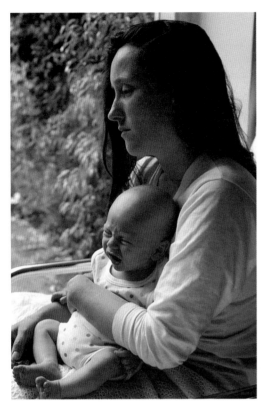

Fig. 20.2 Mother with depression and her baby.

Consequences

Disruption of the normal interaction between mother and child is of chief concern (Fig. 20.2).[22,26] Left untreated, PPD is linked with compromised psychological development and less facial expression in the baby.[27] Infants may face difficulty in achieving the development of normal language and emotional and social skills.[28] Safety issues surrounding the baby and any siblings are of paramount importance. The natural sequelae of the disorder may strain family relationships and ultimately result in a relationship failure.

Management

Biological causes of depression must be ruled out and corrected before commencing any form of psychotherapy. Mild cases may not require psychiatric intervention and can be managed in the community by the general practitioner (GP) and health visitors during postnatal checks.[25] Women with PPD may require referral to specialist mental health services, for example to a mother-and-baby unit (MBU), where patient assessment can take place and mother–baby interactions can be observed, as an in-patient.

Expert advice may be needed on the risks and benefits of using psychotropic medication.[29] Treatment options also include psychosocial and psychological therapies[25,30] (see Table 20A).

Postpartum psychosis

Postpartum psychosis is an acute episode, occurring in 2.2 per 1000 women, presenting in 2–4 weeks after delivery.[31] Its aetiology is unknown but may be related to family history, previous psychosis and hormonal fluctuation (in particular, rapid falls in oestrogen).[31,32] The risk of relapse of schizophrenia is greatest in the first 3 months after parturition.[32] Relapse is clearly of great significance for the neonate, as blunted emotional response and unresponsiveness on the part of the mother can resulting in poor maternal–infant interactions.[32]

Clinical features

Clinical presentations include affective symptoms of mania, depression with or without psychosis and so-called schizoaffective disorder. Clinical features include paranoid, grandiose delusions, confusion, mood changes, insomnia and suicidal ideation.

Treatment

Once medical causes for psychosis have been ruled out, primary assessment should include documentation of delusional ideas and assessment of the risk of harm that the mother poses to herself and her infant. Admission to a specialist MBU for psychiatric assessment may be warranted.[33] Observations should be made of the relationship between mother and child, as well as of the practical abilities of the mother (e.g. breastfeeding technique). The use of psychotropic medication should be tailored to the patient (see next section). Electroconvulsive therapy may bring a quick resolution of symptoms and should be considered in patients who have failed trials of or are intolerant of the side-effects of pharmacotherapy.[31]

Management of mental disorders during pregnancy

Whenever appropriate, colleagues specialising in perinatal psychiatry should be consulted. A stepped care approach is required in the management of women with psychiatric disorders during pregnancy and the puerperium.[29] Adopting this approach can help to reinforce working relationships across the organisations offering care and support to the patient.

Psychopharmacology

Women may require prescribed psychotropic medication for new or existing mental health problems during pregnancy. Conditions may extend from pre-existing prophylactic management of depression, mania or psychosis to new episodes of the aforementioned diagnoses. Clinicians should be aware of the significant risk associated with pharmacological agents used and potential detrimental effects on both mother and developing fetus. This risk of harm, though, has to be balanced against the potential that treatment may reduce the severity of the illness and thereby promote the mental well-being of the mother (see Box 20.6).

The psychiatrist's role is to help guide the patient in deciding the timely and efficient method of treatment for symptom relief while discussing the risk posed to the mother and baby if the illness is left untreated. There is evidence to suggest that depressive disorder is associated with prenatal poor nutrition, smoking, substance misuse and risk of suicide, which may put mother and fetus at risk (Box 20.5).[34,35] Obstetric complications of low birth weight, miscarriage, pre-eclampsia and infants who are small for their gestational age have also been reported in women with untreated prenatal stress and depression.[36,37] Mothers with bipolar disorder and schizophrenia have similar poor maternal and fetal outcomes, during pregnancy.[38]

Box 20.5 Adverse effects of untreated depression during pregnancy

All of the following are more likely if depression is left untreated during pregnancy:

- suicidal ideation
- substance misuse
- hypertension
- pre-eclampsia
- preterm birth
- spontaneous abortion
- intrauterine growth restriction
- low birth weight
- postpartum depression
- neurobehavioural change in the infant.

Women using paroxetine should avoid pregnancy, as paroxetine is associated with cardiac malformations if taken in the first trimester.

Antidepressants

Up to 8% of women use antidepressants during pregnancy.[39] As a broad classification, antidepressants are not attributed to an increased incidence of congenital anomalies.[40] Tricyclic antidepressants (TCAs) offer the lowest known risk profile of any of the antidepressants used during pregnancy and breastfeeding. This is in part because they were the first psychotropic medication prescribed for the treatment of depression and are therefore the most studied.[27] Negligible amounts of TCAs are found in breast milk. Long-term studies of child development following exposure to TCAs have found no difference in IQ, language, mood or temperament when compared with non-exposed children.[41]

Paroxetine has been associated with cardiac malformations such as atrial and ventricular septal defects, when used in the first trimester.[42] Women taking paroxetine who are planning or who have an unplanned pregnancy should be advised to stop taking the drug,[29] as per product prescribing guidelines. Gradual tapering of the medication is advocated due to the risk of withdrawal symptoms in the neonate.[10] Fetal echocardiography should also be considered in those women who have taken paroxetine in early pregnancy.[27]

Selective serotonin reuptake inhibitors (SSRIs) may be considered in the postpartum period, as small but detectable levels are found in infants of breastfed

Box 20.6 Points to consider in the treatment of pregnant women with psychiatric disorders

- Consultation with patient and caregivers
- Discuss side-effects of therapy and risk of remaining untreated (fetal and maternal)
- Monitor pharmacological therapy closely; start at low dose and monitor frequently
- Consider alternative treatment if primary choice not appropriate

mothers. Fluoxetine is regarded as the safest drug in this class.[29] Neonates are particularly susceptible to the side-effects of SSRIs, serotonin-noradrenaline reuptake inhibitors (SNRIs) and TCAs, with a range of associated perinatal symptoms reported (tremors, shaking, irritability).[43,44] These side-effects are, however, considered to be mild and self-limiting.[22,27,28] No serious side-effects have been reported in infants of breastfeeding mothers.[27]

Use of monoamine oxidase inhibitors (MAOIs) during pregnancy and breastfeeding is not advised, as other antidepressants (e.g. the SSRIs, SNRIs and TCAs) are safer and more efficient.[29,44]

Anxiolytics

Benzodiazepine use is associated with a small increase in the incidence rate of cleft palate in the neonate.[27] Studies have also attributed its use during the organogenesis period of the first trimester to the development of pylorostenosis, premature birth and low birth weight.[27] In the postnatal period, benzodiazepines have been shown to be associated with 'floppy baby' syndrome and withdrawal symptoms for the neonate.[29]

Combined use of benzodiazepines with an SSRI such as paroxetine during the third trimester has led to more harmful neonatal symptoms than with paroxetine alone.[19] Benzodiazepine use therefore should be restricted to the low-dose, short-term treatment of extreme anxiety and limited to a maximum of 4 weeks.[44] As low but detectable levels have been found in breast milk, manufacturers advise the discontinuation of benzodiazepines in breastfeeding mothers.[45]

Antipsychotics

Women of child-bearing age taking antipsychotics (e.g. amisulpride, risperidone and sulpride) should be warned of the possible difficulties that may arise when trying to conceive due to raised prolactin levels associated with their use.[29,46,47] When used during the first trimester the conventional antipsychotics – the phenothiazines – carry a small additional adverse risk of congenital abnormalities when compared with the general population (2.4% *v.* 2%).[22] They have a role in the treatment of women with hyperemesis gravidarum during the first trimester, in small dosages (see above).[26] Haloperidol and chlorpromazine use during the third trimester is associated with poor oral feeding and extrapyramidal abnormalities such as neonatal dyskinesia, seizure and restlessness, which may persist for weeks after birth.[5,48] Haloperidol and penfluridol have been reported to result in a twofold increase in low birth weight among infants born at term.[49]

Atypical antipsychotics are generally associated with weight gain, diabetes, sedation and hypertension during pregnancy.[31] Use of the antipsychotics olanzapine, risperidone, clozapine and quetiapine in the first trimester is not associated with increased risk of malformation compared with those not exposed.[50] However, routinely prescribed clozapine and olanzapine carries an increased risk of gestational diabetes in the developing fetus.[29,32] Additionally, clozapine use is attributed to the development of agranulocytosis in breastfed infants, owing to detectable levels in breast milk.[5,32] Sedation and cardiovascular instability in infants who have been breastfed have also been reported. Pregnant women on clozapine should therefore be switched to an alternative drug.[29] The psychiatrist should take into account family history, diabetes and weight when considering the use of olanzapine, due to the risk of gestational diabetes and weight gain.[51]

Guidelines from NICE do not advise the use of clozapine during pregnancy or in the puerperium.[29] Olanzapine has been detectable in breast milk but it is not clear whether reported adverse reactions to the infant are owing to its use. A study by McKenna *et al*[50] grouped several treatments together.

Mood stabilisers

Sodium valproate

The use of sodium valproate is not recommended during pregnancy, and alternative drugs should be considered in women of child-bearing potential.[29] It is associated with the highest rate of major congenital malformations.[52] Neural tube defects occur in 5–9% of all neonates exposed to sodium valproate during the first trimester.[22] Other known abnormalities of the fetus, which are known to be dose dependent, include: growth retardation, heart defects, urogenital malformation, psychomotor slowness and facial dysmorphias.[44,53] The facial dysmorphias can form part of a well-recognised 'fetal valproate syndrome'. They include broad epicanthic folds, flat nasal bridge, small nose and anteverted nostrils.[54] There is an additional associated risk of impaired cognitive development of the infant exposed to valproate *in utero*.[55]

In women in whom there is no alternative, doses should be limited to 1 g/day, in divided doses and in slow-release form.[29] It is advised that 5 mg of folic acid is given concurrently; however, its value in protection has not been well documented.[56]

If a patient has taken lithium in the first trimester of pregnancy, recommend that the patient has an ultrasound scan of the fetus to check for Ebstein's anomaly.

Concerns about the effect of psychotropic medication during the antenatal and postnatal periods should be discussed with patients alongside discussion about the potential risk of relapse of the mental disorder.

Lithium

Lithium is not recommended for routine use during pregnancy, especially during the first trimester, as it has the potential for severe toxicity to mother and increased teratogenic risk to the infant.[29] A recognised congenital malformation in infants born to mothers treated with lithium during pregnancy is Ebstein's anomaly, which consists of the abnormal downward displacement of the cusps of the tricuspid valve. Ultrasonography at 16–18 weeks is recommended in cases of fetal exposure, as the effect has been shown to manifest during the first trimester.[22]

Other neonatal effects reported in infants exposed to lithium include premature birth, macrosomia, 'floppy baby' syndrome and nephrogenic diabetes insipidus.[54]

High levels of lithium are found in breast milk and so its use is contraindicated in breastfeeding women.[44] Women on lithium who are confirmed to be pregnant in the first trimester should be advised to stop taking lithium gradually over 4 weeks.[29] Guidelines from NICE indicates that women at high risk of relapse should consider switching to alternative medication (e.g. an antipsychotic medication), continue with their medication or stop their medication with a view to restarting in the second trimester if not planning to breastfeed.[29]

In those women continuing with lithium, serum levels should be checked every 4 weeks, and then weekly up to 36 weeks gestation.[29,44,51] Doses should be kept at the lower end of therapeutic levels (normal therapeutic window 0.8–1.0 mmol/l),[54] with provision made for adequate fluid intake. Lithium is renally excreted. Glomerular filtration rate (GFR) increases by 50% during pregnancy and returns to pre-pregnancy levels during parturition. Lithium must be titrated in response to the proportional changes in GFR to maintain therapeutic pre-pregnancy serum concentration levels. The mother's mental state should also be monitored owing to risk of relapse.

Carbamazepine and lamotrigine

Women taking carbamazepine or lamotrigine during pregnancy should be advised to consider an alternative (e.g. antipsychotics), owing to the risk of neural tube development such as spina bifida[5] or cleft palate (7.3/1000 *v.* 0.7/1000 in unexposed neonates)[52,56] with exposure during the first trimester.

Low birth weight, microcephaly, cardiovascular malformation, craniofacial anomalies and growth retardation have been noted in infants exposed to carbamazepine *in utero*.[29,44,52] Likewise, adverse neonate outcomes have been recorded with lamotrigine.

Lamotrigine is not advocated in breastfeeding mothers as it is excreted in the breast milk readily and can induce both serious and non-serious dermatological reactions.[29,30] Breastfeeding mothers using lamotrigine should be warned of the potential development of life-threatening Stevens–Johnson syndrome in the infant.[31] If no alternative method of treatment is deemed suitable, lamotrigine levels need to be closely monitored during pregnancy and into the postpartum period, as increased clearance of the drug may influence its efficacy.[54] If it is used in the postpartum period, breastfeeding mothers should be advised that the onset of any infant rash requires immediate medical attention and immediate cessation of lamotrigine.[29]

Electroconvulsive therapy

Electroconvulsive therapy (ECT) should be considered in patients with severe mental illness, with psychotic symptoms, major depressive disorder or strong suicidal urges.[31,57] Women with postpartum psychosis appear to respond more positively to ECT, with resolution of their psychotic symptoms, than do women with psychosis unrelated to pregnancy.[31]

Reported adverse side-effects are few but may include the general effects of ECT – confusion, memory loss, muscle soreness and headache.[57] Fetal bradyarrhythmias and premature uterine contractions and premature labour have been noted to occur in women undergoing ECT during pregnancy.[57]

Please go to p. 281 for this chapter's learning points and recommended reading

Summary

The treatment of women with psychiatric disorders during pregnancy should be patient centred, dependent on the needs and requirements of the patient and carers. The mental health obstetric complications that may occur in patients if psychotropic treatment is withheld need to be balanced against the pharmacological implications that psychopharmacotherapy may have on the mother and infant.

References

1 Dennis CL, McQueen K. The relationship between infant-feeding outcomes and postpartum depression: a qualitative systematic review. *Pediatrics* 2009; **123**: e736–51.

2 O'Keane V, Marsh MS. Depression during pregnancy. *BMJ* 2007; **334**: 1003–5.

3 Kahn DA, Moline ML, Ross RW, *et al*. Major depression during conception and pregnancy: a guide for patients and families. *Postgrad Med* 2001; (spec no):110–1.

4 Ross LE, Dennis CL. The prevalence of postpartum depression among women with substance use, an abuse history, or chronic illness: a systematic review. *J Womens Health (Larchmt)* 2009; **18**: 475–86.

5 Howard LM. Fertility and pregnancy in women with psychotic disorders. *Eur J Obstet Gynecol Reprod Biol* 2005; **119**: 3–10.

6 Bennett HA, Einarson A, Taddio A, *et al*. Prevalence of depression during pregnancy: systematic review. *Obstet Gynecol* 2004; **103**: 698–709.

7 Evans J, Heron J, Francomb H, *et al*. Cohort study of depressed mood during pregnancy and after childbirth. *BMJ* 2001; **323**: 257–60.

8 World Health Organization. *Medical Eligibility Criteria For Contraceptive Use (4th edn)*. WHO, 2010.

9 Costello DM, Swendsen J, Rose JS, *et al*. Risk and protective factors associated with trajectories of depressed mood from adolescence to early adulthood. *J Consult Clin Psychol* 2008; **76**: 173–83.

10 Bunevicius R, Kusminskas L, Bunevicius A, *et al*. Psychosocial risk factors for depression during pregnancy. *Acta Obstet Gynecol Scand* 2009; **88**: 599–605.

11 Gonsalves L, Schuermeyer I. Treating depression in pregnancy: practical suggestions. *Cleve Clin J Med* 2006; **73**: 1098–104.

12 Cohen LS, Altshuler LL, Harlow BL, *et al*. Relapse of major depression during pregnancy in women who maintain or discontinue antidepressant treatment. *JAMA* 2006; **295**: 499–507.

13 Goodwin TM. Nausea and vomiting of pregnancy: an obstetric syndrome. *Am J Obstet Gynecol* 2002; **186S**: 184–9.

14 Kim DR, Connolly KR, Cristancho P, *et al*. Psychiatric consultation of patients with hyperemesis gravidarum. *Arch Womens Ment Health* 2009; **12**: 61–7.

15 Ismail SK, Kenny L. Review on hyperemesis gravidarum. *Best Pract Res Clin Gastroenterol* 2007; **21**: 755–69.

16 Bottomley C, Bourne T. Management strategies for hyperemesis. *Best Pract Res Clin Obstet Gynaecol* 2009; **23**: 549–64.

17 Kametas NA, Nelson-Piercy C. Hyperemesis gravidarum, gastrointestinal and liver disease in pregnancy. *Obstet Gynaecol Reproductive Medicine* 2008; **18**: 69–75.

18 Sheehan P. Hyperemesis gravidarum – assessment and management. *Aust Fam Physician* 2007; **36**: 698–701.

19 Jewell D, Young G. Interventions for nausea and vomiting in early pregnancy. *Cochrane Database Syst Rev* 2003; **issue 4**: CD000145.

20 Henshaw C. Mood disturbance in the early puerperium: a review. *Arch Womens Ment Health* 2003; **6** (suppl 2): S33–42.

21 Bloch M, Rotenberg N, Koren D, *et al*. Risk factors for early postpartum depressive symptoms. *Gen Hosp Psychiatry* 2006; **28**: 3–8.

22 Pearlstein T. Perinatal depression: treatment options and dilemmas. *J Psychiatry Neurosci* 2008; **33**: 302–18.

23 Marcus SM. Depression during pregnancy: rates, risks and consequences—Motherisk Update 2008. *Can J Clin Pharmacol* 2009; **16**: e15–22.

24 Oppo A, Mauri M, Ramacciotti D, *et al*. Risk factors for postpartum depression: the role of the Postpartum Depression Predictors Inventory-Revised (PDPI-R) – results from the Perinatal Depression-Research & Screening Unit (PNDReScU) study. *Arch Womens Ment Health* 2009; **12**: 239–49.

25 Musters C, McDonald E, Jones I. Management of postnatal depression. *BMJ* 2008; **337**: a736.

26 Payne JL. Antidepressant use in the postpartum period: practical considerations. *Am J Psychiatry* 2007; **164**: 1329–32.

27 Misri S, Kendrick K. Treatment of perinatal mood and anxiety disorders: a review. *Can J Psychiatry* 2007; **52**: 489–98.

28 Ward RK, Zamorski MA. Benefits and risks of psychiatric medications during pregnancy. *Am Fam Physician* 2002; **66**: 629–36.

29 National Institute of Health and Clinical Excellence. *Quick Reference Guide: Antenatal and Postnatal Mental Health – The NICE Guideline on Clinical Management and Service Guidance*. NICE, 2007.

30 Dennis CL, Hodnett E. Psychosocial and psychological interventions for treating postpartum depression. *Cochrane Database Syst Rev* 2007; **issue 4**: CD006116.

31 Sit D, Rothchild AJ, Wisner KL. A review of postpartum psychosis. *Womens Health* 2006; **15**: 352–68.

32 Yaeger D, Smith HG, Altshuler LL. Atypical antipsychotics in the treatment of schizophrenia during pregnancy and the postpartum. *Am J Psychiatry* 2006; **163**: 2064–70.

33 Irving CB, Saylan M. Mother and baby units for schizophrenia. *Cochrane Database Syst Rev* 2007; **issue 1**: Art. No.: CD006333.

34 Hallberg P, Sjoblom V. The use of selective serotonin reuptake inhibitors during pregnancy and breast-feeding: a review and clinical aspects. *J Clin Psychopharmacol* 2005; **25**: 59–73.

35 Nonacs R, Cohen LS. Assessment and treatment of depression during pregnancy: an update. *Psychiatr Clin North Am* 2003; **26**: 547–62.

36 Bonari L, Pinto N, Ahn E, *et al*. Perinatal risks of untreated depression during pregnancy. *Can J Psychiatry* 2004; **49**: 726–35.

37 Alder J, Fink N, Bitzer J, *et al*. Depression and anxiety during pregnancy: a risk factor for obstetric, fetal and neonatal outcome? A critical review of the literature. *J Matern Fetal Neonatal Med* 2007; **20**: 189–209.

38 Howard LM, Goss C, Leese M, *et al*. Medical outcome of pregnancy in women with psychotic disorders and their infants in the first year after birth. *Br J Psychiatry* 2003; **182**: 63–7.

39 Andrade SE, Raebel MA, Brown J, *et al*. Use of antidepressant medications during pregnancy: a multisite study. *Am J Obstet Gynecol* 2008; **198**: 194. e1–5.

40 Davis RL, Rubanowice D, McPhillips H, *et al*; HMO Research Network Center for Education, Research in Therapeutics. Risks of congenital malformations and perinatal events among infants exposed to antidepressant medications during pregnancy. *Pharmacoepidemiol Drug Saf* 2007; **16**: 1086–94.

41 Nulman I, Rovet J, Stewart DE, *et al*. Neurodevelopment of children exposed in utero to antidepressant drugs. *N Engl J Med* 1997; **336**: 258–62.

42 GlaxoSmithKline. *Study EPIP083: Bupropion and Paroxetine, Epidemiology Study. Preliminary Report on Bupropion in Pregnancy and the Occurrence of Cardiovascular and Major Congenital Malformation*. GSK Medicine, 2005 (http://download.gsk-clinicalstudyregister.com/files/3493.pdf).

43 Ferreira E, Carceller AM, Agogué C, *et al*. Effects of selective serotonin reuptake inhibitors and venlafaxine during pregnancy in term and preterm neonates. *Pediatrics* 2007; **119**: 52–9.

44 Kohen D. Psychotropic medication in pregnancy. *Adv Psychiatr Treat* 2004; **10**: 59–66.

45 British National Formulary. http://www.bnf.org/bnf/

46 Liu-Seifert H, Kinon BJ, Tennant CJ, *et al*. Sexual dysfunction in patients with schizophrenia treated with conventional antipsychotics or risperidone. *Neuropsychiatr Dis Treat* 2009; **5**: 47–54.

47 Bostwick JR, Guthrie SK, Ellingrod VL. Antipsychotic-induced hyperprolactinemia. *Pharmacotherapy* 2009; **29**: 64–73.

48 Kennedy D. Antipsychotic drugs in pregnancy and breast feeding. *Aust Prescr* 2007; **30**: 162–3.

49 Diav-Citrin O, Shechtman S, Ornoy S, *et al*. Safety of haloperidol and penfluridol in pregnancy: a multicenter, prospective, controlled study. *J Clin Psychiatry* 2005; **66**: 317–22.

50 McKenna K, Koren G, Tetelbaum M, *et al*. Pregnancy outcome of women using atypical antipsychotic drugs: a prospective comparative study. *J Clin Psychiatry* 2005; **66**: 444–9.

51 Newham JJ, Thomas SH, MacRitchie K, *et al*. Birth weight of infants after maternal exposure to typical and atypical antipsychotics: prospective comparison study. *Br J Psychiatry* 2008; **192**: 333–7.

52 Nguyen HT, Sharma V, McIntyre RS. Teratogenesis associated with antibipolar agents. *Adv Ther* 2009; **26**: 281–94.

53 Kini U, Adab N, Vinten J, *et al*. Liverpool and Manchester Neurodevelopmental Study Group. *Dysmorphic features: an important clue to the diagnosis and severity of fetal anticonvulsant syndromes. Arch Dis Child Fetal Neonatal Ed* 2006; **91**: F90–5.

54 Dodd S, Berk M. The safety of medications for the treatment of bipolar disorder during pregnancy and the puerperium. *Curr Drug Saf* 2006; **1**: 25–33.

55 Meador KJ, Baker GA, Browning N, *et al*; NEAD Study Group. Cognitive function at 3 years of age after fetal exposure to antiepileptic drugs. *N Engl J Med* 2009; **360**: 1597–605.

56 Holmes LB, Baldwin EJ, Smith CR, *et al*. Increased frequency of isolated cleft palate in infants exposed to lamotrigine during pregnancy. *Neurology* 2008; **70**: 2152–8.

57 Anderson EL, Reti IM. ECT in pregnancy: a review of the literature from 1941 to 2007. *Psychosom Med* 2009; **71**: 235–42.

58 Taylor D, Paton C, Kapur S. *The Maudsley Prescribing Guidelines in Psychiatry* (11th edn). Wiley-Blackwell, 2012.

Appendix

able 20A Psychotropic drugs in pregnancy and breastfeeding

harmacological gent	1st trimester	2nd trimester	3rd trimester	Breastfeeding	Notes
CAs			Caution*		Lowest known risk during pregnancy;* documented perinatal complications include withdrawal symptoms of irritability, convulsions in fetus, eating and sleeping difficulties at high doses, caution 3rd trimester[45]
Clomipramine	Unsafe[27]	Caution[45]	Caution[45]	Caution[45]	Congenital heart disease.[27] More dangerous in overdose than other antidepressants[45]
mipramine	Caution[45]	Caution[45]	Caution[45]	Caution[45]	More dangerous in overdose than other antidepressants[45]
Amytriptyline	Caution[45]	Caution[45]	Caution[45]	Caution[45]	More dangerous in overdose than other antidepressants[45]
Nortriptyline	Caution[45]	Caution[45]	Caution[45]	Caution[45]	More dangerous in overdose than other antidepressants[45]
Lofepramine	Caution[45]	Caution[45]	Caution[45]	Caution[45]	No more likely to cause death in overdose than SSRIs[45]
SRIs					Increased risk of spontaneous abortions not statistically significant.[11] May be associated with increased risk of PPHN during 2nd half of pregnancy.[22,27] Neonatal behavioural syndrome[22]
Fluoxetine	Caution[29]	Caution[29]	Unsafe[27]	Unsafe[27,45]	Concern over increased risk of persistent pulmonary hypertension of the newborn in 2nd half of pregnancy; high blood pressure at high doses; manufacturer advises avoid[45] as high levels in breast milk reported
Paroxetine	Unsafe[27]	Unsafe[27]	Unsafe[27]	Good[45]	Amounts too small to be hamful[45] expecially for postpartum depression[27]
Sertraline	Good[27]	Good[27]	Good[27]	Good[27,45]	No data for congenital malformation or impaired neurological malformation. Not thought to be harmful in short term use[45]
Escitalopram	Caution[45]	Caution[45]	Caution[45]	Unsafe[45]	Neonatal toxicity in animal studies.[45] Manufacturer advises avoid[45] in breastfeeding
Citalopram	Caution[45]	Caution[45]	Caution[45]	Unsafe – high levels in breast milk	Case of sleep disturbance. Manufacturer advises avoid[45] in breastfeeding; use during pregnancy only if benefits outweigh risks
Fluvoxamine	Caution[45]	Caution[45]	Caution[45]	Unsafe[45]	Manufacturer advises avoid[45] in breastfeeding; use only if benefits outweigh risks
RIs					
Venlafaxine	Caution[27]	Caution[27]	Caution[27]	Unsafe[45]	No increased incidence of birth defects;[22,27] low levels with no adverse outcomes;[27] manufacturer advises avoid[45] in breastfeeding and avoid unless potential benefit outweighs risk
Mirtazapine	Unsafe	Unsafe	Unsafe	Unsafe	Insufficient data on risk. Manufacturer advises avoid
Mood stabilisers					
Lithium	Unsafe[29]	Caution[45]	Caution[45]	Unsafe[29]	Not to use during 1st trimester or perinatally as risk of cardiac malformation and floppy baby; polyhydramnios, diabetes insipidus and foetal goitre in 2nd and 3rd trimesters; not recommended during breastfeeding, plus adverse effect on infant
Valproate	Unsafe[29]	Caution[45]	Caution[45]	Avoid	Not to use during 1st trimester or perinatally. Risk of NTD and foetal valproate syndrome; amount too small to be harmful (BNF)

contd

Table 20A ***contd***

Pharmacological agent	1st trimester	2nd trimester	3rd trimester	Breastfeeding	Notes
Anxiolytics					Do not routinely prescribe. Consider for short-term treatment of extreme anxiety and agitation[29]
Diazepam	Unsafe[29]	Unsafe[29]	Unsafe[29]	Unsafe[29]	Avoid regular use; high dose during late pregnancy ca cause neonatal hypothermia, hypotonia and respirato depression[27,45]
Alprazolam	Unsafe[29]	Unsafe[29]	Unsafe[29]	Unsafe[29]	High dose during late pregnancy can cause neonatal hypothermia, hypotonia and respiratory depression[45]
Lorazepam	Unsafe[29]	Unsafe[29]	Unsafe[29]	Unsafe[29]	High dose during late pregnancy can cause neonatal hypothermia, hypotonia and respiratory depression[45]
Oxazepam	Unsafe[29]	Unsafe[29]	Unsafe[29]	Unsafe[29]	High dose during late pregnancy can cause neonatal hypothermia, hypotonia and respiratory depression[45]
Antipsychotics					
First generation					
Flupentixol	Caution[45]	Caution[45]	Caution[45]	Caution[45]	Manufacturer advises use only if potential benefit outweighs risk; avoid in breastfeeding unless absolute necessary
Haloperidol	Caution	Caution	Unsafe[45]	Unsafe[58]	Preferred low-dose therapy for treatment of schizophrenia;[29] ultrasound may be required during 1st trimester;[22] not to be used as depot in pregnant women;[29] EPS in neonate[45]
Chlorpromazine	Unsafe[27]	Caution	Unsafe[45]	Unsafe	Preferred low-dose therapy for treatment of schizophrenia;[29] Reported risk of non-specific teratogenic effects; EPS reported.[27] Can be used in low dose for antiemetic effect in patients with hyperemesis gravidarum
Second generation					Reported weight gain, diabetes, sedation and hypertension during pregnancy; obstetric complicatio include gestational diabetes, pre-eclampsia and C-section
Aripiprazole	Caution[45]	Caution[45]	Caution[45]	Unsafe[45]	Manufacturer advises use only if potential benefit outweighs risk and avoid in breastfeeding
Clozapine	Unsafe[29]	Unsafe[29]	Unsafe[29]	Unsafe[29]	Congenital anomalies reported. Gestational diabetes, pregnancy-induced hypertension, agranulocytosis and orthostatic hypertension. Manufacturer advises avoid i breastfeeding
Risperidone	Caution[45]	Caution[45]	Caution[45]	Unsafe[45]	No reported congenital malformations;[31] 3rd trimester extrapyramidal effects;[45] manufacurer advises avoid in breastfeeding
Olanzapine	Caution[45]	Caution[45]	Caution[45]	Unsafe[45]	Manufacturer advises use only if potential benefit outweighs risk and avoid in breastfeeding.[45] Neonatal lethargy, tremor and hypertonia reported
Quetiapine	Caution[45]	Caution[45]	Caution[45]	Unsafe[45]	No reported congenital malformations.[31] Manufacturer advises use only if potential benefit outweighs risk and avoid in breastfeeding

BNF, *British National Formulary*; EPS, extrapyramidal side-effects; NTD, neural tube defects; PPHN, persistent pulmonary hypertension of t newborn; TCAs, tricyclic antidepressants; SRIs, serotonin reuptake inhibitors; SSRIs, selective serotonin reuptake inhibitors.

Learning points

- If a contraceptive pill is missed for over 12 hours, patients should be advised to immediately use barrier methods of contraception for the next 7 days.
- Clinicians should consider the possibility of drug interaction when prescribing contraceptives, especially those containing hormonal composites.
- Depo-Provera given as a single intramuscular dose of 150 mg should be considered in psychiatric patients with comorbidities, those on multiple medications and those who misuse drugs and alcohol.
- Care should be taken if there are significant risks of thromboembolic disease.
- Contraceptive choice should reflect patient preference, lifestyle and compliance.
- Discussion of contraceptive choice with patients on long-term medication may involve primary, secondary and community mental health providers.
- Women using paroxetine should avoid pregnancy, as it is associated with cardiac malformations if taken in the first trimester.
- If a patient has taken lithium in the first trimester of pregnancy, recommend that she has an ultrasound scan of the fetus to detect Ebstein's anomaly.
- Concerns about the effect of taking psychotropic medication during the antenatal and postnatal periods should be discussed with patients but should also be balanced against the potential risk of relapse of the mental disorder.

Recommended reading

Callahan TL, Caughley AB. *Blueprints: Obstetrics and Gynaecology* (8th edn). Lippincott, 2009.

Edmonds K (ed.) *Dewhurst's Textbook of Obstetrics and Gynaecology* (8th edn). Blackwell, 2012.

Guillebaud J. *Contraception Today* (5th edn). Informa Healthcare, 2003.

Henshaw C, Cox J, Barton J. *Modern Management of Perinatal Psychiatric Disorders*. RCPsych Publications, 2009.

Royal College of Psychiatrists' website (http://www.rcpsych.ac.uk) for information leaflets for women, their partners and friends on 'Mental health in pregnancy' and 'Severe mental illness following pregnancy'.

21
Cancer

Mark Tuthill and Jonathan Waxman

Written by oncologists, this chapter describes the symptoms of cancers of the lung, breast and gastrointestinal tract, as well as gynaecological, urological, hepatological, neurological and skin cancers. The criteria for referral to specialists are set out and information is provided about chemotherapy, radiotherapy, end-of-life care and oncology emergencies.

Introduction

Cancer affects one in three people during their lifetime and is a leading cause of death in higher-income countries. Many psychiatrists will manage patients with psychiatric illness who are at high risk of developing, or who have been diagnosed and treated for, cancer. This chapter provides essential information for psychiatrists on the presentation of 'red flag' symptoms of cancer, the referral of patients with suspected cancer, the management of common cancers and the recommended screening intervals for the UK national screening programmes for breast, bowel and cervical cancer. Some websites that provide useful information for patients and healthcare professionals are given in Table 21.1. The information in this chapter should be used only as a guide, as clinical practice and recommendations can change.

Cancer is feared by the general population because it is a leading cause of death. However, it is a highly treatable illness:

- many patients with early cancers and some forms of advanced cancer such as lymphoma or testicular cancer will be cured with modern therapies
- outcomes for patients with advanced cancer are continually improving due to advances in drug treatment.

Epidemiology of cancer

Cancer is caused by complex genetic changes which lead to uncontrolled cellular proliferation. These genetic changes may be present at birth or develop as a result of environmental exposures, lifestyle factors and increasing age. Individuals with mental disorders have a high prevalence of tobacco smoking, obesity and high alcohol use, and may have diets low in fresh fruit and vegetables, all of which are associated with an increased risk of developing cancer.

Tobacco smoking is the leading preventable cause of cancer of the lung, head, neck, bowel, mouth, pharynx, pancreas, kidney and bladder. The risk of cancer is proportional to the duration of smoking and number of cigarettes smoked and is enhanced by alcohol consumption, particularly for cancers of the oropharynx, oesophagus and stomach. Smoking cessation or

Table 21.1 Websites that provide useful information on cancer for patients and healthcare professionals

Website	Organisation	Information
www.macmillan.org.uk	Macmillan Cancer Support	Comprehensive information for patients and healthcare professionals about cancer and treatment of cancer, along with leaflets
www.nice.org.uk	National Institute for Health and Clinical Excellence	Current national guidelines on cancer care
www.cancerscreening.nhs.uk	NHS Cancer Screening Programmes	Information about the UK national cancer screening programmes
www.cancer.gov	National Cancer Institute at the US National Institutes of Health	Comprehensive information for patients and healthcare professionals about cancer treatment and management
www.cancerresearchuk.org	Cancer Research UK charity	Detailed information about cancer news, statistics, science and health

reduction in cigarette consumption leads to a significant decline in lifetime risk of developing lung and other smoking-related cancers. Many patients with psychiatric disorders smoke tobacco, so smoking cessation is the most important way to reduce their risk of developing cancer. Detailed information on smoking cessation can be found in Chapter 6.

Alcohol is a carcinogen, and excess consumption significantly increases lifetime risk of cancers of the oral cavity, pharynx, oesophagus, liver, breast, pancreas, stomach and large bowel. Alcohol also causes liver cirrhosis (see Chapter 17), which is an important risk factor for the development of hepatocellular cancer.

Obesity (Chapter 7) is associated with a modestly increased risk of endometrial, bowel, kidney, pancreatic and prostate cancers, and a twofold increase in breast cancer risk. The precise details of the molecular link between cancer and obesity are unclear; however, studies have shown that weight loss in morbidly obese patients reduces the chance of developing cancer.[1] A diet high in fresh fruit and vegetables and low in red meat may reduce an individual's lifetime risk of developing cancer.

Sexually transmitted infection (Chapter 19) with certain subtypes of human papilloma virus (HPV) is strongly associated with the development of cervical cancer. The newly licensed HPV vaccine protects against infection with the most oncogenic strains of the virus and is being offered to all 12- and 13-year-old girls (see 'Cancer screening', below).

The cancer referral pathway

The majority of patients are referred by their general practitioner (GP) to a specialist hospital clinic for investigation of a suspected cancer. Doctors who suspect cancer should refer patients to hospital using a dedicated form within 24 hours of assessment. National guidelines currently require that patients should be seen and assessed by a specialist within 2 weeks of referral.

Patients with symptoms such as *rectal bleeding* or *unexplained iron-deficiency anaemia* may be referred direct for investigations such as colonoscopy or endoscopy without having to see a specialist. If an abnormality is detected, then a direct referral will be made to a specialist for an assessment.

When patients are referred for assessment, they will undergo a detailed clinical examination and urgent investigations. If an abnormality is found at clinical or radiological assessment, then a tissue biopsy will be taken to confirm or exclude cancer. Some services, such

National guidelines currently require that patients should be seen and assessed by a specialist within 2 weeks of referral, although patients with symptoms such as rectal bleeding or unexplained iron-deficiency anaemia may be referred direct for appropriate investigation, without having to see a specialist.

as those for breast cancer, offer a 'one stop' service, which allows patients to have all relevant tests in one day.

Many patients will receive their cancer diagnosis from a surgeon or medical specialist such as a respiratory physician or gastroenterologist. In the UK, all clinicians managing patients with cancer work as part of a multidisciplinary team, which takes overall responsibility for care. Members of that team include oncologists, surgeons, radiologists, medical specialists and specialist nurses. Meetings are usually held weekly and are where all important management decisions are made.

Cancer is usually diagnosed by a tissue biopsy, which requires specialist histological staining. The analysis takes around 7 working days to complete, provides detailed information about the cancer and allows treatment to be planned. Patients diagnosed with cancer undergo 'staging' investigations such as computerised tomography (CT), magnetic resonance imaging (MRI) or ultrasound scanning to assess the local and distant extent of the cancer. Once the diagnosis of cancer and staging are complete, definitive treatment should start within 4 weeks.

After diagnosis, patients may be assigned a specialist nurse to provide guidance and support during treatment. Patients with advanced cancer may be referred to community Macmillan nurses, who usually work from local hospices. Referral to a Macmillan nurse can be made by either the hospital specialist or the patient's GP. After a referral is received, the patient is initially assessed by telephone and a home visit may be arranged. Information about local services is provided, with telephone numbers to call in case the patient becomes unwell in the community.

Referral guidelines for suspected cancer

The symptoms of cancer are non-specific, making the clinical diagnosis difficult. Alarm or 'red flag' symptoms of cancer necessitate urgent investigation and urgent referral to specialist hospital clinics for assessment. They include:

- haematuria
- rectal bleeding
- haemoptysis
- dysphagia.

Nonetheless, it is important to remember that many 'red flag' symptoms can be caused by non-malignant conditions like urinary tract infection or haemorrhoids.

> Many 'red flag' symptoms such as haematuria, rectal bleeding, haemoptysis or dysphagia can be caused by non-malignant conditions. The majority of investigations for suspected cancer will turn out to be normal.

The majority of investigations for suspected cancer will turn out to be normal. Moreover, although 'red flag' symptoms have been widely incorporated into clinical practice, the evidence behind their use is limited. Clinical assessment and judicious use of investigations are an important part of the assessment of patients with suspected cancer. An individual's risk of cancer is related to their age, which is taken into account in the referral guidelines. The clinical recommendations for specialist referral in this chapter are based on current guidelines from the National Institute for Health and Clinical Excellence (NICE), which can be found at http://guidance.nice.org.uk.

Lung cancer

Tobacco smoking causes around 90% of all lung cancer, which is the commonest cause of death from cancer in men and women in the UK. Risk factors for lung cancer include increasing age, a history of cancer (especially head and neck cancer), asbestos exposure and smoking-related lung disease such as bronchiectasis and emphysema. Five-year outcomes in the UK are poor and survival is only 7%. Major reasons for poor outcomes in the UK are a lack of specialist cardiothoracic surgical services, delay in referral and imaging, and the fact that lung cancer affects a disenfranchised population. Patients with lung cancer are underrepresented in political and medical terms as most are too unwell to lobby or create publicity to highlight the need for better treatments. The development of improved services and treatment for lung cancer is a major health priority.

Referral for suspected lung cancer

In a smoker who is 40 years old or more, the following symptoms should prompt urgent referral to a lung cancer specialist:

- persistent haemoptysis
- shortness of breath
- chest pain with a history of asbestos exposure

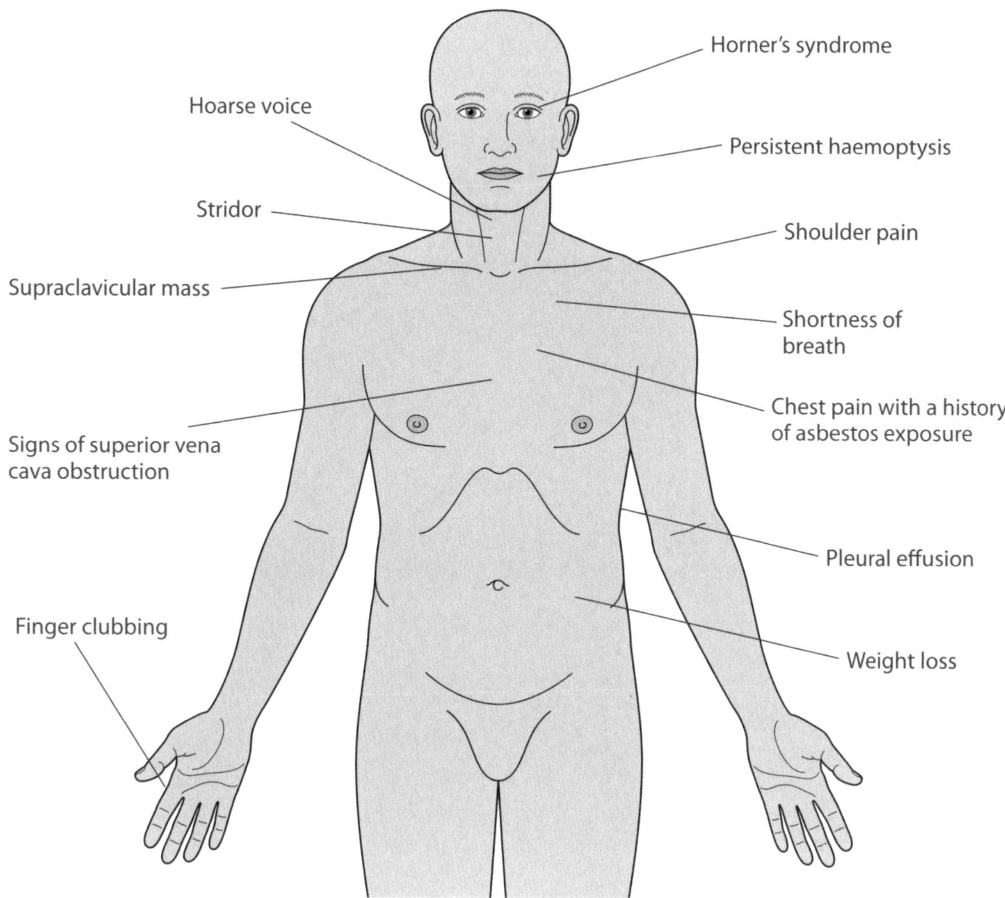

Fig. 21.1 Lung cancer.

- chest or shoulder pain
- voice hoarseness
- weight loss.

Clinical features that suggest lung cancer are:

- pleural effusion
- haemoptysis
- supraclavicular mass
- Horner's syndrome
- stridor
- obstruction in the superior vena cava
- finger clubbing
- cervical or supraclavicular lymphadenopathy.

Patients with clinical signs of stridor or obstruction in the superior vena cava should be immediately referred to hospital for management. Haemoptysis, or symptoms persisting for 3 weeks and over, warrant urgent referral for a chest X-ray and consideration for urgent referral to a hospital specialist.

The management of lung cancer

The clinical behaviour of lung cancer is related to its histological subtype. Non-small-cell lung cancer (NSLC) is potentially curable with surgery and/or chemo-radiotherapy. Small-cell lung cancer (SCLC) disseminates widely and is treated with systemic chemotherapy and consolidation radiotherapy for patients who respond well to chemotherapy. Patients with lung cancer are investigated with CT and positron emission tomography (PET) scanning to look for local or distant spread. Bronchoscopy and thoracoscopy may be used to assess regional lymph-node involvement before surgery. The main surgical procedures for NSLC are lobectomy, bi-lobectomy and pneumonectomy, which are all associated with significant morbidity. Many patients with lung cancer have coexisting emphysema and should undergo lung function tests (see Chapter 13) to ensure that residual lung function will be adequate after surgery. Radiotherapy may be offered to patients who are unsuitable for surgery. Cure rates for radical radiotherapy range up to 15%, and up to 80% for surgery in young patients.

Patients with advanced lung cancer can be treated with chemotherapy or radiotherapy. The median survival for patients with metastatic lung cancer is usually only 6–9 months. Chemotherapy treatments for lung cancer are out-patient procedures, are well tolerated and offer modest improvements in survival and symptom control. Newer oral drugs are available and are increasingly being used instead of chemotherapy. Patients with metastatic lung cancer will usually need palliative care, as the development of liver, bone and brain metastasis is common.

Breast cancer

Breast cancer is the commonest cancer in women: the lifetime risk is around one in nine. Breast cancer outcomes in the UK are generally excellent, with around 80% of women with breast cancer being cured when the condition is detected early and treated with surgery, hormone manipulation, radiotherapy and adjuvant chemotherapy. A reassuring message should be imparted at referral for a breast assessment, as there is a reasonable chance of a benign diagnosis (breast lumps are common) or cancer cure.

Referral for suspected breast cancer

Breast cancer usually presents as a painless breast lump, although slow-growing tumours and small early tumours may be detected by breast screening (Figs 21.2, 21.3; and see below on screening). Risk factors for breast cancer include increasing age, late menopause, strong family history, postmenopausal obesity, late age at first pregnancy, excess alcohol consumption and use of hormone replacement therapy (HRT).

The clinical features that suggest a cancerous breast lump include:

- in a woman aged 30 years and older a discrete hard lump with fixation, with or without skin tethering that persists after menstruation or presents after menopause
- unilateral eczematous or nipple changes not responding to topical treatments

> In the UK, the outcome of breast cancer, when it is detected early, is generally excellent, with around 80% of women being cured.

- new nipple distortion
- unilateral bloody discharge.

Breast cancer is rare in women aged under 30 years and urgent referral of women under 30 is not necessary unless: the lump is enlarging, fixed or hard, or there is concern due to a strong family history of breast cancer. Breast pain without breast changes is not a sign of breast cancer and does not require mammography to exclude breast cancer.

Breast cancer can occur in older men. Those affected present with unilateral firm subareolar mass, with or without nipple distortion or skin changes. Patients are usually seen in 'one stop' clinics that combine radiological, clinical and histological assessments. These clinics aim to produce a diagnosis within a day.

The management of breast cancer

Overall cure rates have improved by 15–20% over the past 15 years because of screening and the widespread use of adjuvant therapy.[2] Advanced breast cancer is sensitive to chemotherapy and hormonal treatments and the median survival of patients with advanced breast cancer has doubled in recent years because of modern treatments.

The primary treatment for breast cancer is lumpectomy and axillary node dissection. Breast cancer

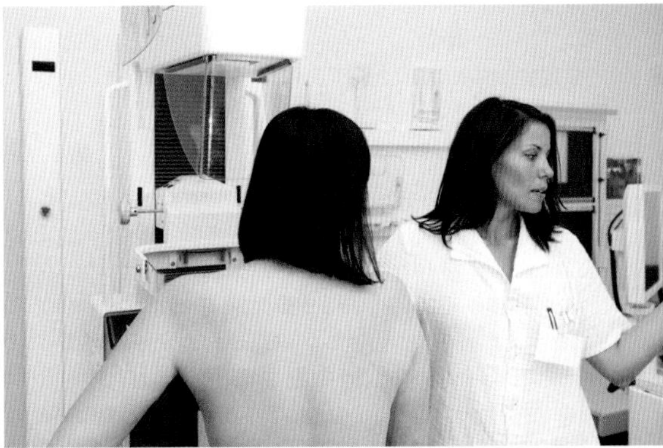

Fig. 21.2 Nurse with young woman having a mammogram.

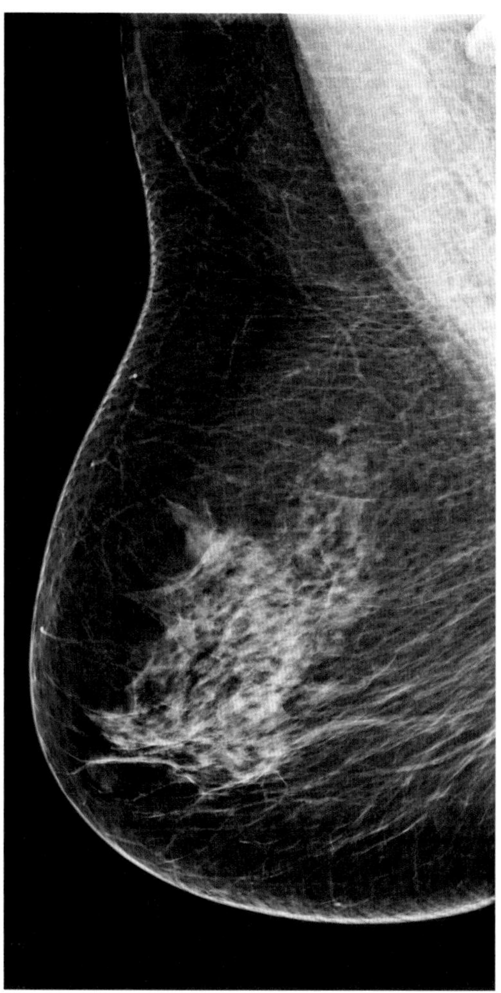

Fig. 21.3 Mammogram of breast with cancer.

surgery is changing, as outcomes after wide local excision and radiotherapy are similar to those achieved with mastectomy.

Sentinel node biopsy is increasingly used to assess axillary lymph nodes. Women with sentinel or clinically involved axillary lymph nodes are offered axillary dissection, which may be complicated by lymphoedema. Women undergoing mastectomy can now be offered immediate breast reconstruction. Radiotherapy after wide local excision reduces the risk of local recurrence.

After surgery, women with oestrogen-sensitive breast cancer are treated with oral tamoxifen for 5 years, which

The antidepressants paroxetine and fluoxetine and antipsychotic medications such as haloperidol inhibit the metabolism of tamoxifen, leading to a reduction in that drug's clinical efficacy; these medications can therefore reduce survival rates from breast cancer. If a patient on tamoxifen requires a psychotropic drug, it is essential to check whether the new or existing psychotropic medication inhibits the liver cytochrome P450 enzyme isoform CYPD6, which metabolises tamoxifen to its active form.[3]

reduces the risk of recurrence and mortality by 30%. Aromatase inhibitors such as anastrozole reduce the chance of recurrence and may be used as an alternative to tamoxifen in postmenopausal women. The current standard is for sequential treatment with both agents, which provides a survival gain over monotherapy.[2] The psychiatrist should be aware that tamoxifen can cause vaginal bleeding, which may be due to endometrial hyperplasia or cancer, and so requires investigation.

Women with axillary lymph node involvement, large or high-grade tumours may be offered adjuvant chemotherapy. Women with HER2-positive breast cancer should receive adjuvant treatment with trastuzumab (Herceptin), which improves survival rates by around 10%.[4]

Ductal carcinoma *in situ* (DCIS) is a non-invasive proliferation of the ductal epithelium which may be diagnosed on mammography. It is considered a pre-malignant condition and treated with surgical excision followed by radiotherapy and tamoxifen.

In psychiatric practice, women with breast cancer and without mental capacity may be difficult to diagnose and treat. Legal advice and court judgments (see Chapter 11) may be needed to manage patients without the mental capacity to consent to investigations and treatment.

Cancers of the upper gastrointestinal tract

Cancers of the upper gastrointestinal tract include those of the oesophagus, stomach and duodenum, biliary tree, liver and pancreas. Symptoms are non-specific and patients tend to present with advanced disease, which limits the overall chance of cure. One of the main risk factors for the development of oesophageal carcinoma is Barrett's oesophagus, where the normal squamous cell lining is replaced by intestinal-type columnar cell lining. Although it has been recommended since 2005 that patients with Barrett's undergo screening, evidence of any improvement in the rate of diagnosis of oesophageal cancer or of a survival benefit is limited.

Gastric cancer is the seventh commonest cancer diagnosed in the UK and is found in around 7000 people each year. Risk factors for gastric cancer include surgery for peptic ulcer (> 20 years ago), dysplasia, atrophic gastritis, intestinal metaplasia and achalasia.

Around 4000 people each year are diagnosed with pancreatic cancer. Most of these patients present with:

- painless obstructive jaundice
- weight loss
- back pain
- cachexia.

The symptoms of pancreatic cancer are non-specific and many patients present with advanced disease. Patients with suspected pancreatic cancer should be referred for an urgent specialist assessment.

Referral for suspected cancer of the upper gastrointestinal tract

Patients *of all ages* with dyspepsia should be referred for urgent endoscopy or specialist assessment if they have:

- dysphagia
- chronic gastrointestinal bleeding
- progressive unintentional weight loss
- persistent vomiting
- iron-deficiency anaemia
- an epigastric mass
- an abnormal barium meal result.

Patients *aged 55 years or more* who have recent-onset dyspepsia should be urgently referred for endoscopy. Patients *under 55 years old*, without these symptoms or signs, do not usually need endoscopy as they have a low risk of developing cancer. Patients with iron-deficiency anaemia and weight loss should be considered for endoscopy. Clinical examination and blood tests for iron-deficiency anaemia should be performed at the initial clinical assessment.

> Patients who have recent onset dyspepsia should be urgently referred for endoscopy (as above).

> The symptoms of cancers of the upper gastrointestinal tract are non-specific and patients tend to present with advanced disease, which limits the overall chance of cure.

The management of cancer of the upper gastrointestinal tract

Surgery is the primary treatment for early oesophageal and gastric cancers. Around 80% of patients with early-stage tumours and 20–30% of patients with more advanced tumours will be cured by surgery. Of all presenting patients, only 30% will be suitable for surgery, and just 30% of these patients will have a potentially curative resection. Computerised tomography and endoscopic ultrasound are used to assess tumour invasion and local lymph node involvement. Pre- or post-operative chemotherapy may be given to reduce the chance of recurrence.

Oesophageal cancer often causes dysphagia, which can be managed by endoscopic stent placement, radiotherapy and/or chemotherapy. Palliative chemotherapy for oesophageal and gastric cancer has modest survival benefits (no more that 2–3 weeks) but does improve quality of life.

Unfortunately, only 14% of patients with pancreatic cancer are suitable for surgical resection, and the majority who do undergo resection will suffer from relapse of the tumour within 2 years. Biliary obstruction is a common complication of pancreatic cancer and is rapidly relieved by endoscopic insertion of a metal biliary stent. Palliative chemotherapy with intravenous gemcitabine is well tolerated and improves quality of life; however, the survival gain is only around 1 month.[5]

Cancers of the lower gastrointestinal tract

After lung and breast cancer, colorectal cancers are the third commonest group. Each year in the UK, colorectal cancer will be diagnosed in around 37 000 people and cause 13 000 deaths. The main risk factors for colorectal cancer are a strong family history of bowel cancer, inflammatory bowel disease, and hereditary conditions such as Peutz–Jeghers syndrome and hereditary non-polyposis coli.

Colorectal cancer develops over many years, first as a polyp or adenoma, which progresses through different stages into an invasive bowel cancer. Adenomas and cancers may cause bleeding that can be detected by screening for faecal occult blood or bleeding that is noticed by patients.

Referral for suspected cancer of the lower gastrointestinal tract

The symptoms of cancer of the lower gastrointestinal tract, including the bowel, are non-specific and current guidelines recommend that it is reasonable to use a period of 'treat, watch and wait' in patients with equivocal symptoms before referral. Patients with symptoms may be directly referred for a colonoscopy by their GP or referred for assessment by a gastroenterologist or colorectal surgeon. Patients should be examined, including a digital rectal examination, before referral. Any patients with a right-sided lower abdominal mass suggestive of bowel cancer or a palpable rectal mass should be urgently referred, irrespective of age. A full blood count may be helpful in diagnosing iron-deficiency anaemia, but urgent referral should not be delayed pending the results.

Referral for urgent assessment and colonoscopy is recommended if:

- patients aged over 40 with rectal bleeding or persistent change in their bowel habit towards looser stools
- patients aged over 60 with rectal bleeding, without anal symptoms, persisting for over 6 weeks
- unexplained iron deficiency in men (haemoglobin level of 11 g/100 ml or below) or non-menstruating women (haemoglobin of 10 g/100 ml or less) should be referred for urgent assessment.

The management of cancer of the lower gastrointestinal tract

Cancers of the large bowel can occur within the colon or rectum and are treated by surgical excision. Tumours within the right or left colon are treated by hemicolectomy. Patients with tumours within the rectum are treated with an anterior resection and may require a stoma. Pre-operative chemo-radiotherapy may be used to shrink rectal tumours to improve the chances of a curative resection. Adjuvant chemotherapy is offered to patients who have a high risk of recurrence after surgery. Patients who develop isolated recurrences within the liver may be offered a potentially curative liver resection. The outlook for patients with metastatic colorectal cancer is improving, and median survival is now over 18 months with modern chemotherapy treatments.

Gynaecological cancer

Cancers of the female genital tract include ovarian cancer, endometrial cancer and cancers of the Fallopian tube and ovary. Endometrial cancer mainly occurs in post-menopausal women. The main risk factors are obesity, unopposed oestrogens and previous or current use of tamoxifen. Ovarian cancer is the most lethal of all the gynaecological cancers and has non-specific symptoms. Many women with ovarian cancer will have had symptoms for months prior to diagnosis, which are often attributed to other conditions, such as irritable bowel disease.

Referral for suspected gynaecological cancer

The symptoms of gynaecological cancer include:

- a change in the menstrual cycle
- post-coital bleeding
- inter-menstrual bleeding
- post-menopausal bleeding
- vaginal discharge.

Vulval cancer develops from vulval intraepithelial neoplasia (VIN); in this pre-malignant phase, it is generally treated with topical creams. Patients should undergo a full pelvic examination and full speculum examination of the cervix if they present with:

- pruritus, which may be thought to be a functional symptom but should not be ignored
- pain
- ulceration

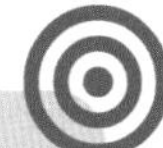

Many women with ovarian cancer will have had symptoms for months prior to diagnosis; these are often attributed to other conditions, such as irritable bowel disease.

- bleeding
- a lump.

If significant abnormalities are detected by clinical examination or cervical smear, then patients should be referred for an urgent gynaecological assessment. Urgent referral for gynaecological assessment is also recommended when:

- a female patient has a palpable abdominal or pelvic mass, not thought to be fibroids (an urgent ultrasound is also required)
- a post-menopausal woman who is not taking hormone replacement therapy (HRT) has vaginal bleeding
- a post-menopausal woman who is taking HRT has unexplained vaginal bleeding which persists after cessation of HRT.

The symptoms of ovarian cancer are non-specific and include:

- lower abdominal pains
- bloating
- constipation
- urinary symptoms
- back pain.

If ovarian cancer is suspected, clinicians must perform an abdominal and pelvic examination and consider referral of the patient to a gynaecologist. Although the tumour marker CA125 is raised in 80% of patients with advanced ovarian cancer, it is not specific for ovarian cancer and is raised in both benign and malignant conditions.

The management of gynaecological cancer

Surgery is the principal treatment for patients with early and advanced forms of ovarian cancer. Chemotherapy is used to treat patients with ovarian cancer, except for those rare patients presenting at the earliest stage of the disease.

Endometrial cancer has an excellent prognosis if detected early and around 80% of patients will be cured by hysterectomy. Adjuvant radiotherapy may be offered to patients who are at high risk of relapse after surgery for endometrial cancer. Cervical intraepithelial neoplasia is managed by complete excision, usually by laser in younger patients. Invasive cervical cancer is treated with hysterectomy. Chemo-radiotherapy is the standard treatment in older patients. Vulval cancer can be treated by both radiotherapy and surgical excision.

> Early endometrial cancer has an excellent prognosis; hysterectomy is curative in around 80% of patients.

Urological cancer

Prostate cancer is the commonest cancer in men and the second most common cause of male cancer death. Prostate and bladder cancer can present with lower urinary tract symptoms or symptoms of advanced cancer such as weight loss or bone pain.

Referral for suspected urological cancer

If patients have lower urinary tract symptoms, perform a digital rectal examination of the prostate and refer for urgent urological specialist assessment if:

- the patient has a hard and irregular prostate, as this may be a sign of prostate cancer and should trigger testing of prostate-specific antigen (PSA)
- a symptomatic patient has a high PSA level.

Note that PSA values increase with age, with benign prostatic hypertrophy or urinary tract infection. In the absence of symptoms, a PSA level that is raised but within a patient's age-specific range does not indicate the need for urgent referral.

Bladder and kidney cancers may present with:

- persistent urinary tract infections
- frank haematuria or unexplained microscopic haematuria in a patient over 50.

These symptoms mandate referral for investigation.

Testicular cancer is the commonest cancer in young men but has an excellent prognosis. Refer for an urgent assessment any patient with:

- a testicular mass
- a swelling within the body of the testis or within the scrotum (that does not transluminate).

> Screening for prostate cancer based on PSA levels has not been shown to have a survival advantage because of the test's lack of specificity. Clinicians should discuss the potential implications of this lack of specificity with their patients before testing.

The management of urological cancer

The management of early prostate cancer depends on the Gleason grading of the tumour, which predicts the clinical outcome. Men with lower-grade prostate cancer, which is confined to the prostate, can safely be managed by 'watchful waiting' and treated in the event of significant increases in PSA values. All 'curative' treatment options for prostate cancer are associated with a significant risk of long-term impotence and urinary incontinence. Younger men with higher grade tumours tend to be offered surgery and older men tend to be offered radiotherapy. Clinical outcomes after both treatments are very similar. Surgery is 'better' for men with higher grade tumours but the survival advantage is very minor.

Patients with advanced prostate cancer can be treated with androgen suppression and the psychiatrist should be aware that this can cause mood changes. Early bladder, kidney and testicular cancers are treated with surgery. Metastatic testicular cancer has an excellent prognosis and high cure rate with modern chemotherapy. Metastatic kidney cancer is managed using drugs such as sunitinib which stop the tumour growing by inhibiting the formation of blood vessels.[6] Palliative chemotherapy for bladder cancer is effective and improves patients' symptoms and overall survival.

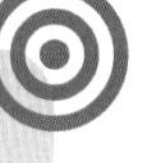

Treatment with androgen suppression can cause mood changes.

Haematological cancer

Cancers of the haematological system comprise acute and chronic leukaemia, lymphoma and myeloma. Patients with haematological cancers can present with:

- fatigue
- fever
- weight loss
- lymphadenopathy (in young people this is common and is often associated with Epstein–Barr virus infection)
- splenomegaly
- infection
- bruising and bleeding.

Referral for suspected haematological cancer

Investigation is recommended for patients with lymph nodes that are increasing in size or over 2 cm in size for 6 weeks or more, especially where this is associated with weight loss or night sweats.

Patients with fatigue should have a full blood count, tests for erythrocyte sedimentation rate (ESR) or C reactive protein (CRP) and a clotting screen.

The management of haematological cancers

The management of acute leukaemia requires intensive chemotherapy to induce remission followed by extensive consolidation treatment. Children with leukaemia have a better prognosis than adults. Higher grade lymphomas have a high cure rate (around 60–80%) with modern chemotherapy. Indolent forms of lymphoma and leukaemia such as B-cell chronic leukaemia can be managed by watchful waiting, and chemotherapy or radiotherapy used in the event of symptomatic progression.

Skin cancer

The incidence of skin cancers is increasing. Skin disorders are difficult to diagnose and clinicians who are unsure of the diagnosis of any skin condition should refer the patient to a specialist.

Skin cancer may be:

- non-melanoma skin cancer – the majority of these are basal cell and squamous cell carcinomas, which are common and cause few deaths
- malignant melanoma (Fig. 21.4) – this is less common but causes 2000 deaths in the UK each year.

The primary treatment for skin cancers is surgical excision, although radiotherapy can be used to treat basal cell carcinoma and squamous cell carcinoma.

Skin disorders are difficult to diagnose. If the diagnosis of any skin condition is uncertain, refer to a specialist. This is particularly important if melanoma is suspected.

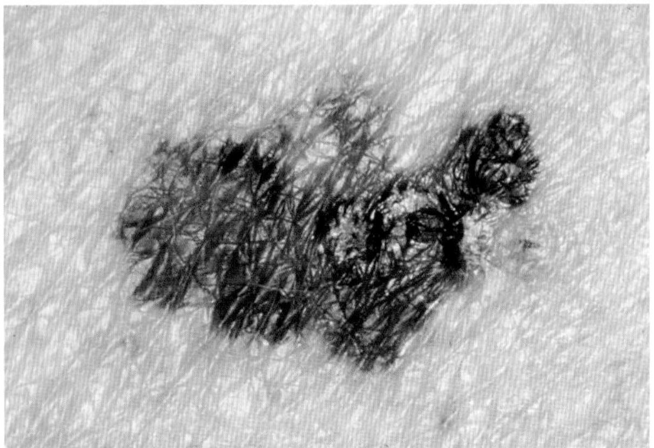

Fig. 21.4 A malignant melanoma.

Referral for suspected skin cancer

The major features that suggest that a pigmented lesion may be a melanoma include:

- a lesion greater than 7 mm or changing in size
- irregular shape or colour
- inflammation or oozing.

Patients with lesions that are suspicious for melanoma should be referred for dermatology assessment. Squamous cell carcinoma presents as a crusty or keratinised lesion. Lesions commonly appear on sun-exposed areas such as the head and back of the hand, and may be indurated and ulcerated.

Head and neck cancer

Smoking and alcohol are strongly associated with the development of head and neck cancer. Cancers of the mouth may present with red and white patches, which may be swollen, painful and bleed, or a new unexplained lump in the neck. Lichen planus is a pre-malignant condition and should be routinely monitored by dentists.

Referral is recommended for patients with:

- a non-healing ulcer
- a new ulcer with unexplained tooth mobility
- a hoarse voice in a smoker aged over 50 years, for whom a chest X-ray will be needed.

Cancer of the head and neck is curable with surgery and chemotherapy and radiotherapy. Treatments are intensive and often leave patients unable to swallow or with a permanent tracheostomy stoma. Patients with head and neck cancers often have considerable comorbidities which are related to excess alcohol consumption and smoking, which complicates treatment.

Cancers of the brain and central nervous system

Brain tumours are common but many clinicians are uncertain about their diagnosis and management. Headaches are a common complaint and can be a common functional component of psychiatric illness. Functional headaches are more commonly frontal, while organic headaches tend to be occipital.

If a brain tumour is suspected, check fundoscopy to look for papilloedema and refer for an urgent neurological assessment any patient with:

- new-onset seizures
- a progressive neurological deficit
- mental changes
- cranial nerve palsy
- unilateral sensorineural deafness
- headache with features of raised intracranial pressure such as vomiting, posture-related headache, drowsiness or pulse-synchronous tinnitus
- non-focal symptoms such as a change in personality
- a history of cancer with new-onset seizures, focal, neurological deficits, persistent headaches, neurological signs or cognitive changes.

The management of primary brain tumours

High grade brains tumours like glioma are treated with surgical debulking followed by radiotherapy with chemotherapy, which afford long-term survival for around 15% of patients. Surgery is rarely curative for brain tumours which infiltrate the brain widely, often making complete resection without significant

> Most patients with a neck cancer will experience dysphagia during their treatment. Remember that many psychotropic and antipsychotic medications can be administered as liquids or via nasogastric feeding tubes.

functional deficit impossible. Patients with slower-growing tumours can have an excellent prognosis and survive for years.

Cancer screening

The UK has established national screening programmes for the early detection of breast, bowel, cervical and colon cancer. Further information about the national screening programmes can be found at www.cancerscreening.nhs.uk. These programmes have been shown to improve outcomes for each cancer. The risk of developing cancer is related to age and the benefits of screening are restricted for economic reasons to certain age groups. If symptoms or signs develop outside recommended screening intervals, the patient should be referred to an appropriate hospital clinic for assessment.

There is no screening mechanism for some cancers, while for others current screening is flawed. For example, there is no clear evidence to support the routine use of PSA for *prostate cancer screening* in asymptomatic men. Those wishing to have a PSA check are encouraged by government dictat to discuss the risks and benefits with their GP, who may consider it appropriate and arrange for PSA testing. Prostate cancer diagnosis requires transrectal ultrasound and biopsy, which is particularly unpleasant; paradoxically, treatment may not be curative and certainly causes side-effects.

Breast cancer screening

Mammographic screening reduces the mortality from breast cancer by around 15% and is offered to all women in the UK aged between 50 and 70. The upper age cut-off is remarkable in that cancers of the breast increase with age, and so screening is of maximal benefit in the aged.

The programme invites women from each general practice in turn, and therefore some women will not receive an invitation until they are 53. Women under 50 years are not offered screening as they have a low incidence of breast cancer, and their higher breast density limits the sensitivity of mammography. Clinicians who are concerned about a patient's family history of breast cancer, or who assess women with symptoms or signs suggestive of breast cancer, should make an urgent referral to a breast clinic.

Cervical cancer screening

The aim of the cervical cancer screening programme is to detect and treat pre-malignant changes or *cervical intra-epithelial neoplasia* (CIN) before cancer develops. The smear test and liquid-based cytology tests are routinely used by GPs to diagnose CIN, which is caused by the sexually transmitted human papilloma virus (HPV).

All women aged 25–64 years are eligible for cervical screening at intervals of 3–5 years, depending on age. The current age intervals are:

- aged 25–50 years – screening at 3-year intervals
- aged 50–64 years – screening at 5-year intervals
- aged over 65 years – screened only if they have not been screened since they were 50 or have had recent abnormal test results.

Patients who are registered with a GP are monitored by the National Health Service (NHS) 'call and recall' system, which tracks investigations and recalls women for screening.

Women who have never been sexually active have a very low risk of developing cervical cancer and may therefore have good reason to decline screening. Vaccination against HPV is offered to all 12- and 13-year-old girls and girls aged 17–18 are eligible for the vaccine as part of a 'catch up' programme. The long-term efficacy of HPV vaccination is unknown and vaccinated women are still advised to attend routine screening. Current vaccines cover around 60% of the oncogenic viruses and there are strong arguments to vaccinate boys as well as girls.

Bowel cancer screening

The UK national bowel cancer screening programme started in 2009 and uses the faecal occult blood (FOB) system to detect early-stage cancers and pre-malignant polyps. Screening is offered to all men and women aged between 60 and 69 years. General practitioners are not directly involved in the programme but do receive copies of all test results.

Individuals eligible for screening receive an invitation letter and leaflet explaining the programme and a testing kit is sent in the post a week later. The majority of people (98/100) will receive normal results; those with abnormal results are offered a colonoscopy, around 50% of which will be normal, while 40% will have polyps detected and 10% will be diagnosed with a cancer.

Cancer treatments

Chemotherapy

Chemotherapy drugs kill cancer cells, which tend to divide more rapidly than healthy normal cells. Chemotherapy is a safe and effective treatment for patients with advanced cancer. It can be used as a *primary curative* medical treatment for patients with advanced cancers such as leukaemia, lymphoma or testicular cancer, or as an *adjuvant treatment* to increase the chance of cure after surgery for breast, bowel, lung and bladder cancer.

Although chemotherapy has side-effects, the majority of patients have a reasonable quality of life during treatment. The common side-effects include fatigue, hair loss, infection, nausea and vomiting, but are manageable with supportive care and specialist advice.

Chemotherapy is usually administered on a specialist out-patient day unit by specialist nurses or in specialist wards. On the day of treatment, patients undergo a clinical assessment by a doctor or specialist nurse. A semi-permanent intravenous line called a Hickman or Groshong line may be inserted to allow administration of complex chemotherapy regimens over several days. These lines are usually managed by specialist nurses and must be urgently removed if they become infected.

Before chemotherapy is given, all the common and potentially serious side-effects will be explained and the patient asked to sign a consent form. An information sheet is provided, as the list of potential side-effects is difficult to remember. Macmillan Cancer Support is a charity for patients with cancer (www.macmillan.org.uk) and provides excellent information leaflets about cancer treatment. Many cancer centres provide a 24-hour help-line for patients who become unwell in the community, and allow medical professionals to make hospital referrals directly to an oncologist. Many hospitals are introducing 'acute oncology' services for the management of patients who require hospital admission.

Around 1–2% of patients taking the atypical antipsychotic clozapine are at risk of developing agranulocytosis, which can be fatal. The benefits of continuing clozapine during chemotherapy may outweigh the risks of changing to another antipsychotic medication. If planning to prescribe clozapine during chemotherapy, it is essential to inform the clozapine monitoring service and obtain permission to prescribe clozapine 'off licence'. If there is any doubt about the patient's consent or the permission given to prescribe treatment with clozapine during chemotherapy, it is advisable to seek the opinion of a second-opinion approved doctor, under the relevant mental health legislation. It is important to establish good communication between the psychiatric team, the patient and the treating oncologists, as all parties must be aware of the risks associated with concomitant treatment with clozapine during chemotherapy.

Adjuvant treatments

Adjuvant treatments are used to reduce the risk of recurrence for patients with breast, lung and bowel cancer. The risk of recurrence after surgery is estimated using clinical factors such as tumour grade, number of involved lymph nodes and tumour size. Oncologists may use web-based applications such as 'Adjuvant On-line' to predict the risk of recurrence after surgery. The information is provided in a pictorial format that patients can more easily understand. The potential benefits of adjuvant treatment have to be weighed against the treatment toxicities and the knowledge that many patients will receive unnecessary treatment.

Radiotherapy

Radiotherapy treatment uses high-energy radiation to destroy cancer cells. It is a specialist treatment and not every hospital is able to give it, so patients may need to travel to a specialist centre. It can be used as a primary treatment for cancers of the cervix, endometrium, bladder, prostate, lung, anus and skin and is a very good palliative treatment for pain.

Radiotherapy is prescribed in dosages denoted in the SI unit gray (commonly as centigrays) and the total dose is divided into 'fractions'. Before treatment starts, the patient will have a 'planning scan' and the treatment process will be explained. Sometimes marks or tattoos are used to allow the radiotherapy machines to be set up to treat the same area each time.

The side-effects of radiotherapy are fatigue, hair loss, nausea and vomiting, skin inflammation and irritation. Swallowing or eating may be affected if the mouth or throat is treated. Long-term side-effects include a risk of the development of secondary cancers, skin changes, infertility, vaginal stenosis, dysphagia, bladder problems and coronary heart disease after radiation to the left side of the chest.

Palliative care and end-of-life pathways

Many patients with cancer will have complex medical and social needs. The focus of palliative or supportive care is to allow patients with advanced cancer to have a good quality of life. The patient's GP has an important role in managing this care. Community Macmillan nurses and district nurses may visit patients at home. If symptoms cannot be controlled in the community, a hospice admission may be arranged. Where possible, arrangements will be made to follow a patient's wishes to die at home or within a local hospice.

Oncology emergencies

Patients with both early and particularly with advanced cancer may develop serious complications requiring emergency treatment. This section covers some of the most common and potentially serious complications that arise in patients with cancer. Other serious complications, such as raised intracranial pressure, stridor, obstruction of the bowel or ureters, are not covered. Emergencies such as neutropenic sepsis or radiotherapy burns are potentially serious complications of treatment. Complications like spinal cord compression and hypercalcaemia may be directly caused by the cancer.

Although many patients will present to their GPs or directly to their oncology service, atypical presentations of new or recurrent cancers do occur. Patients may present to multiple healthcare professionals before a diagnosis is established. Patients suspected of having potentially serious medical conditions arising from a cancer should be referred for an urgent specialist assessment. Prompt diagnosis and treatment are essential, as delays increase morbidity and mortality. Although many psychiatrists may not feel confident in their general medical and examination skills, they should remember that all will have examined many hundreds or even thousands of patients during their careers. Psychiatrists should therefore feel confident that they will be able to detect major physical or neurological abnormalities. If the patient's history and/or examination findings warrant urgent referral, then persistence on the part of the referrer may be required, as some physicians can be reluctant to receive a referral directly from a psychiatrist.

Neutropenic sepsis

Neutropenic sepsis is a common complication of chemotherapy for both early and advanced cancer. The risk of infection after chemotherapy is highest 7–10 days after chemotherapy treatment. The symptoms of neutropenia are non-specific but usually manifest as flu-like. Patients receiving chemotherapy are given detailed verbal and written instructions about what to do if a fever or symptoms of sepsis develop.

Neutropenic sepsis responds quickly to emergency treatment with broad-spectrum intravenous antibiotics such as tazocin. If neutropenic sepsis is suspected, an urgent referral should be made for a medical assessment at an emergency department. Untreated, the death rates from neutropenic sepsis approach 30%.

Spinal cord compression

Spinal cord compression may be caused by extrinsic compression of the spinal cord by a tumour or compression of the vertebral canal by vertebral collapse. It results in decreased blood flow, ischaemia and infarction of the spinal cord. Bony metastasis is a frequent cause of cord compression, occurring commonly in breast, prostate, lung, kidney, bladder and bowel cancer, melanoma, myeloma and lymphoma.

Pain is the principal symptom of spinal cord compression and is often present for months before clinically significant neurological impairment occurs. The pain is often worse at night and may be made worse by coughing or straining. Lumbar back pain is relatively common, whereas thoracic or cervical back pain is relatively uncommon. Pain within the thoracic or cervical spine should arouse suspicion of spinal cord compression or other potentially serious organic pathology, particularly if there is a history of previous breast or prostate cancer.

Complete compression of the spinal cord causes a reduction in skin sensation below the level of compression, and a corresponding bilateral loss of power. Partial cord compression causes a partial loss of sensation and power below the level of the lesion. Lesions below the level of the spinal cord give rise to a cauda equina syndrome, which is characterised by sciatic pains, loss of anal tone, urinary and faecal incontinence, and weakness of the gluteal muscles.

Patients with suspected cord compression should be referred for an immediate MRI scan to confirm or exclude the diagnosis. These examinations should be performed on the same day of referral. Plain X-rays and CT scanning may be used to look for vertebral collapse but should not delay MRI scanning. The initial management of spinal cord compression is high-dose steroids (usually dexamethasone 8 mg twice daily) and consideration for urgent radiotherapy or neurological decompression.

A 'rule of thirds' applies to the prognosis after spinal cord compression: one-third will recover, one-third stay the same and one-third deteriorate. Only a small proportion of paralysed patients walk again after treatment for spinal cord compression, whereas 90% of mobile patients retain their mobility. Radiotherapy is usually given over 5 days (20 gray in five fractions). Surgical decompression should be performed only at specialist centres and is associated with better outcomes than radiotherapy.

Hypercalcaemia

Hypercalcaemia occurs in around 5–10% of patients with cancer. Benign conditions such as hyperparathyroidism are common and should be considered in the differential diagnosis. Hypercalcaemia arises a result of factors that are secreted by the tumour and is common in breast cancer, myeloma and lung cancer. The symptoms of hypercalcaemia include constipation, anorexia, nausea, polyuria, dehydration, confusion, lethargy and weakness, and overlap with the symptoms of psychiatric illness. The treatment is rehydration with intravenous fluids and bisphosphonate drugs such as zoledronic acid or pamidronate.

Superior vena cava obstruction

Superior vena cava obstruction (SVCO) occurs due to extrinsic compression and/or thrombosis of the vein. It causes swelling of the neck, face and upper torso, and distension of the veins of the neck and upper torso. If severe, it can lead to headache and papilloedema. It is usually diagnosed using CT.

Management depends on tumour type. Chemotherapy can be used for patients with chemotherapy-sensitive cancers such as small-cell lung cancer or lymphoma. Patients with non-small-cell lung cancer or other tumours may have a metal stent inserted radiologically, which provides rapid relief of symptoms. Most patients are started on corticosteroids and may be considered for radiotherapy. Thrombosis is treated with anticoagulation.

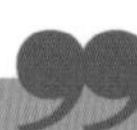

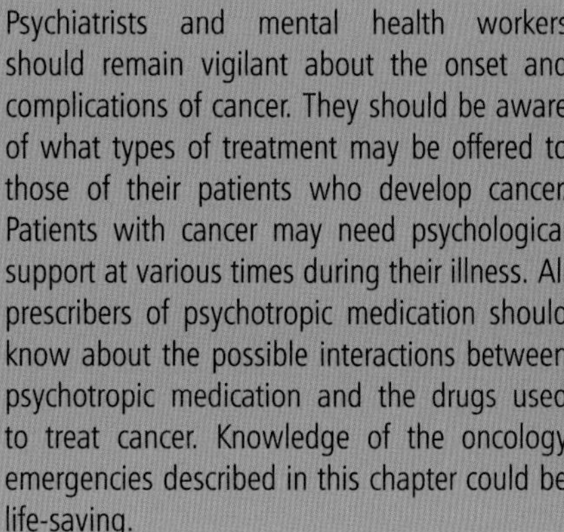

Summary

Psychiatrists and mental health workers should remain vigilant about the onset and complications of cancer. They should be aware of what types of treatment may be offered to those of their patients who develop cancer. Patients with cancer may need psychological support at various times during their illness. All prescribers of psychotropic medication should know about the possible interactions between psychotropic medication and the drugs used to treat cancer. Knowledge of the oncology emergencies described in this chapter could be life-saving.

References

1 Sjostrom L, Narbro K, Sjostrom CD, *et al.* Effects of bariatric surgery on mortality in Swedish obese subjects. *N Engl J Med* 2007; **357**: 741–52.

2 Early Breast Cancer Trialists' Collaborative Group (EBCTG). Effects of chemotherapy and hormonal therapy for early breast cancer on recurrence and 15-year survival: an overview of the randomised trials. *Lancet* 2012; **365**: 1687–717.

3 Kelly CM, Juurlink DN, Gomes T, *et al.* Selective serotonin reuptake inhibitors and breast cancer mortality in women receiving tamoxifen: a population based cohort study. *BMJ* 2010; **340**: c693.

4 Slamon D, Eiermann W, Robert N, *et al.* Adjuvant trastuzumab in HER2-positive breast cancer. *N Engl J Med* 2011; **365**: 1273–83.

5 Burris HA 3rd, Moore MJ, Andersen J, *et al.* Improvements in survival and clinical benefit with gemcitabine as first-line therapy for patients with advanced pancreas cancer: a randomized trial. *J Clin Oncol* 1997; **15**: 2403–13.

6 Motzer RJ, Hutson TE, Tomczak P, *et al.* Overall survival and updated results for sunitinib compared with interferon alfa in patients with metastatic renal cell carcinoma. *J Clin Oncol* 2009; **27**: 3584–90.

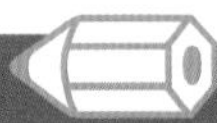

Learning points

- Smoking cessation is the most important way to reduce the risk of developing cancer.
- Many patients with early cancers and some forms of advanced cancer such as lymphoma or testicular cancer will be cured with modern therapies.
- Breast cancer outcomes are excellent. Around 80% of women with early breast cancer are cured with surgery, hormone manipulation, radiotherapy and adjuvant chemotherapy.
- Adjuvant chemotherapy and hormone treatments are used to reduce the risk of recurrence for patients with breast, lung and bowel cancer.
- An individual's risk of cancer is related to their age, which should be taken into account when considering a referral.
- The evidence behind the use of the 'red flag' symptoms of cancer is limited.
- Testicular cancer is the commonest cancer in young men.
- National guidelines currently require patients with suspected cancer to be seen and assessed by a specialist within 2 weeks of referral.
- Patients with symptoms such as rectal bleeding or unexplained iron-deficiency anaemia may be referred direct for investigations without first having to see a specialist.
- Tobacco smoking causes around 90% of all lung cancer, which is the commonest cause of death from cancer in men and women in the UK.
- Some forms of psychotropic medication can reduce the efficacy of tamoxifen (used to treat breast cancer) by inhibiting its conversion to its active form, by causing the inhibition of the liver cytochrome P450 enzyme isoform CYPD6.
- Gastric cancer is the seventh commonest cancer diagnosed in the UK (diagnosed in around 7000 people each year).
- Early endometrial cancer has an excellent prognosis. Hysterectomy is curative in around 80% of patients.
- Screening for prostate cancer with PSA levels has not been shown to have a survival advantage because of the test's lack of specificity.
- Androgen suppression for advanced prostate cancer can lead to mood changes.
- If the diagnosis of any skin condition is uncertain, refer to a specialist, especially if a melanoma is suspected.
- Benefits of continuing clozapine during chemotherapy may outweigh the risks of changing to another antipsychotic medication.
- Pain within the thoracic or cervical spine should arouse suspicion of spinal cord compression or other potentially serious organic pathology, particularly if there is a history of breast or prostate cancer.
- Symptoms of hypercalcaemia include constipation, anorexia, nausea, polyuria, dehydration, confusion, lethargy and weakness, and may overlap with symptoms of mental illness.
- Spinal cord compression may be caused by bony metastases, occurring commonly in breast, prostate, lung, kidney, bladder and bowel cancer, and melanoma, myeloma and lymphoma.
- Patients with suspected spinal cord compression should be referred for an urgent MRI scan to confirm or exclude the diagnosis.

Section III

Psychiatric specialties and physical health

22
Alcohol

Ed Day and Sanjay Khurmi

Most users of alcohol do so 'responsibly' and so are spared the harmful acute and chronic effects on body systems that are described in this chapter. Physical signs often become apparent in those dependent on alcohol, but widely available blood tests can be used to monitor the impact of alcohol on individuals who do not show obvious signs of resultant ill health. Also described are standardised screening questionnaires, advice on when to refer to specialised services and management of the neurological consequences of alcohol withdrawal.

Introduction

Alcohol-related problems are highly prevalent in the UK, with an estimated 38% of men and 16% of women aged between 16 and 64 suffering from an alcohol use disorder.[1] The harm related to alcohol has increased over the past three decades, with deaths from alcoholic liver disease doubling in the UK since 1980.[2] Excessive use of alcohol has consequences for both the individual and society, with the estimated annual cost to the National Health Service (NHS) of alcohol-related harm alone totalling £1.7 billion.[3] The potential physical health complications are numerous and varied, and alcohol consumption has been associated with more than 60 different types of physical disorder.[4] The mortality rate of heavy drinkers is at least twice that of the normal population.

Alcohol is a small molecule that is soluble in both water and lipids. Its toxic effects may be caused directly by alcohol or by its metabolic by-products, and every organ system in the body may be affected. Definitions of hazardous, harmful, dependent and binge drinking are given in Table 22.1 (adapted from UK Government guidance).[5]

Acute alcohol intoxication produces a steady progression through euphoria to incoordination, ataxia, stupor, coma and death; intoxicated individuals are also at increased risk of soft-tissue injuries, fractures, head injuries and other trauma. Withdrawal effects can follow a bout of acute intoxication and vary widely in severity. Weakness, faintness, sweating and insomnia can occur within a few hours of blood alcohol levels beginning to decline, accompanied by a coarse tremor. In chronic heavy drinkers more severe withdrawal symptoms occur after 12–36 hours, and include generalised tonic–clonic seizures in 5–15% or cardiac dysrhythmias secondary to electrolyte imbalance or alcoholic cardiomyopathy. Delirium tremens is characterised by gross tremor, severe agitation, disorientation, confusion, sweating, tachycardia, delusional beliefs and visual hallucinations. These symptoms may last for up to 7–10 days and may ultimately lead to death.

Table 22.1 Categories of alcohol use

Term	Definition
Hazardous drinking	Drinking alcohol in excess of recommended healthy limits: • adult women should not regularly drink more than 2–3 units of alcohol a day • adult men should not regularly drink more than 3–4 units of alcohol a day • pregnant women or women trying to conceive should avoid drinking alcohol; if they do drink, they should not drink more than 1–2 units of alcohol once or twice a week and should not get drunk.
Harmful drinking	Drinking alcohol at levels that lead to significant harm to physical and mental health, or at levels that may be causing substantial harm to others. Examples include liver damage or cirrhosis, substantial stress or aggression in the family, or loss of employment. Women who regularly drink over 6 units a day (or over 35 units a week) and men who regularly drink over 8 units a day (or 50 units a week) are at highest risk of such alcohol-related harm.
Dependent drinking	Alcohol dependence is characterised by a loss of control over one's drinking, and is usually associated with unsuccessful attempts to cut down or control use. Alcohol is drunk in larger amounts or over a longer period than was intended, and considerable time is spent in obtaining and using alcohol, or recovering from its effects. This leads to a reduction in other social, occupational or recreational activities, but use continues despite the alcohol-related problems. Physical tolerance to alcohol and a withdrawal syndrome on reduction or cessation of use are usually present.
Binge drinking	Drinking too much alcohol over a short period of time (e.g. over the course of an evening). It is typically this kind of drinking that leads to drunkenness. People who become drunk are much more likely to be involved in an accident or to be assaulted, to be charged with a criminal offence, or to contract a sexually transmitted disease. Women are more likely to have an unplanned pregnancy. Trends in binge drinking are usually identified in surveys by measuring those drinking over 6 units a day for women or over 8 units a day for men. In practice, many binge drinkers are drinking substantially more than this, or drink this amount rapidly, which leads to the harm linked to drunkenness.

One unit = 8 g alcohol. To calculate number of units, multiply the volume of the drink in millilitres by its percentage alcohol by volume (ABV), and divide by 1000: 1 pint of 5% lager contains (568 x 5)/1000 = 2.8 units. Adapted from HM Government, 2007.[5]

Systemic effects of alcohol misuse

Cardiovascular system

Population-based studies suggest a 'J-shaped' relationship between alcohol consumption and the risk of coronary heart disease, with a 20–40% lower rate among drinkers compared with non-drinkers. Thus, 'low risk' alcohol consumption (up to 3 units per day) protects middle-aged men against coronary heart disease. However, above 3 units per day in men and 2 units in women, mortality from all causes increases as alcohol consumption increases.[6]

Alcohol is a common cause of reversible hypertension, and this association is independent of age, body weight and smoking. It occurs in up to 25% of those drinking at a 'harmful' level, and a significant proportion of the excess deaths attributable to alcohol are attributable to cardiovascular problems.

Heavy alcohol consumption increases the risk of cardiac dysrhythmias such as supraventricular tachycardia

> Drinking to excess can have undesirable social consequences as individuals are more likely:
>
> - to be involved in an accident
> - to be assaulted
> - to be charged with a criminal offence
> - to contract a sexually transmitted disease.
>
> Additionally, women are more likely to have an unplanned pregnancy.

and atrial fibrillation. 'Holiday heart syndrome' refers to an association between heavy alcohol consumption in a binge pattern and rhythm disturbances in a person with no other clinically evident heart disease. The patient is likely to describe palpitations, or possibly shortness of breath and loss of consciousness if the ventricular response is very rapid. Chronic 'harmful' drinkers are at greater risk of all forms of stroke (thrombo-embolic, haemorrhagic and subarachnoid haemorrhage). Alcoholic dilated cardiomyopathy is probably a direct toxic effect of alcohol, and both men and women are susceptible.

Respiratory system

High levels of intoxication with alcohol lead to the depression of vital centres in the central nervous system, and ultimately to respiratory failure and stupor. Aspiration pneumonia is a serious consequence of being under the influence of alcohol, and obstructive sleep apnoea can occur as a result of the muscle relaxant properties of alcohol. Alcohol dependence and associated nutritional deficiencies lead to a weakening of various pulmonary defence systems and an increased rate of pulmonary infections, including tuberculosis.

Gastrointestinal system

Stomatitis in the lips and glossitis in the tongue can be secondary to alcohol toxicity, particularly when there is a deficiency of vitamins B and C. Prolonged exposure to alcohol leads to chronic inflammation of the oral mucosa and an increased risk of pre-cancerous lesions. Chronic consumption at 'harmful' levels may lead to smooth muscle dysfunction and altered oesophageal sphincter tone, resulting in gastroesophageal reflux and oesophagitis (usually presenting as heartburn).

Alcohol misuse in conjunction with heavy smoking is associated with carcinoma of the oesophagus. Frequent vomiting may result in tears of the mucosa of the cardioesophageal junction (the Mallory–Weiss syndrome), leading to heavy bleeding. Alcoholic gastritis occurs in more than 80% of dependent alcohol users. A combination of damaged small bowel permeability and autonomic neuropathy may lead to poor small bowel functioning, diarrhoea and malabsorption.

Hepatobiliary system

Steady alcohol consumption leads to the development of fatty change in the liver (steatosis), which is present in 90% of heavy drinkers and is usually asymptomatic. In about 30–40% of heavy drinkers this progresses to alcoholic hepatitis, which may present with pain in the right hypochondrium, jaundice or fever. This is the active phase of alcoholic liver disease, in which an inflammatory process destroys liver cells, leaving a diffuse fibrosis with nodules of regenerating liver cells (cirrhosis). Cirrhosis develops in 8–30% of drinkers with a 10- to 20-year history of daily heavy drinking, but susceptibility varies between individuals.

The risk of developing cirrhosis increases steeply with consumption of more than 3 units of alcohol per day, and other risk factors include female sex, obesity, poor nutrition, type 2 diabetes and hepatitis C infection. Twin studies suggest that there is also a genetic component to disease risk.

Alcohol consumption is a major cause of both acute and chronic pancreatitis, which usually presents initially with severe abdominal pain, followed later by nausea and vomiting. The intensity and frequency of acute attacks usually decrease with abstinence and may stop altogether. Complications include pseudocysts, bile duct stenosis and thrombosis of the portal vein or splenic artery. Chronic inflammation can disrupt either the endocrine or the exocrine functions of the pancreas, leading to diabetes mellitus or malabsorption with steatorrhoea and malnutrition.

Central and peripheral nervous systems

The energy content of alcohol is relatively high and can account for a significant proportion of the calorific intake of dependent drinkers. Poor diet leads to nutrient deficiencies, which are often compounded by malabsorption due to alcohol-induced gastrointestinal, liver or pancreatic damage. The brain depends on an adequate supply of glucose both as an energy source and as a donor of carbon fragments for protein, neurotransmitter and lipid biosynthesis. Glucose utilisation depends on vitamin B and a breakdown in this metabolic process can lead to brain damage. Hypoxia, electrolyte imbalance or hypoglycaemia associated with intoxication or withdrawal may also combine with the direct toxic effect of alcohol to produce long-term damage to the brain.

Wernicke's encephalopathy is traditionally thought of as a disorder of acute onset characterised by nystagmus, abducent and conjugate gaze palsies, ataxia of gait and a global confusional state, in various combinations.[7]

The classical triad of nystagmus/gaze palsy, ataxia and confusion occurs in less than 10% of those with Wernicke's encephalopathy. It is wise to consider the diagnosis in anyone with a history of heavy alcohol consumption and ophthalmoplegia, ataxia, acute confusion, memory disturbance, unexplained hypotension, hypothermia, coma, or unconsciousness because if untreated, Wernicke's encephalopathy leads to death in up to one in five cases and Korsakoff's psychosis in 85% of the survivors, one in four of whom will require long-term institutionalisation.

Carl Wernicke first described the disorder in 1881, when he recorded disturbances of eye movement, ataxia of gait, polyneuropathy and mental changes, including apathy, decreased attention span and disorientation in time and space. Sergei Korsakoff gave an account of the amnestic syndrome that now bears his name in 1887, when he described a range of features, including delirium and characteristic loss of recent memory with confabulation but with relative preservation of other intellectual functions. Wernicke–Korsakoff syndrome is now considered to be a unitary disorder comprising acute Wernicke's encephalopathy which proceeds in a proportion of cases to Korsakoff's psychosis.[7]

Post-mortem studies have demonstrated typical lesions of Wernicke's encephalopathy in 1.4% of patients examined, and in those misusing alcohol this figure is as high as 35%.[8] However, the pathology of Wernicke's encephalopathy may not be associated with the classical clinical triad in up to 90% of patients.[9] Therefore, it has been suggested that a presumptive diagnosis of Wernicke's encephalopathy should be made for any patient with a history of alcohol dependence who may be at risk. This includes anyone showing evidence of ophthalmoplegia, ataxia, acute confusion, memory disturbance, unexplained hypotension, hypothermia, coma or unconsciousness. Untreated, Wernicke's encephalopathy leads to death in up to 20% of cases,[9] or Korsakoff's psychosis in 85% of the survivors (of whom 25% will require long-term institutionalisation).[10]

Between 50% and 80% of people with chronic alcohol use disorders experience mild to severe cognitive deficits.[11] The clinical and neuropsychological features of alcohol-related brain damage (ARBD) are well described, and the deficits appear to centre on visuospatial coordination, memory, abstract thinking and learning new information, with general knowledge, over-rehearsed information and verbal skills largely spared.[12] Attempts have been made to describe the unique features of 'alcoholic dementia',[13] but there is a lack of evidence linking any specific neuropathology with heavy alcohol intake.[14] A range of potential factors have been implicated in the causation of ARBD, including direct alcohol neurotoxicity, thiamine deficiency, traumatic brain injury, familial alcoholism, childhood psychopathology, age and education.[11]

Epileptic seizures frequently occur in the context of heavy drinking with pre-existing epilepsy, brain damage secondary to trauma or other factors, or the use of prescribed or illicit drugs. Alcohol withdrawal seizures are diagnosed only when these other potential causes are ruled out, and are often a marker of severe alcohol dependence. They are usually short, generalised tonic–clonic seizures that occur up to 48 hours after the last drink, although multiple fits may occur over the course of 1–6 hours. They can present without other signs of alcohol withdrawal, and may occur at a very high blood alcohol level if it has recently fallen from an even higher level. The presence of either partial seizures or status epilepticus suggests the presence of structural brain lesions.

Peripheral neuropathy is very common in heavy alcohol users, and may range from subjective symptoms of paraesthesia to a severe distal sensory and motor neuropathy. The pathological mechanism is probably a combination of vitamin deficiency and direct alcohol toxicity. Coexisting autonomic neuropathy may contribute to hypotension and gastrointestinal motility problems. Other rare conditions associated with nutritional deficits in alcohol dependence include Marchiafava–Bignami syndrome, central pontine myelinolysis and alcoholic amblyopia, a painless bilateral loss of vision in association with alcohol misuse.

Short, generalised tonic–clonic seizures occurring up to 48 hours after the last drink are often a marker of severe alcohol dependence. If partial seizures or status epilepticus occurs, look for the presence of a structural brain lesion.

Effective treatment of alcohol withdrawal should prevent seizures. If a seizure occurs, review the dose of prescribed benzodiazepines. Patients with a structural brain lesion or an epileptogenic focus on an EEG need treatment with long-term anticonvulsants.

Musculoskeletal system

Trauma is commonly associated with alcohol intoxication; additionally, reduced calcium absorption and a variety of endocrine abnormalities lead to an increased risk of osteoporosis in heavy drinkers. Proximal myopathy is associated with chronic alcohol use, and this leads to weakness and muscle wasting.

Endocrine system

Down-regulation of the pituitary–gonadal axis secondary to alcohol dependence leads to gonadal atrophy. In men this is associated with gynaecomastia and testicular atrophy, and impotence occurs in up to half. Increased levels of circulating oestrogen secondary to liver failure may also contribute to the problem. Women experience amenorrhoea, subfertility and recurrent abortion.

An alcoholic pseudo-Cushing's syndrome may develop due to excessive glucocorticoid production, leading to the characteristic 'moon' facial appearance, obesity and hypertension. Glucose intolerance occurs in up to 40% of alcohol-dependent individuals and there is an association with type 2 diabetes (although possibly a J-shaped dose–response curve, as low alcohol consumption may have protective effects against diabetes). Depleted liver stores of glycogen and altered glucocorticoid secretion also lead to frequent episodes of hypoglycaemia.

Skin

There is a distinct, alcohol-related form of psoriasis that affects up to 15% of alcohol misusers.

Physical examination

General appearance and observation

Alcohol dependence may be suggested by neglect of personal appearance. Acute intoxication with alcohol can be accompanied by an ataxic gait, drowsiness, slurred speech and a smell of alcohol on the breath. An ataxic gait associated with other symptoms should alert the examiner to the possibility of Wernicke's encephalopathy. Alcohol-related injuries may be apparent, especially soft-tissue injuries such as bruising. Excess sweating, tremor and agitation support the diagnosis of alcohol withdrawal.

Inspect the hands for signs of alcoholic liver disease (palmar erythema, leukonychia) and other nutritional deficits (koilonychia). A flapping tremor of the hands may be suggestive of hepatic encephalopathy. Nutritional deficiency is also associated with a tongue that is smooth and often described as erythematous or 'beefy' (glossitis). A moon-shaped facial appearance could indicate alcohol-induced pseudo-Cushing's syndrome. Nystagmus and bilateral lateral rectus or conjugate gaze palsies are found in Wernicke's encephalopathy, reflecting cranial nerve involvement of the oculomotor, abducens and vestibular nuclei.

Inspection of the chest and abdomen may expose further signs of alcoholic liver disease, including spider naevi, abdominal ascites or engorged superficial veins indicative of portal hypertension. Spider naevi are telangiectases that consist of a large arteriole from which radiate numerous small vessels. They are found in the distribution of the superior vena cava. Ascites is an abnormal collection of fluid in the peritoneal cavity, and is detected by testing for shifting dullness.

Cardiovascular and respiratory system

Alcohol is a common cause of reversible hypertension and measurement of the pulse may reveal atrial fibrillation or other arrhythmias.

Gastrointestinal system

There are three morphological types of damage in alcoholic liver disease (ALD):

- *fatty liver (alcohol steatosis)* – usually asymptomatic, although patients may complain of right hypocondrial pain; examination occasionally reveals an enlarged, smooth, firm liver
- *alcoholic hepatitis* – asymptomatic or presents with right hypochondrial pain, jaundice and heptomegaly; an arterial bruit is heard over the liver in half of cases
- *alcoholic cirrhosis* – which may present with all the features of chronic liver disease (see Table 22.2).

Pancreatitis can present with an acute abdomen (rigidity, rebound tenderness and guarding). The patient typically struggles to find a comfortable position, but may find relief by sitting forwards (the 'jack-knife position'). Chronic pancreatitis may be evident on examination by epigastric tenderness and occasionally a mass.

Table 22.2 Signs of chronic and decompensated liver disease on physical examination

	Chronic liver disease	Decompensated liver disease
Face	Parotid enlargement	Foetor hepaticus
	Facial flushing	Jaundice
Hands and body	Palmar erythema	Asterixis ('liver flap')
	Telangiectasia	Peripheral oedema
	Liver palms	
	Finger clubbing	
	Leukonychia	
	Spider naevi	
	Loss of body hair	
	Gynaecomastia	
	Muscle wasting	
Central nervous system	Ophthalmoplegia	Encephalopathy
	Nystagmus	
Cardiovascular system	Dysrhythmias	
	Hypertension	
Abdomen	Ascites	Ascites
	Hepatomegaly	Prominent veins on abdominal wall
	Splenomegaly	
Genitourinary	Testicular atrophy	

Central and peripheral nervous systems

Proximal myopathy is associated with chronic alcohol use, leading to weakness and muscle wasting. Characteristically the patient will have difficulty standing from the sitting position. Peripheral neuropathy is very common in heavy alcohol users, with sensory loss in the lower extremities (and the hands in severe cases). In addition to distal atrophy and weakness, deep tendon reflexes maybe decreased or absent, and glossiness and thinness of skin of the lower legs are also common findings (see p. 307, Fig. 22.1).

Investigations for assessment, diagnosis and monitoring

Investigations may be useful in the assessment, diagnosis and monitoring of alcohol use disorders, but there is no single test that serves all three purposes with complete accuracy. Box 22.1 lists those tests that are useful to clarify the results of the history and physical examination. Box 22.2 lists some other useful tests.

Screening for hazardous or harmful alcohol use

The most cost-effective method of screening for excessive drinking in primary care or general psychiatric settings is the use of standardised questionnaires.[16] The CAGE questionnaire and the Michigan Alcohol Screening Test (MAST) have now largely been replaced by the Alcohol Use Disorders Identification Test (AUDIT), which provides a brief measure of alcohol consumption, alcohol-related problems and symptoms of dependence. It is short and has relatively high sensitivity (92%) and specificity (93%). Other, even briefer instruments have developed from the AUDIT, including the Fast Alcohol Screening Test (FAST; four items), the AUDIT-C (three items) and the Paddington Alcohol Test (PAT; four items). The shorter tools have lower sensitivity and specificity but are easier to use in routine clinical practice. A NICE review has covered the evidence base for these tools.[17]

Treatment progress

Biochemical markers are useful in the clinical management of alcohol use disorders, principally to monitor treatment progress. These commonly include breath alcohol concentration and blood tests such as the erythrocyte mean cell volume (MCV) and liver enzymes such as alanine and aspartate aminotransferase (ALT and AST) and gamma-glutamyltransferase (GGT). As

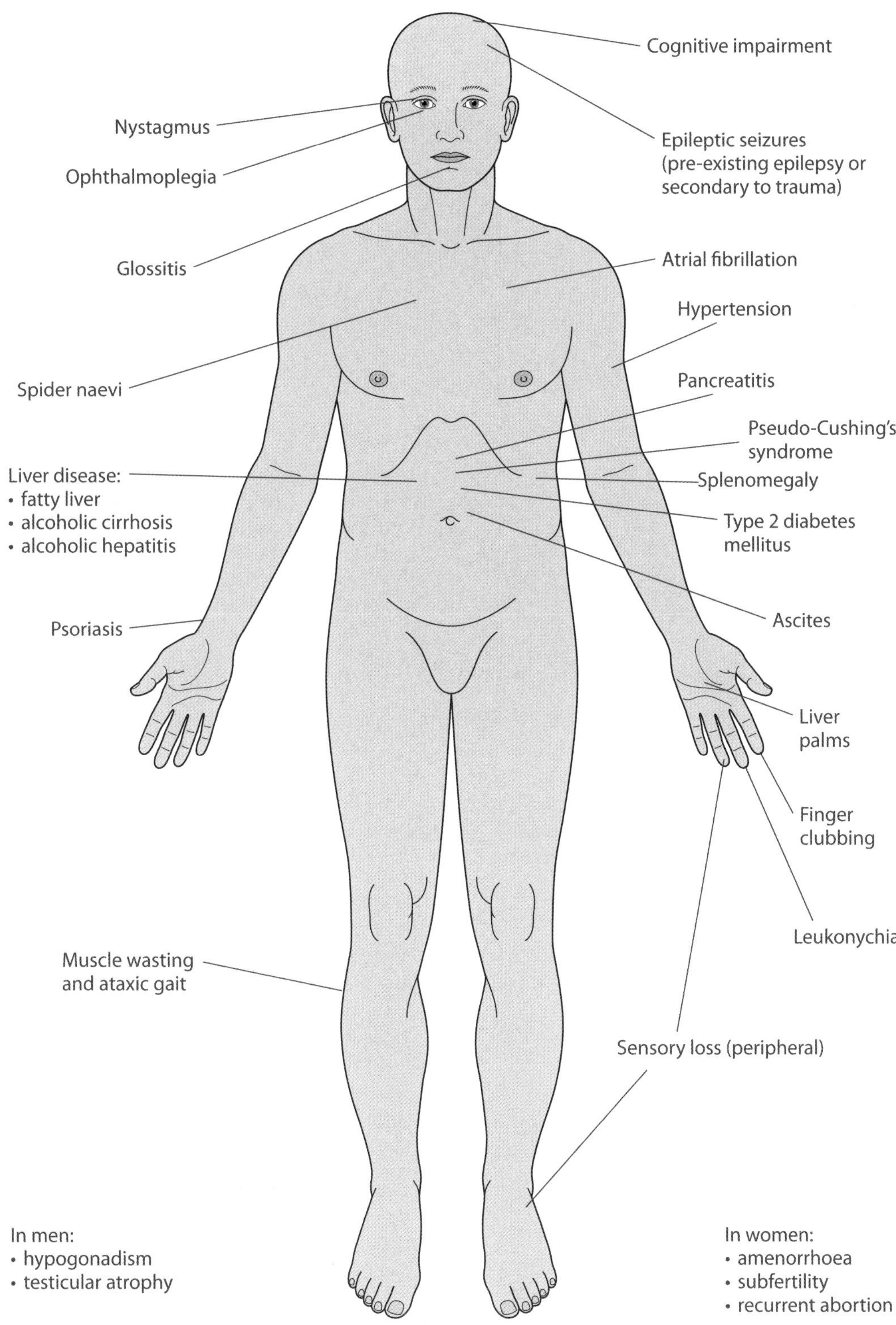

Fig. 22.1 Physical effects of alcohol misuse.

Box 22.1 Tests that are useful to clarify the results of the history and physical examination

- *Blood pressure and pulse* Exclude alcohol-related hypertension or arrhythmia
- *Electrocardiogram (ECG)* Important to diagnose arrhythmia and exclude ischaemia, infarction or hypertrophy
- *Chest X-ray* May be useful to confirm the development of pneumonia (including aspiration pneumonia) and tuberculosis, or to look for evidence of cardiac enlargement or pulmonary congestion associated with alcoholic cardiomyopathy
- *Blood tests* (see section on screening, below) Full blood count (to assess anaemia and hazardous drinking, which will be indicated by a raised mean corpuscular volume); urea and electrolytes (potassium must be checked if there is arrhythmia)
- *Liver function tests* Assess severity of liver disease
- *Clotting function* (e.g. international normalised ratio) Disrupted in liver failure
- *Thyroid function* To evaluate a differential diagnosis of arrhythmia

Box 22.2 Investigations useful to elucidate alcohol misuse in specific circumstances

- *Pregnancy test* This may alter guidance about alcohol consumption or treatment strategies
- *Echocardiography* This may be necessary to assess potential cardiac chamber enlargement associated with cardiomyopathy, valvular disease or reduced systolic function
- *Computerised tomography (CT) of the brain* This should be performed on all alcohol-dependent patients with a new onset of seizures or partial seizure, status epilepticus or a clear history of significant head trauma.[15]
- *Magnetic resonance imaging (MRI) or electroencephalography (EEG)* These investigations may be reserved for patients with no specific findings on CT examination of the brain, but who are at high risk for structural abnormalities (e.g. following a partial or prolonged seizure). The EEG should be carried out more than 48 hours after the seizure, but a routine EEG is likely to be normal in patients with alcohol-related seizures without epilepsy

carbohydrate-deficient transferrin (CDT) is unaffected by liver disease (relative to liver enzymes), it was initially hoped that it would prove useful in the detection of alcohol use disorders. However, the sensitivity is lower than first thought, although it may be useful in detecting relapse in alcohol-dependent patients in treatment.

In practice, tests are rarely used in isolation, and the sensitivity of combined tests is greater than that of any individual test alone.

When to refer patients who misuse alcohol

The conditions discussed below are all likely to require immediate referral to an acute medical service.

Acute liver failure

Rapid deterioration of liver function leads to encephalopathy and altered mental state, as well as coagulopathy (international normalised ratio > 1.5) in someone with no history of cirrhosis.

Hepatic decompensation

This occurs in patients with a history of liver disease of more than 6 months, as well as encephalopathy, jaundice, hepatic foetor, ascites and peripheral oedema.

The psychiatrist should take a history and examine the patient, and organise liver function tests.

Referral to a liver specialist should occur when:

- liver dysfunction is chronic (>6 months) and unexplained (i.e. tests of liver function are abnormal for ALT, AST, GGT, alkaline phosphatase)
- when the liver dysfunction is irreversible (e.g. in hepatitis C)
- when there is persistent abnormal synthetic function (i.e. raised bilirubin, low albumin, prolonged international normalised ratio)
- when the patient has taken a paracetamol overdose. See Chapter 17 on hepatology.

Acute upper gastrointestinal haemorrhage

Vomiting bright red blood (haematemesis) or production of black stools (melaena) is a medical emergency. Patients with severe bleeding are likely to require surgery and may experience circulatory shock (i.e. systolic pressure less than 100 mmHg, postural hypotension, pulse over 100 beats per minute). Where possible, blood should be taken for full blood count, urea and electrolytes, liver function tests and clotting tests (international normalised ratio, INR). Group and save/cross-match 4 units, and establish intravenous access using the largest gauge needle possible. Plasma expanders may help to prevent worsening of shock. (See p. 436 for differential diagnosis of the collapsed patient.)

Consideration for liver transplantation in those with alcoholic liver disease

Alcohol-related cirrhosis has become an increasingly common indication for liver transplantation in the past 20 years. There is no evidence of increased rates of post-operative complications in this group and survival rates are comparable to those of patients with cirrhosis of other aetiologies. Despite this, patients with alcohol-related cirrhosis are probably underrepresented on transplant waiting lists, and there is often uncertainty about which patients to refer and when to refer them.

People who are still actively drinking are not candidates for referral. A period of abstinence demonstrates commitment and will help to protect a scarce resource (a donated liver), as well as allowing the liver the chance to recover (thus potentially removing the need for the operation). There is still uncertainty over what period of abstinence is necessary. The Liver Advisory Group of UK Transplant has made recommendations to standardise criteria accepted by the UK liver transplant units for the assessment, listing and follow-up of patients where alcohol has contributed to the liver disease. These are summarised in Box 22.3.

Box 22.3 Recommendations for transplantation for patients with alcohol-related liver disease

Assessment by a specialist in substance misuse should consider risk factors associated with relapse to drinking and advise the transplant team on follow-up requirements to prevent this.

A fixed period of abstinence (usually 6 months) may help to predict abstinence after transplant, and some candidates for transplant will improve with abstinence such that transplantation is no longer indicated.

It is crucial to stress the importance of complete abstinence at all times, before and after the operation. The patient should be told that a return to alcohol consumption while on the waiting list will result in removal from the list.

Factors that preclude listing for a transplant because of a high likelihood of poor graft outcome include:

- alcoholic hepatitis, diagnosed by the clinical syndrome of acute jaundice and coagulopathy
- more than two episodes of non-compliance with medical care with no satisfactory explanation
- return to drinking following specialist assessment and advice (including removal from the list if found to be drinking while listed)
- concurrent or consecutive illicit drug use (except occasional cannabis use).

Predictors of liability to alcohol use following transplant are not currently recommended because of the inconsistent evidence base.

Following listing, the patient will be asked to sign an agreement that they will not drink after the transplant and will comply with follow-up.

Follow-up for alcohol use should be separate from and additional to the transplant follow-up and should be carried out by specialists in substance misuse.

The same process of assessment and listing should be applied to patients where alcohol has contributed to the progression of another chronic liver disease.

Alcohol contributes to the progression of hepatitis C recurrence and the safest approach is to advise all such patients to abstain totally from alcohol.

Source: Liver Advisory Group alcohol guidelines.[18]

What should happen in the community?

Alcohol detoxification

Steady consumption of alcohol over a period of time can lead to neuroadaptation and tolerance to its effects. A characteristic alcohol withdrawal syndrome then occurs when alcohol levels in the blood fall (Table 22.3).

Detoxification is the process of achieving an alcohol-free state as quickly and as comfortably as possible. Detoxification can occur in the home, on an out-patient or day-patient basis, or within a supported residential facility. A commonly used model of home detoxification involves daily visits from a psychiatric nurse trained to

Table 22.3 Alcohol withdrawal syndrome

Time after cessation of drinking	Symptoms
3–12 hours	Weakness
	Faintness
	Insomnia
	Tremor
	Sweating
8–48 hours	Illusions and fleeting hallucinations
	Seizures
	Cardiac dysrhythmias
> 72 hours	Gross tremor
(delirium tremens)	Tachycardia
	Sweating
	Raised temperature
	Insomnia
	Agitation
	Restlessness
	Confusion
	Disorientation
	Delusions
	Hallucinations

assess withdrawal and monitor for complications. Any prescribing or medical care is provided by a consultant-led team or on a shared-care basis with a general practitioner. The support of reliable family or friends is also important. For people without a home or without the support of friends or relatives, a community-based facility is a safe alternative to in-patient care.[19]

The following steps are important in preparing for the detoxification process:[19]

- giving information about the nature of withdrawal symptoms and what to expect during detoxification
- assessing the stage of change and refreshing care plans accordingly
- discussing practical issues such as childcare arrangements, time off work and travel
- identifying a friend or relative to provide support
- arranging for follow-up, including a discussion of whether the service user wishes to take disulfiram or other medication after detoxification
- planning daily activities for the weeks immediately after detoxification.

When medication is used to treat uncomplicated alcohol withdrawal, chlordiazepoxide is recognised as the gold standard. Diazepam has been used as if equivalent to chlordiazepoxide, although theoretically it has greater dependence-forming potential. Chlordiazepoxide is taken four times a day with the initial *daily total dose* around 100–200 mg, gradually reduced over 5–10 days. The patient should be encouraged to eat regularly and drink plenty of fluids.

Follow-up is important after detoxification, as a range of problems may occur 3–6 months after alcohol cessation. These include depression, anxiety, anhedonia, fatigue, sleep disturbances, craving for alcohol, headaches, and autonomic and metabolic dysfunction. These prolonged symptoms have been described as a 'protracted alcohol withdrawal syndrome' and they are associated with an increased rate of relapse to drinking.

Even though donor livers for liver transplantation are a scarce resource, alcoholic liver disease is not a contraindication. A period of abstinence may demonstrate commitment to recovery and can restore liver function, obviating the need for transplant. Do not refer for liver transplant assessment if the person is actively drinking.

Prophylaxis of Wernicke–Korsakoff syndrome

A flowchart for the assessment and management of Wernicke's encephalopathy is shown in Fig. 22.2. It is reasonable to recommend oral thiamine 50 mg four times per day for well nourished patients with no history of poor diet and no neuropsychiatric symptoms or signs of Wernicke's encephalopathy.[20] However, evidence suggests that in the most vulnerable patients the total absorption of thiamine is reduced to less than one-third of that in healthy people, and it is clear that oral preparations cannot be relied upon to treat patients at high risk of Wernicke's encephalopathy (particularly if medication compliance is also a problem). Therefore, the choice is between intravenous or intramuscular thiamine therapy.

'At risk' patients in the community should be given intramuscular thiamine, and this could be administered in a number of locations, including a general practice surgery, an accident and emergency department, an out-patient clinic, or day hospital, provided facilities to deal with anaphylactic reactions are available.[21] Patients at risk should receive intramuscular thiamine once a day for a minimum of 3 days.[8] Intramuscular Pabrinex® has a lower incidence of anaphylactic reactions than the intravenous preparation at 1 per 5 million pairs of Pabrinex® ampoules, which is far lower than the rate with many frequently used drugs that carry no special warning in the *British National Formulary*.[8,22]

The interface between community and in-patient settings

Alcohol detoxification

The majority of episodes of alcohol withdrawal occur with no complications, but careful monitoring is always recommended. Since withdrawal seizures and delirium tremens are likely to recur during further withdrawal episodes, if such a history is elicited, careful consideration should be given to the location of any future detoxification.

The need for admission to a medically managed in-patient facility depends on both social and medical risk factors. Homeless or socially isolated people may need supported accommodation to achieve detoxification, but not necessarily in an acute medical or psychiatric bed. Hospital admission is highly likely to be required if any of the following are present:

- seizures or delirium tremens at or around the time of assessment
- high levels of alcohol consumption combined with a history of seizures or delirium tremens
- coexisting misuse of other drugs (e.g. heroin, cocaine or benzodiazepines)
- recent head injury with loss of consciousness
- risk factors for/features of Wernicke's encephalopathy (see Fig. 22.1)
- illnesses requiring medical or surgical treatment (e.g. liver decompensation, pneumonia, cardiovascular failure)
- conditions requiring psychiatric admission (suicidal intent, severe anxiety or depression, psychotic illness).

Such cases require careful monitoring of pulse rate, blood pressure, temperature, level of consciousness, mental state and electrolytes.

> Detoxification in the community is safe and effective but hospitalise if: history of seizures or delirium tremens; co-existing misuse of drugs; risk factors for Wernicke's encephalopathy; or illness requiring treatment, such as depression or psychosis, liver decompensation, heart failure or pneumonia.

The likelihood of additional problems increases as the severity of withdrawal increases; they are often treated according to standard therapy. For example, where paranoid thoughts are a feature of withdrawal an antipsychotic might be the treatment of choice, and seizures may be treated with an anti-epileptic medication.

Wernicke–Korsakoff syndrome

Patients with a history of alcohol misuse and symptoms or signs suggestive of Wernicke's encephalopathy should be admitted to hospital for treatment (see Fig. 22.1). This should include two ampoule pairs of Pabrinex® (containing 500 mg thiamine) three times a day for 2–3 days, followed by one pair daily until improvement in the symptoms stops. It may be necessary to correct a low level of magnesium or other vitamins (e.g. niacin, vitamin B6, folate or vitamin B12).

Pharmacotherapy for relapse prevention

The 6 month period after alcohol detoxification is a high-risk period for lapse or relapse back to regular alcohol consumption. Therefore, consideration should be given to offering pharmacotherapy (using either acamprosate or oral naltrexone) in combination with an individual psychological intervention (e.g. cognitive–behavioural therapies, behavioural therapies or social network and environment-based therapies) focused specifically on alcohol misuse.[24] Alternatively, disulfiram may be considered for patients who have a goal of abstinence but for whom acamprosate and oral naltrexone are not suitable, or for those who prefer disulfiram and understand the relative risks of taking the drug. Oral naltrexone does not currently have UK marketing authorisation for this indication, and so informed consent should be obtained and documented. A full assessment should be conducted before the patient starts treatment with pharmacotherapy, as outlined above in the section on physical examination.

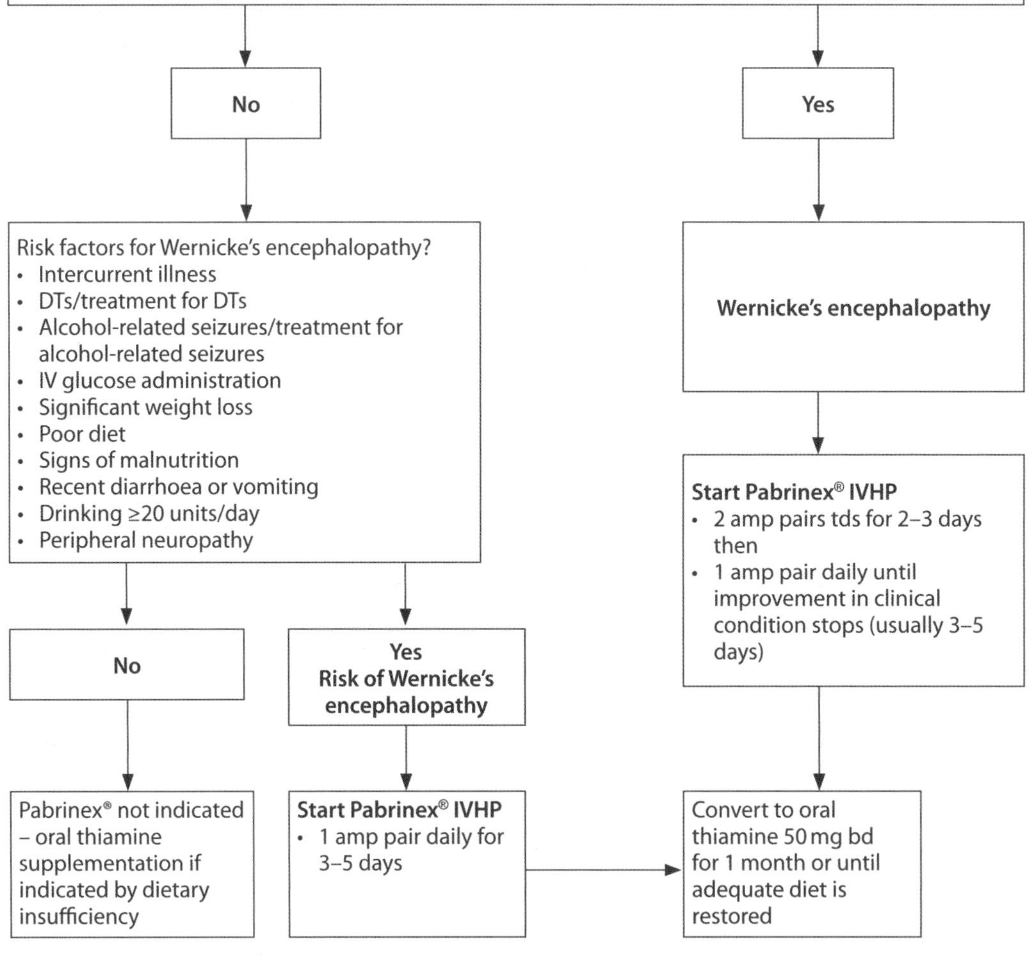

Fig. 22.2 Flowchart for the assessment and management of Wernicke's encephalopathy. Source: Day *et al*, 2010.[23] amp, ampoule; bd, twice per day; DTs, delirium tremens; IV, intravenous; IVHP intravenous high-potency; tds, three times per day.

Acamprosate treatment should be started as soon as possible after detoxification, at a dose of 1998 mg (666 mg three times a day), unless the patient weighs less than 60 kg (in which case the maximum dose is 1332 mg per day). It is usually prescribed for up to 6 months, but can be used for longer with those who benefit from the drug and who want to continue with it. Prescribing should continue if the patient returns to alcohol but stopped if drinking persists for 4–6 weeks. The patient should stay under monthly supervision for 6 months, and at reduced but regular intervals if the drug is continued after 6 months. Routine use of blood tests to monitor treatment is unnecessary, but should be considered for monitoring recovery of liver function and as a motivational aid for patients.[24]

Oral naltrexone is also started after detoxification, commencing at 25 mg per day but aiming for a maintenance dose of 50 mg per day. The patient should be given an information card about its impact on opioid-based analgesics. The usual length of treatment, level of supervision and monitoring arrangements are the same as for acamprosate, but it is worth noting that naltrexone has been associated with acute liver failure when prescribed at doses of 300 mg or more per day. If patients feel unwell they should be advised to stop the oral naltrexone immediately.[24]

Disulfiram treatment should start at least 24 hours after consumption of the last alcoholic drink. It is usually prescribed at a dose of 200 mg per day, but if this dose is taken regularly for at least a week and does not cause a sufficiently unpleasant reaction when combined with alcohol, consider increasing the dose in consultation with the patient. Liver function tests, urea levels and electrolytes are essential before the patient starts disulfiram to assess for liver or renal impairment; the drug is contraindicated in pregnancy and in patients with a history of severe mental illness, stroke, heart disease or hypertension. Review is required at least every 2 weeks for the first 2 months, then monthly for the following 4 months. Ideally, a family member or carer who is properly informed about the use of disulfiram should oversee the administration of the drug. The patient and family should be warned about the interaction between disulfiram and alcohol (which may also be found in food, perfume, aerosol sprays and so on), the symptoms of which may include flushing, nausea, palpitations and, more seriously, arrhythmias, hypotension and collapse. There is also the rare possibility of the rapid and unpredictable onset of hepatotoxicity, so patients should be advised that if they feel unwell or develop a fever or jaundice, they should stop taking disulfiram and seek urgent medical attention.[24]

Antidepressants, including selective serotonin reuptake inhibitors (SSRIs) and long-term courses of benzodiazepines should not be given routinely for the treatment of alcohol misuse alone.

Management of alcohol-related seizures

Alcohol dependence is associated with poor seizure control in patients with epilepsy. This may be due to the stimulant effect of alcohol, alcohol withdrawal, poor compliance with and enhanced metabolism of anti-epileptic medication, and altered pattern of sleep. There is a difference between preventing seizures, treating a patient during a seizure and preventing recurrent seizures. Effective treatment of alcohol withdrawal will prevent seizures, so a seizure should prompt a review of the doses of benzodiazepines being used.

Alcohol withdrawal seizures are usually self-limiting, but fast-acting benzodiazepines such as lorazepam reduce the chances of further seizures occurring. Doses of benzodiazepines up to 60 mg diazepam equivalent administered orally in divided doses are helpful in attenuating an initial seizure and preventing recurrence in the first 24 hours.[15] Anti-epileptics such as phenytoin, carbamazepine and valproic acid appear to be effective in preventing primary alcohol withdrawal seizures, but their beneficial effects are not increased when combined with longer-acting benzodiazepines. They have not been shown to be effective and safe in preventing recurrent alcohol withdrawal seizures. The risks and benefits must be carefully weighed up in patients whose compliance with medication is variable, as rapid withdrawal of drugs such as phenytoin may increase the risk of seizure. Patients with a known structural brain lesion or an epileptogenic focus on EEG should be treated with long-term anticonvulsant therapy.

References

1 Department of Health. *Alcohol Needs Assessment Research Project*. Department of Health, 2005.

2 Leon DA, McCambridge J. Liver cirrhosis mortality rates in Britain from 1950 to 2002: an analysis of routine data. *Lancet* 2006; **367**: 52–6.

3 Prime Minister's Strategy Unit. *Alcohol Harm Reduction Strategy for England*. Cabinet Office, 2004.

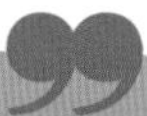

Summary

'Low-risk' alcohol consumption (up to 3 units per day) protects middle-aged men against coronary heart disease, but mortality from all causes increases as alcohol consumption increases above 3 units per day in men and 2 units in women. Alcohol misuse or dependence is associated with a wide range of serious physical health problems. The toxic effects of alcohol may be caused directly by alcohol or by the by-products of its metabolism, and every organ system in the body may be affected. The mortality rate of heavy drinkers is at least twice that of the normal population. A range of screening tools are available for detecting excessive alcohol consumption in non-specialist settings, and physical examination and investigations are an important part of management. There are a number of alcohol-related consequences that are genuinely life-threatening (e.g. delirium tremens, acute liver failure, and acute upper gastrointestinal haemorrhage), and others that merit further investigation and treatment (e.g. chronic liver failure, Wernicke–Korsakoff syndrome).

4 Anderson P, Gual A, Colom J. *Alcohol and Primary Health Care: Clinical Guidelines on Identification and Brief Interventions.* Department of Health of the Government of Catalonia, 2005.

5 HM Government. *Safe. Sensible. Social. The Next Steps in the National Alcohol Strategy*. Department of Health/ Home Office, 2007.

6 Royal Colleges of Physicians, Royal College of Psychiatrists and Royal College of General Practitioners. *Alcohol and the Heart in Perspective: Sensible Limits Reaffirmed: Report of a Joint Working Group (CR42).* Royal College of Physicians, 1995.

7 Victor M, Adams RD, Collins GH. *The Wernicke–Korsakoff Syndrome and Related Neurological Disorders Due to Alcoholism and Malnutrition.* F. A. Davis Company, 1989.

8 Thomson AD, Marshall J. The treatment of patients at risk of developing Wernicke's encephalopathy in the community. *Alcohol Alcohol* 2006; **41**: 159–67.

9 Harper CG, Giles M, Finlay-Jones R. Clinical signs in the Wernicke–Korsakoff complex: a retrospective analysis of 131 cases diagnosed at necropsy. *J Neurol Neurosurg Psychiatry* 1986; **49**: 341–5.

10 Cook CCH. Prevention and treatment of Wernicke–Korsakoff syndrome. *Alcohol Alcohol* 2000; **35** (suppl 1): 19–20.

11 Bates ME, Barry D, Dowden SC. Neurocognitive impairment associated with alcohol use disorders: implications for treatment. *Exp Clin Psychopharmacol* 2002; **10**: 193–212.

12 Lishman WA. Wernicke's encephalopathy. In *Organic Psychiatry: The Psychological Consequences of Cerebral Disorder* (3rd edn): 575–85. Blackwell Science, 1998.

13 Oslin DW, Cary MS. Alcohol-related dementia: validation of diagnostic criteria. *Am J Geriatr Psychiatry* 2003; **11**: 441–7.

14 Joyce EM. Aetiology of alcoholic brain damage: alcoholic neurotoxicity or thiamine malnutrition? *Br Med Bull* 1994; **50**: 99–114.

15 Rathlev NK, Ulrich AS, Delanty N, *et al.* Alcohol-related seizures. *J Emerg Med* 2006; **31**: 157–63.

16 Drummond C, Ghodse H, Chengappa S. Use of investigations in the diagnosis and management of alcohol use disorders. In *Clinical Topics in Addiction* (ed E Day): 113–29. RCPsych Publications, 2007.

17 Jackson R, Johnson M, Campbell F, *et al. Screening and Brief Interventions for Prevention and Early Identification of Alcohol Use Disorders in Adults and Young People.* ScHARR Public Health Collaborating Centre, University of Sheffield, 2010 (http://www.nice.org.uk/nicemedia/live/13001/49007/49007.pdf).

18 Liver Advisory Group. *Alcohol Guidelines: UK Liver Transplant Group Recommendations for Liver Transplant Assessment in the Context of Alcohol-related Liver Disease.* Liver Advisory Group, 2005 (http://www.organdonation.nhs.uk/ukt/about_transplants/organ_allocation/pdf/liver_advisory_group_alcohol_guidelines-november_2005.pdf).

19 Raistrick D, Heather N, Godfrey C. *Review of the Effectiveness of Treatment for Alcohol Problems.* National Treatment Agency for Substance Misuse, 2006.

20 Thomson AD, Cook CCH, Touquet R, *et al*. The Royal College of Physicians' report on alcohol: guidelines for managing Wernicke's encephalopathy in the accident and emergency department. *Alcohol Alcohol* 2002; **37**: 513–21.

21 Scottish Intercollegiate Guidelines Network. *The Management of Harmful Drinking and Alcohol Dependence in Primary Care.* SIGN, 2003.

22 Thomson AD, Cook CCH. Parenteral thiamine and Wernicke's encephalopathy: the balance of risks and perception of concern. *Alcohol Alcohol* 1997; **32**: 207–9.

23 Day E, Callaghan R, Kuruvilla T, *et al.* Pharmacy-based intervention in Wernicke's encephalopathy. *Psychiatrist* 2010; **34**: 234–8.

24 National Institute for Health and Clinical Excellence. *Alcohol-Use Disorders: Diagnosis, Assessment and Management of Harmful Drinking and Alcohol Dependence*. Clinical Guideline 115. NICE, 2011.

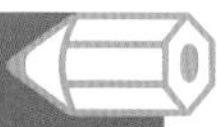

Learning points

- Alcohol-related hypertension occurs in up to 25% of those drinking at a 'harmful' level, and a significant percentage of the excess deaths attributable to alcohol are attributable to cardiovascular problems. Alcohol use in conjunction with tobacco smoking leads to an increased risk of oral and oesophageal cancers.
- Fatty change in the liver (steatosis) is present in 90% of steady drinkers, and in about 30–40% of heavy drinkers this progresses to alcoholic hepatitis. Cirrhosis develops in 8–30% of drinkers with a 10- to 20-year history of daily heavy drinking, but susceptibility varies between individuals.
- The risk of developing cirrhosis increases steeply with consumption of more than 3 units of alcohol per day. Other risk factors include female sex, obesity, poor nutrition, type 2 diabetes and hepatitis C. Twin studies suggest that there is also a genetic component to disease risk.
- Wernicke's encephalopathy carries significant levels of mortality and morbidity, but is easily prevented. However, the pathology may not be associated with the classical clinical triad (nystagmus, abducent and conjugate gaze palsies, ataxia of gait, and a global confusional state) in up to 90% of patients.
- A presumptive diagnosis of Wernicke's encephalopathy should be made for any patient with a history of alcohol dependence and evidence of ophthalmoplegia, ataxia, acute confusion, memory disturbance, unexplained hypotension, hypothermia, coma or unconsciousness.
- Between 50 and 80% of people with chronic alcohol use disorders experience mild to severe cognitive deficits.
- Alcohol-related seizures are usually short generalised tonic–clonic seizures that occur up to 48 hours after the last drink, and can present without other signs of alcohol withdrawal. The presence of either partial seizures or status epilepticus suggests structural brain lesions.
- Glucose intolerance occurs in up to 40% of individuals with alcohol dependence and there is an association with type 2 diabetes (although possibly a J-shaped dose–response curve, as low alcohol consumption may have protective effects against diabetes).
- Key investigations in those with harmful alcohol use include blood pressure, pulse, ECG and blood tests.
- Computerised tomography of the brain should be performed on all patients with alcohol dependence with new onset of seizures or a partial seizure, status epilepticus or a clear history of significant head trauma. Magnetic resonance imaging or electroencephalography may be reserved for patients with negative head findings on CT but at high risk for structural abnormalities (i.e. following a partial or prolonged seizure).
- The most cost-effective method of screening for excessive drinking in primary care or general psychiatric settings is the use of standardised questionnaires such as the Alcohol Use Disorders Identification Test (AUDIT), which are short and have relatively high sensitivity (92%) and specificity (93%).
- Hepatic decompensation is a potential reason for referral for specialist medical assessment, and may present with encephalopathy, jaundice, hepatic foetor, ascites and peripheral oedema. The psychiatrist should take a history, examine the patient and organise some liver function tests. The patient should be referred to a liver specialist when there is persistent abnormal synthetic function (i.e. raised bilirubin, low albumin, prolonged INR).
- Vomiting bright red blood (haematemesis) or production of black stools (melaena) is a medical emergency.

23

Drug misuse

Ed Day and Sanjay Khurmi

Illicit drugs cause a range of physiological effects, and can ultimately lead to a state of dependence which is often associated with a decline in physical and mental health. This chapter describes the signs and symptoms of the commonly used drugs of misuse, and the features of withdrawal. It also covers the physical signs and laboratory tests that may be used to monitor dependent individuals, drug and metabolite testing, how to reduce the risk of accidental overdose and when to refer to other services.

Introduction

Man has been consuming natural compounds with sedative, stimulant or euphoriant properties for thousands of years. Three broad categories of psychoactive substances are highlighted in Tables 23.1 and 23.2. The effect that each will have depends on the amount used and the frequency with which it is taken, the route (swallowed, smoked, sniffed, injected), the user's past experience with this or other substances, and a variety of other factors. There is a current trend towards taking combinations of drugs, and this can alter the risks and benefits of each of them. Most substances produce some form of initial pleasure for the individual, and this may develop into a degree of 'necessity' or 'addiction' and a loss of personal control over use of the substance.

Opioids

Most physical problems associated with the use of illicit opioids such as heroin come not from the drug itself. Once people become dependent, maintaining a supply of opioids is often a full-time occupation, and they often neglect their physical health.

Acute administration of opioids causes feelings of euphoria and well-being, followed by drowsiness and poor concentration ('gauching'). Large doses can cause depression of the respiratory centres and respiratory arrest, but tolerance develops rapidly with repeated doses. Once physical dependence has developed, a characteristic opioid withdrawal syndrome occurs when use is reduced or stopped. This peaks after 3–4 days, although mild symptoms, including insomnia, may persist for several weeks.

Heroin not only suppresses appetite but also the cough reflex, increasing the risk of respiratory problems, including aspiration pneumonia. There is a strong link between injecting heroin and tuberculosis, due to the physiological effects of the drug on cell-mediated immune response, the environment and the risk behaviours of drug users.

Table 23.1 Symptoms and signs of intoxication

Opioids	Stimulants	Benzodiazepines
Symptoms		
Apathy	Excessive activity	Relaxation
Sedation	Difficulty sitting still	Drowsiness and sleep
Psychomotor retardation	Poor appetite	Mild euphoria
Impaired attention	Limited or no sleep	Light-headedness
Impaired judgement	Irritable and argumentative	Lack of facial expression or animation
Disinhibition	Anxious	Flat affect
Interference with personal functioning	Euphoria and increased energy	
	Hypervigilance	
	Grandiose beliefs/actions	
	Paranoid ideation	
	Auditory, visual or tactile illusions	
	Hallucinations with intact orientation	
Signs		
Drowsiness	Dilated pupils	Slurred speech
Slurred speech	Dry mouth and nose	Muscle incoordination
Pupillary constriction	Runny nose	Ataxia
Decreased level of consciousness	Chronic sinus/nasal problems	Seizures
	Nose bleeds	
	Tachycardia	
	Increased blood pressure	
	Repetitive stereotyped behaviours	

Stimulants

Intoxication with stimulant drugs such as cocaine or amphetamine produces elevated mood and increased alertness and self-confidence. As the dose increases, there may be restlessness, rapid speech, muscle twitching, nausea, vomiting and irregular respiration. Large doses promote ataxia, insomnia and hyperthermia, and extreme hypertension may lead to cerebral haemorrhage and stroke. The beneficial mental effects of use and the depressant nature of withdrawal tend to promote binges. Large or frequent doses over 24–48 hours may lead to grand-mal seizures, and longer periods of use lead to malnutrition, vitamin deficiencies, weight loss, exhaustion and dental problems.

Stimulant use is associated with both acute and chronic cardiovascular problems,[1] including myocardial ischaemia and infarction, hypertension and accelerated atherosclerosis, aortic dissection, myocarditis, dilated and hypertrophic cardiomyopathy and arrhythmias.

Cocaine is rapidly absorbed by either nasal snorting or inhaling, increases the oxygen demand of the heart (by increasing blood pressure and heart rate) and reduces oxygen delivery (by coronary spasm). The risk of acute myocardial infarction is highest within the first hour of use.

Methylenedioxymethamphetamine (MDMA; 'ecstasy')

Ecstasy enhances sensory perceptions and can produce states of altered consciousness and visual illusions, in combination with tachycardia, dry mouth, dilated pupils and facial muscle stiffness. Tiredness, muscle aching and headache may be present 24 hours after taking the drug. Some occasional users of ecstasy have died as a consequence of taking only one tablet. The cause of death is variable, but hyperthermia is a characteristic feature.

Table 23.2 Key features of withdrawal syndromes

Opioids	Stimulants	Benzodiazepines
Sweating	Fatigue	Sweating
Gooseflesh	Psychomotor retardation or agitation	Insomnia
Flushing	Increased appetite	Weakness
Low-grade fever	Insomnia or hypersomnia	Tinnitus
Running eyes and nose		Dizziness
Sneezing		Muscle twitching
Yawning		Psychomotor agitation
Dilated pupils		Headache
Shivering		Tremor
Psychomotor agitation		Tachycardia
Pains in muscles, bones and joints		Postural hypotension
Tachycardia		Palpitations
Hypertension		Anorexia
Nausea		Nausea
Vomiting		Abdominal discomfort
Abdominal discomfort		Diarrhoea
Diarrhoea		
Insomnia		

Hypnotics and sedatives

Benzodiazepines

The benzodiazepines produce anxiolytic, hypnotic, anticonvulsant and muscle relaxant effects. The development of tolerance and a dependence syndrome can lead to unpleasant discontinuation (withdrawal) effects. The pattern is variable and the time course depends on the half-life of the benzodiazepine involved. The physical effects are combined with a wide range of neuropsychiatric complications and perceptual disturbances in all modalities, often leading to considerable disability. In high-dose users, there is a risk of seizures during acute withdrawal, which can be particularly problematic with concurrent alcohol dependence.

Barbiturates

Barbiturate misuse is now relatively rare, but intoxication is associated with a high risk of respiratory depression or arrest.

Cannabis

Mild intoxication with cannabis (Fig. 23.1) produces a feeling of light-headedness, often accompanied by ringing in the ears. In addition to a feeling of exhilaration and lightness of the limbs, there may be psychomotor overactivity, with rapid speech or else a lethargic state approaching stupor. The user may wake with fatigue or generalised aches and pains.

Psychomotor impairment caused by cannabis may lead to an increased risk of road traffic accidents. Cannabis can precipitate hypertension and worsen symptoms of coronary artery disease; subtle memory and attention deficits may persist after periods of chronic intoxication.

Other drugs of misuse

Lysergic acid diethylamide (LSD)

In addition to its hallucinogenic properties, LSD has a sympathomimetic action. Tachycardia, hypertension, pyrexia and dilated pupils occur shortly after ingestion.

Alkyl nitrites ('poppers')

Used for their euphoric and relaxant properties, alkyl nitrites have a vasodilatory effect that leads to the rapid onset of palpitations, tachycardia, hypotension, flushing, sweats, headache and dizziness.

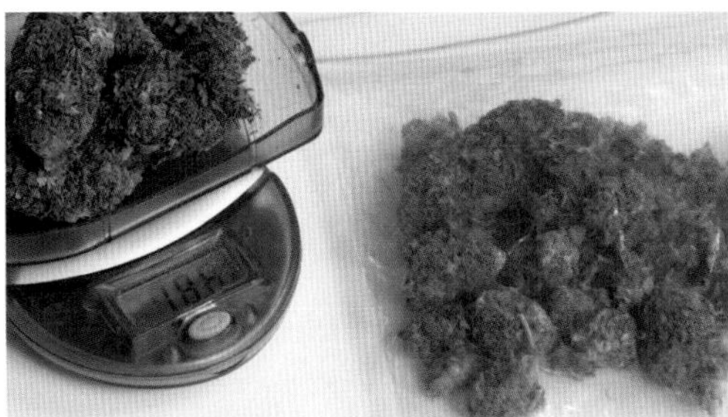

Fig. 23.1 Weighing marihuana to sell

Gamma-hydroxybutyrate (GHB)

This has been used to treat depression, alcohol dependence, insomnia, narcolepsy and as a general anaesthetic in obstetric procedures. It is misused for its euphoric effects, and use has been increasing in the past decade. GHB receptors can be found in many brain areas, mainly in the hippocampus and cortex. At low concentrations in the central nervous system (CNS), it mediates dopamine release from GHB receptors (leading to euphoria), but as GHB levels rise, stimulation of GABA-B receptors leads to a decrease in dopamine release and to sedative and hypnotic effects.

Ketamine

Ketamine-provoked sensations are dose related and characteristically dissociative. Lower doses produce a pleasant feeling of floating in a 'magical world' ('K-land'), whereas higher doses may lead to a feeling of complete sensory detachment similar to an out-of-body experience ('K-hole'). Other symptoms may include dizziness and decreased seizure threshold, neuromuscular disturbances (muscle rigidity, slurred speech, loss of coordination, numbness, polyneuropathy, diplopia and nystagmus), and autonomic disturbance, respiratory and cardiac arrest at high doses.

Solvents

Intoxication with solvents produces similar physical features to sedative or hypnotic drugs. Regular users may have nasal or perioral sores, and sudden death can occur due to asphyxia or cardiac arrhythmia on exercise.

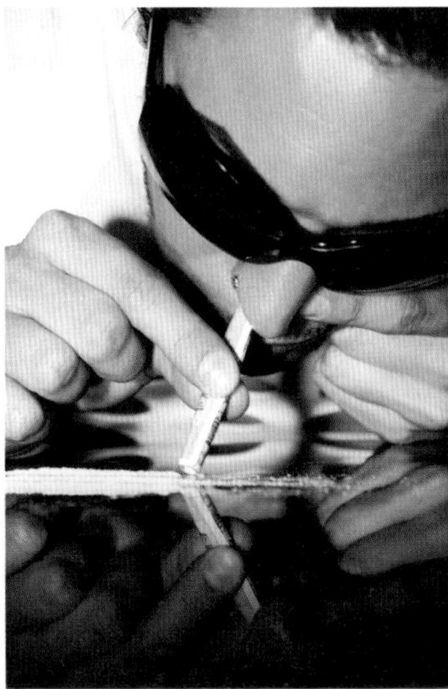

ig. 23.2 Snorting ocaine powder

Routes of use

Inhalation, smoking, chasing

Chronic bronchitis has been associated with smoking cannabis, and histopathological changes that precede the development of lung malignancy may also occur. The risk of developing cancers of the oral cavity, pharynx and oesophagus is increased.

Inhaling cocaine (Fig. 23.2) predisposes users to infection of the upper respiratory tract, including sinusitis and septal abscesses. Acute respiratory symptoms develop within minutes to hours of cocaine use. The commonest problems are a cough accompanied by the production of black sputum, chest pain (sometimes with shortness of breath), haemoptysis and an exacerbation of asthma.[2] Thermal injury resulting in reactive airways disease is possible, as is barotrauma such as pneumothorax and pneumomediastinum. A syndrome called 'crack lung' has been described, and usually occurs within the first 48 hours of smoking cocaine. It is recognised by the combination of chest pain, cough with haemoptysis, shortness of breath and bronchospasm. It appears to be caused by a hypersensitivity pneumonitis, and itchiness, fever and pulmonary and systemic eosinophilia are also present.

As mentioned above, the risk of pulmonary tuberculosis (including drug-resistant cases) appears to be increased among drug users as a result of crowded living conditions, delays in diagnosis, poor adherence to treatment, and the prevalence of HIV infection or AIDS.

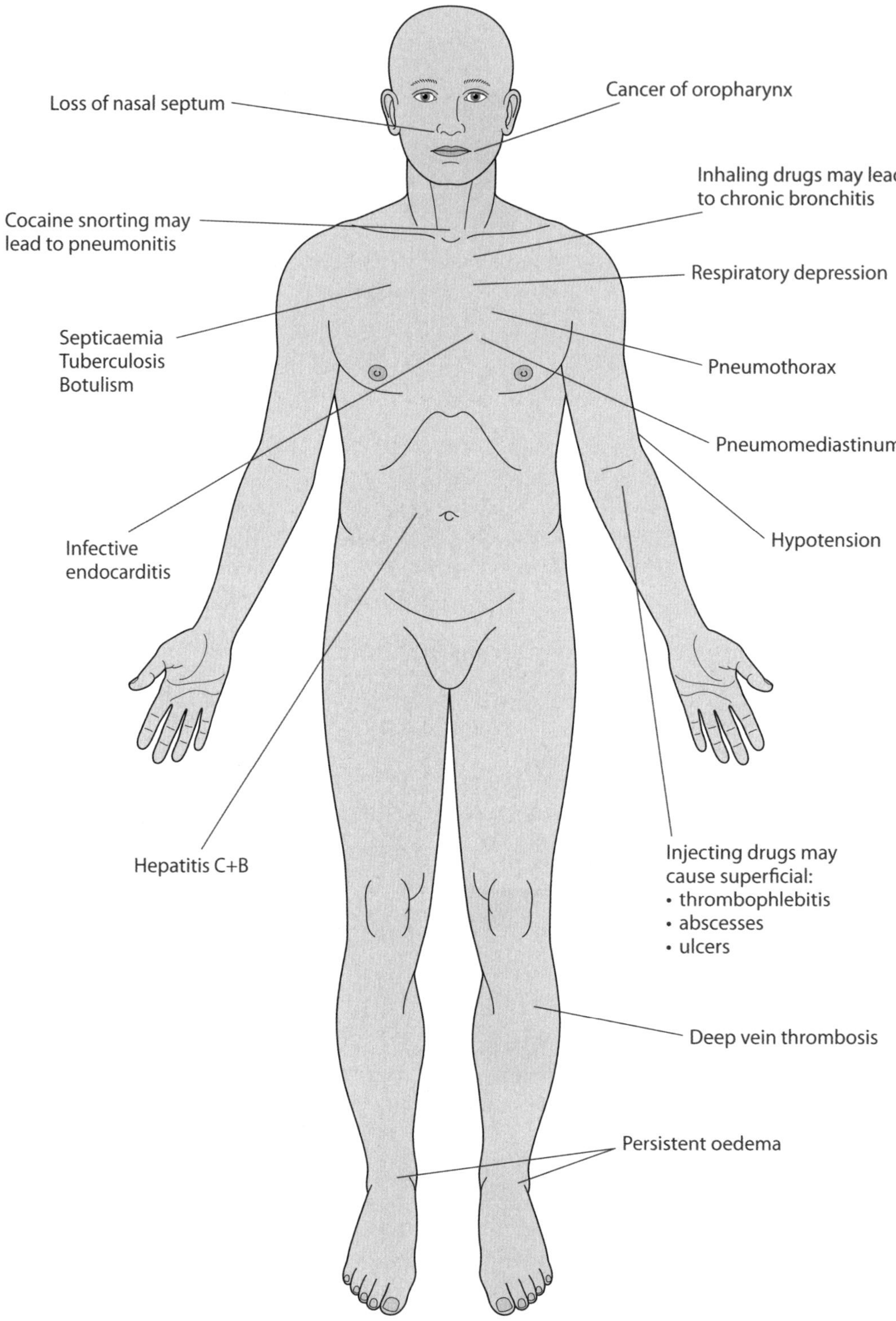

Fig. 23.3 Complications of drug misuse.

Intravenous or intramuscular injection

Many of the deleterious physical effects of illicit drugs are a direct result of injecting (Fig. 23.4). Opioids, amphetamines, cocaine and benzodiazepines can be injected, and this mode of administration is common when supplies of a drug are limited. The drive towards 'harm reduction' aims to reduce the adverse health consequences of injecting drug use by encouraging the employment of safer techniques and equipment, and ultimately to substitute it with another mode of drug administration.

Blood-borne viruses

The greatest public health concern relating to injecting arises from the transmission of blood-borne bacterial and viral infections via shared equipment. In the UK, approximately one in every 65 injecting drug users (IDUs) is infected with HIV, but this figure is low in comparison with hepatitis C, where best estimates suggest that approximately half of IDUs are infected (albeit with wide geographical variation in rates – between 30% and 80% of past and current IDUs may be infected).[3] The commonest route of transmission of hepatitis C is by sharing blood-contaminated needles or injecting equipment. As only 20% develop hepatitis, most acute infections fail to be diagnosed. The virus persists in 85% of cases and virtually all patients with chronic infection develop some inflammatory liver changes. Severity ranges from slowly progressive, low-grade inflammation to chronic active hepatitis. About 20% of those chronically infected develop cirrhosis, and 25% of these may develop hepatocellular carcinoma. These complications can take 20–30 years to develop.[4]

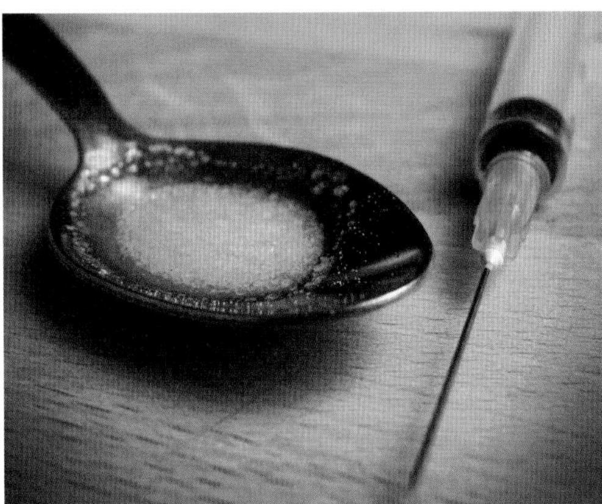

Fig. 23.4 Illicit drug prepared for injection

Transmission of hepatitis B continues among IDUs even though there is an effective vaccine. Hepatitis B is transmitted both parenterally and sexually. The incubation period varies from 6 weeks to 6 months, with a spectrum of severity between subclinical infection and fatal hepatic necrosis. Only 30% of adult cases appear to result in jaundice and many go unrecognised. About 5% of those infected become chronic carriers of the virus, and around 15–25% of carriers may develop an active hepatitis which progresses to cirrhosis. Chronic hepatitis B carriers with liver disease are at increased risk of developing hepatocellular carcinoma. (See Chapter 18 on blood-borne viruses.)

Infective endocarditis

Infective endocarditis has an estimated incidence of 1.5–3.3 cases per 1000 IDUs per year. Right-sided endocarditis is more frequent (over 50% of cases involve the tricuspid valve) and may cause pulmonary pathology, including abscesses.[5]

Skin

Cutaneous adverse effects of injecting are common. Repeated injection of drugs and adulterants using unsterile, contaminated equipment leads to the development of hyperpigmented 'tracks' along the path of veins. Inflammation of the veins (thrombophlebitis), local infections, abscesses, ulcers and septicaemia are all common. Collapse of surface veins in the limbs can lead to persistent oedema. Necrotising fasciitis is a rare but severe manifestation, usually associated with subcutaneous injection. It is associated with a high rate of mortality and amputation.

Overdose

Opioid overdose can result from simultaneous use of more than one drug and by fluctuations in the purity of a drug bought on the street. It often follows a period of abstinence, when tolerance to the drug's respiratory depressant effects falls. The effects of opioid overdose are slow, shallow breathing, low blood pressure, reduced

> Infective endocarditis is diagnosed in up to 20% of IDUs hospitalised with fever, so a low index of suspicion is required.

levels of consciousness and ultimately coma and death. However, these effects can be rapidly reversed by the antagonist naloxone, and some treatment services have now started to train service users to administer naloxone in an emergency to a fellow IDU who has accidentally overdosed (see below).[6]

Vascular system

Other consequences of injecting drug use include botulism, tetanus and deep vein thrombosis. The repeated trauma of venepuncture, local infections and the irritating qualities of the drugs and adulterants are the main cause of superficial and deep-venous thrombosis, and the latter is a complication particularly associated with injecting in the femoral vein. The femoral vein is easy to locate and it may be the last accessible vein. Injection marks in the groin are less visible than those in other sites, and some users report a quicker or better drug effect.

Drug interactions and polypharmacy

Regular users of psychoactive drugs rarely use them in isolation. For example, up to two-thirds of people who take cocaine combine it with alcohol; the combination is thought to prolong cocaine's euphoric effect and to decrease its unpleasant consequences, such as agitation and dysphoria. This may be partly due to the formation of a third active compound, ethylbenzoylecgonine (commonly known as cocaethylene), which has similar behavioural pharmacology and psychomotor stimulant effects to cocaine but higher levels of toxicity.[7] Both cocaine and cocaethylene inhibit catecholamine reuptake into nerve terminals, but the half-life of cocaethylene is four times longer than that of cocaine, and so cocaine-related symptoms may continue long after the drug was last used.

Nicotine is the second most commonly combined drug with cocaine. Most patients with cocaine-induced myocardial infarction also smoke cigarettes, and it is suggested that the simultaneous use of cocaine and tobacco may enhance coronary vasospasm. It is not unusual to find normal coronary arteries on cardiac catheterisation after cocaine-induced myocardial infarction, and many such patients smoke more than 20 cigarettes per day.

Combining cocaine and heroin in the same syringe creates a 'speedball'; this accounts for 12–15% of cocaine-related patient presentations to emergency departments in the USA. Cocaine's stimulant effects wear off quicker than the sedating effects of the heroin, leading to a high risk of delayed respiratory depression.

> Combining cocaine and alcohol can increase the risk of cardiovascular problems, liver damage, injuries and death (see p. 328, cocaine and chest pain).

Illicit drugs are often mixed with both inert and active substances either to increase the apparent quantity of the street drug or to enhance its effect. Such adulterants are likely to increase the risk of adverse effects, including respiratory, vascular and systemic problems. Active substances known to be used are local anaesthetics, other stimulants such as amphetamine, caffeine, methylphenidate or strychnine, LSD, phencyclidine (PCP), and benzodiazepines. Bulking agents may include talc, ascorbic acid, chalk, brick dust, cornstarch and lactose.

Physical examination

The findings on physical examination vary according to the drug(s) of misuse and the method of administration. The examination should focus on the patient's complaints, while bearing in mind the general sequelae of the patient's drug(s) of choice outlined in the following paragraphs.

General appearance

The general appearance of the patient may give valuable clues to a diagnosis of illicit drug misuse. Acute intoxication with illicit drugs may be indicated by an unsteady (ataxic) gait, drowsiness, slurred speech and restlessness or poor concentration. Neglect of personal appearance and weight loss commonly occur in patients dependent on illicit drugs. Observation of the hands and fingers may show signs of infective endocarditis such as clubbing, Osler's nodes and Janeway lesions.

General observation

Pupillary dilation (mydriasis) can indicate opioid withdrawal or acute intoxication with stimulants or LSD. Pupillary constriction (miosis) occurs after recent opioid use. Red eyes (dilation of conjunctival blood vessels) occur with cannabis and solvent misuse. Nystagmus can indicate intoxication with sedative hypnotics. Lacrimation, rhinorrhoea and profuse sweating should alert the examiner to the possibility of opioid withdrawal. Occasional snorting of drugs may produce congestion of the nasal mucosa, and this may become nasal septum ulceration or even perforation with more prolonged use. Solvent misuse is suggested by the characteristic breath odour or traces on the cuffs of jackets, on lapels, handkerchiefs, rags or plastic bags or bottles.

Basic observations

Hypertension is found in cases of acute intoxication with stimulants and LSD. Intravenous drug use can lead to septicaemic shock accompanied by significant hypotension and other systemic features. Tachycardia is found in withdrawal from opioids and benzodiazepines, or intoxication with stimulants, ecstasy or LSD. Pyrexia is associated with acute intoxication with ecstasy, LSD and infections related to drug use.

Skin

It is important to examine the sites of injecting drug use for complications secondary to poor technique, unhygienic use and highly irritant adulterants found in street drugs. Early in the career of an injector, the common sites used are those that are accessible and are easily hidden. Frequently, the veins of the arms are used, but as access to these becomes more difficult through sclerosis, other sites are sought, including the feet, groin, neck, toes and eventually fingers. It is important to inspect any areas that are used and to be aware that tattoos may hide needle 'track marks'. Scarring from abscesses may also be visible.

Frequent findings at injection sites include cellulitis (inflammation of the skin), abscesses and thrombophlebitis (inflammation of the veins). Lymphangitis may also occur, characterised by red blushes and streaks in the skin corresponding to the inflamed and infected lymphatic system. When peripheral veins are sclerosed, the user may inject into subcutaneous tissue and muscle, leading to necrotising fasciitis. Initially this causes cellulitis with loss of sensation over the affected area, but as the problem develops there may be pain, purple/black skin discoloration, blistering bullae and systemic features.

Other rare findings include gangrene and mycotic aneurysms. Mycotic aneurysms are caused by micro-organisms in the vessel wall, and the diagnosis should be considered whenever a mass is encountered over a major vessel in an IDU. The clinical findings often include a tender, pulsatile mass overlying an artery, but in some cases it can appear as a non-pulsatile mass and be mistaken for a cutaneous abscess. Most cases involve the femoral artery following groin injection.

Box 23.1 Some physical tests to perform for patients who misuse drugs

- Height, weight and body mass index – to assess the extent of any malnutrition
- Blood pressure and pulse – to exclude cocaine-related hypertension or arrhythmia
- Electrocardiography (ECG) – to diagnose arrhythmia and exclude ischaemia, infarction or hypertrophy (see also the notes about prolonged QTc interval below)
- Chest X-ray – may be useful to confirm the development of pneumonia (including aspiration pneumonia) and tuberculosis
- Tests of lung function, including peak flow, forced expiratory volume (FEV) and forced vital capacity (FVC) – may be useful in assessing the extent of drug-related pulmonary damage
- Blood tests – full blood count (for anaemia, hazardous drinking); urea and electrolytes (potassium must be checked if there is an arrhythmia)
- Tests of liver function and clotting function (e.g. INR, international normalised ratio) – to assess severity of liver disease
- Tests of thyroid function – for differential diagnosis of cardiac arrhythmia
- Pregnancy test
- HIV, hepatitis B and C – refer to Chapter 18 for appropriate tests
- Echocardiography – to show any enlargement of the cardiac chamber associated with cardiomyopathy, valvular disease or reduced systolic function
- Computerised tomography (CT) of the brain – performed on all dependent patients with new onset seizure or partial seizure, status epilepticus or a clear history of significant head trauma[8]
- Magnetic resonance imaging (MRI) or electroencephalography (EEG) – reserved for patients with negative head CT but at high risk for structural abnormalities (i.e. following a partial or prolonged seizure). ECG should be carried out >48 hours after the seizure. ECG is likely to be normal in patients with alcohol-related sezures without epilepsy.

Cardiovascular system

Tachycardia may be secondary to recent stimulant use, and a new cardiac murmur can suggest a pulmonary embolus, infective endocarditis or hypertrophic cardiac changes. A parasternal heave may be evident in patients with multiple small emboli.

Respiratory system

Acute intoxication with opioids and consumption of large amounts of barbiturates and stimulants will lead to a suppression of the respiratory rate. Breathlessness may indicate an infection of the lower respiratory tract, with the clinical signs of dullness to percussion, crackles, bronchial breathing and occasionally pleural rub. Pleural rub and breathlessness occur in pulmonary embolism secondary to intravenous drug use, usually accompanied by haemodynamic changes (hypotension and tachycardia), raised jugular venous pressure and occasionally changes in heart sounds.

Gastrointestinal system

Hepatitis secondary to intravenous use may present with hepatomegaly and jaundice. Opioid dependence commonly leads to constipation, which may present as mild abdominal tenderness and a faecally loaded colon on the left side. There is usually a mass of faeces felt on rectal examination.

Box 23.2 Factors influencing the time window of detection of a drug

- Bodily substance tested
- Sensitivity of testing method
- Amount of drug use
- Frequency of drug use
- Interaction between drugs
- Urine pH
- Metabolic rate
- Body mass
- Age
- Overall health
- Drug tolerance

Table 23.3 Approximate duration of detectabilit of drugs in urine

Drug or its metabolite	Duration of detectabilit
Amphetamines, including methylamphetamine and ecstasy	2 days
Cocaine metabolites	2–3 days
Heroin, morphine, codeine, dihydrocodeine, propoxyphene	2 days
Methadone (maintenance dosing)	7–9 days
Buprenorphine and metabolites	8 days
Benzodiazepines	
Ultra-short acting (half-life 2 hours), e.g. midazolam	12 hours
Short acting (half-life 2–6 hours), e.g. triazolam	24 hours
Intermediate acting (half-life 6–24 hours), e.g. temazepam, chlordiazepoxide)	2–5 days
Long acting (half-life 24 hours e.g. diazepam, nitrazepam)	>7 days
Cannabis	
Single use	3–4 days
Moderate use (3 times per week)	5–6 days
Heavy use (daily)	20 days
Chronic heavy use (more than 3 times a day)	Up to 45 days

Source: Adapted from *Drug Misuse and Dependence: UK Guidelir on Clinical Management.*[10]

Investigations and monitoring

Tests useful to clarify the results of the patient's history and physical examination are listed in Box 23.1.

Drug testing

Drug tests may be used:

- for screening
- to make the initial diagnosis of substance misuse
- to gauge drug exposure over time
- to determine the efficacy of treatment
- to measure compliance with a prescribed medication.

ox 23.3 Four possible interpretations of a drug est result

rue positive
ven where drug use is correctly identified, a screening est may not indicate the specific drug or the dose, me or route of drug administration.

rue negative
ven where the test correctly indicates that drugs have ot been recently used, drug elimination times vary, nd a negative test could result from a sample taken oo long after drug consumption.

alse positive
ests recognise all compounds, including metabolites, elonging to a particular class of drug. Legal seudoephedrine in cough medicine and illegal mphetamine are chemically similar and may lead to false positive interpretation. Passive drug exposure e.g. to cannabis) may have a similar effect.

alse negative
negative finding in a patient known to have recently aken the drug may occur if the sensitivity of the nalytical procedure is set above the limit of detection f the drug, or if another substance interferes with he analysis (e.g. aspirin interferes with some assays of rine).

The choice of body fluid or hair to test is determined by the nature of the suspected drugs and the potential time window of substance use (Box 23.2). Blood and, to a lesser degree, saliva give the best measurement of primary drugs, whereas metabolites in urine provide a longer time frame of assessment (Table 23.3). Hair grows at 1 cm per month and so may provide an indication of substance use over several months.

The mechanism of collection and need for supervision of samples are also important. There is good concordance (63–92%) between self-report and urine testing.[9] However, this depends on the substance, the population under study and the circumstances of the test. Over-reporting of drug use is as common as under-reporting.

The standard procedure for screening for drugs of misuse is a two-step process:

- an initial automated immunoassay – this will identify only the class of drug, such as opioid or benzodiazepine
- chromatography – to confirm the presence of a specific drug in a sample.

Box 23.4 Summary of key physical assessment points in community drug treatment services

- Presenting symptoms
- Past medical issues – operations, injuries, hospital admissions
- Drug-related complications (e.g. abscesses, venous thrombosis, septicaemia, endocarditis, constipation)
- Accidental or deliberate overdose
- Current or past infection with blood-borne viruses
- Assessment of risk for blood-borne viruses– previous injecting, sharing, homemade tattoos
- Immunisation against hepatitis B
- Tests for hepatitis B and C
- Contraception history and cervical screening
- Menstrual and pregnancy history
- Sexual health and sexually transmitted infections
- Oral health
- Allergies or sensitivities

Source: Adapted from *Drug Misuse and Dependence: UK Guidelines on Clinical Management.*[10]

Interpreting the results of a drug test for clinical use can be complicated, as compounds from the same drug class may have common metabolic end-products; for example, morphine is a metabolite of both heroin and codeine, whereas dihydrocodeine has its own distinct metabolic pattern.

When interpreting test results, bear in mind that no screening test is perfect (Box 23.3).[11]

The more information the clinician can gather prior to sample collection, the better.

'Chain of custody' refers to the procedure ensuring that an identified sample was provided by a specified individual and is crucial if the result is to be used in court. Such procedures usually require the collection of a urine sample witnessed by a designated member of staff and written confirmation of its validity from the individual producing the sample.

The probability of detection increases with the frequency of drug use and urine testing, but it is worth

Infrequent drug use (e.g. once a month) is difficult to detect whichever testing frequency is used.

remembering that infrequent drug use (e.g. once a month) is difficult to detect whatever testing frequency is used.[12] The benefits of more frequent testing are greatest with moderate drug use, and clinicians are most likely to be interested in the mid-range, intermittent-to-regular users. Detection times for drugs in urine do not seem to vary consistently with drug dosage. A urinalysis schedule of 3 days per week seems the most efficient to pick up illicit cocaine or heroin use,[12] but the cost of conducting such frequent tests would be prohibitive for most services and is recommended only in exceptional circumstances, or as part of a time-limited contingency management programme.

Methadone and the electrocardiogram

Methadone has a relatively good safety profile but it has been associated with prolongation of the QT segment of the electrocardiogram (ECG), defined as a rate-corrected QTc interval of 450 ms or greater.[13] This may increase the risk of torsades de pointes, a ventricular tachycardia with the potential to cause sudden death. The effect is dose dependent and is due to delayed repolarisation. Clinical scrutiny should increase if other risk factors for torsade de pointes are present, such as:

- pre-treatment QT prolongation
- hypokalaemia
- structural heart disease
- co-prescription of cytochrome P450 inhibitors
- methadone dose greater than 100 ml/day

It is important to evaluate any patient receiving methadone who has unexplained syncope or generalised seizures. Ideally, an ECG should be recorded before the patient starts methadone. QT prolongation occurs within weeks of starting treatment, and if a repeat ECG shows an increased QTc interval (Fig. 23.5), long-term risk of torsade de pointes is increased (Fig. 23.6).[13]

What should happen in the community?

The UK guidelines for the management of drug misuse highlight the importance of opportunistic assessment of physical health problems in illicit drug users (Box 23.4).[10] It is important to elicit a history of illicit injecting drug

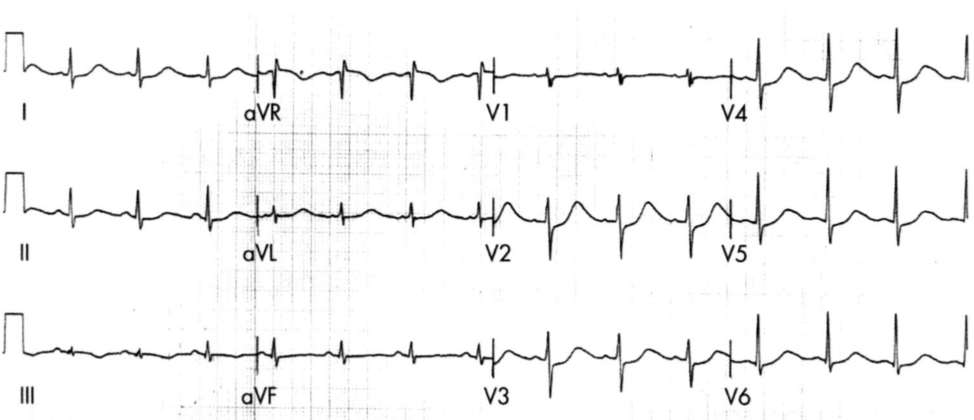

Fig. 23.5 An electrocardiogram showing a long QTc at 619 ms.

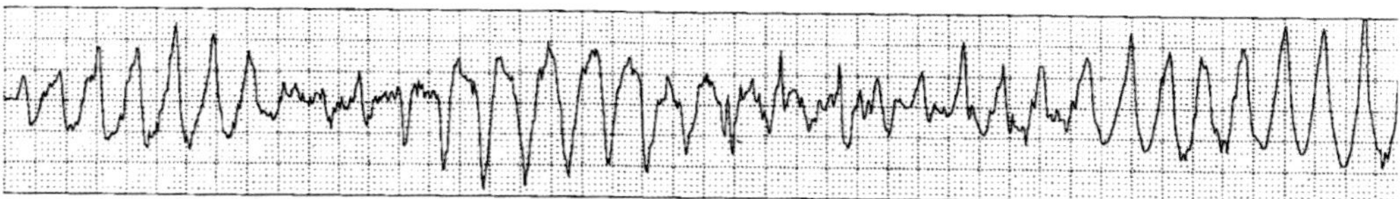

Fig. 23.6 An electrocardiogram showing torsades de pointes.

use, as relatively simple interventions (outlined below) may reduce the risk of morbidity or mortality.

Advice on harm reduction

A common harm-reduction strategy includes provision of clean needles, syringes and other injecting paraphernalia, often in exchange for used equipment.

Hepatitis B vaccination

This can prevent hepatitis B and its complications, including liver cancer and cirrhosis.

Reducing drug-related deaths

Fatal heroin overdose is partly responsible for the 6- to 20-fold increase in mortality for injecting drug users, compared with age- and gender-matched non-drug users.[14] Most opioid-related deaths result from accidental overdose and at least 50% of opioid users report overdosing at some point.[6]

Non-fatal overdose may lead to physical health problems, including pulmonary oedema, pneumonia, rhabdomyolysis (muscle breakdown from prolonged pressure on limbs during coma), renal failure and physical injuries from falls, burns or assault.

Reducing the risk of accidental overdose

A variety of measures have been proposed:

- Assess those at greatest risk (e.g. those who regularly inject drugs; individuals dependent on opioids, alcohol or benzodiazepines; those who have recently lost their opioid tolerance, such as after detoxification or imprisonment).
- Provide education to all drug users and their families on the risk of overdose and how to respond effectively, including advice on the dangers of combining drugs, especially alcohol and benzodiazepines.
- Educate new patients prescribed buprenorphine or methadone, and use supervised consumption arrangements in the initial stages of treatment.
- Alert all patients to the need for satisfactory home storage arrangements, particularly when there are children in the house.

A high proportion of overdoses are witnessed and yet medical help is often not sought. The presence of bystanders such as peers or family has been seen as an opportunity for intervention while awaiting the arrival of emergency medical care.[15] Other users/friends/family can be trained in what to do if they see someone overdose. Naloxone, an opioid antagonist that reverses the effects of opioids on the brain and thus restores breathing, is associated with transient withdrawal symptoms such as gastrointestinal disorders, aggressiveness, tachycardia, shivering, sweating and tremor. Peers can administer this life-saving treatment[16] and a growing evidence base supports the distribution of naloxone to intravenous drug users as part of a training package.

When to refer to other services

Some medical conditions are more prevalent or severe in individuals with drug dependence.[17] Acute infections associated with injecting may merit immediate action, whereas other infections represent a significant public health risk, notably HIV, hepatitis B or C, sexually transmitted diseases and tuberculosis. Chronic diseases such as diabetes, asthma, hypertension or seizure disorders are common in this population and periods of drug use may interfere with their adequate management (Box 23.5).

Conditions that may require acute medical admission

Acute infective complications of injecting

Endocarditis

A diagnosis of endocarditis should be considered in any patient who has recently injected and who has a fever or

Box 23.5 Referral to specialist medical services

Referral to specialist medical services may be needed where:

- there is acute infection associated with injecting
- infection represents a significant public health risk (especially HIV, hepatitis B or C, sexually transmitted diseases and tuberculosis)
- a chronic disease (e.g. diabetes, asthma, hypertension, seizure) affects management.

Extended periods of treatment with substitution medication such as methadone may provide an opportunity for screening and treatment of physical disorders.

new heart murmur. Typical clinical features include fever, shortness of breath, pleuritic chest pain and cough. A murmur may not be present.

Soft-tissue infections

Abscesses and cellulitis involve inflammation of skin, subcutaneous tissue and muscle.[17] Cellulitis may require treatment with intravenous antibiotics and an abscess might need incision and drainage.

Necrotising fasciitis

This rare *Streptococcus pyogenes* infection from a contaminated needle should be considered when pain at an injection site is more severe than expected from the redness or warmth at the site. It spreads rapidly and can cause death from overwhelming sepsis within days, with little evidence of inflammation. Oedema, fever, a drop in blood pressure, and a high white blood cell count are additional clues. Treatment includes extensive debridement and intravenous antibiotics.

Botulism

This infection, caused by the neurotoxin of *Clostridium botulinum*, may be linked to batches of contaminated heroin. It causes loss of muscle tone, including respiratory muscle weakness, and so has a significant mortality rate if not treated with antitoxin.

Acute-onset chest pain and stimulant use

ECG changes induced by cocaine are common.[1] Cocaine may induce a myocardial infarction with typical ST-segment elevation. Cardiac troponin levels will be raised but may be normal for 12 hours. Admission to hospital is imperative. Cocaine use may also induce severe hypertension, seizures, intracerebral haemorrhage and aortic dissection.

Health professionals should recognise that novel illicit drugs emerge often and these new drugs may have detrimental effects on both physical and mental health.

Vascular trauma and deep-vein thrombosis

Injecting into the femoral vein leads to a number of complications, including sepsis and deep-vein thrombosis. A swollen limb in an intravenous drug user can be challenging to investigate and treat, as soft-tissue pathology and problems with venous access hamper ultrasonography and venography.[18] The optimum strategy is not clear and rates of recurrence of deep vein thrombosis are high.

Hepatitis C infection

Treatment of chronic HCV infection aims to achieve sustained eradication of the virus (defined as the persistent absence of HCV RNA in serum 6 months or more after completing antiviral treatment) and to prevent progression to cirrhosis, hepatocellular cancer, and decompensated liver disease.[4] Antiviral therapy for chronic hepatitis C is currently recommended for patients over 18 years old with elevated serum levels of alanine transaminase (ALT), positive tests for hepatitis C virus antibody and serum hepatitis C virus RNA, and no contraindications for treatment. The decision as to whether a person with mild chronic hepatitis C should be treated immediately or should wait until the disease has reached a moderate stage ('watchful waiting') should be made by the patient after consultation with a hepatologist.

Combination therapy, comprising peginterferon alfa-2a or alfa-2b and ribavirin, is recommended in mild chronic hepatitis C. The duration of treatment varies according to the licensed indications of the chosen drug, the genotype of the virus, the initial viral load, the response to treatment and the treatment regimen chosen. Treatment may last up to 48 weeks, depending on genotype. Adverse effects are common with combination therapy, with approximately 75% of patients experiencing one or more problems. Low mood is a particular problem but antidepressants are effective in patients at risk of, or who develop, depression during treatment.

Patients are closely monitored for treatment toxicity, including full blood count, renal function testing, liver function tests (including ALT level) and thyrotropin level.

References

1 Kloner RA, Rezkalla SH. Cocaine and the heart. *New Engl J Med* 2003; **348**: 487–8.

Summary

Drug misuse has adverse consequences on various body systems that put individuals at risk of developing life-threatening infections, cardiac dysrhythmia and lung disease. In addition, the initial experience of a 'high' is soon replaced by dependence, when maintaining a supply of illicit drugs such as opiates becomes a full-time occupation to avoid the physical and mental consequences of withdrawal.

2 Haim DY, Lippmann ML, Goldberg SK, *et al.* The pulmonary complications of crack cocaine. A comprehensive review. *Chest* 1995; **107**: 233–40.

3 Health Protection Agency. *Shooting Up – Infections Among Injecting Drug Users in the UK 2007. An Update 2008*. HPA, 2008.

4 National Institute for Health and Clinical Excellence. *Peginterferon Alfa and Ribavarin for the Treatment of Mild Chronic Hepatitis C*. NICE Technology Appraisal Guidance. NICE, 2006.

5 Contoreggi C, Rexroad VE, Lange WR. Current management of infectious complications in the injecting drug user. *J Subst Abuse Treat* 1998; **15**: 95–106.

6 Strang J, Kelleher M, Best D, *et al.* Emergency naloxone for heroin overdose. Should it be available over the counter? *BMJ* 2006; **333**: 614–5.

7 McCance EF, Price LH, Kosten TR, *et al.* Cocaethylene: pharmacology, physiology and behavioural effects in humans. *J Pharmacol Exp Ther* 1995; **274**: 215–23.

8 Rathlev NK, Ulrich AS, Delanty N, *et al.* Alcohol-related seizures. *J Emerg Med* 2006; **31**: 157–63.

9 Darke S. Self-report among injecting drug users: a review. *Drug Alcohol Depend* 1998; **51**: 253–63.

10 Department of Health (England) and the devolved administrations. *Drug Misuse and Dependence: UK Guidelines on Clinical Management*. Department of Health (England), the Scottish Government, Welsh Assembly Government and Northern Ireland Executive, 2007.

11 Wolff K, Welch S, Strang J. Laboratory investigations for assessment and management of drug problems. In *Clinical Topics in Addiction* (ed E Day): 130–148. RCPsych Publications, 2007.

12 Crosby RD, Carlson GA, Specker SM. Simulation of drug use and urine screening patterns. *J Addict Dis* 2003; **22**: 89–98.

13 Krantz MJ, Martin J, Stimmel B, *et al.* QTc interval screening in methadone treatment. *Ann Intern Med* 2009; **150**: 387–95.

14 Advisory Council on the Misuse of Drugs. *Reducing Drug Related Deaths*. TSO (The Stationery Office), 2000.

15 Strang J, Darke S, Hall W, *et al.* Heroin overdose: the case for take-home naloxone. *BMJ* 1996; **312**: 1435–6.

16 Dettmer K, Saunders B, Strang J. Take home naloxone and the prevention of deaths from opiate overdose: two pilot schemes. *BMJ* 2001; **322**: 895–6.

17 Center for Substance Abuse Treatment. *Medication-Assisted Treatment for Opioid Addiction in Opioid Treatment Programs*. Treatment Improvement Protocol (TIP) Series. Substance Abuse and Mental Health Services Administration, 2005.

18 Syed FF, Beeching NJ. Lower-limb deep-vein thrombosis in a general hospital: risk factors, outcomes and the contribution of intravenous drug use. *Q J Med* 2005; **98**: 139–45.

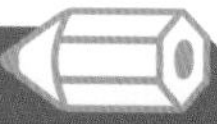

Learning points

- Most physical problems associated with the use of illicit opioids come not from the drug itself but from the pattern of use (e.g. injecting drugs increases the risk of spread of blood-borne viruses such as hepatitis B and C, and HIV).
- Accidental opioid overdose is a significant cause of death in young people.
- Stimulant drugs such as cocaine and amphetamine are often used in large quantities in a binge pattern, increasing the risk of cardiovascular problems such as myocardial infarction and stroke.
- Psychiatrists should be aware of the increasing use of less familiar drugs such as gamma-hydroxybutyrate (GHB) and ketamine, as the physical effects of intoxication or withdrawal can be difficult to manage.
- Smoking or 'chasing' drugs produces low-grade lung trauma, and increases the risk of pulmonary infection; an extreme syndrome called 'crack lung' may occur within the first 48 hours of smoking, possibly caused by a hypersensitivity pneumonitis.
- There is an association between intravenous drug use and tuberculosis.
- Consideration should always be given to potential interactions between illicit (and prescribed) drugs. Combining drugs can lead to the production of another active compound that may have higher toxicity than the parent drugs (e.g. the production of cocaethylene from alcohol and cocaine).
- Key findings on physical examination that would suggest more detailed investigation include infected injection sites, cardiac murmurs and a raised temperature or blood pressure.
- Change in the length of the QTc interval on the ECG may be significant after starting methadone.
- The choice of body substance to test for drugs is determined by the nature of the suspected drugs and the potential time window of substance use. Blood and, to a lesser degree, saliva give the best results, whereas metabolites in urine provide a longer time frame. Hair provides the longest time window for analysis.
- 'Chain of custody' refers to the procedure adopted to ensure that an identified sample was provided by a specified individual, and is crucial to consider if the test results are going to be used as evidence in court.
- The probability of detection of a drug increases with the frequency of drug use and urine testing – infrequent drug use (e.g. once a month) is difficult to detect whatever testing frequency is used.
- Systematic training of intravenous drug users in the basic management of accidental overdose, combined with the provision of take-home naloxone, may reduce the rate of drug-related deaths.
- Vaccination against hepatitis B is an important public health measure.
- The use of combined peginterferon alfa and ribavirin now allows the sustained eradication of the hepatitis C virus and the prevention of progression to cirrhosis. However, patients require support to cope with the significant physical and mental side-effects of the treatment.

24

Physical aspects of mental illness in children and adolescents

Gordon Bates

This chapter discusses the potential physical problems associated with psychiatric conditions with their onset in childhood. It includes physical comorbidities as well as the physical conditions that can be mistaken for mental health diagnoses. In addition, it outlines the importance of physical examination, regular growth checks and the investigation of deteriorating function or 'skill loss' in young people. It also gives an overview of the potential physical complications of the most commonly prescribed psychotropic drugs used in childhood.

Introduction

Young people not only differ from adults in their size, physiology and cognitive ability (among others) but they also suffer from distinct physical and mental illnesses and display them in a range of ways. Historically, these distinctions led to the establishment of the clinical specialties of paediatrics and child and adolescent psychiatry, which today have separate training requirements from general adult medicine and general adult psychiatry. The two broad categories of mental disorder seen by child psychiatrists are neurodevelopmental and psychiatric disorders.

Neurodevelopmental disorders

'Neurodevelopmental disorder' is the term given to the wide range of conditions that affect emotional and behavioural development and learning, which have their onset in childhood. These include:

- attention-deficit hyperactivity disorder (ADHD)
- autism spectrum disorder (ASD)
- Tourette's syndrome
- developmental coordination disorder (also known as dyspraxia in the UK)
- dyslexia
- dyscalculia
- generalised intellectual disability.

Our knowledge of these conditions has rapidly expanded over the past 10 years and they represent a significant and growing proportion of the work of child psychiatrists.

Neurodevelopmental disorders tend to cluster both in individuals and in families. If a child has one of these diagnoses, there is a substantially greater chance than the base population rate that they will have a second neurodevelopmental disorder. However, comorbidity and co-occurrence are specifically excluded in the ICD-10 and DSM-IV classification systems, for research reasons.[1,2] There are also higher rates of physical illness, particularly neurological conditions, in young people with neurodevelopmental disorders. This partly explains the converse observation that there is an excess of mental health problems seen in young people with neurological illness. In the epidemiological study in the Isle of Wight, 44% of children with structural brain abnormalities and 29% of children with idiopathic epilepsy were found to have a psychiatric disorder. Background rates for healthy children and children with non-cerebral chronic illness were 7% and 12%, respectively.[3]

Child psychiatrists working in neurodevelopmental clinics must be able to recognise a range of comorbid neurological conditions within the neurodevelopmental disorders. Many clinicians work with or alongside community or developmental paediatricians in order to hone their skills or seek help when necessary.

The two most common neurodevelopmental disorders are ASD and ADHD.

Autism spectrum disorders

'Autism spectrum disorder' is the umbrella term for autistic disorder, Asperger syndrome and pervasive developmental disorders, a term that is preferred by most clinicians and patients' families, although it is not mentioned in ICD-10 or DSM-IV. It refers to a group of conditions characterised by functional impairments in three domains:

- language problems, ranging from subtle semantic and pragmatic deficits to no useful speech
- social problems, ranging from aloof lack of interest in others to overformal, stilted relationships
- preference for sameness, manifest in repetitive motor activities or developmentally inappropriate and excessive special interests.

The wider diagnosis affects probably 1% of children.

There are high rates of physical illness in children with ASD (Box 24.1). These rates are greater than in those with associated intellectual disability; they vary from 7% to 37%,[4] depending upon the intelligence of the population under scrutiny and how assiduously the clinicians investigate. The relationship of the medical condition to the genesis of the autism varies. For example, in Rett syndrome all affected children will have ASD; in others, autistic symptoms may co-occur but full diagnostic criteria for autism are not met by the majority of physically affected children. It is helpful for families to know if there is an additional physical illness, to assist their understanding of the cause of the autism, explain previously unexplained symptoms and inform treatment and prognosis.

Other health problems include joint pains, sleep problems and toileting problems, from constipation to diarrhoea, which may be most important to the child and family. Management of these conditions is beyond the scope of this chapter but clinicians who regularly treat children with ASD should have some basic management strategies for them. Neoprene splints (as used for example by athletes) can be helpful for joints that have become painful due to ligamentous laxity. Sleep hygiene and melatonin can significantly improve family life disrupted by sleep deprivation. Exploration and management of toileting problems and faddy diets will help some individuals.

> ADHD can delay attainment of educational, social and personal organisational skills, so that affected children frequently have poor relations with peers and reduced academic achievement.

Attention-deficit hyperactivity disorder

The DSM-IV criteria for ADHD include the presence of developmentally inappropriate levels of impulsiveness and overactivity and/or inattention. The condition affects approximately 5% of children. The popular use of this term has meant that it has practically superseded the more restrictive but more reliable ICD-10 diagnosis of hyperkinetic disorder in routine clinical use. Hyperkinetic disorder requires the presence of symptoms in all three clusters of hyperactivity, inattention and impulsive symptoms, occurring in more than one environment (e.g. school or clinic). Most British clinicians will diagnose and treat only hyperkinetic disorder but still use the term ADHD.

Children with ADHD have a variety of impairments because of their delayed attainment of educational, social and personal organisational skills. They frequently have poor, more conflictual peer relations and reduced academic achievement, even when intelligence is taken into account. Continuing ADHD is a major risk factor for teenage and adult substance misuse, depression and anxiety as well as conduct disorder and later criminality. It has a huge individual and societal burden. In England and Wales, children with ADHD place a significant cost on health, social and education services, reaching £23

Box 24.1 Physical conditions associated with autism spectrum disorder (ASD)

Genetic syndromes
Angelman syndrome
CHARGE association
De Lange syndrome
Down syndrome
Fragile X syndrome
Goldenhar syndrome
Hypomelanosis of Ito
Joubert syndrome
Lujan–Fryns syndrome
Moebius syndrome
Neurofibromatosis 1
Noonan syndrome
Peroxisomal disorders
Untreated phenylketonuria
Rett syndrome
Smith–Magenis syndrome
Sotos syndrome
Tuberous sclerosis
Velocardiofacial syndrome (CATCH-22)
Williams syndrome

Endocrine disorders
Hypothyroidism
Pituitary deficiency

Prenatal and postnatal infections
Rubella
Herpes simplex encephalitis
Cytomegalovirus
Toxoplasmosis

Toxins
Fetal alcohol syndrome
Fetal cocaine exposure
Fetal valproate exposure
Lead poisoning
Thalidomide embryopathy

Sensory impairments
Visual impairment
Hearing impairment

Brain disorders
Cerebral palsy
West syndrome
Lennox–Gastaut syndrome

million for initial specialist assessment and £14 million annually for follow-up care, excluding medication.[5]

Attention-deficit hyperactivity disorder can be difficult to diagnose and requires a detailed and comprehensive assessment, which includes evaluation of academic and social functioning. Recent guidance from the National Institute for Health and Clinical Excellence (NICE) provides a helpful set of minimum standards.[5] The assessment must include a physical health check in which a series of alternative or contributing diagnoses must be considered (Box 24.2). Since ADHD is best considered as a heterogeneous final common pathway, the list includes comorbid conditions as well as directly causative conditions, for which treatment of the underlying illness will resolve the ADHD symptoms.

Continuing ADHD is a major risk factor for teenage and adult substance misuse, depression and anxiety as well as conduct disorder and later criminality.

Psychiatric disorders

Affective and anxiety disorders

Affective and anxiety disorders are common conditions in childhood. Prevalence rates are debatable but figures of 2–5% for affective disorder and 8–10% for anxiety disorder are generally accepted.[6] Depression can present from middle childhood and its prevalence increases into adolescence. Symptoms are similar to those in adulthood: sustained low mood, reduced energy and changes in sleep and appetite. Anxiety disorders can present from an early age but may take more child-specific forms, such as separation anxiety and simple phobia. They can also complicate ASD.

Children frequently somatise their anxiety and distress, particularly in the forms of abdominal pain

Box 24.2 Physical conditions presenting with symptoms of attention-deficit hyperactivity disorder

Major systemic illness
Cardiac disease
Pulmonary disease
Renal disease
Iron deficiency and anaemia

Hormonal disorder
Hypothyroidism
Hyperthyroidism

Sensory impairments
Visual impairment
Hearing impairment

Brain disorders
Epilepsy (absence and complex partial)
Complex migraine
Hydrocephalus
Brain tumours
Acquired brain injury

Behavioural phenotypes
Fragile X
Turner syndrome
William syndrome
XXY syndrome
XYY syndrome

Neurological disease
Neurofibromatosis I
Tuberous sclerosis
Sydenham's disease
Paediatric autoimmune neuropsychiatric disorders associated with *Streptococcus* infection
Tourette's syndrome

Sleep disorders
Narcolepsy
Sleep deprivation
Obstructive sleep apnoea
Restless leg syndrome

Toxins
Fetal alcohol syndrome
Prenatal cocaine exposure
Maternal smoking
Environmental lead

Medication
Anticonvulsants (e.g. phenobarbitone)
Sedative antihistamines
Benzodiazepines

and headache. New symptoms should be treated on their own merits and must not be *assumed* to be part of the mental health presentation. The author has been caught out by thyroid disease emerging in a teenage girl complaining of anxiety and tiredness.

The majority of the physical conditions that form the differential diagnosis of anxiety and depression are those which arise in adulthood (covered in Chapter 26).

Early-onset psychosis

Early-onset schizophrenia can be split into:

- VEOS – 'very-early-onset schizophrenia', with symptoms occurring before the age of 12 years
- AOS – 'adolescent-onset schizophrenia', with documented major signs of schizophrenia emerging in the teenage years.

There are only one or two cases of VEOS in every 100 000 children.[7] Boys appear more likely to be affected than girls. The clinical picture is usually of insidious onset of hallucinations and disorganised thinking. Accurate mental state evaluation can be difficult because, typically, these children have a lower IQ than the general population and have complex premorbid problems, including social impairments and speech and language deficits. Significant affective symptoms, particularly mood swings, are common both in the premorbid stage and as a comorbid feature.

Although AOS is more common than VEOS, again accurate epidemiological data are sparse. Gillberg *et al* suggested a prevalence rate across the teenage population of 0.23%.[8] There is a sharp increase in the frequency of diagnosis from about age 13 and a gradual increase each year until 18. In general, the onset is

Neurodegenerative conditions rarely present with psychotic symptoms only, so any movement disorder such as tremor or dystonia should be carefully evaluated. Regression or loss of practical skills is more suggestive of a neurodegenerative condition.

more acute and as many girls are affected as boys. Intelligence does not appear to differ from the normal population. The clinical features are much closer to adult presentations, with prominent auditory hallucinations, delusions and thought disorder. Mood instability is common; obsessional symptoms can occasionally occur.

The most common organic cause for psychotic symptoms in young people is recreational drug use. Cannabis, stimulants (amphetamines, cocaine and ecstasy) and hallucinogens (LSD, 'magic mushrooms' and mescaline) can all directly induce psychotic phenomena, as can prescribed medication, particularly steroids and anticholinergics. The symptoms of drug intoxication are usually short-lived, lasting only a few days after drug use.

Box 24.3 shows other physical causes that should be considered and investigated further if the whole clinical presentation is suggestive. Neurodegenerative conditions rarely present with psychotic symptoms only, so any movement disorder such as tremor or dystonia should be carefully evaluated. Ideally, this should be prior to antipsychotic medication use. The observation of significant regression or skill loss can also aid in the distinction between a psychosis and neurodegenerative disorders. The loss of practical physical skills is more suggestive of a neurodegenerative condition.

Box 24.3 Physical conditions to consider in the differential diagnosis of childhood-onset schizophrenia or skills loss

Epilepsy
Complex partial seizures
Lennox–Gastaut syndrome
Landau–Kleffner syndrome
Chronic spike-waves with slow-wave sleep (CSWSWS)

Hormonal disorders
Hypo- and hyperthyroid states

Infections
Neurosyphilis
AIDS encephalopathy
Subacute sclerosing panencephalitis

Toxins
Lead and heavy metals

Medication
Steroids
Anticonvulsants
Psychotropic drugs

Brain structural abnormalities
Cerebellar lesions idiopathic and after surgery
Ventricular enlargement
Cavum septum pellucidum

Mucopolysaccharidoses
Hurler syndrome
Sanfilippo syndrome

White-matter diseases
Adrenoleukodystrophy
Metachromatic leukodystrophy
Multiple sclerosis

Autoimmune conditions
Systemic lupus erythematosus
Anti-NMDA receptor encephalopathy (see Clinical pearl on next page)

Basal ganglia disorders
Huntington's chorea
Wilson's disease
Fahr's disease

Genetic
Velocardiofacial syndrome (CATCH-22)
Rett syndrome
Lesch–Nyhan disease

Ceroid-lipofucinosis
Batten disease
Speilmeyer–Vogt disease

Loss of skills

Although not a diagnosis in itself, loss of skills in children can be very serious and needs careful evaluation (Box 24.4). The term 'regression' is also used but can also mean a child's return to more immature behaviours such as thumb-sucking and clinginess and is usually viewed as more psychologically driven. In clinical practice, it is important to distinguish between the practical abilities that a child has previously demonstrated but can no longer achieve and those they choose not to use. For example, the complete loss of speech is more worrying than selective mutism. It can also be helpful to obtain previous schoolwork from teachers for comparison purposes.

Goodman recommends that organic causes be considered and appropriate referrals and investigations instigated if a child meets one or more of the following criteria:[9]

- progressive loss of well-established linguistic, academic or self-help skills, with performance well below previous levels even when the child seems content, motivated and not preoccupied
- emergence of other features suggestive of a brain disorder, such as seizures, visual impairment, tremor or postural disturbance
- risk factors for relevant genetic or infectious diseases, (e.g. father with Huntington's disease, mother with AIDS).

If the above features are present, the child should be assessed by a community paediatrician or paediatric neurologist for a neurodegenerative disorder or other organic cause. The list of possibilities closely resembles that for an early-onset psychosis, so the lists are combined in Box 24.3.

Anti-NMDA receptor antibody encephalopathy is a recently described condition which has attracted a great deal of interest among paediatric neurologists but is not yet well known. Children and adults present with new-onset epilepsy, personality change, skill loss and a movement disorder. Initially found in women with ovarian cancer, there appear to be other triggers for this autoimmune condition which targets the N-methyl-D-aspartate (NMDA) receptor. Diagnosis is by blood test and the condition responds to steroids, immunosuppressants and plasmaphoresis (see p. 193).

Box 24.4 Skills loss

Skills loss is an important sign and symptom but one which requires careful unpacking with several questions:

- Is the skill loss pervasive?
- Does it occur in all situations and with all people?
- Can't the child perform the skill, or won't the child?
- Is it progressive or skill specific (e.g. bed wetting)?
- Are there other physical symptoms: epilepsy, motor weakness or movement disorders?

Child abuse

Child abuse may take the form of physical, sexual and/or emotional abuse or neglect. Fabricated or induced illness (previously known as Munchausen syndrome by proxy) usually involves all forms except sexual abuse, which should be considered separately. Child abuse is not a psychiatric diagnosis in itself but is included in this chapter because it can have significant mental health consequences in both childhood and adulthood and because children with disabilities are more vulnerable. Abuse provokes great anxiety in all healthcare professionals and under UK government guidance all of us have a responsibility to pass on any child protection concerns to local social services (see Recommended reading).

Child abuse is a culturally determined construct, which varies by society and era. While the margins may be blurred for some forms of corporal punishment, severe physical abuse of children at the hands of parents and carers is a serious problem, as the recent high-profile UK cases of Victoria Climbié and Baby Peter demonstrate. The annual mortality rate for physical abuse is 1 in 10 000 children.

Physical abuse has multiple causative factors and in specific cases some of the reasons can only be inferred. A set of risk factors has been described and these tend to be cumulative. Children are more at risk if they are aged under 3 years or are the first born. They tend to have 'difficult' temperaments, meaning they are non-compliant, sleep poorly and are hard to soothe. Abusive parents or carers are often young adults and have been abused themselves as children. Men are more likely to abuse than women, particularly if they are not the child's father. Poor impulse control and substance misuse in carers are other risk factors. Major mental illness in the

Risk factors for child abuse include the child being under 3 years of age or the first born, with a tendency to be non-adherent, a poor sleeper and hard to soothe. Abusive parents are often young adults, are more likely to have been abused in childhood, to be male, particularly if not child's father, to exhibit poor impulse control and to be a substance misuser. Major mental illness in the carer is rare.

carer is rare. Unfortunately, institutional care settings such as residential homes and schools for children with disabilities also place children at risk. It is important to 'think the unthinkable' in all cases because child abuse occurs in all social classes and cultures.

Child physical abuse is more likely to be presented to and detected by general practitioners and in accident and emergency (A&E) departments than by mental health professionals (Fig. 24.1). Establishing and documenting a clear history is a priority. Delays in the presentation of a child with physical injury, inconsistencies in the explanation of its acquisition or unusual vagueness should raise suspicion and prompt further enquiry.

Bruises on the ears, chin, neck or buttocks are worrying, particularly if they are in a configuration that suggests they were caused by a hand. A more thorough examination may also reveal small round cigarette burns, adult-size bite marks or a torn tongue frenulum. Other concerning physical findings are retinal haemorrhages or a subdural haematoma. General practitioners and A&E should have systems in place that flag up regular attendees. This may indicate physical abuse or inadequate supervision as part of neglect.

The possibility of sexual abuse should be considered in young people presenting with recurrent urinary tract infections or sexually transmitted disease or pregnancy in those too young to consent legally. Some children develop wetting or soiling as a strategy to deter the abuser. More intimate examination should only ever be performed by a senior paediatrician, or forensic medical examiner with the necessary skills and experience. This is generally done after referral to a statutory authority (i.e. social services).

Neglect can be picked up by a wide range of people, including educational staff. In child psychiatry clinics, the routine use of some form of school liaison should highlight features like limited school attendance, poor hygiene and unwashed clothes. Short stature and limited growth will be picked up by regular monitoring and the use of growth charts (see below). Other worrying signs are rocking, head-banging and language delay. These can be caused by chronic understimulation. The presence of more than one sign increases the likelihood of neglect and chronic understimulation.

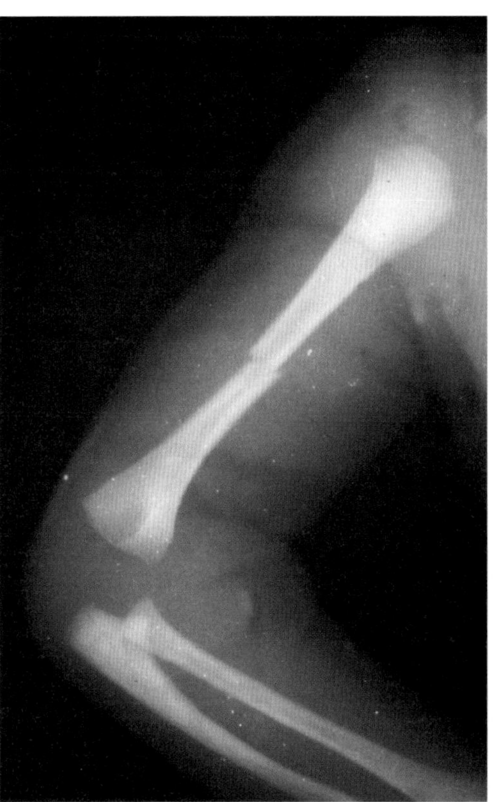

Fig. 24.1 Transverse fracture humerus, infant, non-accidental injury.

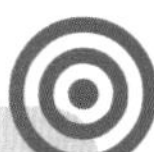

Signs suggestive of physical abuse include:

- bruising to the ears, chin, neck or buttocks, especially if suggestive of a handmark
- cigarette burns, adult-size bite marks or a torn tongue frenulum
- retinal haemorrhages or subdural haematoma.

Physical examination

Child psychiatrists vary as to whether they will routinely carry out physical examinations. Their reasons vary from lack of experience and confidence to more theoretical reservations about physical contact with children with whom they have a psychotherapeutic relationship. If children have physical symptoms it is mandatory that they have a physical examination as part of a medical assessment to identify or exclude possible organic pathology. General practitioners and paediatricians will perform this as a matter of course. Some child psychiatrists will undertake a physical examination and others will refer the child to the relevant specialist, although such deferring of responsibility risks delay or, worse, the child having no physical examination.

Arguably, all psychiatrists should have a minimum set of physical examination skills. Important information can be gathered which does not require great skill or training. The observation of play or walking can reveal more than would a formal neurological examination. Routine recording of height and weight and plots of the data on growth charts are essential in many conditions ranging from failure to thrive and eating disorders to stimulant-treated ADHD. Abnormal head circumference can be a useful pointer to autistic disorder, some behavioural phenotypes or raised intracranial pressure. Unexplained bruising can suggest physical abuse at home or at school. A targeted neurological examination does require training and interpretation but is invaluable in the evaluation of possible neurodevelopmental disorders.

Demonstrating physical signs

Eliciting soft motor signs (detailed below) during a physical examination is extremely satisfying and useful. First, it is a tangible physical finding over and above a good history. It also occurs commonly enough in neurodevelopmental clinics that it becomes reinforcing: you continue to perform physical examinations and improve your skills because you find something. Finally, it can act as an external validator; clinical history taking can have many biases but a good physical sign is hard to dispute, even by the most sceptical parent, educational psychologist or anti-medical model team member!

Growth charts

Most British residents should be familiar with the Department of Health parent-held record (the 'red book') either as parents or as children themselves. Certainly, all doctors will have had the value of the growth charts they contain instilled into them during their basic paediatric training. There is current controversy as to which population data-set is most accurate and appropriate for comparison, owing to the increasing size of British children and the difference between the early growth of bottle-fed versus breast-fed babies.

A paediatric growth chart is a basic grid on which growth information is plotted against chronological age and then compared with population averages for boys or girls (Fig. 24.2). Three pieces of essential information are recorded on growth charts: height, weight and head circumference. Head circumference is often not routinely measured or plotted beyond 18 months of age but is well worth checking on at least the child's first visit to a neurodevelopmental clinic.

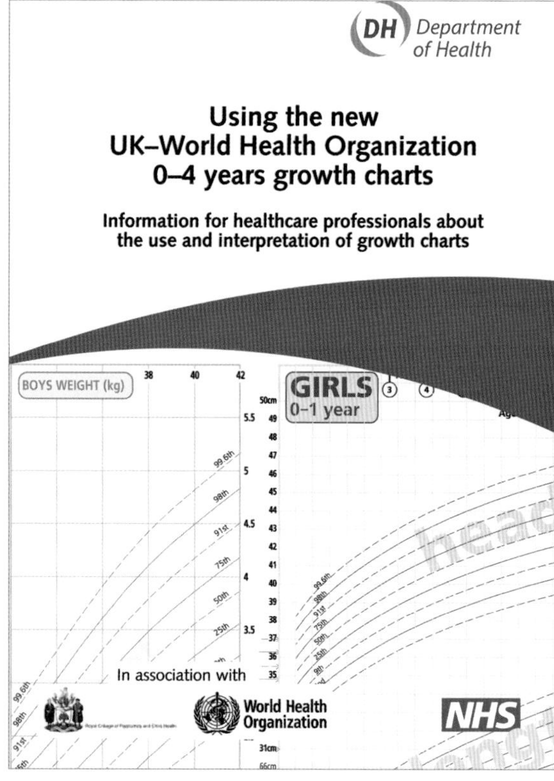

Fig. 24.2 Growth charts and information on their use are available on the website of the Royal College of Paediatrics and Child Health (www.rcpch.ac.uk).

Clinicians routinely record height and weight at each hospital or clinic visit. The growth chart is used as a tool to monitor growth as well as to establish how a child's height and weight compare with those of their peers. On the graph, rising coloured or dotted lines mark the standard growth trajectory of the 'average' child (50th percentile) and to demarcate the top and bottom 10% of the population (10th and 90th percentiles). Tracking height and weight over time enables clinicians to see if young people are losing or gaining weight more rapidly than expected. Deceleration or plateauing of height gain is also of concern. There are many physical conditions as well as mental health conditions that can cause these changes, but with more subtle conditions the growth chart can be the first indicator of ill health or an unsuspected eating disorder.

There are several conditions that are linked to short stature such as Turner and Noonan syndromes and Cornelia de Lange syndrome. Early excessive growth is seen in fragile X syndrome and Sotos syndrome. Obesity is a feature of Prader–Willi and Cohen syndromes.

Abnormalities of head circumference can suggest other developmental syndromes, although the most common association is paternal head circumference. Macrocephaly is found in Sotos syndrome and the mucopolysaccharidoses, which include Hunter, Hurler and Sanfilippo syndromes. Microcephaly is seen in fetal alcohol syndrome and Rett syndrome.

Neurological examination

A full description of a paediatric neurological examination is beyond the scope of this chapter. There are several excellent introductory accounts, such as that by Devlin.[10] Three aspects are important: examination of the skin for neurocutaneous syndromes; disorders of movement and posture; and examination for so-called 'soft signs'.

Neurocutaneous syndromes

The examination of the skin of a young person is important but most children or teenagers are unlikely to wish to strip for a full examination unless absolutely necessary. I usually ask the child or the parent if they have any funny rashes or patches of skin that are abnormally dark or do not go brown in the sun. I would then follow up any positive responses (see Table 24.1).

Disorders of movement or posture

It should be possible to pick up abnormalities of movement or posture through the history or direct observation. Engaging the child in play can also help to elicit movement signs. Ball play with smaller children or just watching the child walking along a short stretch of corridor can be instructive. Once the movement type is identified, you can consider the differential diagnoses (see Table 24.2).

Soft motor signs

Soft motor signs are common in children with neurodevelopmental disorders. They are described as 'soft' because more judgement is required in their interpretation. Since many of the signs are found in normally developing younger children, the assessor will

Table 24.1 Neurocutaneous conditions

Condition	Skin lesions	Associated developmental conditions
Neurofibromatosis (type 1)	Café-au-lait spots; axillary or inguinal freckling; violet neurofibromas	Epilepsy; dyslexia and dyspraxia; speech and language problems; attention-deficit hyperactivity disorder (especially the 'inattentive' subtype); excess anxiety and depression
Tuberous sclerosis	Areas of hypopigmentation; Shagreen patches; acne-like facial butterfly rash (adenoma sebaceum); periungal fibroma (adolescents)	Epilepsy; autism spectrum disorder; attention-deficit hyperactivity disorder
Hypomelanosis of Ito	Whorls and linear areas of hypopigmentation following dermatomes	Intellectual disability; epilepsy; autism spectrum disorder

Table 24.2 Abnormal patterns of movement in neurodevelopmental disorders

Movement abnormality	Associated developmental disorder
Pyramidal signs/ spasticity	Mitochondrial encephalomyopathy with lactic acidosis and stroke-like episodes (MELAS), moyamoya disease, cerebral autosomal dominant arteriopathy with subcortical infarcts and leukoencephalopathy (CADASIL)
Pyramidal signs and ataxia	Adrenoleukodystrophy, metachromatic leukodystrophy, autosomal dominant and recessive spinocerebellar degeneration, vitamin E deficiency, Abetalipoproteinaemia
Dystonia	Glutaric aciduria type 1, branched-chain amino acid disorders (methylmalonic and propionic acidaemia), Wilson's disease, Niemann-Pick disease type C, drug toxicity (antipsychotics)
Chorea	Huntington's chorea, Sydenham's chorea (post-streptococcal), drug toxicity, systemic lupus erythematosus (SLE), Wilson disease, glutaric aciduria type 1, choreoacanthocytosis, methylmalonic and propionic acidaemias, mitochondrial encephalomyopathies
Ataxia	Pelizaeus–Merzbacher disease, GM1 and GM2 gangliosidosis, Friedrich's ataxia, autosomal dominant and recessive spinocerebellar degeneration, juvenile Gaucher disease, Refsum disease, ataxia/telangiectasia, ataxia/occulomotor apraxia, Joubert syndrome
Repetitive or paroxysmal	*Tics*: Tourette's syndrome or paediatric autoimmune neuropsychiatric disorders associated with streptococcal infection (PANDAS) *Handwringing*: Rett syndrome *Panting*: Joubert syndrome *Laughter and jerky limbs*: Angelman syndrome
Myoclonus or myoclonic epilepsy	Subacute sclerosing panencephalitis, mitochondrial encephalomyopathy with ragged red fibres, Unverricht–Lundborg disease, Lafora disease, mucolipidoses (sialidosis, galactosialidosis), juvenile Gaucher disease, hereditary dentatorubral-pallidoluysian atrophy (DRPLA), new-variant Creutzfeldt–Jacob disease

Adapted from Devlin, 2003.[10]

need to be aware of the standard evolution of these signs with age. Soft signs do not disappear overnight and so do not have the ease of the more categorical 'hard' signs, such as tendon reflexes, which are usually the domain of the developmental paediatrician or paediatric neurologist.

Soft signs are not diagnostic of a particular disorder; nor are they specific to functional problems. Nevertheless, when several soft signs are elicited or they are excessive they can suggest that practical problems of function are likely. Fine motor problems can be responsible for academic problems with writing. Gross motor deficits cause clumsiness (dyspraxia), which is linked to peer-group rejection for boys and a particularly poor outcome when it complicates ADHD. If soft signs cluster on the dominant side (for most, the right-hand side), then they can be considered as a more sinister 'localising sign' and investigation may be required.

Two useful tests for eliciting soft signs are sequential finger opposition and Fog's test.[11] In sequential finger opposition, the child is asked to touch each finger of the same hand to their thumb in turn, first one way, then the other. The examiner will note the ease with which the task is performed (any child over the age of 5 should be capable of the task) and observe the other hand, which should be left in the lap. In most children between the ages of 5 and 10, mirror movements will be seen. The hand that the child is not exercising will echo the movements of the tested hand. The mirror movements or *synkinesias* can be inhibited by direct effort, so the child

Soft signs clustering on the dominant side are potential 'localising signs' that may warrant investigation.

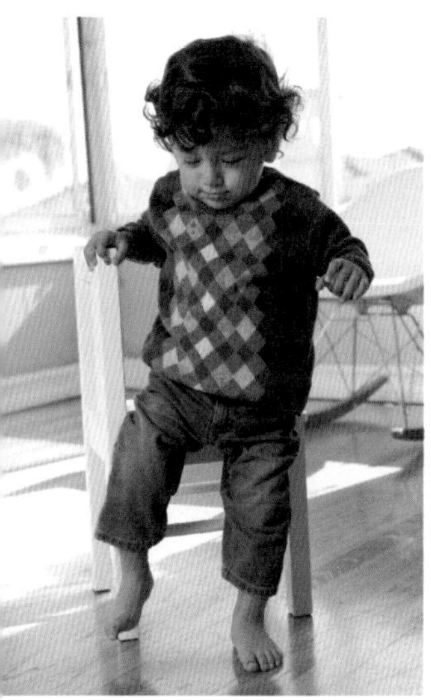

g. 24.3 Normal 1-year-old taking eps and using arms to balance.

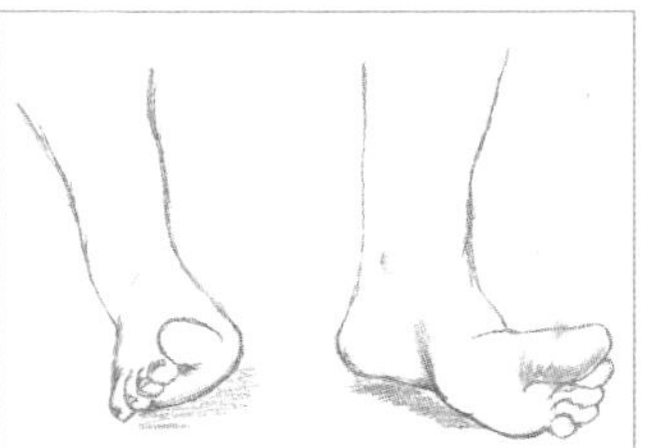

Fig. 24.4 Fog's test part 1 – walking with ankle eversion.

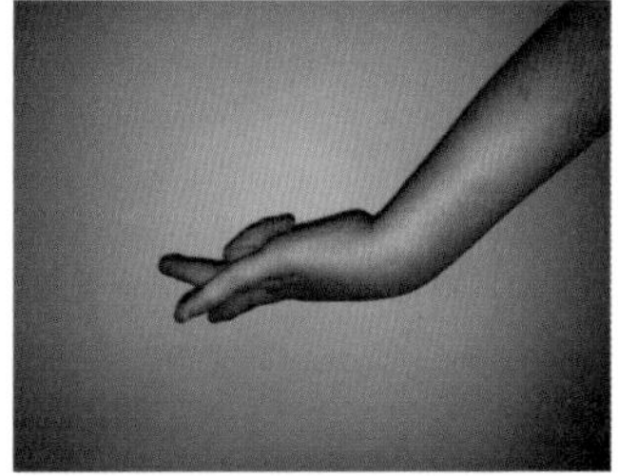

Fig. 24.6 Detail of hand demonstrating synkinesia or mirror movement.

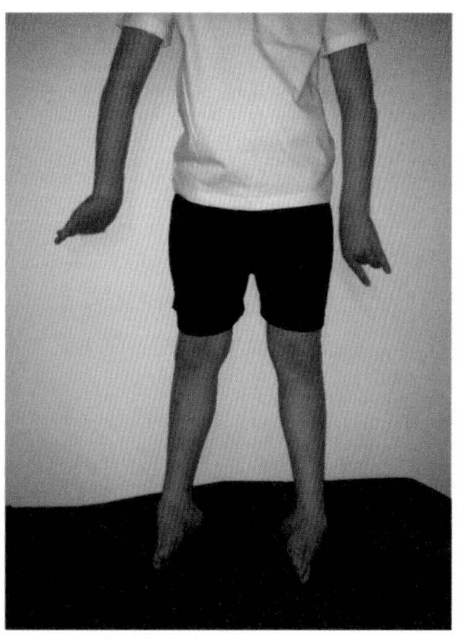

Fig. 24.5 A positive Fog's test with accessory movements.

should not be alerted to the movements. Typically, the test will be performed more accurately and with fewer extraneous movements on the dominant side before the age of 10–12. After this age, most children will be able to perform the task equally well with both hands and without any synkinesia. The persistence of mirror moves into the teen years is common in children with neurodevelopmental disorders. In clinic, this sign can be usefully demonstrated to parents to help engagement and to corroborate a neurodevelopmental diagnosis. A normal 1-year-old child walking is shown in Fig. 24.3.

Fog's test is usually performed as part of a sequence of observed walks in clinic. The child should be asked to walk on tiptoes and then on their heels, and then on the outside and then on the inside of their feet. The final two manoeuvres form Fog's test. Children over the age of 7 should be able to walk on tiptoes or heel walk without posturing of their upper limbs. Unilateral posturing can be caused by cerebral palsy. Bilateral posturing over the age of 7 is a positive soft sign and is more common in those with neurodevelopmental disorders.

Children over 12 should be able to perform Fog's test without posturing of their upper limbs. Below 12, walking on the outside of the feet (Fig. 24.4) is likely to cause decorticate posturing (arms internally rotated and hands supinated) (Figs 24.5 and 24.6). Walking on the inside of the feet will cause decerebrate posturing (arms externally rotated and hands pronated). It is easier to observe than to describe. Again, persistence beyond the cut-off is suggestive of some form of neurodevelopmental disorder.

Psychotropic medications used in childhood

There has been a steady rise in the use of medication in childhood psychiatric disorders. There are several reasons for this. First, increasing research in the area has led to a larger evidence base upon which to make treatment decisions that involve medication. Secondly, there are newer medications or formulations, which are better tolerated by children. Probably most importantly, there have been attitudinal changes within society at large and among psychiatrists in particular about the appropriateness of prescribing drugs for young people.

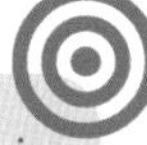

Persistence of mirror movements into the teen years is common in children with neurodevelopmental disorders.

Using psychotropic medication requires that the prescriber is aware of the risks as well as the potential benefits. Risks may include diversion to other family members or ingestion as part of an act of deliberate self-harm, as well as the physical side-effects that are more usually considered.

Psychostimulants

Psychostimulants have been used in the treatment of ADHD for decades. In the UK the two licensed drugs are methylphenidate and dexamphetamine. They act mostly by increasing dopaminergic transmission and activity, particularly in the frontal cortex. Stimulants have been studied for so long and on so many occasions that the side-effects are well described and well known (Table 24.3).

Most side-effects are dose related and subject to individual variation. Many diminish within a week or two of starting treatment and almost all will cease on discontinuation. Where side-effects do persist, most become more tolerable with dose reduction. The two principal categories of physical side-effects of concern are the effects both on growth and on the cardiovascular system.

Weight loss and growth

Stimulants are believed to suppress height and weight through appetite reduction and by direct effects on growth hormone. As a result, it is routine practice to monitor height and weight at review. Excessive weight loss or suppression of normal growth in height can be a reason for discontinuation or dose reduction.

The recent Multimodal Treatment study of children with ADHD (MTA) 3-year follow-up clarified the size of the effect.[12] The subgroup of 65 children who were never medicated in the study were larger than the subgroup of 88 children who were consistently treated (and closely monitored). At the 3-year mark, there was an average difference of 2 cm and 2.7 kg. The growth suppression was greatest in the first year and approached zero by the third year.

There are a number of ways to tackle stimulant-induced weight loss. The most obvious approach is to reduce the dose or stop the medication. In clinical practice this can be problematic, as the symptoms of ADHD will resurface. An alternative strategy is to change children's eating habits. Possibilities include allowing children to eat high-energy snacks throughout the day and/or ensuring breakfast and the evening meal are high calorie and outside of the stimulant side-effect window of 4–10 hours, depending on the preparation, and in extremis the use of dietary supplement drinks. Dietitians can be helpful in teaching parents that the principles of adult healthy eating such as a low-fat diet and no snacking do not apply to children with such high-energy needs.

Cardiovascular effects

Stimulants cause small but measurable increases in heart rate and blood pressure. This has been

Table 24.3 Side-effects of stimulants

Common	Uncommon	Rare
Appetite suppression	Weight loss or restricted growth	'Overfocus'
Sleep disturbance	Worsening of tics	Restricted attention
Abdominal pain	Irritability	Hallucinations
Transient tearfulness	Thought disorder	
Anxiety and depression	Neutropenia	
Behavioural rebound		
Headache		
Significantly raised blood pressure		
Tachycardia		
Skin picking and nail biting		
Skin rashes		

acknowledged for many years, though there has been recent concern about the dangers of sudden death with stimulants. Two recent decisions by North American regulators received publicity in the British press. Both related to the evaluation of the risk of serious cardiac events for those taking stimulants. The Canadian and US regulators subsequently overturned their positions on Aderall® (a dexamphetamine salt preparation) and methylphenidate, respectively. The differing opinions expressed by those on the committees related to the dearth of useful evidence as much as the professional background of the assessors.

Most of the US data come from post-marketing surveillance and the Adverse Event Reporting System of the Food and Drug Administration (FDA), a system similar to the British 'yellow card' arrangement. These approaches have recognised inadequacies that lead to underreporting of adverse events. Nevertheless, the estimated annual sudden death rate on stimulants is 0.25 per 100 000 based on the FDA data.[13] This compares with the background rate of between 0.6 and 6 annual sudden cardiac deaths per 100 000 of the general population.[14]

A Florida study, using a more rigorous design, retrospectively analysed 10 years of health insurance data cross-linked to death registry information and found no cardiac deaths, sudden or otherwise, in 42 612 person-years of stimulant use.[15] The researchers found a background rate in the state of 4 sudden cardiac deaths per 100 000 per year. From the current literature it does not appear that stimulants significantly increase the risk of sudden cardiac death in children.

The NICE guidance[5] has given clear standards about the required clinical assessment necessary before initiating drug therapy:

- full mental health and social assessment
- full history and physical examination, including:
  - assessment of history of exercise syncope, undue breathlessness and other cardiovascular symptoms
  - heart rate and blood pressure (plotted on a centile chart)
  - height and weight (plotted on a centile chart)
  - family history of cardiac disease
- an electrocardiogram (ECG) if there is a medical or family history of serious cardiac disease, a history of sudden death in young family members or abnormal findings on cardiovascular examination.

Stimulants can adversely affect heart rate and blood pressure, raising concerns about the danger of sudden death. Where evidence is available, sudden death due to stimulants seems to be similar to 'background' rates of sudden death.

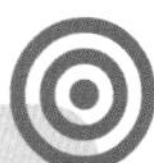

The chance of abnormal cardiac events is increased by a family history of cardiac arrhythmias or syncope. It is reasonable to request an ECG prior to treatment in these circumstances or if the child complains of palpitations.

Antidepressants

In 2003, the UK Committee for the Safety of Medicines decided that the only antidepressant with the data showing the right balance of safety against efficacy for teenage depression was fluoxetine.[16] The main safety concern related to the possibility of increased suicidal thinking or acts in adolescents treated with selective serotonin reuptake inhibitors (SSRIs). While this issue remains controversial for adolescents as well as adults, most clinicians accept the possibility of behavioural activation in the early stages of SSRI treatment for depression. It is pragmatic to discuss these risks with patients and their parents and to regularly review patients treated for depression. Child psychiatrists in the UK will use fluoxetine as the first-line agent but will use other drugs for moderate and severe depression if they encounter treatment resistance or significant side-effects.

Another SSRI, sertraline, has a licence for obsessive–compulsive disorder in youth. The side-effects of SSRIs in young people are similar to those experienced by adults. Conventionally, a half dose is given in the first week and a full adult dose thereafter, to reduce initial behavioural activation and anxiety.

There are occasions when other antidepressants are useful: when there are side-effects; when other treatments fail; or when treatment is for a sleep or tic disorder. Given concerns about the effect of tricyclic antidepressants on cardiac conductivity it is desirable to arrange for an ECG to look for arrhythmias and QT prolongation. This becomes particularly important when doses above 1 mg/kg are being taken.

Atypical antipsychotics

Prescriptions of atypical antipsychotics for young people are on the increase in the UK. They are used in teenagers at conventional or near conventional adult doses for the treatment of psychosis. At lower doses they also have a role in the treatment of tic disorder and the aggressive behaviour and temper outbursts seen in autism, although in the UK they do not have a licence for this. They are also used in the short-term management of anxiety and in combination with benzodiazepines in protocols for rapid tranquillisation.

The side-effects of atypical antipsychotic medications with young people are similar to those experienced by adults and include:

- neuromotor adverse effects – extrapyramidal side-effects (EPSE), akathisia, tardive and withdrawal dyskinesias and neuroleptic malignant syndrome
- weight gain and metabolic adverse effects
- prolactin-related effects
- sedation
- blood dyscrasias
- cardiac effects, such as postural hypotension and QT prolongation.

For child psychiatrists, the two most concerning adverse responses to atypical antipsychotic treatment apart from movement disorders are the weight gain and raised prolactin levels.

Weight gain

Compared with adult patients there is less evidence to inform practice, but it seems clear that young people with psychiatric illness do have an increased rate of obesity.[17] Excessive weight gain is not only stigmatising and associated with low self-esteem but is now known to have long-term risks due to its links to glucose and lipid abnormalities and cardiovascular complications (see Chapter 7). The causes of the weight gain are multiple and interrelated but the atypical antipsychotics can play a major role. Correll's work has shown that the relative impact of the atypical antipsychotics on weight is in roughly the same ranking order as for adults but the size of the effect is greater.[18] However, risperidone appears to have a greater impact on weight gain in young people than in adults.[19] Other useful findings from the literature include the fact that, when used in combination, stimulants do not substantially reduce the weight-gain effect of atypical antipsychotics,[20] while the addition of a mood stabiliser will exaggerate the weight gain.[21]

The association between antipsychotic medication and adverse metabolic consequences such as dyslipidaemia, hyperglycaemia, diabetes and the metabolic syndrome has been established by large-scale studies of adults. The evidence for a link is less robust for children and adolescents, but Correll's ongoing prospective paediatric safety study and the growing number of case reports describing children and adolescents developing diabetes while on antipsychotic treatment suggest that this is a real phenomenon deserving of attention.[18]

> Ongoing prospective studies report children and adolescents developing diabetes while on antipsychotic treatment.

Prolactin levels

Both typical and atypical antipsychotic medications can raise prolactin levels in the blood. Hyperprolactinaemia can cause a range of adverse effects, from breast symptoms, like tenderness, enlargement and galactorrhoea, to sexual side-effects such as reduced libido and menstrual disturbance. These are embarrassing symptoms and need specific enquiry. The relationship is complex as the actual levels do not correlate with the presence of symptoms or their severity. Young people with very high prolactin levels should be assessed for the possibility of pituitary tumours, hyperthyroidism, renal failure, pregnancy or oral contraceptive use even if the level is expected to be high because they are taking antipsychotics. The blood test should be done on a fasting specimen taken before the morning antipsychotic dose, owing to the effects of food, exercise and stress.

Antipsychotic medications cause a dose-dependent increase in blood prolactin levels. The effect is greater in adolescents than in adults. Usually the blood level will reduce towards the normal range over months of treatment and return to normal on discontinuation. The relative risk of an individual medication causing hyperprolactinaemia is the same as for adults. Risperidone has the greatest risk and aripiprazole the lowest of the atypical antipsychotics.

If a patient has symptomatic hyperprolactinaemia the response is straightforward: reduce the dose or swap to a lower-risk medication. There is more uncertainty around the management of asymptomatic hyperprolactinaemia. Some have raised the possibility that high serum levels of prolactin in young people may reduce bone density, delay sexual maturity and increase the risk of breast cancer or benign prolactinomas. The current evidence base remains unclear and even in the litigation-conscious USA, the guidelines do not require routine monitoring of prolactin levels.[21]

Professional development

Clinicians interested in developing skills in the physical aspects of children's mental health will have to ensure that they regularly perform a physical examination after they have taken the history. They will also need to read widely and invest in some reference books. Paediatric neurology can be daunting for beginners, with its seemingly endless list of eponymic syndromes and acronymic investigations. A good starting point would be Devlin's review of paediatric neurological examination,[10] a standard textbook like the one by Aicardi,[22] and a book with pictures to assist in identifying the syndromes associated with dysmorphism.[23] I would also strongly recommend *A Handbook of Neurological Investigations in Children*,[24] which provides the names of relevant investigations, from imaging to blood testing, for the rare and unusual disorders mentioned in the chapter.

Summary

This chapter has described the importance of being aware of and identifying physical health problems that can affect children and adolescents who present to child and adolescent psychiatric services. The differential diagnosis is given for the physical conditions to consider in those with autism spectrum disorder, attention-deficit hyperactivity disorder and if there is childhood onset of schizophrenia or skills loss. There are tips on how to conduct a physical examination, as well as information on the use of psychotropic drugs in children.

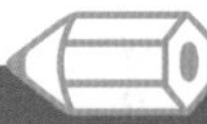

Learning points

- Neurodevelopmental disorders usually occur with other disorders: psychiatric, physical and neurodevelopmental.
- Psychiatric and neurodevelopmental disorders are frequently found in those with brain-based neurological disorders.
- A physical health check should be mandatory for all those with autism and ADHD.
- Child psychiatrists must develop competence in physical examination skills and know when to refer.
- It is common for children and adolescents with depression and anxiety to present with physical symptoms like abdominal pain or sickness.
- Physical causes such as drug intoxication and neurodegenerative conditions should always be considered for early-onset psychosis, particularly in those under 12 years old.
- Neurodegenerative conditions rarely present with psychotic symptoms in isolation. Look for epilepsy, visual loss and movement disorder or a family history.
- Cigarette burns and bruising to ears, the chin, neck or buttocks should alert clinicians to the possibility of child abuse.
- Growth charts should be used in all neurodevelopment clinics.
- Soft motor signs such as Fog's test and sequential finger opposition are a useful marker of neurodevelopmental disorder.
- Use of psychotropic medication in children is on the increase in UK practice and most other high-income countries.
- Stimulants can cause weight loss and reduce final adult height by 2 cm on average.
- An ECG is required before commencing stimulants in a child with a family history of sudden cardiac death.
- Atypical antipsychotics cause weight gain, hormonal disruption and changes in fat metabolism in children as well as adults.

References

1 World Health Organization. *The ICD-10 Classification of Mental and Behavioural Disorders* (10th revision) (ICD-10). WHO, 1992.

2 American Psychiatric Association. *Diagnostic and Statistical Manual of Mental Disorders* (4th edn, text revision) (DSM-IV-TR). APA, 2000.

3 Rutter M, Graham P, Yule W. *A Neuropsychiatric Study in Childhood*. Clinics in Developmental Medicine Nos 35/36. Heinemann, 1970.

4 Fombonne E, du Mazaubrun C, Cans C, Grandjean H. Autism and associated medical disorders in a French epidemiological study. *J Am Acad Child Adolesc Psychiatry* 1997; **36**: 1561–9.

5 National Institute for Health and Clinical Excellence. *Diagnosis and Management of Attention-Deficit/Hyperactivity Disorder (ADHD) in Children, Young People and Adults*. NICE, 2008.

6 Costello EJ, Mustillo S, Erkanli A, *et al.* Prevalence and development of psychiatric disorders. *Arch Gen Psychiatry* 2003; **60**: 837–44.

7 Gillberg C, Steffenburg S. Outcome and prognostic factors in infantile autism and similar conditions: A population-based study of 46 cases followed through puberty. *J Autism Development Disord* 1987; **17**: 273–87.

8 Gillberg C, Wahlstrom J, Forsman A, *et al.* Teenage psychoses: epidemiology, classification and reduced optimality in the pre-, peri- and neonatal periods. *J Child Psychol Psychiatry* 1986; **27**: 87–98.

9 Goodman R. Brain disorders. In *Child and Adolescent Psychiatry* (4th edn) (eds M Rutter, E Taylor): 241–60). Blackwell Science, 2002.

10 Devlin A. Paediatric neurological examination. *Adv Psychiatr Treat* 2003; **9**: 125–34.

11 Fog E, Fog M. Cerebral inhibition examined by associated movements. In *Minimal Cerebral Dysfunction* (eds M Bax, R MacKeith): 52–7. Spastic International Medical Publications, 1963.

12 Swanson JM, Elliot GR, Greenhill LL, *et al.* Effects of stimulant medication on growth rates across 3 years in the MTA follow up. *J Am Acad Child Adolesc Psychiatry* 2007; **46**: 1015–27.

13 Rappley MD, Moore JW, Dokken D. ADHD drugs and cardiovascular risk. *New Engl J Med* 2006; **354**: 2296.

14 Berger S, Dhala A, Freiderberg D. Sudden cardiac death in infants, children and adolescents. *Pediatr Clin North Am* 2004; **46**: 221–34.

15 Winterstein AG, Gerhard G, Shuster J, *et al.* Cardiac safety of central nervous system stimulants in children with attention deficit/hyperactivity disorder. *Pediatrics* 2007; **120**: e1494–501.

16 Committee for the Safety of Medicines. *Selective Serotonin Reuptake Inhibitor (SSRI) Antidepressants – Findings of the Committee on Safety of Medicines (CSM)*. CSM, 2004.

17 Patel NC, Hariparsad M, Mathias-Akthar M, *et al.* Body mass indexes and lipid profiles in hospitalized children and adolescents exposed to atypical antipsychotics. J Child Adolesc Psychopharmacol 2007; 17: 303–11.

18 Correll CU, Carlson HE. Endocrine and metabolic adverse effects of psychotropic medications in children and adolescents. *J Am Acad Child Adolesc Psychiatry* 2006; **45**: 771–91.

19 Safer DJ. A comparison of risperidone-induced weight gain across the age span. *J Clin Psychopharmacol* 2004; **24**: 429–36.

20 Aman MG, Binder C, Turgay A. Risperidone effects in the presence/absence of psychostimulant medication in children with ADHD, other disruptive behavior disorders and subaverage IQ. *J Child Adolesc Psychopharmacol* 2004; **14**: 243–54.

21 Correll CU. Antipsychotic use in children and adolescents: minimizing adverse effects to maximise outcomes. *J Am Acad Child Adolesc Psychiatry* 2008; **47**: 9–20.

22 Aicardi J. *Diseases of the Nervous System in Childhood* (3rd edn). MacKeith Press, 2009.

23 Jones KL. *Smith's Recognizable Patterns of Human Malformation*. Saunders, 2005.

24 King MD, Stephenson JBP. *A Handbook of Neurological Investigations in Children*. MacKeith Press, 2009.

Recommended reading

HM Government. *Working Together to Safeguard Children: A Guide to Inter-Agency Working to Safeguard and Promote the Welfare of Children*. TSO (The Stationery Office), 2006.

25

Forensic psychiatric services

Irene Cormac

This chapter outlines the physical health needs of adult offenders who have a mental disorder and describes the physical healthcare services that are needed in forensic psychiatric services. Topics covered in this chapter include the physical health of prisoners, health risks associated with restraint, common injuries in forensic psychiatric settings and dealing with a death in custody.

Introduction

Forensic psychiatric services (FPS) provide assessment and treatment for offenders with mental disorders and for those involved in civil or criminal legal proceedings.[1] In the UK, the National Health Service (NHS) provides most FPS; others are provided by the private sector or charitable organisations. Forensic psychiatric services are delivered in the community, in police custody, the courts and penal establishments, and in secure psychiatric settings. In-patients are normally detained under the mental health legislation pertaining to the country where the patient is detained. Patients who have *not* offended or been convicted of any offence may receive treatment in FPS if they cannot be managed safely elsewhere.[1]

Security

Forensic psychiatric settings

In FPS, security levels vary from high, medium and low to open or community facilities. In England and Wales, the Ministry of Justice (MoJ) determines whether a penal or psychiatric facility meets MoJ standards for at least one or more of these levels of security. In FPS, the level of security must be deemed to be sufficient to prevent the escape of patients who are convicted prisoners, prisoners on remand, unsentenced prisoners or patients detained under a hospital order with a restriction imposed under relevant mental health legislation that pertains to the jurisdiction where the patient is detained.

The three main forms of therapeutic security are classified as physical, procedural and relational.[2]

Physical security is provided by fences, buildings, locks, keys, alarm systems, seclusion facilities, observation systems (e.g. cameras and 'line of sight' with mirrors and observation windows) and communications systems (e.g. short-wave radios). Fittings and furnishings are strengthened and furniture may be fixed in.

Procedural security is maintained using security policies and procedures, management systems and governance. There will be policies and procedures for searches, for entry and exit arrangements for patients, visitors and staff, for the movement of people and goods to and from secure areas, management of the environment, and use

Security in secure settings is the responsibility of everyone. Intelligence from incidents and information provided by staff and others can help to compile a risk assessment of a group of patients or prisoners, as well as the risks of individuals.

of restraints such as handcuffs. Clinical staff are trained to use elements of procedural security such as personal searches ('rub down' and 'intimate' body searches), use of seclusion, breakaway techniques, control and restraint techniques, de-escalation and management of violence and aggression, with or without the use of physical restraint or medication. The type and quantity of personal belongings may be restricted by policy. Routine searches may be regularly made for contraband, weapons, means of self-harm or materials that could be used in hostage-taking, assault or escape attempts.

Relational security depends upon the development of therapeutic relationships between staff and patients. In FPS, requirements for relational security vary between clinical areas, with locally set requirements for the number of staff, gender mix and ratio of qualified to unqualified staff.

Penal establishments

Forensic psychiatric services may provide in-reach psychiatric services to the courts and prisons and receive patients from them. Security levels in penal establishments in England and Wales vary according to the level of danger presented by prisoners and the importance of preventing escape. Each prisoner is allocated to a 'personal' risk category and must not be assigned to a lower category of prison security than this. For men, there are three 'closed' prison categories (A, B and C) and one 'open' prison category (D):

- Category A prisons are 'maximum secure' prisons for highly dangerous prisoners who must not be allowed to escape.
- Category B prisons detain those who do not require maximum security, but for whom escape needs to be made very difficult.
- Category C prisons detain those who cannot be trusted in 'open' conditions but who are unlikely to try to escape.
- Category D prisons are 'open' prisons where some prisoners can be granted access to the community.

There are four similar categories of prison for women, and for penal establishments detaining young offenders and juveniles. Prisoners may become mentally disordered and require transfer to an in-patient FPS with appropriate security provision.

The information on categories of penal establishment in the UK has been adapted from the UK DirectGov website (www.direct.gov.uk).

Physical health of offenders with a mental disorder

In FPS, the physical health risks of patients are similar to the physical health risks of the prison and psychiatric populations. The health of prisoners is worse than that of the general population. A national longitudinal survey in the UK of 1457 newly sentenced prisoners found high rates of social, psychological and physical health problems.[3] These were more severe in adult prisoners (aged 21 and over), female prisoners and those sentenced to less than 12 months' imprisonment. These problems included:

- unemployment (37%)
- lack of qualifications (46%)
- unstable accommodation (15%)
- drug misuse in the year before custody (cannabis 54%, crack cocaine 32% and heroin 31%)
- drinking >2x the recommended safe limits (36%)
- at least one long-standing physical disorder (27%)
- poor psychological health (psychosis 10% and personality disorder 61%).[3]

Another review of the health of prisoners found high rates of physical morbidities, such as epilepsy (2%) and sexually transmitted diseases (17% in female prisoners, 15% in male), as well as high rates of intravenous use of illicit drugs in the previous month (21% in females, 14% in males) and cigarette smoking (75–80%).[4]

Alcohol misuse and dependence have been found in 18–30% of male prisoners and in 30–60% of female prisoners.[5] This review found that 10–48% of male prisoners and 30–60% of female prisoners were likely to misuse drugs or to be dependent on drugs.[5] Prisoners with severe dependence on cannabis or cocaine were found to have an increased risk of developing psychoses, highlighting the importance of addiction services in prisons.[6] Among drug users in prison who injected drugs, the prevalence of antibodies to HIV (0.5%), hepatitis C (31%) and hepatitis B (20%) suggested

Staff must be aware that prisoners are more likely to be infected with blood-borne viruses and sexually transmitted diseases than people in the general population.

that blood-borne viruses are transmitted in prisons by sharing non-sterile injecting equipment.[7]

Although illegal in many countries, non-consensual and consensual sexual activity (mainly homosexual) is known to take place in prisons between inmates, and with staff.[8] Without access to latex protection, prisoners may make makeshift devices in an attempt to practise safe sex.[9] The risk of sexual violence and coercion is greater in overcrowded prisons and in prisons with gang cultures.[8] Other high-risk practices common in prisons are tattooing, blood pacts and violence where the skin is pierced. Staff providing care for prisoners or former prisoners should be aware that prisoners are more likely than the general population to be infected with HIV, hepatitis C, hepatitis B and sexually transmitted diseases.

The health of male prisoners aged over 60 years has been shown to be worse than that of younger prisoners, with high rates of cardiovascular disease (20%), osteoarthritis (13%), diabetes mellitus (8%) and chronic obstructive pulmonary disease (7%).[10]

In prisoners with a mental disorder, the physical health risks associated with imprisonment are compounded by the physical health risks that are associated with various mental disorders and their treatment.

Settings for the delivery of forensic psychiatric services

Criminal court

In the UK, many FPS provide screening services to the courts to detect mental disorders in prisoners awaiting trial and also provide advice to the courts so that people who need mental healthcare can be diverted into appropriate health services. There is normally little time or opportunity to detect physical illness. However, staff should alert the custody staff if they have concerns about a detainee's health.

In penal establishments, if there are concerns about the physical or mental health of a prisoner, it is essential to liaise with the healthcare staff.

In custody

Forensic psychiatrists and team members may assess people detained in police custody. If physical health problems are detected or suspected, staff should advise that appropriate medical care should be provided.

In prison, prisoners normally reside in cells in prison house blocks or wings. Segregation units are used to isolate prisoners who are disturbed, violent or under special restrictions. However, prisoners who are unwell may be transferred to the healthcare block or receive care from the healthcare centre while remaining resident in a house block. Since 2005, the responsibility for providing healthcare in prisons has been transferred to NHS providers in England.[11]

If a patient's physical or mental health deteriorates as a result of a mental disorder (e.g. refusal to eat or drink due to severe psychosis or eating disorder; see p. 125), a prisoner may need urgent transfer to a general hospital or transfer to a psychiatric unit for treatment. In England, the procedures and issues which should be taken into account are described in a good practice procedure guide for the transfer of adult prisoners to and from hospital under sections 47 and 48 of the Mental Health Act.[12]

Medical records

In penal establishments, health professionals will find it useful to check the inmate medical record and other prison records for health problems, significant events (e.g. suicide attempts, hospital transfer) and medical history. Medical records may be requested by the police and the courts; if there is any doubt over whether or not this might breach medical confidentiality it is best to seek advice from senior colleagues and/or a medical defence organisation.

Community

In the community, patients should register with a general practitioner and with a dentist. Staff from FPS should promote healthy lifestyles, exercise and a healthy diet, and may assist with monitoring of physical health parameters such as weight and the side-effects of psychotropic medication.

In-patient settings

Medium secure units mainly admit male prisoners with severe mental illness who are either charged with, or are convicted of, serious violent crimes.[13] Most NHS medium secure units aim for a length of stay of 2 years. High secure services and many private FPS provide long-term psychiatric care. A study in a high secure hospital found that 54% of patients had one or more physical health comorbidities, as well as high rates of tobacco smoking, weight gain and obesity.[14] Since 2007, the three high secure hospitals in England have become totally smoke-free for patients and staff.

Physical health services for in-patients in forensic psychiatric services

Commissioners and management should ensure that physical health services in FPS meet the standards set in current guidelines from the National Institute for Health and Clinical Excellence and standards set for primary care services in the community, such as the Quality and Outcomes Framework standards for primary care (www.qof.ic.nhs.uk). The budget for physical health services may be used to employ staff directly and for service-level agreements with providers for health services, such as haematology. A sample set of standards for routine physical healthcare is presented in Box 25.1.

Box 25.1 Standards for routine physical healthcare

Physical healthcare services

- An initial physical health assessment on admission
- Routine physical health reviews at pre-set intervals
- Chronic disease management
- Access to emergency healthcare and health promotion

A healthy environment

- Adequate food and fluids
- Access to fresh air and exercise facilities at regular intervals
- Adequate washing, bathing and toilet facilities

Physical healthcare plans

- Physical healthcare plans should be reviewed regularly
- On transfer to other forensic psychiatric services or penal establishments, discharge summaries and plans should include physical healthcare plans

Source: adapted from Cormac & Walsh.[15]

Delivery of services

Physical health services should be designed to meet the needs of the patient population. Information should be collected on the demographics, health risks and prevalence of chronic and acute diseases in the patient population. Patients will need access to a range of health services, including primary care, secondary care and services provided by healt care professionals allied to medicine (see Chapters 3, 4 and 5).

A range of clinicians may deliver physical health services, including psychiatrists, general practitioners (GPs), general and psychiatric nurses, visiting hospital specialists and clinical nurse specialists. These staff can be directly employed by the FPS or by local providers, who contract to deliver services in the forensic psychiatric unit.

Attending general hospital

In FPS, it is costly to provide escorts to manage risk and maintain security when patients attend general hospitals, especially if several escort staff are needed or if a patient is admitted to a general hospital. To make best use of resources, GPs should be involved in making the referral to specialists whenever possible. Costs can be reduced by arranging for local specialists to undertake clinical sessions in the FPS or by using technology to reduce 'out of grounds' visits. For example, telemedicine services can provide remote access to consultants via video-link, for routine and emergency consultations.

Investigations

Contracts or service-level agreements should be arranged with local providers for haematology, biochemistry and bacteriology services. Electrocardiography should be available for routine and emergency use. It is helpful if arrangements can be made for a cardiologist to check the accuracy of automated reports from ECG machines. Radiology services are normally provided by local general hospitals. Systems should be in place to monitor

If a patient collapses or appears to be unconscious, be aware that a patient in FPS may be the victim of an assault or may be feigning injury to trap unwary staff into a vulnerable position.

investigation results so that appropriate and timely action can be taken.

Emergency physical healthcare

In in-patient units, staff should be able to respond rapidly (within 3 minutes) to emergency calls for resuscitation.[16] A first-aid kit must be kept on each ward. Medical and nursing staff should receive appropriate training in resuscitation techniques. Resuscitation equipment should be kept close to clinical areas. Physical and procedural security may impede access by the emergency services, so in a medical emergency it is essential to avoid delay in calling for an ambulance, and to liaise with the security team.

Acute illness

Doctors and nursing staff with appropriate training can triage and treat acute conditions. The *Oxford Handbook of General Practice*[17] and the website GP Notebook (www.gpnotebook.co.uk/homepage.cfm) are useful resources.

Chronic diseases

In the community, most people with chronic diseases are treated by primary care services and similarly patients in FPS should have access to primary care. In in-patient settings, GPs, practice nurses and nurse specialists can be employed directly or under service-level agreements. Nursing staff should have a range of skills that enable them to undertake, for example, wound care, cervical screening, infection control, immunisation and monitoring of patients with chronic conditions (e.g. asthma, diabetes and epilepsy).

Other healthcare services

Arrangements should be made for patients to have access to health services such as dentistry, ophthalmology, audiology, optometry, retinal screening for patients with diabetes, dietetics, weight management, speech and language therapy (dysphagia services), chiropody, physiotherapy, infection control, health promotion and disease prevention. The roles of health professionals allied to medicine are described in Chapter 5.

Physical disabilities

Physical disabilities may not necessarily reduce the risks that an offender may pose, so patients with mobility and other health problems may remain in FPS. In-patient FPS should provide ground-floor accommodation in a quiet, settled environment for those with disabilities, and aim to reduce risks posed to sick patients by the behaviour of fellow patients. Staff should have expertise in physical healthcare and have the necessary equipment to care for those with physical disabilities (e.g. King's Fund beds, hoists and wheelchairs).

Routine monitoring and detection of changes in physical health

Many in-patient FPS are geographically isolated so it is essential to monitor and detect changes in baseline measurements of physical health parameters as soon as possible. See Chapter 4 for role of nurses in routine mentoring. In general hospitals, modified early-warning systems (MEWS) are used to measure, record and monitor physical health parameters. These measurements include pulse rate, respiratory rate, oxygen saturation, blood pressure, peak flow, urine output and fluid intake. MEWS measurements systems have defined limits or normal ranges to which are allocated a numerical score, also known as a 'patient at risk' score (PAR score). When MEWS or PAR scores exceed certain levels, this should prompt staff to take appropriate action such as increased frequency of observations or to call for medical assistance. (See Table 31.3, p. 423.)

Medication monitoring

Pharmacists can assist psychiatrists and clinical teams with effective and appropriate monitoring of psychotropic medication, according to Maudsley guidelines.[18] Weight should be measured and recorded monthly or more frequently, to check for weight gain or unintended weight loss. The role of the pharmacist in mental health settings is outlined in Chapter 5.

Physical health review

Physical health reviews should take place at least annually. In-patient services should have facilities for physical examinations, including the appropriate equipment (see Chapters 9 and 10).

Care plans can be used to manage routine physical healthcare. It is advisable to prepare care plans in advance for use in case of sudden deterioration in a patient's physical condition.

Communication

Systems should be developed to ensure effective and reliable communication between health professionals. Contemporaneous entries should be made in patients' healthcare records. If separate computer systems are used by mental health professionals and by primary healthcare services, it is best if clinicians have access to both systems. Letters or copies of the GP notes can be entered directly into psychiatric records. Mental health professionals should be prepared to provide up-to-date health information that is needed by other health professionals.

Governance

Standards for physical healthcare services should be established and monitored to ensure consistent delivery of care across FPS. Protocols, procedures and standardised recording forms may improve the quality of service delivery and enable services to be audited. Committees are often used to manage services; these might include drugs and therapeutics, medical devices, resuscitation and audit committees. Untoward events and 'near misses' should be monitored and addressed by clinical governance.

Box 25.2 Injuries in forensic psychiatric services

Trauma and injuries

- Punching walls – fractured metacarpals
- Kicking walls – fractured metatarsals
- Head-banging – contusions, laceration of scalp, pain, concussion

Laceration

- Check for underlying tissue damage
- Test for movement, sensation and perfusion
- Check for areas without sweating that indicate nerve damage
- Objects may be inserted into wounds or wounds may be reopened
- Blood loss can be life-threatening if a cut is kept open under water

Bites and needle-stick injuries

- Human bites easily become infected (Chapter 30)
- Needle-stick injuries may transmit blood-borne viruses (see p. 248 for management)
- Consider using retractable needles

Assault

- Non-accidental injuries may be attributed to falls, e.g. in a shower
- Sexual assault may lead to injury and infection

Challenges in FPS with the management of injury and illness

Patients may self-harm by various means including cutting, head-banging, punching and kicking walls (Box 25.2). Although a patient may describe their injuries as accidental, for example due to a 'fall in the shower', staff should consider the possibility that they may instead be the victim of an assault.

In the controlled environment of an FPS, although there are fewer opportunities for patients to obtain medication to take as an overdose, a patient might secrete their own medication or take medication obtained from others. Staff should be aware of the type and severity of injuries that require referral to the accident and emergency department.

On admission, patients may be addicted to drugs or alcohol, and develop an acute withdrawal reaction. Urgent treatment may be necessary (see Chapters 22 and 23).

Patients may refuse food and liquids, medication or routine monitoring with the aim of being transferred to a general hospital, where escape might be easier to effect. It is essential to have close liaison between clinical teams and security staff, as well as the hospital's physical health services, to ensure that security, safety and the physical health of patients are maintained in in-patient FPS. (See p. 408 for the assessment of nutritional compromise in eating disorders.)

Healthy environment

Diet and nutrition

The UK government recommends that at least five portions of fruit or vegetables should be eaten per day and at least two portions of oily fish should be consumed per week. In institutions, main meals should contain less than 15 g of fat and desserts less than 10 g of sugar, with a daily salt intake no more than 6 g; 'healthy options' should be marked on the menu.[19] Patients who have difficulty eating or swallowing (dysphagia) may need texture-modified meals or high-calorie meals. Catering departments and dietitians should work together to ensure that the menu provides a nutritious and healthy diet, which meets the needs of patients and meets NICE guidelines on obesity.[20]

In FPS, the consumption of confectionery and sugar-containing drinks may substantially increase daily calorie intake.[21] Patients should be encouraged to be moderate in their purchases of food, especially 'take-away' meals, which have a high calorie, fat and salt content. Patients should have free access to drinking water, unless there is a risk of polydipsia.

Box 25.3 Physical health reviews

A physical health review should be undertaken with the patient's consent, ideally in the first 24 hours after admission and at least annually thereafter:

- Obtain information about current health, symptoms, medical history, lifestyle and health screening
- Undertake a physical examination relevant to the patient's history and current complaints; note any injuries
- Review medication, including history of allergies
- Arrange physical investigations
- Take action to address clinical needs (e.g. diet, fluids, medication)

If a patient declines a health check, note the reason in the clinical record. Record the level of consciousness, appearance, gait, movements, nutritional state and level of hydration, as a minimum.

Source: Cormac & Walsh, 2009.[15]

Physical activity

The benefits of physical activity with recommendations for improving fitness are described in Chapter 8. In FPS, security restrictions will affect access to recreational areas and exercise facilities. Nevertheless, FPS should provide patients with access to at least 30 minutes of moderate-intensity exercise at least five times per week, to meet government guidelines.[22] In secure settings, patients can exercise more easily if gym equipment is available for use on wards under the supervision of trained staff.

Tobacco smoking

Chapter 6 contains information on smoking cessation in psychiatric settings. Before admission to a smoke-free hospital, patients should be informed in advance that smoking is not allowed. Smoking cessation services should be provided for all new patients who are smokers.

Transfers and discharge

Admission to in-patient FPS

Before a patient is transferred to an FPS it is important to check for physical health conditions. General nurses can provide invaluable assistance to the admitting clinical team by making a pre-admission physical health assessment together with recommendations and arrangements for physical healthcare in the forensic unit before admission (Box 4.1, p. 35).

The ward doctor, GP and ward nurses should be informed in advance about the physical health status of a new patient. Physical health risks should be identified as soon as possible (Box 25.3). Standardised recording forms can be used for a functional enquiry about symptoms, a physical examination on admission and the annual physical health review.

Transfer to general hospital from FPS

Appropriate levels of security must be maintained while a patient receives physical healthcare outside the secure perimeter. Clinical and security teams must follow agreed policies and procedures for leave of absence. A risk assessment will inform decisions about the type of transport required, whether physical restraints such as handcuffs should be worn (or carried) and the number, gender and training of escorting staff.

Patients may need urgent transfer to a general hospital, so it is advisable to prepare in advance a draft 'leave of absence' form and a risk assessment for each patient, for use in the event of an emergency transfer to a general hospital. For admission to a general hospital, it is helpful to liaise with the admitting team about the security requirements as well as providing information about current medication and monitoring (e.g. if the patient is taking clozapine).

Discharge or transfer

Discharge or transfer arrangements should include information about physical health needs and arrangements. For patients in the community, information should be provided on community services that support and encourage healthy living. All patients should be encouraged to register with a GP and should be offered a physical health review at least annually.

Before transfer of a patient from FPS to a penal establishment, it is essential to liaise with the receiving healthcare services about the patient's physical health and invite appropriate staff from the prison to a discharge planning meeting, an 'after-care planning' meeting or a section 117 meeting.[23] In England, a coordinator for the care programme approach should be identified, or an equivalent care coordinator.[24]

Challenges in forensic psychiatric services

Management of a potentially violent or violent patient

Guidelines from NICE should be followed for the management of violence and aggression, including the use of rapid tranquillisation.[16] Prescribers of rapid tranquillisation must be familiar with the use of benzodiazepines, the antagonist flumazenil, as well as the use of antipsychotic, antimuscarinic and antihistamine medications. The effects of rapid tranquillisation will be affected by the state of arousal of the patient and their physical state, such as dehydration and intoxication with alcohol or illicit drugs (see Box 26.6, rapid tranquillisation p. 365).

Physical restraint can cause fatalities if not properly applied (Box 25.4). Research by Parkes and Carson[25] has shown that if a person is restrained in a prone or supine position on the floor, their vital capacity and forced expiratory volume can be significantly reduced compared with a standing position. If the restraining persons lean with their body weight on the back of a person being restrained who is lying face downwards, this can cause a reduction in lung function of 24–27%.[25]

In the UK, NICE recommends that:[16]

- One team member should lead the team through the 'physical intervention'.
- The team leader 'should be responsible for protecting and supporting the head and neck, where required', and should 'ensure that the airway and breathing are not compromised and that vital signs are monitored'.

Box 25.4 Factors known to increase the risk of death from restraint

Patient factors

- Obesity
- Prolonged struggle
- Use of illicit drugs
- Respiratory disease, cardiovascular disease, trauma
- Difficulties in communicating distress due to intellectual disabilities or speech problems

Incorrectly applied restraint techniques or restraint techniques that may impede respiration

- Obstruction to the mouth or nose with a gag or tape restricting air entry, with increased risk if the patient struggles or is obese
- Neck holds that are applied with compression of carotid arteries or trachea
- Restraint in the prone position with pressure or weight pressing on the patient's back (e.g. people leaning on the back of a prone patient)
- Restraint in prone position with arms held or handcuffed behind the back or if both arms and legs are tied together behind the patient's back while the patient is prone (this is known as 'hobble-tying')
- Restraint in a sitting or kneeling position when the patient is forced to flex from the waist and lean forwards (especially high risk with an obese patient)
- If clothing is used to tie a patient, this can lead to accidental strangulation

Source: Based on Paterson *et al*, 2003[26] and Parkes & Carson, 2008.[25] See also Fig. 25.1.

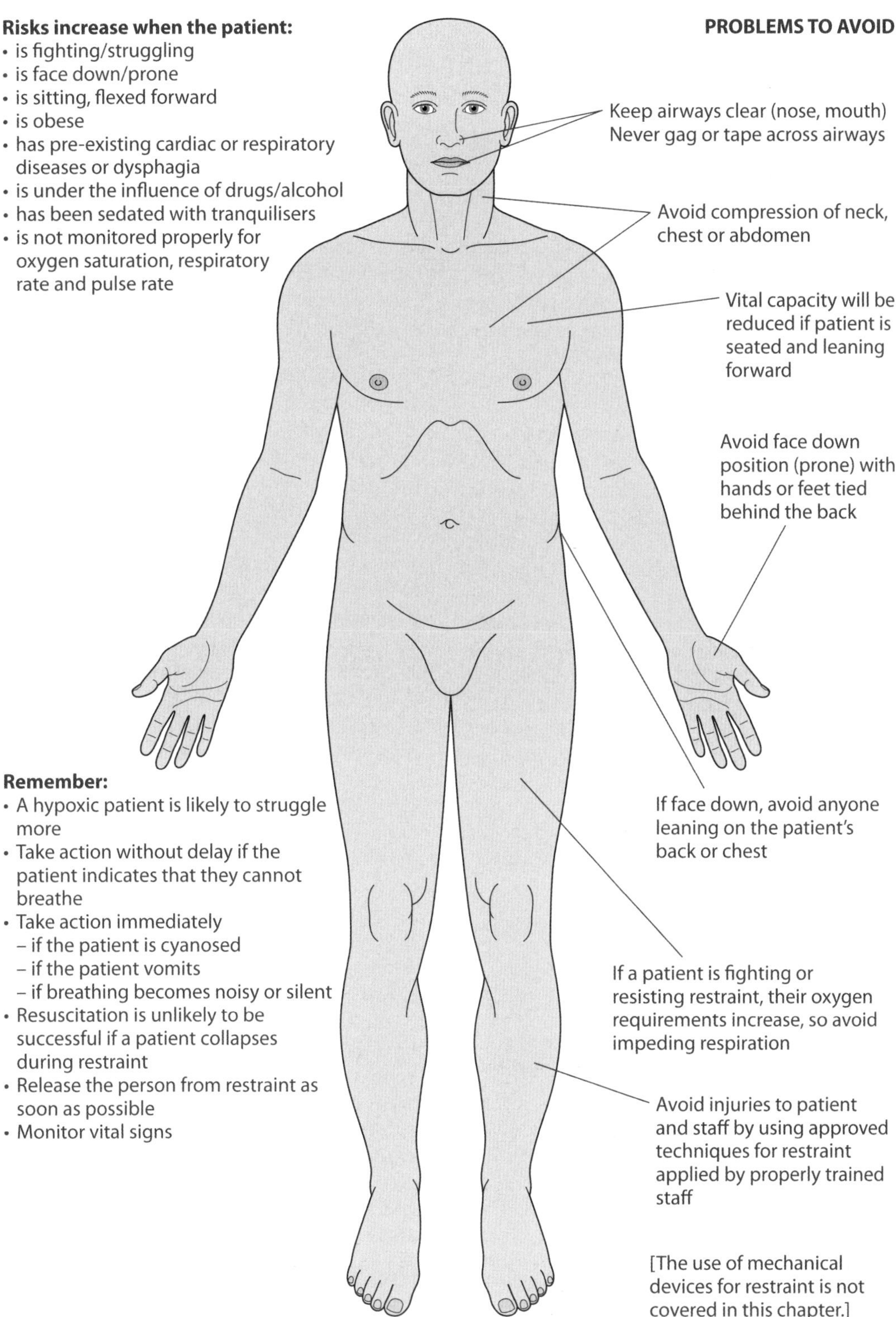

Risks increase when the patient:
• is fighting/struggling
• is face down/prone
• is sitting, flexed forward
• is obese
• has pre-existing cardiac or respiratory diseases or dysphagia
• is under the influence of drugs/alcohol
• has been sedated with tranquilisers
• is not monitored properly for oxygen saturation, respiratory rate and pulse rate
PROBLEMS TO AVOID
Keep airways clear (nose, mouth)
Never gag or tape across airways
Avoid compression of neck, chest or abdomen
Vital capacity will be reduced if patient is seated and leaning forward
Avoid face down position (prone) with hands or feet tied behind the back
Remember:
• A hypoxic patient is likely to struggle more
• Take action without delay if the patient indicates that they cannot breathe
• Take action immediately
– if the patient is cyanosed
– if the patient vomits
– if breathing becomes noisy or silent
• Resuscitation is unlikely to be successful if a patient collapses during restraint
• Release the person from restraint as soon as possible
• Monitor vital signs
If face down, avoid anyone leaning on the patient's back or chest
If a patient is fighting or resisting restraint, their oxygen requirements increase, so avoid impeding respiration
Avoid injuries to patient and staff by using approved techniques for restraint applied by properly trained staff
[The use of mechanical devices for restraint is not covered in this chapter.]

Fig. 25.1 Physical restraint.

The more that a patient struggles, the greater will be their oxygen requirements. If a patient collapses during restraint, resuscitation is unlikely to succeed.

- At no time should direct pressure be applied to the neck, thorax, abdomen or pelvic areas.
- If possible, a pulse oximeter should be used to check oxygen saturation.
- Any injuries sustained during physical restraint should be documented and treated as necessary. It is not unusual for complaints to be made later.

Seclusion

Seclusion is defined as 'the supervised confinement of a patient in a room, which may be locked'.[23] It should be used only to contain severely disturbed behaviour that is likely to cause harm to others.[23] Seclusion rooms must have adequate ventilation and heating, and if possible en-suite toilet and washing facilities, including oral healthcare and sanitary supplies as needed. Bedding and clothing should be changed regularly. It may be necessary to use 'strong' bedding and clothing that cannot be torn by the patient. Nutritious finger food and adequate amounts fluids must be provided. A patient's level of consciousness should be recorded using the AVPU system (Alert, responds to Verbal commands, responds to Pain, Unresponsive) (Box 4.3, p. 360).

Box 25.5 Checks to make on a patient held in seclusion

The local or NHS trust seclusion policy and procedures should be followed, but the following are good practice.

- If a patient is sedated, check pulse, blood pressure, respiration rate and level of consciousness at pre-set intervals. Record findings on the hospital observation chart
- A patient who stays in the same position may have collapsed, become unconscious or died. Staff must observe and record their observations of the movement of the patient at pre-set intervals, even when the patient is asleep
- Call for urgent assistance if a patient does not move, if it is suspected that the patient is unconscious, or if vital signs are outside the normal range of the parameters set by the MEWS or 'patient at risk' score (see Chapter 30)

Checks to make when a patient is in seclusion are summarised in Box 25.5.

Death in custody

The coroner in England and Wales (in Scotland, the procurator fiscal) must be informed if a death occurs in prison, in custody, in a 'detained' patient, if the death is violent, unnatural, sudden, or without a known cause. Deaths of patients in secure FPS fall into the category of 'death in custody'.[27] The coroner's officer (procurator fiscal) should be contacted immediately. Following a death in custody, the scene of the death must be left untouched, exactly as it was when the body was found, or where the patient died. This includes leaving endotracheal tubes and other medical equipment *in situ*.

In England and Wales, the coroner's officer is usually a police officer and the officer will attend the scene and make preliminary enquiries about the death. The coroner will decide whether a post-mortem examination is necessary, whether the death can be registered and whether the body can be cremated or buried. Death certificates can be issued by the coroner to allow disposal of the body. The coroner may decide to hold an inquest. The staff involved in the patient's care may be asked to provide written statements and to attend the inquest to give oral evidence. In most cases it is wise to seek legal representation and to prepare to be questioned under oath. For further information see the Medical Protection Society factsheet.[27]

After the death of an in-patient, fellow patients and staff may appreciate support. Patients often hear rumours about a deceased patient's death, and can have fantasies and fears about the cause of death. Patients may believe that the deceased patient was murdered by staff or was killed by poisonous medication. Patients may fear becoming the next one to die, especially if they take the same medication as the deceased patient. The death may raise issues to do with a patient's index offence, especially if it involved killing. Patients may fear dying in custody. It is important to ask how patients are feeling because otherwise these issues may linger. A religious ceremony and support groups can relieve tension, give comfort and enable patients and staff to resolve grief.

Legal matters

Patients in FPS may be experienced in dealing with legal issues relating to mental health legislation. However, they may not have attended to civil matters such as making an advanced decision or a statement of wishes. Patients may want to make a will or grant a lasting power of attorney. Their financial affairs may need to be managed by the Court of Protection. Chapter 11 covers the legislation pertaining to mental capacity and mental health.

Addictions

In an abstinent patient, reinstatement of previous patterns of addiction can be dangerous. Drug-related mortality was found to be seven times higher in the 2 weeks following leaving prison.[28] Ex-smokers taking clozapine who transfer from a non-smoking environment to an environment where smoking is allowed may recommence smoking. Smoking tobacco leads to liver enzyme induction, thus reducing plasma levels of clozapine, so the patient who starts smoking again may need to take an increased dose. The reverse is true when smokers taking clozapine stop smoking.[14]

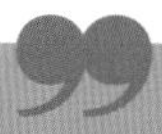

Summary

Physical healthcare in FPS and in penal establishments should be delivered to the same standard as healthcare in the community. The transfer of patients between penal and psychiatric settings should be carefully coordinated to ensure the transfer of necessary information on physical health as well as information on mental health and risk issues. In FPS healthcare, professionals from all disciplines should be aware of the security requirements operating in penal establishments and in forensic psychiatric settings.

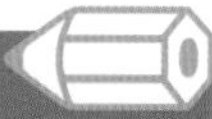

Learning points

- The physical health of prisoners is worse than that of the general population, with higher rates of addiction, infection with blood-borne viruses and at least one long-standing physical disorder in about a quarter of adult prisoners.
- About 75–80% of prisoners smoke.
- The three main types of security are physical, relational and procedural.
- Long-stay in-patients have high rates of inactivity, obesity, diabetes and tobacco-smoking.
- General practitioners should be involved in planning of referral to specialists to reduce the number of referrals to general hospitals.
- Regular monitoring of physical health parameters will allow a deterioration in health to be recognised more easily.
- Physical health reviews should be undertaken at least annually, using standard systems and recording forms.
- Prepare leave-of-absence pro formas and risk assessments in advance in case emergency admission is need to a general hospital.
- Management of violence and aggression should be undertaken according to NICE guidelines.[16]
- Ensure the patient's airway and breathing are not impaired during physical restraint.
- Deaths in FPS are treated as deaths in custody and the coroner or procurator fiscal must be informed.
- On discharge, ensure information is provided on the patient's physical health to the healthcare centre in the penal establishment or to the patient's GP in the community.
- Advise patients and staff about the risks of reinstatement of addictions.
- If a patient who is taking clozapine gives up smoking, the dose of clozapine will need to be reduced, and *vice versa*, if a non-smoking patient starts to smoke tobacco.

References

1 Cormac I, Launer M. *Forensic Psychiatric Services*. Royal College of Psychiatrists, The Princess Royal Trust for Carers, 2005 (http://www.rcpsych.ac.uk/PDF/ForensicPsychiatric.pdf).

2 Kennedy HG. Therapeutic uses of security: mapping forensic mental heath services by stratifying risk. *Adv Psychiatr Treat* 2002; **8**: 433–43.

3 Stuart D. *The Problems and Needs of Newly Sentenced Prisoners: Results from a National Survey*. Ministry of Justice Research Series 16/08. Ministry of Justice, 2008.

4 Marshall T, Simpson S, Stevens A. *Health Care in Prisons: A Health Care Needs Assessment*. Department of Public Health and Epidemiology, University of Birmingham, 2000.

5 Fazel S, Bains P, Doll H. Substance abuse and dependence in prisoners: a systematic review. *Addiction* 2006; **101**: 181–91.

6 Farrell M, Boys A, Bebbington T, *et al*. Psychosis and drug dependence: results from a national survey of prisoners. *Br J Psychiatry* 2002; **181**: 393–8.

7 Weild A, On G, Bennett D, *et al*. Prevalence of HIV, hepatitis B, and hepatitis C antibodies in prisoners in England and Wales: a national survey. *Com Dis Pub Health* 2000; **3**: 121–6.

8 Gears S. *Sex, Sexual Violence and Coercion in Men's Prisons*. University of Witwatersrand, South Africa, 2001 (http://www.csvr.org.za/docs/correctional/sexsexualviolence.pdf).

9 Mahon N. New York inmates' HIV risk behaviours: the implications for prevention policy and programs. *Am J Pub Health* 1996; **86**: 1211–5.

10 Fazel S, Hope T, O'Donnell I, *et al*. Health of elderly male prisoners: worse than the general population, worse than younger prisoners. *Age Ageing* 2001; **30**: 403–7.

11 de Viggiani N, Orme J, Powell J, *et al*. New arrangements for prison health care. *BMJ* 2005; **330**: 918.

12 Department of Health. *Good Practice Procedure Guide: The Transfer and Remission of Adult Prisoners under s47 and s48 of the Mental Health Act*. Department of Health, 2011.

13 Coid J, Kahtan N, Gault B, *et al*. Medium secure forensic psychiatry services: comparison of seven English health regions. *Br J Psychiatry* 2001; **178**: 55–61.

14 Cormac I, Brown A, Creasey S, *et al*. A retrospective evaluation of the impact of total smoking cessation on psychiatric in-patients taking clozapine. *Acta Psychiatr Scand* 2010; **121**: 393–7.

15 Cormac I, Walsh M. Physical health standards in forensic psychiatric services. In *Physical Health in Mental Health, Final Report of a Scoping Group (Occasional Paper 67)*: 39–43. Royal College of Psychiatrists, 2009.

16 National Institute for Health and Clinical Excellence. *Violence: The Short-Term Management of Disturbed/Violent Behaviour in Psychiatric In-Patient Settings and Emergency Departments (Clinical Guidelines CG25)*. NICE, 2005.

17 Simon C, Everitt H, van Dorp F. *The Oxford Handbook of General Practice*. Oxford University Press, 2009.

18 Taylor D, Paton C, Kapur S. *Maudsley Prescribing Guidelines* (10th edn). Blackwell, 2009.

19 Department of Health. *Better Hospital Food Programme*. Department of Health, 2010.

20 National Institute for Health and Clinical Excellence. *Obesity: The Prevention, Identification, Assessment and Management of Overweight and Obesity in Adults and Children*. NICE, 2010.

21 Harper S, Ferriter M, Cormac I. Impact of the increase in state benefits on the pattern of expenditure by patients in a high secure hospital. *Ment Health Rev J* 2008; **13**: 4–7.

22 Department of Health. *At Least Five a Week: Evidence on the Impact of Physical Activity and Its Relationship to Health: A Report of the Chief Medical Officer*. Department of Health, 2004.

23 Department of Health. *Code of Practice: Mental Health Act 1983*. TSO (The Stationery Office), 2008.

24 Department of Health. *Care Programme Approach*. Department of Health, 2008.

25 Parkes J, Carson R. Sudden death during restraint: do some positions affect lung function? *Med Sci Law* 2008; **48**: 137–41.

26 Paterson B, Bradley P, Stark C, *et al*. Deaths associated with restraint use in health and social care in the UK. *The results of a preliminary survey. J Psychiatr Ment Health Nurs* 2003; **10**: 3–15.

27 Medical Protection Society. Factsheet on reporting deaths to the coroner. MPS, 2011 (http://webarchive.nationalarchives.gov.uk/+/www.dh.gov.uk/en/Managingyourorganisation/Workforce/Leadership/Healthcareenvironment/DH_4116450).

28 Bird SM, Hutchinson SJ. Male drugs-related deaths in the fortnight after release from prison: in Scotland, 1996–99. *Addictions* 2003; **98**: 185–90.

26

General adult psychiatry

David Osborn

This chapter outlines the more common physical conditions encountered in general adult psychiatry, and how to assess and manage these in both in-patient and community settings. The focus is on severe mental illnesses such as schizophrenia and bipolar disorder. The different practical strategies are described for improving the assessment and monitoring of physical health, at both an individual and a service level.

Introduction

General adult services should work closely with primary care services to ensure good physical healthcare is provided for their patients. This requires commitment, especially when demands on psychiatrists are increasing. The trend towards functional organisation of adult psychiatric services brings opportunities and difficulties in the provision of coherent physical healthcare for this at-risk population. While primary care is the natural setting for routine assessment of physical health, general adult psychiatrists must recognise that there are many situations in which they are responsible for their patients' physical health, either because a patient is unable or unwilling to attend the general practitioner (GP), or because the psychiatrist is the principal medical officer.

General adult services provide care in various settings, including community mental health settings, out-patient clinics, depot and clozapine clinics, general and specialist in-patient services and in the home, with crisis teams. The chronicity and fluctuating nature of many severe mental illnesses often results in patients being transferred between teams and lack of continuity can create pitfalls in both mental and physical healthcare.

Every new patient should be screened for current physical symptoms. This should include a review of the patient's medical history and any relevant family medical history. An organic aetiology is more likely with:

- pre-existing physical conditions
- a family history of the condition
- neurological symptoms or abnormal endocrine tests
- abnormal visual perceptions such as illusions
- disturbance within the cognitive examination
- treatment resistance.

Physical conditions associated with adult mental disorders

Physical conditions may present with symptoms of depression before the underlying condition has been diagnosed (examples are given in Box 26.1). Some endocrine and neurological conditions, including disorders of the thyroid,

Every new patient should be screened for current physical symptoms.

epilepsy and multiple sclerosis, are the most likely to present with psychiatric symptoms. These conditions have replaced syphilis, which is now largely of historical interest, at least in terms of psychiatric disorder.

Medication for physical diseases that may contribute to poor mental health include parenteral steroids, the acne treatment isotretinoin and agents used to increase dopamine levels in Parkinson's disease, such as L-dopa.

It is also important to note that chronic diseases, cancer and terminal illness increase the risk of developing a depressive disorder (see Box 26.2 for examples) and a psychotic disorder (Box 26.3).

Severe mental illnesses

People with schizophrenia and bipolar disorder are more likely to die prematurely from physical causes than from suicide. In particular, there is a two- to threefold greater risk of cardiovascular disease (including myocardial infarctions) compared with the general population, especially when they are young.[1] The number of cardiovascular deaths occurring among people with severe mental illness aged under 70 is six to seven times greater than the number of suicide deaths; the reasons for this excess are complex. Large cohort studies have used multivariate analysis to show that increased cardiovascular risk is not simply explained by increased rates of smoking or by social deprivation.[1] Unhealthy lifestyle, including poor diet and lack of exercise, probably contributes. In addition, the stress associated with mental disorders may have a direct impact on cardiovascular health. Long-term stress has been shown to affect the hypothalamic–pituitary–adrenal axis with a subsequent increase in cardiometabolic problems such as diabetes and dyslipidaemia.[2]

Cardiovascular disease

Guidance from the National Institute for Health and Clinical Excellence (NICE) on the treatment of bipolar disorder and schizophrenia emphasises the importance of screening for cardiovascular risk factors.[3,4] This includes measuring and recording at least annually:

- plasma lipid levels
- blood glucose level

Box 26.1 Physical conditions that can present with symptoms of depression

- Endocrine disorders: hypothyroidism, hyperparathyroidism, Addison's disease, Cushing's syndrome
- Substance misuse: alcohol, amphetamines, cannabis, cocaine, anabolic steroids
- Infections: neurosyphilis, HIV infection
- Toxins: pesticides (e.g. organophosphates)
- Medication side-effects: beta-blockers, barbiturates, benzodiazepines, calcium channel blockers, statins, isotretinoin (accutane), opiates
- Cancer: pancreatic cancer, bowel cancer, cerebral tumour

Box 26.2 Physical conditions that may lead to developing depression

- Chronic diseases: chronic heart disease, diabetes mellitus
- Neurological disorders: epilepsy, head injury, multiple sclerosis, Parkinson's disease, stroke
- Infections: infectious mononucleosis, influenza, tuberculosis
- Autoimmune disease: systemic lupus erythematosus
- Genetic disorders: haemochromatosis, Huntington's disease

Box 26.3 Conditions that can cause psychotic symptoms

- Endocrine: Cushing's syndrome, hyperthyroidism, hypothyroidism (myxoedema), hypoglycaemia
- Substance misuse: alcohol, amphetamines, cannabis, cocaine, LSD, anabolic steroids
- Infections: HIV/AIDS, Lyme disease, malaria, neurosyphilis
- Medication side-effects: anti-epileptic medication, corticosteroids, L-dopa, mefloquine (larium; antimalarial drug), proton pump inhibitors, psychotropic medication
- Cancer: cerebral tumour
- Neurological: epilepsy, head injury, multiple sclerosis, Parkinson's disease, stroke
- Autoimmune disease: systemic lupus erythematosus

- blood pressure
- smoking status
- weight
- body mass index
- waist size.

While *fasting* samples are ideal for diagnosing diabetes, *random* samples are good enough for the ongoing monitoring of serum cholesterol and glucose in the absence of abnormal findings. Screening and management require collaboration between primary and secondary care. Service issues that result from this collaboration are discussed below.

Cancer

There is conflicting evidence on rates of cancer in people with serious mental illness. One study failed to show an association between schizophrenia, bipolar disorder and cancer, apart from a slight increase in respiratory tumours, explained by smoking.[1] Other research has found increased rates of colonic and breast cancer in people with schizophrenia, yet a decreased risk of respiratory tumours.[5] Others have suggested that families of those with schizophrenia might be protected from cancer.[6,7] Cancer screening programmes (see Chapter 9) are relevant to all patients, whether in primary care, in secondary care or in psychiatric services.

People with schizophrenia and bipolar disorder are six to seven times more likely to die prematurely from physical causes than from suicide.

People with schizophrenia have increased levels of smoking, obesity, diabetes and dyslipidaemia and possibly hypertension.

Other mental illnesses: depression and anxiety

People with more common mental disorders less frequently receive joint primary and secondary care. The general adult psychiatrist still has an educational role regarding the physical impact of these illnesses, through liaison with primary care. A patient's physical illnesses should not be overshadowed by anxiety and depressive disorder, as these mental disorders increase a patient's risk of premature death, especially from cardiovascular disease. General practitioners should therefore ensure adequate physical screening is provided, appropriate to the patient's age group.

Conversely, depression and anxiety are common sequelae of serious physical conditions, such as brain tumours and genitourinary complaints.[8] Depression also increases the risk of cardiovascular disease but has been described as one of the least understood cardiovascular risk factors.[9] People with depression are 25–60% more likely to suffer a heart attack in the 10 years after diagnosis than is someone in the general population in a given 10-year period. For those who develop heart disease, the prognosis is significantly worsened by comorbid depression.[10] After 6 months, the mortality rate of those who are depressed is more than three times[11] and at six years more than twice as high as that of patients with heart disease who have not developed depression.[12]

These risks are not restricted to depressive illnesses. A large UK database study showed that *panic disorder* is a risk factor for ischaemic heart disease; with those aged under 50 years and people with a panic disorder having a 40% greater chance of experiencing a myocardial infarction.[13]

Panic disorder provides a clinical dilemma, since the disorder may closely mimic cardiovascular symptoms, even in the absence of demonstrable myocardial ischaemia. A careful history will usually distinguish between panic and ischaemic pain:

- panic attacks classically present with an awareness of the heart beat and fear of a heart attack
- myocardial events usually present with crushing central chest pain, accompanied by signs of sympathetic activity, including sweating and pallor.

However, the distinction may not be clear and whenever chest pain is a prominent feature of the presentation, a diagnosis of panic disorder should not be made before an urgent review, including an ECG, in an accident and emergency setting.

Those with *generalised anxiety disorders* also have increased risks for all-cause and cardiovascular mortality, and the risk is greater when anxiety and depression occur in the same individual.[14]

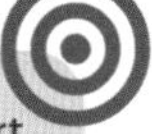

People with depression are more likely to have a heart attack in the 10 years following diagnosis. For those who develop heart disease, the prognosis is significantly worsened by comorbid depression.

Risk factors for physical illnesses

Smoking, diabetes, obesity and dyslipidaemia are all more common in people with severe mental illnesses.[15] Although the evidence in this field is of variable epidemiological quality, there are now enough studies to be confident. One of the larger studies revealed increased levels of hypertension, dyslipidaemia and elevated glucose levels among people with schizophrenia compared with the general population.[16]

Cardiovascular risk is further compounded by a diet low in fibre and high in fat, alongside levels of exercise that are significantly lower than in the general population, and lower even than those of people from other deprived social groups.[17,18] In other words, most of the common risk factors for poor physical health cluster in people with severe mental illness.

Effects of psychotropic medication

General adult psychiatrists must be familiar with the adverse effects of the medications they prescribe. Before taking any psychotropic medication, patients should have an assessment of their physical health and health risk factors.[19]

Metabolic effects

Second-generation antipsychotic medications are associated with weight gain and increased glucose and lipid levels,[20] although whether this is due to drugs alone is debatable.[21] National and international guidelines recommend regular monitoring of patients taking these drugs.[4,20] Before initiating antipsychotic medication, always check baseline body mass index (BMI), as well as lipid and glucose levels (fasting preferred) and repeat at 3 months and then annually, or more often if abnormal values emerge. The psychiatrist must ensure these investigations are arranged for patients both in the community and in in-patient settings. Box 26.4 summarises advice on physical monitoring for patients on antipsychotic medication.

Cardiac arrhythmia

Some antipsychotic drugs can increase the risk of serious cardiac arrhythmia, usually through prolongation of the

Sexual side-effects are unacceptable to adults of all ages. Routinely enquire about them, especially if prescribing first-generation antipsychotic medications, risperidone or amisulpride.

Box 26.4 Physical health monitoring of patients on antipsychotic medication

Take a physical history, including current symptoms and conditions

Choose an antipsychotic agent least likely to exacerbate existing problems:

- weight gain less likely with amisulpride, quetiapine, aripiprazole
- sexual problems less likely with quetiapine, clozapine and aripiprazole

Baseline investigations

- Body mass index and/or waist circumference
- Glucose
- Lipids, including total and high-density lipoprotein cholesterol
- Prolactin
- ECG for those at risk of sudden death (check family history), on high doses, on combinations of antipsychotics or on specific agents (see text).

Repeat monitoring

- Repeat all above at 4 weeks, at 3 months and then annually, or more frequently if abnormalities or changes are detected
- Olanzapine and clozapine deserve special attention to weight gain

Check for

Extrapyramidal side-effects, especially with first-generation antipsychotics, risperidone and amisulpride

Optimal practice

Use a side-effect rating scale such as the Liverpool University Neuroleptic Side-Effect Rating Scale (LUNSERS)[22] (which does not include metabolic effects) or the Antipsychotic Non-Neurological Side-Effects Rating Scale (ANNSERS).[23]

Valuable resource: Physical Health Check tool, available for free download from Rethink Mental Illness (www.rethink.org).

QT interval on the ECG. An ECG is recommended for patients when:

- considering treatment with sertindole, ziprasidone and thioridazine
- the patient has a personal or family history of cardiac disease, especially sudden, unexpected, unexplained death under 40 years when a cardiac arrhythmia is the likely cause
- the dose of antipsychotic medication is higher than recommended in the *British National Formulary*[24]
- more than one antipsychotic medication is prescribed concurrently (see pp. 152, 153).

Hyperprolactinaemia

Levels of prolactin are frequently raised by most first-generation and some second-generation antipsychotic medications (especially risperidone and amisulpride) because they are potent antagonists of dopamine-2 (D_2) receptors, which can cause unwanted effects:

- in men:
  - erectile dysfunction, decreased libido and ejaculatory problems, including retrograde ejaculation or failure to ejaculate
  - at higher prolactin levels, mammary hypertrophy and galactorrhoea
- in women:
  - low libido
  - failure of both arousal and orgasm
  - oligomenorrhoea or amenorrhoea
  - mammary hypertrophy and galactorrhoea at higher prolactin levels.

Sexual side-effects should be discussed with patients routinely.

A baseline prolactin measurement should be performed at initiation of, and 3 months after starting, antipsychotic medication, and again after another 3 months. If abnormal, or if antipsychotic doses are changed,[25] it should be repeated at 3-month intervals. If hyperprolactinaemia is identified and problematic, antipsychotic medications with less impact on prolactin should be used, such as olanzapine or quetiapine.

Anticholinergic effects

The tricyclic antidepressants and some first-generation antipsychotics have anticholinergic (antimuscarinic) side-effects, which can exacerbate pre-existing prostatic symptoms and constipation.

No one wants to gain weight. Intervene early with people taking clozapine and olanzapine to avoid increased calorie intake that occurs with these drugs.

Gastrointestinal effects

Selective serotonin reuptake inhibitors (SSRIs) should be prescribed with caution for patients with a propensity for upper gastrointestinal bleeding, such as those with a history of acid indigestion requiring medical treatment on more than one occasion.[26]

Lithium

The narrow therapeutic/toxic ratio for lithium requires regular monitoring of serum concentrations. This is now remunerated in the UK primary care General Medical Services contract. Side-effects may involve most body systems but the emergence of neurological signs such as tremor, ataxia, dysarthria, nystagmus and convulsions are ominous and potentially fatal. Shared care requires the communication of these important test results, as well as any relevant physical health problems, between different services, although this is by no means routine current practice.

Choice of medication when physical problems are identified

Table 26.1 indicates which medications (categorised as antipsychotics, mood stabilisers and antidepressants) are less likely to exacerbate physical problems as well as those worth avoiding. When patients are established on medication regimens, the clinician must discuss the risks and benefits of changing drugs, in terms of both physical and mental health.

Service provision

The role and responsibility of adult psychiatrists in the provision of physical healthcare (Box 26.5) varies according to the treatment setting. In the community, most patients should be registered with a GP. The consensus is that primary care should therefore undertake the majority of physical health assessments and interventions.

Table 26.1 Choice of psychotropic medication for patients with a raised body mass index, cardiovascular disease or diabetes

	Mood stabilisers	Antidepressants	Antipsychotics
Raised body mass index			
Recommended	Lamotrigine	Selective serotonin reuptake inhibitors	Haloperidol
Problematic	Lithium, sodium valproate	Tricyclics, mirtazepine	Olanzapine, clozapine
Cardiovascular disease			
Recommended	Lamotrigine, sodium valproate	Sertraline, mirtazepine	Amisulpride, flupentixol, quetiapine
Problematic	Lithium	Tricyclics	Clozapine, pimozide
Diabetes			
Recommended	Lithium, carbamazepine	Selective serotonin reuptake inhibitors, including sertraline	Amisulpride, haloperidol, aripiprazole
Problematic	Sodium valproate	Monoamine oxidase inhibitors, tricyclics, mirtazepine	Olanzapine, clozapine

However, the psychiatrist has a role in ensuring that physical healthcare has been provided, and should take steps to address any gaps or omissions. In in-patient settings, where many patients are detained compulsorily, the psychiatrist has greater responsibility for the assessment and management of physical health problems. These should be performed within the doctor's clinical competence, and support requested from specialists and/or primary care as and when necessary. It is important to ensure that documentation regarding allergies, significant health problems and treatment is completed. Agreement should be reached locally on how best to achieve this.

Box 26.5 Interventions to improve physical health services for people with mental health problems

When driving forward the agenda to improve physical health services for people with mental health problems, local clinicians may focus on interventions such as:

- specialist smoking cessation nurses for people with severe mental illness
- weight-management programmes
- well-being support nurses
- cardiovascular screening clinics
- targeting people in clozapine clinics or those not seen in primary care
- in-patient programmes to increase physical activity
- healthy catering options in psychiatric units
- peer support (service users who have quit smoking or changed lifestyle can be the most inspiring educators)

In-patient settings

Assessment

All psychiatric in-patients require a careful physical assessment as part of their admission process. This should include:

- screening for current physical health problems
- targeted physical examination (this is often overlooked; it should be guided by the physical history, which is usually omitted from most psychiatric textbooks and so rarely taken,[27] despite most physical diagnoses being made from a history rather than examination)
- appropriate investigations and nursing observations.

The contents of a good physical assessment are detailed in Chapter 9, but an important element involves obtaining the dates and results of previous physical investigations. Single measures of blood pressure, BMI and blood tests are sometimes revealing, but they are

Most physical diagnoses are made from a history, rather than an examination.

always more relevant in the longitudinal context of previous findings. When the clinical record is missing, the quickest way to obtain such results is from the GP or even the local biochemistry or haematology laboratory; this requires careful planning well before clinic or community appointments, particularly if there is no access to paper or electronic records. This role can be performed by clinic or secretarial staff supporting busy clinicians.

Often, the most basic issues act as barriers to physical health assessments on in-patient units. Ward managers should ensure there is adequate, functioning medical equipment that is easily available and regularly maintained. The Royal College of Psychiatrists has provided a list of appropriate equipment.[28]

Regular audits of rates of physical examination will help to highlight patterns and to derive solutions.

Patients refusing assessments and rapid tranquillisation

It is not uncommon for patients to refuse a physical examination when they are admitted to a psychiatric hospital. This may be driven by anxiety or paranoia, or frustration with being admitted compulsorily, particularly when insight is lacking.

This provides a challenge to the ward team, particularly if a patient is agitated, distressed or even dangerous. Such patients may be more at risk of physical health problems, especially if there is a need to restrain them or administer medication against their will (see Chapter 25). It is essential to obtain baseline observations such as respiratory rate, pulse and level of alertness, gait and absence of gross neurological deficits. If it is necessary to administer rapid tranquillisation, in the absence of a previous physical assessment, patients must be carefully physically monitored over the following 24 hours, including pulse, blood pressure, airway and respiratory rate. Guidance on rapid tranquillisation from NICE[29] is summarised in Box 26.6. Adequate and functioning resuscitation equipment must be available, as should a pulse oximeter.

Box 26.6 Rapid tranquillisation

- Use verbal de-escalation throughout
- Move to place of safety
- Assess risks of procedures to patient's physical health, including underlying physical conditions, cardiovascular and respiratory collapse, drug interactions, oversedation and loss of therapeutic relationship
- Use minimum effective doses of medications – check previous prescriptions
- Use oral drugs first – lorazepam plus an oral antipsychotic for a psychotic patient. If this fails, use an intramuscular agent (consider lorazepam and if the patient is psychotic also consider haloperidol). Use intravenous agents only in exceptional circumstances after consultation with a senior colleague
- Monitor the patient's vital signs closely after medication. Record pulse rate, blood pressure, respiratory rate, hydration and temperature at intervals agreed by the team, and at increased frequency if the patient is sedated. Frequency should be intensive (every 5–15 minutes) for the first hour, especially if: the patient is sedated or asleep; doses are higher than the recommended maximum; alcohol or illicit drugs have been used; an intravenous route has been used; there is a pre-existing relevant medical disorder

Regular monitoring of physical health

After the initial physical assessment, ongoing monitoring of physical health is easily overlooked, yet it is essential, especially in people who have been prescribed a new medication regimen. For those who initially declined physical assessments and investigations, these should be reoffered at regular intervals.

Observation charts should be reviewed regularly and procedures should be devised to facilitate regular review of basic physical measurements. Weight should be recorded at set intervals throughout admission, weekly for patients starting treatment with antipsychotic medication likely to cause weight gain and monthly for those on stable medication regimens. For those prescribed antipsychotic medication, fasting lipid and glucose measurements should be repeated at least monthly, especially in the first few months of a new treatment regimen.

After the acute admission, the physical health check (PHC) is a valuable adjunct to the assessment of in-patients.[30] It is no substitute for a medical physical examination, but it prompts attention to all bodily systems. The PHC is discussed further in the section on 'Community settings' below.

Physical interventions

When physical problems are detected, the psychiatric team needs to judge the most appropriate method for addressing them. When physical conditions are beyond the competence of the psychiatric team, more specialised help is required. For patients who can leave in-patient units, the most sensible option is often to arrange a review in primary care, accompanied by a member of staff where possible.

A range of medical in-reach services can be very helpful for long-stay patients, especially for those in rehabilitation wards who require an annual review of their overall physical health, of an equivalent standard to that provided in primary care, and including screening for relevant cancers and cardiovascular risk factors.

This can be more difficult to arrange now that mental health trusts are both geographically and organisationally separate from general hospital services. Service-level agreements should include arrangements for access to relevant specialist medical care. Trusts may arrange for primary care input to wards to ensure psychiatric in-patients receive appropriate and regular physical health reviews. This is a particular issue for patients who are admitted to adult psychiatric wards for prolonged periods. Teams must ensure that regular physical assessment:

- is tailored to the individual's physical health needs, age and medication
- includes sexual health and contraceptive advice for those who are sexually active (Chapters 19 and 20)
- includes similar health screening services available to the general population –
  - cervical screening for women aged 25–49 every 3 years
  - cervical screening for women aged 50–64 every 5 years
  - breast screening for women aged 50–70 every 3 years
  - patients over 50 should be screened for early signs of cancer such as weight loss, ongoing fatigue, prostatic symptoms such as difficulties urinating, and worrying bowel symptoms, including changes in bowel habit or rectal bleeding.

Addressing physical risk factors in in-patient units

The in-patient admission can be an opportunity to offer lifestyle education and interventions to people with mental illnesses. Wards must ensure that risk factors such as obesity and diabetes are not worsened by an admission. This includes the provision of healthy dietary options and access to physical exercise, which often requires creative solutions in more restricted environments. Many wards devise individual or group interventions to improve well-being. Ideally, a ward champion should be nominated who can coordinate exercise and health promotion programmes and maintain momentum after initial enthusiasm has faded.

> Smoking status affects plasma clozapine levels. Check for side-effects or decreased efficacy in those who change their smoking status in either direction.

Smoking

Smoking in UK in-patient units has been one of the greatest challenges of recent years,[31] and most psychiatric units in England and Wales are required to be smoke-free. In some units, outside smoking areas are provided, but where patients are unable to leave the unit appropriate support must be provided. In effect, detained patients are often subjected to enforced smoking cessation and many staff are uncomfortable with this.[31]

All patients must have access to smoking cessation support and a range of nicotine replacement and other pharmacological adjuncts to aid cessation. Specific interventions are discussed in Chapter 6.

Smoking induces hepatic enzymes, which breakdown clozapine and so affect plasma levels. For the smoker, this creates two problems:

- on admission to a 'no smoking' in-patient unit, enzyme induction will cease and less clozapine will be metabolised, leading to increased plasma levels for the same oral dose and increased side-effects such as sedation, hypersalivation and fits
- on leaving the unit, if the patient recommences smoking, enzyme induction will also recommence, leading to lower plasma clozapine levels, decreasing the therapeutic action of the drug, which may lead to re-emergence of psychotic symptoms.

Plasma clozapine levels must be monitored and the dose adjusted.

Ward staff should be trained in smoking cessation; it is best to have a ward 'champion' to lead this work. In our own local service, local commissioners funded a smoking cessation nurse to provide specialist in-reach help for both patients and staff. When support of this nature is lacking, it can be difficult to maintain the smoking agenda, with the competing pressures exerted on busy acute psychiatric wards.

Community settings

For most patients under the care of a community mental health team, the GP provides their physical care. Guidelines from NICE on bipolar disorder and schizophrenia state that the GP should provide screening for cardiovascular risk factors, including glucose, lipids, smoking status and hypertension.[4] Importantly, the GP is expected to communicate the results of this screening to the care coordinator and/or psychiatrist. In practice, this step is often lacking, leaving the psychiatric team uncertain whether appropriate care has been provided. Although the NICE guidelines emphasise cardiovascular care, this should not be to the exclusion of other illnesses; for example, respiratory disease is common in schizophrenia[32] and oral health is frequently poor.[33]

Once physical risk factors such as abnormal lipids are detected, any intervention should follow general guidance for the general population.[34]

The community psychiatric team is expected to ensure that an annual physical health screen has occurred in general practice and to intervene if not. This might involve arranging or supporting visits to the GP, or providing physical assessment and screening within the team. Full documentation is important to ensure that screening is conducted in accordance with best practice.

Rates of physical screening in community settings

Provision of physical health screening for people with severe mental illness is often incomplete in both primary and secondary care. In one primary care study, involving 195 people with schizophrenia, screening for basic cardiovascular risk factors was disappointing and well below similar audits in the general population:[35]

- 40% had no record of a blood pressure measurement in the previous 3 years
- 60% had no record of weight
- only 13% had received a lipid assay.

The UK Prescribing Observatory for Mental Health (POMH-UK) has prioritised the monitoring of these risk factors in people taking antipsychotic medication through a national audit cycle. It studied almost 2000 people under the care of community assertive out-reach teams.[36] At baseline and re-audit 1 year later, after feedback (in parentheses):

- 26% of patients had a blood pressure recording (1 year later, this was 43%)
- 17% had a BMI recorded (34%)
- 28% had a glucose level recorded (38%)
- 22% had a lipid measurement (35%).

There may be many barriers to the provision of regular screening. First, some staff in community teams are not clinically trained, while others have variable interest and confidence in the provision of physical healthcare.[37] Some mental health professionals are concerned that they are insufficiently aware of the latest guidelines for intervening if abnormalities are found. Equipment can be a problem too; community team bases are often housed in non-clinical settings, with inadequate access to properly functioning equipment.

Improving physical healthcare in community teams

The provision of screening in community settings can be improved by close liaison with primary care. This is of particular importance with respect to communication of test results. One practical method for improving communication is for care coordinators to request that all recent results are faxed/emailed on a pro forma (listing relevant tests) before regular reviews under the care programme approach.

Regular case-note audit can identify people who have not received screening, so that special screening clinics can be organised, perhaps run by nurses alongside existing clozapine clinics. The identification of local champions can promote this policy. This is not a major burden if the programme is targeted at the people who do not access physical monitoring in primary care. People without GPs should be encouraged to be registered. They should be provided with lists of local GPs and supported in booking a registration appointment at a practice.

Some local NHS trusts have devised innovative shared-care protocols for monitoring people prescribed antipsychotic medication. A general principle of these protocols is that the *initial prescriber* provides *initial screening* (as described in Box 26.4) and primary care provides ongoing monitoring. Ideally, all equipment for

Regular case-note audit can identify people who have not received screening, so they can be referred to specialist screening clinics, alongside existing clozapine clinics.

taking physical measurements and blood tests should be available in all community and out-patient settings. However, where resources are lacking, this might involve the patient visiting the community team's base or attending a local hospital phlebotomy clinic with a blood form, with results copied to the GP to act on any abnormal findings. Assessments in the community could also better address physical health by including the PHC tool mentioned above.[30] This relatively brief instrument addresses current physical problems, lifestyle and behaviour, family history and common side-effects, as well as screening for common cancers, sexual health and dental care. The PHC can be completed by non-clinical staff, in collaboration with the service user. It is concise, suitable for all community settings (including day centres) and acts as a useful trigger if physical health problems are identified. It is highly recommended and free to download (see Box 26.4).

Well-being services

Community interventions for improving physical health in those with severe mental illness require ongoing commitment and resources. Smoking cessation requires intensive support but there is evidence that exercise and dietary interventions may need to be sustained over years. A randomised controlled trial of free fruit and vegetables in Scotland for people with severe mental illness showed promising short-term gains but they were lost after 12 months.[38]

Behavioural weight management programmes can be effective but there is insufficient evidence that pharmacological approaches to weight gain are effective.[39] The Wellbeing Support Programme has shown some positive outcomes. This programme is nurse-led and provides six or more sessions for people with severe mental illness in the community. Improvements were seen in diet, physical activity and self-esteem but changes in weight were more variable.[40]

People with severe mental illness are just as interested in their physical health as the general population.[41] However, the evidence suggests that if we are to improve their health, we need to invest in longer-term supportive programmes rather than 'quick fixes'. Such interventions require sufficient funding. The nurses in the Wellbeing Support Programme were funded by the pharmaceutical company Lilly, but where such support is lacking, service managers need to argue the case for local, sustained funding for similar initiatives. This can easily be argued at NHS trust level with the current well-being agenda as well as prioritisation of health inequalities in disadvantaged groups. People with severe mental illness constitute one of the most marginalised and deprived groups in any primary care trust's catchment area, and commissioners may be responsive to creative projects targeting this group. In our own locality, trusts have funded specialist smoking cessation nurses, well-being nurses and a well-being fair for people with mental health problems. Similar projects, in different guises, exist across the country.

> Maintain and review the well-being agenda in teams. Enthusiasm often fades, but early detection of physical health problems allows timely remedies.

Newer community teams and transitions between teams

In the UK, most services now include a range of specialist community mental health teams, including early intervention services for psychosis, crisis resolution/home treatment teams and assertive outreach teams. All these teams must liaise with GPs regarding physical healthcare, but patients also flow between these teams, as well as other specialist and general services, including rehabilitation, intensive-care units, day hospitals and out-patient settings.

Each service is usually provided by a distinct team, and patient flow between teams can impede ongoing monitoring of physical health and physical screening. Managers who oversee these services must devise methods to identify who has taken responsibility for baseline and ongoing physical assessments. This requires administrative systems to record all physical measurements clearly in the clinical notes. These

Box 26.7 Abnormal findings on physical assessment for recording in discharge summaries

- Existing medical disorders
- Baseline and discharge values for: weight and/or waist circumference; blood pressure; glucose; lipids; blood pressure; prolactin; ECG
- Summary of physical interventions provided (including medications and behavioural therapy)
- Ongoing healthcare needs (e.g. further smoking support, dietary advice, weight reduction)

Box 26.8 Improving physical healthcare in psychiatric teams

Clinical notes require:

- physical assessment forms
- investigation charts for sequential physical measurements and blood tests
- a physical health section in clinical summaries and care plans.

Staff issues:

- provide training in: basic screening and use of equipment; smoking cessation and nicotine replacement therapy; healthy lifestyle, including diet and exercise
- identify physical health champions in teams.

Service issues:

- place physical health and well-being on the NHS trust's management agenda
- identify an NHS trust manager as a well-being lead
- liaise with those who fund the service to design new initiatives
- regularly review medical equipment
- implement frequent local audit cycles of rates of physical assessment and monitoring
- engage with joint national initiatives (e.g. POMH-UK's audit of cardiovascular monitoring)
- regularly review progress and boost efforts when momentum falters.

results should be accessible to all teams, which can be difficult if teams hold separate case notes. Transfer of physical health information should be easier with the new electronic patient records. However, mental health managers must prioritise physical health when electronic records are designed.

Care plans, discharge notes and summaries should all have physical sections to record this information and the action plan after transition between teams. These documents should include the sections listed in Box 26.7.

Box 26.8 summarises actions which may be successful in improving suboptimal physical healthcare at individual and service levels.

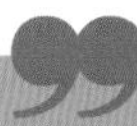

Summary

People with severe mental illnesses suffer gross inequalities in their physical health, contributing to premature mortality. They have raised levels of risk factors for a range of physical health problems, including smoking, diet, exercise and obesity, sometimes exacerbated by antipsychotic medication. The choice of medication should be guided by agreeing which side-effects are most important to avoid for the individual.

Ongoing monitoring of physical health is usually the responsibility of primary care, but psychiatrists should ensure that people prescribed antipsychotic medications receive baseline monitoring of physical measurements, including weight, lipid levels, blood pressure and glucose levels, with the GP providing follow-up. Close communication between GPs and psychiatrists is the key to good physical care.

A range of services and equipment are required to address the poor physical health of people who use general adult psychiatry services. Some, such as regular weight monitoring, are inexpensive but require energy and ongoing commitment. Others are more expensive, such as employing specialist workers in teams, but without these the physical health of people in adult services may remain poor.

References

1. Osborn DPJ, Levy G, Nazareth I, *et al*. Relative risk of cardiovascular and cancer mortality in people with severe mental illness from the United Kingdom's General Practice Research Database. *Arch Gen Psychiatry* 2007; **64**: 242–9.
2. Dinan TG. Schizophrenia and diabetes 2003: an expert consensus meeting. Introduction. *Br J Psychiatry* 2004; **184** (suppl 47): s53–4.
3. National Institute for Health and Clinical Excellence. *The Management of Bipolar Disorder in Adults, Children and Adolescents, in Primary and Secondary Care*. Clinical Guideline 38. NICE, 2006.
4. National Institute for Health and Clinical Excellence. *Schizophrenia: Core Interventions in the Treatment and Management of Schizophrenia in Primary and Secondary Care (Update)*. CG82. NICE, 2009.

5 Hippisley-Cox J, Vinogradova Y, Coupland C, *et al.* Risk of malignancy in patients with schizophrenia or bipolar disorder. *Arch Gen Psychiatry* 2007; **64**: 1368–76.

6 Grinshpoon A, Barchana M, Ponizovsky A, *et al.* Cancer in schizophrenia: is the risk higher or lower? *Schizophr Res* 2005; **73**: 333–41.

7 Dalton SO, Laursen TM, Mellemkjær L, *et al.* Risk for cancer in parents of patients with schizophrenia. *Am J Psychiatry* 2004; **161**: 903–8.

8 Osborn DPJ, King MB, Weir M. Psychiatric health in a sexually transmitted infections clinic: effect on re-attendance. *J Psychosom Res* 2002; **52**: 267–72.

9 Wulsin LR. Does depression kill? *Arch Intern Med* 2000; **160**: 1731–2.

10 Schulz R, Beach SR, Ives DG, *et al.* Association between depression and mortality in older adults: the Cardiovascular Health Study. *Arch Intern Med* 2000; **160**: 1761–8.

11 Frasure-Smith N, Lesperance F, Talajic M. Depression following myocardial infarction: impact on 6-month survival. *JAMA* 1993; **270**: 1819–25 [correction in *JAMA* 1994; **271**: 1082].

12 Glassman AH, Bigger JT, Gaffney M. Psychiatric characteristics associated with long-term mortality among 361 patients having an acute coronary syndrome and major depression: seven-year follow-up of SADHART participants. *Arch Gen Psychiatry* 2009; **66**: 1022–9.

13 Walters K, Rait G, Petersen I, *et al.* Panic disorder and risk of new onset coronary heart disease, acute myocardial infarction, and cardiac mortality: cohort study using the general practice research database. *Eur Heart J* 2008; **29**: 2981–8.

14 Phillips AC, Batty D, Gale C, *et al.* Generalised anxiety disorder, major depressive disorder, and their comorbidity as predictors of all-cause and cardiovascular mortality: the Vietnam Experience Study. *Psychosom Med* 2009; **71**: 395–403.

15 Osborn DPJ, Wright CA, Levy G, *et al.* Relative risk of diabetes, dyslipidaemia, hypertension and the metabolic syndrome in people with severe mental illnesses. Systematic review and metaanalysis. *BMC Psychiatry* 2008; **8**: 843.

16 McEvoy JP, Meyer JM, Goff DC, *et al.* Prevalence of the metabolic syndrome in patients with schizophrenia: baseline results from the Clinic Antipsychotics Trials of Intervention Effectiveness (CATIE) schizophrenia trial and comparison with national estimates from NHANES III. *Schizophr Res* 2005; **80**: 19–32.

17 Samele C, Patel M, Boydell J, *et al.* Physical illness and lifestyle risk factors in people with their first presentation of psychosis. *Soc Psychiatry Psychiatr Epidemiol* 2007; **42**: 117–24.

18 Osborn DPJ, King MB, Nazareth I. Physical activity, dietary habits and coronary heart disease risk factor knowledge amongst people with severe mental illness: a cross-sectional comparative study in primary care. *Soc Psychiatry Psychiatr Epidemiol* 2007; **42**: 787–93.

19 Osborn D, Phelan P. Psychotropic prescribing. In *Physical Health in Mental Health (Occasional Paper OP67)*: 55–61. Royal College of Psychiatrists, 2009.

20 Marder SR, Essock SM, Miller AL, *et al.* Physical health monitoring of patients with schizophrenia. *Am J Psychiatry* 2004; **161**: 1334–49.

21 Smith M, Hopkins D, Peveler RC, *et al.* First- v second-generation antipsychotics and risk for diabetes in schizophrenia: systematic review and meta-analysis. *Br J Psychiatry* 2008; **192**: 406–11.

22 Day JC, Wood G, Dewey M, *et al.* A self-rating scale for measuring neuroleptic side-effects: validation in a group of schizophrenic patients. *Br J Psychiatry* 1995; **166**: 650–3.

23 Ohlsen RI, Williamson RJ, Yusufi B, *et al.* Interrater reliability of the Antipsychotic Non-Neurological Side-Effects Rating Scale (ANNSERS). *J Psychopharmacol* 2008; **22**: 323–9.

24 Joint Formulary Committee. *British National Formulary*. British Medical Association and Royal Pharmaceutical Society, various years (http://bnf.org/bnf/index.htm).

25 Peveler RC, Branford D, Citrome L, *et al.* Antipsychotics and hyperprolactinaemia: clinical recommendations. *J Psychopharmacol* 2008; **22** (suppl): 98–103.

26 Paton C, Ferrier IN. SSRIs and gastrointestinal bleeding. *BMJ* 2005; **331**: 529–30.

27 Osborn DPJ, Warner JP. Assessing the physical health of psychiatric patients. *Psychiatr Bull* 1998; **22**: 695–7.

28 Royal College of Psychiatrists. *Physical Health in Mental Health (Occasional Paper 67)*. RCPsych, 2009.

29 National Institute for Health and Clinical Excellence. *CG25 Violence: SPC Chart for Rapid Tranquillisation.* NICE, 2005.

30 Rethink. The Physical Health Check. Rethink, 2008 (http://www.rethink.org/how_we_can_help/research/service_evaluation_and_outcomes/physical_health_check/physical_health_chec.html).

31 Ratschen E, Britton J, McNeill A. Implementation of smoke-free policies in mental health in-patient settings in England. *Br J Psychiatry* 2009; **194**: 547–51.

32 Himelhoch S, Lehman A, Kreyenbuhl J, *et al.* Prevalence of chronic obstructive pulmonary disease among those with serious mental illness. *Am J Psychiatry* 2004; **161**: 2317–9.

33 McCreadie RG, Stevens H, Henderson J, *et al.* The dental health of people with schizophrenia. *Acta Psychiatr Scand* 2004; **114**: 306–10.

34 National Institute for Health and Clinical Excellence. *Lipid Modification.* Clinical Guideline 67. NICE, 2008.

35 Roberts L, Roalfe A, Wilson S, *et al.* Physical health care of patients with schizophrenia in primary care: a comparative study. *Fam Pract* 2007; **24**: 34–40.

36 Barnes TRE, Paton C, Cavanagh M-R, *et al*, on behalf of the UK Prescribing Observatory for Mental Health. A UK audit of screening for the metabolic side effects of antipsychotics in community patients. *Schizophr Bull* 2007; **33**: 1397–401.

37 Wright C, Osborn DPJ, Nazareth I, *et al.* Prevention of coronary heart disease in people with severe mental illnesses: a qualitative study of patient and professionals' preferences for care. *BMC Psychiatry* 2006; **6**: 16.

38 McCreadie R. Editorial. *Acta Psychiatr Scand* 2006; **114**: 221–2.

39 Faulkner G, Cohn T, Remington G. Interventions to reduce weight gain in schizophrenia. *Cochrane Database Syst Rev* 2007; **issue 1**: CD005148.

40 Smith S, Yeomans D, Bushe CJ, *et al.* A well-being programme in severe mental illness. Reducing risk for physical ill-health: a post-programme service evaluation at 2 years. *Eur Psychiatry* 2007; **22**: 413–18.

41 Osborn DPJ, King MB, Nazareth I. Participation in cardiovascular risk screening by people with schizophrenia or similar mental illnesses: a cross-sectional study in general practice. *BMJ* 2003; **326**: 1122–3.

Learning points

- Always screen for both physical symptoms and physical signs when assessing a psychiatric patient.
- Endocrine and neurological disorders often present with mental health problems.
- Suspect organic causes when there is a coexisting medical disorder, an abnormal cognitive state or if the patient is unresponsive to treatment.
- Relative to the general population, people with severe mental illnesses are more at risk of, and two to three times more likely to die from, cardiovascular disease, which is much more common than suicide.
- Depression and anxiety predispose to acute cardiovascular events.
- Severe depression at least doubles the likelihood of dying after a heart attack.
- Antipsychotic medication can increase weight, and may increase lipid and glucose abnormalities. All patients should be screened for these at baseline. Consider an ECG too.
- Choose antipsychotic medications which are less likely to cause weight gain in overweight patients. Quetiapine, amisulpride and aripiprazole are better.
- People with severe mental illnesses attend screening appointments almost as frequently as the general population.
- Smoking affects plasma clozapine levels. Stopping or restarting smoking can affect drug efficacy as well as side-effects.
- The patient's physical condition must be monitored carefully after rapid tranquillisation, especially if the patient appears at all sedated.
- Up-to-date, functioning medical equipment must be available in all in-patient settings. Equipment for screening should also be available in community settings.
- Include physical healthcare in care plan meetings and liaise with the GP beforehand to obtain the results of recent physical health tests.
- Record all baseline and subsequent physical measurements in discharge summaries. Also list any physical interventions, including drugs and behavioural interventions.
- Interventions for smoking, obesity, diet and exercise can be successful in people with severe mental illnesses, but require commitment.

27

Intellectual disabilities

Geoff Marston and David Perry

People with intellectual disabilities are vulnerable to preventable health inequality and many are dependent on other people. This chapter describes various government and independent initiatives that aim to promote the physical health of this group. It covers the documents that can be used to advise clinicians and to shape delivery of services. It discusses the common health problems that go hand in hand with intellectual disability, barriers to identifying physical health problems and how to improve communication and clinical skills sufficiently to be able to conduct a physical examination.

Introduction

Over recent decades there have been various influences on health services for people with an intellectual disability (PWID). Chief of these has been the move from institutional care – where annual check-ups by medical officers were common practice – to community care, delivered by general practitioners (GPs) and community disability teams (CIDTs); also known as community learning disability teams.

There has also been a dramatically increased life expectancy, especially for those with more severe intellectual disability. Between 2001 and 2021, the population of PWID aged over 60 is expected to increase by 36%.[1] It can be expected that increasingly complex physical health problems will be seen, related to having an intellectual disability and being elderly.

Finally, there is better understanding of physical health problems in this group, as genetic research and epidemiological surveys have increased clinicians' knowledge; they have also increased patients' and carers' expectations of better management of health problems.

Health inequality

People with an intellectual disability are some of the most vulnerable members of our society[2,3] and are often dependent on others for their support. Generally, they are of low socioeconomic status, with only 17% in paid work; have poor coping strategies; and are often excluded from society as 5% are without family or friends. Moreover, 23% experience physical and 47% verbal abuse. These factors coupled, with difficulties in communicating needs and accessing resources, have led to significant health inequalities.

People with intellectual disability are 58 times more likely to die before the age of 50 than the rest of the population[4] and overall mortality rates are 3 times higher for people with moderate to severe intellectual disability; they also have higher rates of preventable deaths. There are a number of factors, discussed below, that might contribute to this, including the possibility of clinicians missing physical health problems because they dismiss behaviours that could be communicating illness or pain as solely due to the intellectual disability ('diagnostic overshadowing'). In some cases there may also be therapeutic negativism or nihilism, with clinicians pursuing neither investigations nor vigorous treatment, for a variety of reasons (Box 27.1).

Over the past decade, there have been a variety of government and independent initiatives and inquiries that have shaped thinking and service delivery:

- The 2001 White Paper *Valuing People* promoted the concept of health facilitation and health action planning for people with intellectual disability.[5]
- The progress review in *Valuing People Now* (2009) reaffirmed the need to improve healthcare for people with intellectual disabilities.[6]
- *Death by Indifference* (a 2007 report from the charity MENCAP) documented six deaths in the National Health Service (NHS) in general hospitals, highlighting the discrimination that people with intellectual disabilities face when receiving care.[7] A 5-year follow up report concludes there are areas of good practice, but inequitable care and avoidable deaths continue.[8]
- The report of a subsequent inquiry, *Healthcare for All* (2008), gave a number of action points to address health and equality that were expected to shape training of health staff, including psychiatry and other areas of medicine.[9]
- The Disability Discrimination Act 2005, now incorporated into the Equality Act 2010, states that 'reasonable adjustments' should be made to accommodate people with disability into mainstream services and clinics.
- The Mental Capacity Act 2005, implemented in England and Wales in 2007, provides a clear legal framework for 'best interest' decision-making for people who lack mental capacity (see Chapter 11). Amendments to the 1983 Mental Health Act introduced 'deprivation of liberty safeguards' (DoLS) into the Mental Capacity Act, to ensure that those who lack mental capacity and are deprived of liberty in care or in hospital but are not subject to mental health legislation are also subject to review and external scrutiny.
- the reports into Sutton and Merton Primary Care Trust (2007) and Cornwall Partnership NHS Trust (2006) highlighted poor standards of care that people with intellectual disability can face within specialist intellectual disability health services.[10,11]

Box 27.1 Possible reasons not to treat physical disorders of PWID appropriately

- Lack of capacity/consent (decisions should be based on Mental Capacity Act 'best interest' – see Chapter 11)
- Inability to understand communication
- Behavioural difficulties
- Potential distress investigations might cause (again, decisions should be based on Mental Capacity Act 'best interest')
- Resources/rationing (e.g. what is best use of a bed on an intensive-care unit?)
- Behaviours are dismissed as solely due to level of intellectual disability (diagnostic overshadowing)

Always consider physical causes for behavioural disturbance in people with limited communication.

Various documents that can guide clinicians and commissioners of services in the provision of more equitable services for people with intellectual disability include:

- *Green Light for Mental Health* (2005 and revised in 2009) aims to develop better access to mainstream psychiatric services[12]
- *Services for People with Learning Disabilities and Challenging Behaviour or Mental Health Needs* (2007)[13] from the Department of Health and *Challenging Behaviour: A Unified Approach* (2007),[14] produced jointly by the Royal College of Psychiatrists and the British Psychological Society
- *Dementia and People with Learning Disabilities* (2009),[15] produced jointly by the Royal College of Psychiatrists and the British Psychological Society, which sets out care pathways and good standards of care for people with a intellectual disability and dementia.

What are the common physical health problems for people with intellectual disability?

Epidemiological studies show high rates of physical and mental health problems in people with an intellectual disability, compared with the general population.[2,3,16–18]

Common conditions are listed below:

- *Sensory impairment.* Around 20–30% of adults with PWID have moderate visual impairment and 1.5% have severe visual impairment or are blind; some 10–40% of PWID are reported to have significant hearing loss.
- *Epilepsy.* Overall, epilepsy is up to 20 times more prevalent than in the general population, with rates increasing with the degree of intellectual disability.[19] Thus, while the prevalence in the general population is 0.5–1%, in those with moderate intellectual disability (IQ 50–35) it is about 15%, rising to 30% in those with severe and profound intellectual disability. A number of factors such as brain injury and specific genetic syndromes (e.g. tuberous sclerosis, Rett syndrome and Angelman syndrome) influence these rates.
- *Eating disorders*
  - Obesity. Up to 68% of PWID are overweight, often owing to poor access to good diet and low levels of physical activity; 80% fall below national standards of activity, compared with 53–64% of the general population.
  - Pica (eating non-food substances). This can be related to a number of factors, including genetic conditions (e.g. Prader–Willi syndrome) and some mineral deficiencies.
  - Underweight. People with intellectual disability are more likely to be underweight than the general population. Classic anorexia is not commonly seen, although atypical patterns of eating can occur. This may be associated with pervasive developmental disorders, where individuals can develop quite extreme 'food fads' which significantly restrict diet. Body weight may be hard to sustain, especially if combined with hyperactivity.
- *Gastro-oesophageal reflux disorder (GORD).* This may affect up to 50% of institutionalised patients with an intellectual disability. Over 60% have *H. pylori* infection, which can result in gastritis (6–20%) and cancer (1%). Testing for *H. pylori* should be routine in those with symptoms of reflux, vomiting or loss of appetite, especially if they live in a group setting.
- *Dysphagia.* The prevalence of swallowing difficulty in children and adults with an intellectual disability varies from 36%, based on case-load pathology from speech and language therapists, to 73% in an in-patient population survey[20] About 5–8% of adults in the community and 36% in a hospital population have dysphagia.[21,22] A low index of suspicion is essential, as unrecognised dysphagia (Box 27.2) can lead to complications, including respiratory infections and ultimately death.
- *Respiratory disease.* This is the commonest cause of death in people with intellectual disability (46–52%, compared with 15–17% in the general population). It is important that vulnerable people have flu vaccinations.
- *Constipation.* This common complaint, affecting up to 69% of institutionalised people with severe intellectual disability, is often related to poor diet, limited exercise and side-effects of medication. Constipation can be a factor in challenging behaviour and increased seizures.
- *Polypharmacy and inappropriate use of medications.* Psychotropic medication is prescribed for up to 60% of those with PWID. Carers need to be aware of the potential side-effects of each medication. Some psychotropic medications must be closely monitored, such as atypical antipsychotics, lithium and some anti-epileptic drugs. As a minimum, medication should be reviewed annually.
- *Dentition.* Dental health is generally poor in PWID,[9] owing to problems in accepting support or attending to self-care (teeth-brushing), poor nutrition, limited access to specialised dental care, high use of medication which can cause xerostomia, and a subjective complaint of dry mouth due to a lack of saliva.
- *Endocrine dysfunction.* Hypothyroidism affects 12% of those with intellectual disability, compared with 0.1% of the general population. Those with Down syndrome, congenital rubella or Turner's syndrome are at particular risk.

Box 27.2 Signs suggesting dysphagia

- Coughing and choking when eating food
- Sweating while eating
- Wet gurgling voice
- Agitation around mealtimes
- Certain foods that cannot be swallowed
- Special preparation needed for food and drinks (e.g. chopped/mashed)
- Several attempts to swallow
- Long time taken over meals
- Recurrent unexplained chest infections

Consider referral for specialist speech and language assessment (see pp. 55–56).

- *Accidental injury*. Excess mortality from accidents has been reported, with a standardised mortality ratio (SMR) of 3.73 among people with severe intellectual disability.[9] Drowning had an SMR of 29 and falls an SMR of 6. Falls are common and may be linked to neurological conditions and medication.
- *Infectious disease*. Hepatitis A and B may be more common within institutionalised care. Vaccinations should be considered for people living and working within group home or other institutional settings, particularly for people with severe intellectual disability, as there is more likely contact with body fluids and risk of challenging behaviour such as biting.
- *Osteoporosis*. This may be more prevalent in people with an intellectual disability, perhaps related to poor diet and exercise but also a number of medications such as anti-epileptic medication.
- *Cancer*. Overall, fewer people with intellectual disability die of cancer than in the general population (12–18% *v.* 26%), but they have a higher proportion of gastrointestinal cancer (48–59% v. 25%).
- *Coronary heart disease*. This is a leading cause of death (14–20%). Almost 50% of people with Down syndrome have congenital heart defects.

Genetic conditions with specific medical health problems

A number of genetic conditions have an increased risk of specific medical problems. The Contact a Family (CAF) directory (www.cafamily.org.uk) can provide helpful information on a number of disorders. Two important examples in this regard are discussed below.

Down syndrome

Down syndrome affects one in 600 births in the UK. Thanks to medical advances, the average life expectancy is now 55 years. Those with the syndrome have higher rates of congenital cardiac problems, hearing impairment (narrow external auditory meatus and recurrent otitis media), visual disorders (cataracts and keratoconus), hypothyroidism, leukaemia, atlanto-axial instability, oesophageal atresia, depression and dementia. Regular health checks recommended by the Down Syndrome Association (www.downs-syndrome.org.uk) are shown in Table 27.1.[23]

Genetic conditions may have certain health problems linked to them. Awareness gives the opportunity for preventive health education and screening.

Tuberous sclerosis

Tuberous sclerosis is an autosomal dominant condition that affects roughly one in 7000 births. It leads to problems with cell growth and is diagnosed on the basis of a number of major and minor physical features. One characteristic is growths (sometimes called 'tubers'), which can cause multiple system dysfunction, with involvement of the heart, lungs, eyes, skin, brain and kidney. Some growths can become malignant or bleed, so acute physical health changes should be investigated thoroughly (see Table 27.2) and regular checks should be made on renal function (ultrasound scan and urea and electrolytes), heart (echocardiogram and ECG), lung (chest

Table 27.1 Recommended health checks for people with Down syndrome

Frequency	Checks to make
Monthly	Breast (supported/self-examination) Weight (if obese)
Annually	Review of medication, weight, teeth
Every 1–2 years	Vision, hearing, psychological status (especially for those over 40)
Every 2–3 years	Routine blood tests and thyroid function tests (done more frequently if problems are found)

Table 27.2 Warning signs for urgent investigation and specialist referral in tuberous sclerosis

Feature	Action
Increased seizures or signs of raised intracranial pressure	Brain scan
Haematuria or abdominal pain	Kidney scan
Signs of congestive cardiac failure or swollen ankles or shortness of breath on exertion or fainting (not related to seizure)	Electrocardiogram, echocardiogram

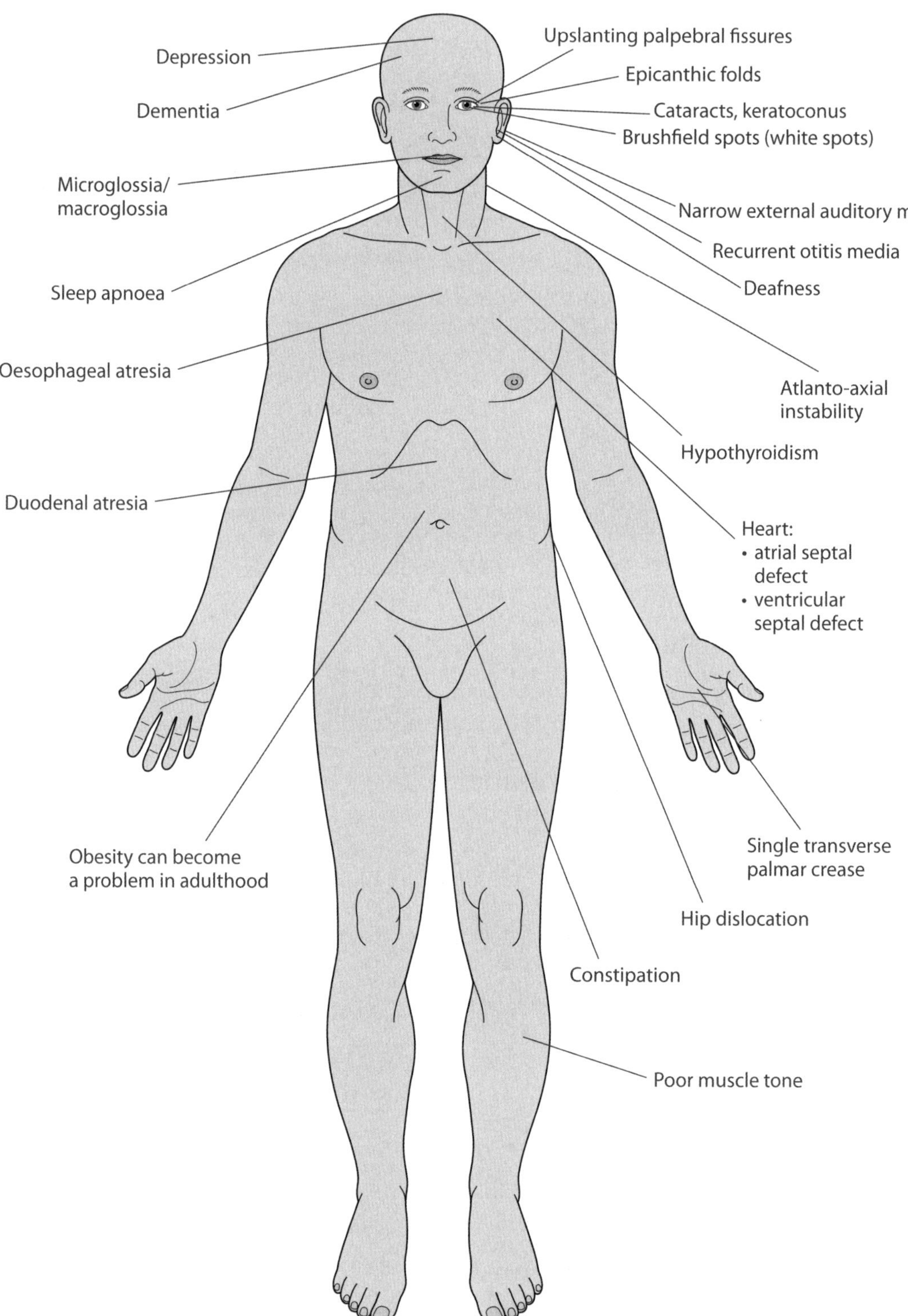

Fig. 27.1 Down syndrome.

Sensory processing difficulties may alter the way people with autism-spectrum disorder perceive and respond to pain (e.g. they may tolerate a fractured leg but not light touch).

X-ray and computed tomography) and brain (computed tomography and/or magnetic resonance imaging).

National tuberous sclerosis clinics are run throughout the country. Details can be found through the Tuberous Sclerosis Association's website (www.tuberous-sclerosis.org).

Epilepsy affects up to 70% of patients with tuberous sclerosis and can be difficult to manage.

Recognising and treating physical health problems in PWID

Health professionals can expect to see high rates of health problems in PWID. However, many problems still go unrecognised, for a number of reasons (Box 27.3).

Awareness

One major barrier to recognition is lack of awareness, which can be overcome by education. Sharing epidemiological data and other syndrome-specific health information with significant others such as service users, carers, care organisations, local GPs and general hospitals is essential. The impact of the inquiry 'Healthcare For All' may yet influence the training of UK health professionals from undergraduate level upwards by emphasising the needs of PWID.

Communication

People with intellectual disability may have significant problems with verbal communication and struggle to link cause and effect, for example pain in the abdomen being linked to intra-abdominal pathology. Often, non-verbal communication gives clues to symptoms. For example, banging on an ear could indicate earache or be a response to auditory hallucinations; rectal digging could be a response to constipation or threadworm; rubbing the sternum might indicate problems with reflux or GORD. By appreciating these possibilities, 'diagnostic overshadowing', where behaviours are dismissed as solely due to level of intellectual disability, may be avoided. Be aware that some people, particularly those with pervasive developmental disorders, may have difficulties with sensory integration, which may result in pain being experienced in different ways – for example, a light touch may be 'excruciating' but a broken leg could be tolerable for many days.

Access issues

Once a problem is suspected, the next barrier to healthcare is accessibility. Many PWID find GP surgeries or out-patient departments intimidating places and some refuse to attend or cooperate with health professionals. This is particularly so in people with more severe intellectual disability and pervasive developmental

Box 27.3 Barriers to identifying the physical health problems of people with intellectual disability

Patient-related factors

- Cognitive ability and health literacy
- Communication (related to level of intellectual disability)
- Phobia/anxiety
- Pervasive developmental disorder
- Sensory impairment

Service-related factors

- Poor site accessibility
- Flexibility of appointment systems
- Environmental issues (ward/clinic layout, signage, etc.)
- Availability of user-friendly information (picture leaflets, etc.)

Clinician-related factors

- Education (continuing professional development) around the needs of PWID
- Personal communication skills
- Ignorance of legislation (Mental Capacity Act, etc.)
- Attitude

Carer-related factors

- Education (training issue for paid carers)
- Own cognitive abilities and health literacy
- Attitude

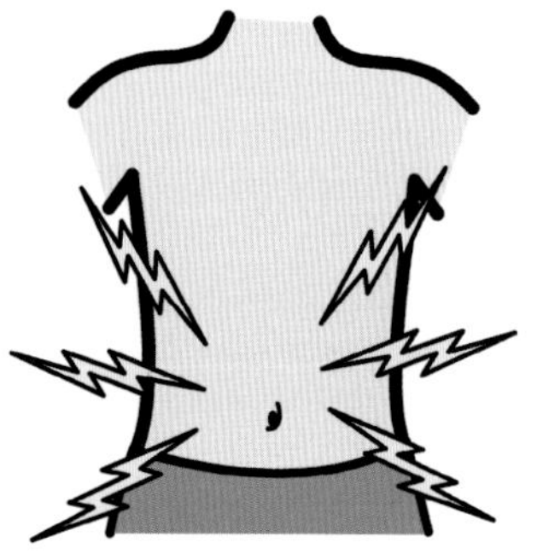

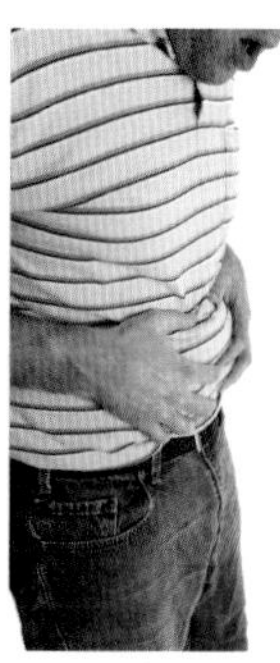

Fig. 27.2 Communication aids for people with intellectual disabilities. People with intellectual disabilities may need symbols and pictures to help communicate their pain or problem – in this case, stomach ache. Every person will have their own preference for communication aid (© Widgit Software 2002–2012, with permission).

disorders. There are, though, ways to make visits less anxiety-provoking:

- Offer the first appointment of the clinic to a person with intellectual disability so that they will not have to wait long.
- Offer more time, perhaps even a double session.
- Offer picture leaflets and user-friendly information before the first appointment (Table 27.3).
- Offer 'trial runs' so that the person can visit the building, meet reception staff and access facilities in a gradual manner.
- Use local intellectual disability teams, who may have 'health facilitators' who can support appointments and communication with professionals.
- In some areas, user groups have trained their own 'health buddies', where more able PWID support those less able and provide education to peers and professionals.
- Ensure clinical environments are fit for purpose check there is enough space, wide corridors for chairs, noise baffling and quieter areas to wait in, with good signage, and check that the facility is on an easily accessible transport route.

Take time to think about your local service provision and identify ways in which it might be improved.

Personal skills

Once in the clinic room, there are ways in which the clinician can act that will help PWID to report their problems, or at least participate in a meaningful way:

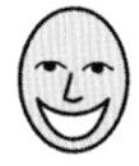 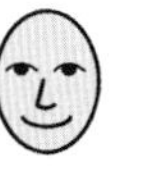 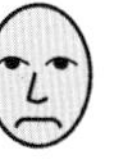 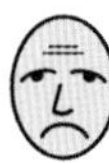 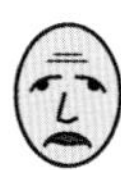 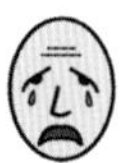

Fig. 27.3 A severity of symptoms scale (© Widgit Softwar 2002–2012, with permission.

- Talk to the patient, even if they have a profound intellectual disability.
- Be aware of sensory impairments and pervasive developmental disorders (which may affect tolerance of boundary issues and eye contact).
- Use simple language, gesture and other non-verbal prompts.
- Have pens and paper available to draw diagrams.
- Offer user-friendly information about medication and procedures (see Table 27.3).
- Have pictures available (but note that people may relate differently to line drawings/cartoon-like images and photographic images; Fig. 27.2); it can be useful to have a severity of symptoms scale available during consultations (Fig. 27.3).
- Use a digital camera to create your own picture bank.
- Ask the person to repeat back their understanding, as PWID often acquiesce or say yes to everything.
- Listen to what the carers have to say.
- Consider physical examination (even if limited) as PWID may allow a psychiatrist to do something they would not let the GP or other professional do.
- Use outcome measures/observation forms for carers to provide objective evidence of treatment response.

Compliance and consent

The final barrier to diagnosis is difficulty in obtaining physical investigations or conducting procedures. Some PWID will not have the capacity to make informed decisions, but this should not exclude them from appropriate investigation and interventions. The Mental Capacity Act (MCA) *Code of Practice* gives clear guidance on making decisions on behalf of people who lack capacity (see also Chapter 11).[24] This should be done through the process of a formally documented 'best

> Be creative with the way you communicate. Everyone is different.

Table 27.3 Websites and resources for user-friendly information

Website	Organisation	Resources available
www.easyhealth.org.uk	Website sponsored by the charity Mencap	Leaflets and videos on various aspects of health
www.ld-medication.bham.ac.uk	University of Birmingham	User-friendly leaflets and MP3 downloads on medication
www.changepeople.co.uk	CHANGE, a human rights organisation for people with intellectual disabilities	Health picture bank and other resources
www.intellectualdisability.info	Collaboration between St George's Hospital Medical School and the Down Syndrome Association	Covers many areas of care for people with intellectual disabilities
www.google.co.uk	Google search engine	Variety of images that can be downloaded subject to copyright issues
www.booksbeyondwords.co.uk	Beyond Words	Range of picture books to facilitate communication with people with intellectual disabilities

interests' discussion with 'significant others' involved in the person's care. Where there is no clear advocate for a PWID, it may be necessary to involve an independent mental capacity advocate (IMCA), who can liaise widely and provide reports to help decision-making. In a minority of cases, such as unresolved conflicting views between carers and clinicians, the Court of Protection may need to be involved.

What is being done in primary care to address the health needs of PWID?

The 2001 White Paper *Valuing People* introduced the concept of 'health facilitation' for PWID and recommended that everyone with intellectual disabilities have a health action plan to highlight their needs. This directive has been widely interpreted on a local basis.

In 2005, GPs in England were encouraged to develop systems to identify PWID on their practice lists; keeping such a register entitled a payment from primary care trusts under the Quality and Outcomes Framework (QOF). There are many other areas of QOF incentive payments indirectly linked to the needs of PWID, including mental health, epilepsy, thyroid disorders, obesity and general screening, such as cervical cytology and breast examinations.

In 2008, the Department of Health took steps to offer further incentives for GPs in England to provide more developed services for PWID. These 'directed enhanced services' (DES) agreements can be claimed if practice staff: attend specialist intellectual disability training covering a number of prescribed areas, offer annual health checks, and keep accurate data on PWID registered with local social services and health teams. Many examples of templates for recording and focusing health checks exist, such as those developed in Cardiff.[25]

What is being done in secondary care to address the health needs of PWID?

The Mencap report *Death by Indifference* highlighted shortcomings in the quality of care provided to PWID in hospital settings.[7] The report of a subsequent inquiry, *Healthcare for All*, offered a number of recommendations to address these issues (Box 27.4).[9] These now influence commissioners and affect quality ratings for acute trusts.

In a number of regions, significant steps have been taken to improve hospital experiences for PWID. Key to many of these developments has been liaison links between local intellectual disability teams, patients, local authority partnership boards and key stakeholders (such as modern matrons) within hospitals.

Once links are established and visions and values are owned by acute NHS trusts, it is possible to work on a number of areas to improve quality of care. These could include:

- intellectual disability awareness training at induction for all new clinical staff
- user involvement in staff induction training
- information packs, including details such as health problems in PWID, capacity assessments and service contacts available on all wards
- agreed care pathways for PWID
- communication tools for PWID available on all hospital wards
- agreed liaison links with local intellectual disability services
- routine assessments for PWID to identify care resources needed during stay (e.g. single room, 1:1 support)
- auditing of initiatives which support patients with intellectual disability.

Many NHS trusts have developed a patient 'hospital passport' and health action plan (see Fig. 27.4). With permission, these can be adapted to suit local need, saving time and resources.

Box 27.4 Recommendations from *Healthcare for All*

- The Department of Health to amend core standards to make explicit the need to make 'reasonable adjustments' to service delivery for vulnerable groups in accordance with the Equality Act 2010.
- The Department of Health should direct primary care trusts to secure health services that make 'reasonable adjustments' for PWID through direct enhanced services (DES).
- Develop confidential enquiry into premature deaths in PWID.
- Ensure an undergraduate and postgraduate clinical training curriculum includes mandatory training in intellectual disability.
- Better monitoring of services for PWID by health organisations.
- Develop data-sets in the Department of Health to monitor how trust boards are demonstrating 'reasonable adjustment' for health services for those with intellectual disability.
- All trusts to involve users and carers in developing services as required under section 242 of the National Health Service Act 2006.
- Reasonable adjustments be made by trusts to support users and carers in decision-making.
- Primary care trusts to identify the needs of PWID as part of their joint strategic needs assessments.

Department of Health, 2008.[9]

People with intellectual difficulties as psychiatric in-patients

People with intellectual difficulties may be admitted to both general mental health services and to specialist intellectual disability mental health services, depending on local provision and clinical need. Physical health issues must be carefully considered at pre-admission assessments and any needs clearly identified in care plans. Common problems to consider are epilepsy, restraint and the side-effects of medication.

- *Epilepsy.* Stress, psychotropic medication and other factors may increase the likelihood of seizures. An epilepsy care plan and clear advice to clinical teams about managing seizures and status epilepticus should be available;
- *Restraint.* People with an intellectual disability may have significant medical contraindications to certain types of restraint. For example, people with Down syndrome may have atlanto-axial instability; cerebral palsy may lead to malformations of the chest and spine. High rates of physical or sexual abuse mean restraint can lead to emotional distress in some individuals. Restraint risks need to be assessed and documented carefully. Some types and positions of restraint may need to be avoided or safe modifications agreed (see Chapter 25).
- *Medication side-effects.* These may not be reported by PWID even though they may actually be more sensitive to them. Ensure that potential side-effects are monitored carefully and that side-effects such

Beware of increased sensitivity to medication side-effects. Where possible go 'low and slow' when introducing medication.

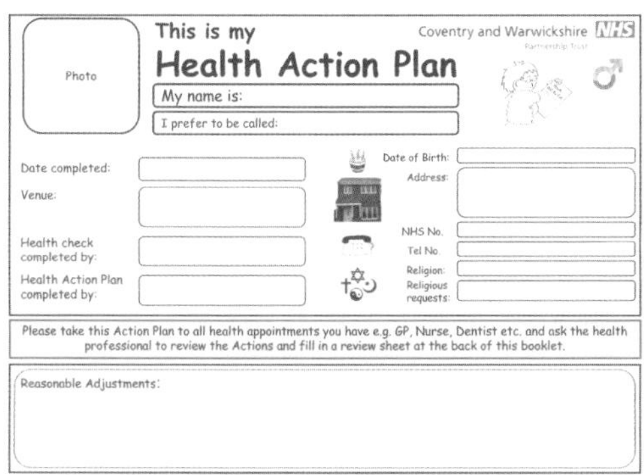
This is my
Health Action Plan
Coventry and Warwickshire NHS Partnership Trust

Photo

My name is:

I prefer to be called:

Date completed:

Venue:

Health check completed by:

Health Action Plan completed by:

Date of Birth:

Address:

NHS No.

Tel No.

Religion:

Religious requests:

Please take this Action Plan to all health appointments you have e.g. GP, Nurse, Dentist etc. and ask the health professional to review the Actions and fill in a review sheet at the back of this booklet.

Reasonable Adjustments:

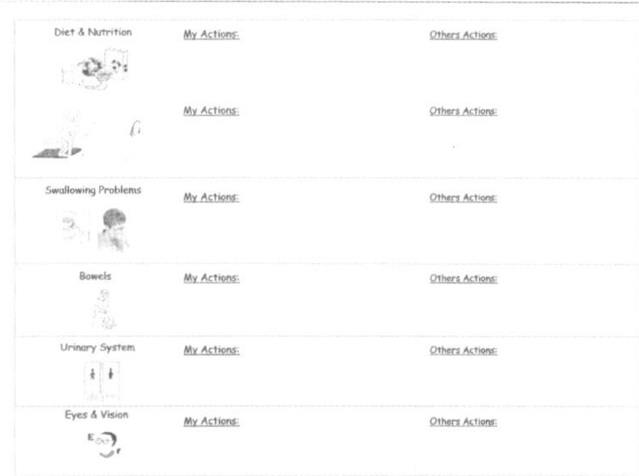
Diet & Nutrition	My Actions:	Others Actions:
	My Actions:	Others Actions:
Swallowing Problems	My Actions:	Others Actions:
Bowels	My Actions:	Others Actions:
Urinary System	My Actions:	Others Actions:
Eyes & Vision	My Actions:	Others Actions:

Fig. 27.4 Example of a hospital health action plan. Coventry and Warwickshire Partnership NHS Trust.

as akathisia are not misinterpreted as challenging behaviour. Extrapyramidal side-effects may affect mobility in those with existing cerebral palsy. Watch also for constipation and treat appropriately, as this may lead to challenging behaviour.

People with an intellectual disability on general units may need one-to-one nursing support. Staff teams may need a clear line of advice and support from local intellectual disability teams. Units would benefit from the same information and care pathway systems as discussed for use in acute hospitals. The Royal College of Psychiatrists' Centre for Quality Improvement has developed an accreditation process, including audit tools, for assessing admission services for PWID, the AIMS-LD.[26]

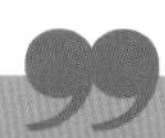

Summary

People with intellectual disability are a vulnerable group, often marginalised and disadvantaged. They suffer poorer health outcomes, sometimes due to preventable reasons such as poor clinical care and challenges accessing health services.

Health professionals should improve their knowledge of potential health issues and ensure they make 'reasonable adjustments' to their working practice and services. Education of themselves, their patients and their carers is essential. Some simple suggestions include putting an intellectual disability-related topic in the personal development plan; at service development meetings, always asking 'What about people with an intellectual disability?'; ensuring that intellectual disability is in the text of any policy documents; making use of local intellectual disability partnership boards, which can support local health initiatives through their subgroups; finding out what your local intellectual disability strategy is and establishing who leads on implementation; and getting to know your local intellectual disability team.

Small changes and good communication do make a difference to patients and their carers.

References

1 Davidson PW, Prasher VP, Janicki MP. *Physical Health, Intellectual Disabilities and the Aging Process*. Blackwell Publishing, 2003.

2 South East Regional Public Health Observatory. *Learning Disabilities and Health*. SEPHO, 2008 (www.sepho.org.uk/viewResource.aspx?id=12117).

3 Emerson E, Baines S, Allerton L, *et al*. *Health Inequalities and People with Learning Disabilities in the UK: 2011*. Improving Health and Lives: Learning Disabilities Observatory, 2011.

4 Hollins S, Attard MT, Von Fraunhofer N, *et al*. Mortality in people with learning disability: risks, causes, and death certification findings in London. *Dev Med Child Neurol* 1998; **40**: 50–6.

5 Department of Health. *Valuing People: A New Strategy for Learning Disability for the 21st Century*. Department of Health, 2001.

6 Department of Health. *Valuing People Now: A New Three-Year Strategy for People with Learning Disabilities*. Department of Health, 2009.

7 Mencap. *Death by Indifference*. Mencap, 2007.

8 Mencap. *Death by Indifference: 74 Deaths and Counting*. Mencap, 2012.

9 Michael J. *Healthcare for All: Independent Inquiry into Access to Healthcare for People with Learning Disabilities*. Department of Health, 2008.

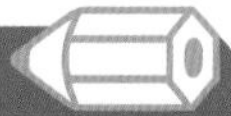

Learning points

- People with an intellectual disability have higher rates of mental and physical health problems. There is often interplay between the two.
- The most common types of physical illness leading to mortality or morbidity may be different from those seen in the general population.
- A person with an intellectual disability is 58 times more likely to die before the age of 50 than the general population.
- Identification of illness and access to appropriate healthcare can be poor, for a number of patient- and clinician-centred reasons, as well as environmental/service-driven reasons.
- All health professionals and services have a legal duty of care to make 'reasonable adjustments' to accommodate people with disability, including intellectual disability.
- A lot of information and good resources are available on the internet to support health professionals.
- Good communication skills and education are essential to improving health outcomes for this vulnerable patient group.
- It is within every professional's power to improve knowledge and skills by adding an intellectual disability-related topic to their personal development aims (e.g. the General Medical Council: www.gmc-uk.org/learningdisabilities).

10 Healthcare Commission. *Investigation into the Service for People with Learning Disabilities Provided by Sutton and Merton Primary Care Trust.* Healthcare Commission, 2007.

11 Commission for Social Care Inspection and the Healthcare Commission. *Joint Investigation into Services for People with Learning Disabilities at Cornwall Partnership Trust.* Healthcare Commission, 2006.

12 Cole A, Gegory M. *Green Light for Mental Health: How Good are Your Mental Health Services for People With Learning Disabilities? A Service Improvement Toolkit.* Foundation for People with Learning Disabilities, 2004 (http://www.learningdisabilities.org.uk/publications/green-light/).

13 Department of Health. *Services for People with Learning Disabilities and Challenging Behaviour or Mental Health Needs: Guidance on Commissioning Adult Learning Disability Health Services, Good Practice.* Department of Health, 2007.

14 Royal College of Psychiatrists, British Psychological Society. *Challenging Behaviour: A Unified Approach* (College Report CR144). Royal College of Psychiatrists, 2007.

15 British Psychological Society, Royal College of Psychiatrists. *Dementia and People with Learning Disabilities* (College Report CR155). Royal College of Psychiatrists, 2009.

16 Prasher VP, Janicki MP. *Physical Health in Adults with Intellectual Disabilities.* Blackwell, 2002.

17 McGuire BE, Daly P, Smyth AF. Lifestyle and health behaviours of adults with an intellectual disability. *J Intellect Disabil Res* 2007; **51**: 497–510.

18 Messent PR, Cooke CB, Long J. Daily physical activity in adults with mild and moderate learning disabilities: is there enough? *Disabil Rehabil* 1998; **20**: 424–7.

19 Trimble M. *Learning Disability and Epilepsy: An Integrative Approach.* Clarius Press, 2003.

20 Leslie P Crawford H, Wilkinson H. People with a learning disability and dysphasia: a Cinderella population? *Dysphagia* 2009; **24**: 103–4.

21 Hickman J, Jenner L. ALD and dysphagia: issues and practice. *Speech Language Ther Practice* 1997; autumn: 8–11.

22 Chadwick DD, Joliffe J. A descriptive investigation of dysphagia in adults with intellectual disabilities. *J Intellect Disabil Res* 2008; **53**: 29–43.

23 Prasher VP, Smith P. *Down Syndrome and Health Care.* Kidderminster BILD Publications, 2002.

24 Public Guardian Office. *Mental Capacity Act 2005 Code of Practice.* TSO (The Stationery Office), 2007.

25 Baxter H, Lowe K, Houston H, *et al.* Previously unidentified morbidity in patients with intellectual disability. *Br J Gen Pract* 2005; **56**: 93–8.

36 Royal College of Psychiatrists' Centre for Quality Improvement. Accreditation for Inpatient Mental Health Services for Learning Disability Services (AIMS-LD). Royal College of Psychiatrists, 2009 (http://www.rcpsych.ac.uk/quality/qualityandaccreditation/psychiatricwards/aims/whygetaccredited/aims-ld.aspx).

28 Liaison psychiatry

Elspeth Guthrie and Ayanangshu Nayak

Liaison psychiatry bridges the gap between mental and physical health services. This chapter describes the adverse effects of comorbid mental health problems in people with physical disorders. It details how to recognise delirium and alcohol problems (as well as other conditions) in general hospital settings and the assessment of mental capacity, all topics that can arise in many areas of psychiatric practice.

Introduction

Liaison psychiatry is the specialty that focuses upon the diagnosis, treatment and management of patients with concurrent physical and mental health problems, and primarily upon psychological problems which develop secondary to mental health problems that arise in the context of physical illness; examples include delirium after surgery, post-traumatic stress disorder after a road traffic accident, and the onset of diabetes in a patient with schizophrenia.

Most liaison psychiatry services are hospital-based, although some offer out-patient treatment or provide outreach and supervision to primary care. Some liaison services are disease-focused (e.g. psycho-oncology services) but the majority provide a generic service to any patient with any type of mental health problem in the general hospital setting. General hospitals are recommended to have liaison psychiatry services that are flexible and responsive to the needs of the acute hospital.[1,2]

Evidence base

Details of the efficacy of consultation liaison work and the consultation process are given in a Dutch guideline on consultation psychiatry.[3] A number of meta-analyses and randomised controlled trials have shown that collaborative care models are effective in improving outcome in patients with physical and psychological problems.[4–9] Antidepressants and psychological treatments are effective in treating depression in patients with chronic physical illness.[10] Several meta-analyses have reported the value of using both psychological treatment and antidepressants in patients with medically unexplained symptoms.[11–13]

Psychiatric consultation in general hospitals and nursing homes is effective in improving clinical outcome,[14,15] although there is no evidence for the efficacy of a single-visit psychiatric evaluation.[16,17] Screening for psychopathology in selected populations followed by consultation and liaison activities is probably more effective than providing consultation only on request.[15,18,19] There are also indications that liaison activities have a positive effect on patients and result in greater satisfaction.[20–23]

Prevalence of mental health problems in the general hospital

The prevalence of mental illness in patients admitted to an acute medical setting is approximately 28%, but a further 40% have subclinical symptoms of anxiety or depression.[24] For older adults in general hospital, the rates of depression and anxiety are even higher, with over half suffering from some kind of mental health problem.

Mental health problems often go unrecognised in the general hospital setting.[25] Detection and treatment of comorbid mental health problems in general hospital patients is important as comorbidity is related to a much poorer physical outcome, even after controlling for severity of disease. Even patients with subclinical psychological symptoms ('mild' symptoms of anxiety and depression) have a poorer health outcome than those without psychological symptoms.[24]

The adverse effects of comorbid mental health problems in people with physical illness are summarised in Box 28.1.

Mental health problems often go unrecognised in general hospital patients. Failure to recognise comorbid mental health problems may lead to poorer physical outcome.

Box 28.1 Adverse effects of comorbid mental health problems in people with physical illness

- Increased length of stay[26,27]
- Increased healthcare costs[28]
- Increased mortality[29–31]
- Increased rate of suicide[32]
- Increased use of urgent care[33]
- Poorer quality of life[34]
- Higher rates of complications and more invasive procedures[30,35]
- Increased symptom burden[26]

Box 28.2 Common mental health problems in th general hospital setting

- Psychological reaction to physical illness
- Delirium
- Dementia
- Acute disturbance
- Self-harm
- Alcohol-related problems
- Medically unexplained symptoms
- Feigned or fabricated illness
- Mental health problems in pregnancy
- Severe mental illness

In addition, liaison psychiatrists are commonly called up to assess capacity.

Common mental health problems in the general hospital setting

Liaison mental health services see a wide range of different mental health problems in the general hospital setting. The most common of these are listed in Box 28.2. Depressive or anxiety disorders are very common reasons for referral to liaison services, followed by organic disease states such as delirium and dementia.

Psychological reaction to physical illness

Anxiety disorders and depression are common in patients with physical illness and can arise from a myriad of causes, such as difficulty in adjusting to the physical condition and problems in dealing with the losses that the physical condition has caused. Depression may occur as a side-effect of medical treatment, such as steroids or interferon, or secondary to social problems that arise because of the illness, notably financial pressures that arise through the patient's inability to work. The stress of illness may result in the break-up of a previously fragile relationship.

People with a history of psychiatric problems will be particularly vulnerable to depression in the context of life stress such as a hospital admission. Many other factors may contribute, either singly or in combination, to the development of anxiety and depression in people who become physically ill.

Depression may occur as a result of medical treatment; following social problems secondary to the physical illness; or from a relationship break-up.

Certain physical conditions, usually those that involve the brain, have been linked with higher rates of mental health problems than other chronic physical disease states. However, one of the most important determinants of how people react to and cope with illness is not the illness itself, but how they perceive it. Leventhal's self-regulation model of health and illness is a useful framework for understanding people's response to illness.[36] Illness representations are considered to be multidimensional, comprising five main components:[36]

- *identity* – the label or name given to the condition and accompanying symptoms
- *cause* – ideas about the perceived cause of the condition, which may or may not be based upon biomedical evidence
- *time-line* – the predictive belief about how long the condition will last
- *consequences* – individual beliefs about the consequence of the condition and how this affects people physically and socially
- *curability/controllability* – beliefs about whether the condition can be cured or kept under control.

Delirium

Delirium is a complex neuropsychiatric syndrome with an acute onset and fluctuating course. It is characterised by:

- clouding of consciousness and cognitive dysfunction
- a range of levels of alertness, from somnolent to hyper-alert
- hallucinations, delusions and illusions – these are more common in activated patients
- agitated behaviour and delirium – these are more likely in somnolent patients, among whom the condition is more likely to go undetected.

Delirium occurs in about 15–20% of all general admissions to hospital and in up to 60% of admissions of elderly patients. The detection and management of delirium in the general hospital setting are, overall, very poor. Patients are often misdiagnosed and are thought to have functional psychosis because they are 'seeing things', although visual hallucinations are often characteristic of an organic pathology.

Treatment should be aimed at symptomatic relief and treatment of the underlying causes of the delirium. Antipsychotics help with a range of symptoms and are effective in patients who are hyper- or hypo-active.[37] Several 'best practice' guidelines have been developed, a useful review of which is provided by Leentjens and Diefenbacher,[38] and treatment options have been reviewed by Bourne *et al.*[39]

Dementia

Dementia is characterised by:

- insidious onset of global impairment of intellectual functioning
- progressive course over months or years
- disturbed memory
- disorientation in time, place and person
- language deficits
- reduced judgement
- altered emotional control, social behaviour and motivation
- interference with personal activities of daily living such as washing, dressing, eating and personal hygiene.

Approximately 35% of elderly people admitted to an acute general ward will be suffering from dementia and a further 20% will have mild cognitive impairment.[40]

Patients with dementia are particularly vulnerable in general hospitals. They are highly susceptible to environmental change and may find it difficult to communicate their needs, for example regarding toileting or pain relief. Patients with dementia are at high risk of delirium.

There is good evidence that better management of dementia in hospital can result in improved function and shorter stays.[19]

Medical wards are receiving increasing numbers of young patients with alcohol-related cognitive impairment. They are often admitted to hospital following an acute medical event such as a fit or head injury, undergo an alcohol withdrawal regimen and are then found to have severe cognitive difficulties.

Of elderly people admitted to general hospital, about 35% will have dementia and another 20% will have mild cognitive impairment. Those patients are highly susceptible to environmental change and are at risk of delirium. They may find it difficult to communicate their needs. Better management of dementia in hospital can result in improved function and shorter stays.

Wernicke–Korsakoff syndrome is thought to be due to deprivation of thiamine resulting from decreased intake and absorption, affecting neurons in the midbrain or thalamus. Usually secondary to alcohol misuse, it characteristically has a rapid onset following weeks of heavy drinking. The signs include confusion, unsteadiness, nystagmus, memory disturbance, hypothermia, hypotension and coma. High-dose thiamine or high-potency vitamins should be given to all patients thought to have alcohol-related problems. Parenteral administration is essential in those suspected of any likely cognitive impairment or Wernicke–Korsakoff syndrome. The risk of an allergic reaction is low but resuscitation equipment and adrenaline should be available to treat an untoward reaction. A quarter of patients with Korsakoff syndrome are left with severe memory problems, both anterograde and retrograde deficits. Confabulation commonly occurs but procedural memory remains relatively intact. Such patients can be very difficult to manage on medical wards. These alcohol-related conditions are discussed in more detail in Chapter 22.

Acute disturbance

Less than 5% of patients in the acute medical setting become acutely disturbed.[41] Males are more likely than females to become disturbed but there is no age differential – acute disturbance is equally common in patients above and below the age of 65 years. In most cases, aggressive behaviour is directed towards staff rather than other patients.

Although the prevalence of disturbed behaviour on acute wards is relatively low, it consumes a disproportionate amount of resources. Additional staff are required and expert knowledge of using sedation in physically unwell people is also important.

Box 28.3 Assessment after self-harm

- Age and sex
- Domestic and family situation
- Financial situation
- Intent
- Motivation
- Measures to avoid discovery
- Attitudes towards living or dying
- Mental illness, including different symptoms
- Substance misuse
- Persistent suicidal ideation
- Previous episodes of self-harm

Box 28.4 Potential psychological functions of repeated self-harm

- Environmental (communicative)
- Drive management (suicidality)
- Affect regulation (anger)
- Interpersonal control (boundaries)

Source: Suyemoto, 1998.[46]

Self-harm

Self-harm is one of the top five reasons for attendance at a hospital emergency department in the UK. Approximately a third will then be admitted to an acute medical ward. Eighty per cent of those who attend the emergency department after an episode of self-harm will have taken an overdose, and the other 20% attend for self-injuries such as cutting, burning or jumping from a height. Some will have made serious (possibly near-fatal) attempts to harm themselves.

All should receive a detailed psychosocial assessment as soon as they are physically well enough to cooperate; the risk of further self-harm or suicide while an in-patient should be considered very seriously. Care should be taken to work closely with the medical or surgical team as well as the ward staff, in terms of both monitoring and the treatment offered.

Some of the important factors to assess in a patient following an episode of self-harm are shown in Box 28.3 and some of the psychological functions of attempted self-harm are shown in Box 28.4.

The *method* of self-harm should not be confused with *intent*. In this context it is useful to remember that self-harm in the elderly is more likely to be a failed suicide attempt than is self-harm in younger patients.[42,43] Detailed assessment of previous episodes and their respective circumstances is useful in evaluating the future risk of self-harm. There are many validated scales for the assessment of this risk following self-harm, but accurate prediction of future self-harm is often not possible.[44] There is some evidence that risk increases with increasing comorbid symptoms[45] and also with social and relationship difficulties. Risk of repeated self-harm is highest following discharge and falls steadily up to around 6–12 months. However, an elevated risk of suicide persists for many years.

According to the National Confidential Inquiry into Suicide and Homicide by People with Mental Illness,[47] there was a small increase in the number of suicides in UK in the 5 years up to 2005, although notably the number of in-patient suicides (mainly in the psychiatric units) fell. Change in the physical environment (such as reducing ligature points) and increased staff awareness may be responsible for this.

In addition to identifying high-risk patients, risk assessment should be used to focus interventions where necessary, leading to a risk management programme incorporating multi-agency working, such as social and psychiatric services working together with the acute hospital departments.

Alcohol-related problems in the general hospital setting

Approximately 20% of all male patients admitted to acute medical wards will have alcohol-related problems; currently the prevalence is approximately 5% for women. There is good evidence that detection followed by a brief alcohol intervention results in significant reductions in alcohol consumption after discharge.[48,49] The same is true for people attending emergency departments with alcohol-related problems, where brief interventions reduce levels of alcohol consumption at 6 months, as well as reducing re-attendance at the emergency department.[50]

Repeated detoxifications may increase craving[51] and increase the risk of alcohol-related seizures.[52] Staff responsible for acute medical wards should work closely with liaison psychiatry services to develop coherent policies regarding alcohol detoxification so that people are given the most suitable treatment for their particular alcohol history.

Referrals for assessments of mental capacity

All doctors should be able to assess a person's mental capacity to consent to medical treatment. The Mental Capacity Act 2005 has helped to clarify the legal framework for patients where capacity may be impaired. Under this Act, people have capacity if they are able:

- to comprehend information relevant to the decision
- to retain the information for long enough to make the decision
- to use the information and evaluate it to arrive at a choice
- to communicate their decision.

In most cases in acute medical settings, the determination of capacity is straightforward, particularly in patients with delirium or severe dementia. It is not uncommon, however, for complex scenarios to arise where the determination of capacity is more difficult, particularly where it is possible that subtle mental health problems (such as depression) may be affecting a person's ability to make a choice, for example to end life-saving treatment. In these cases, the opinion of a consultant liaison psychiatrist is essential to ensure the best interests of the patient are being carefully considered.

Hospital staff on acute wards may occasionally need to prevent a patient who is confused from leaving the ward in order to protect that patient from harm. The Mental Capacity Act 'deprivation of liberty' safeguards were introduced through the Mental Health Act 2007. The safeguards apply to patients aged 18 or over who suffer from a mental disorder or disability of mind and who lack capacity to give informed consent to arrangements made for their care and for whom deprivation of liberty is in their best interests in order to protect them from harm (for further information see Chapter 11 on legal issues).

Medically unexplained symptoms

Patients with medically unexplained symptoms (MUS) are relatively rare in the general in-patient hospital setting because of the high costs involved

Box 28.5 Common functional somatic syndromes

- Irritable bowel syndrome
- Functional dyspepsia
- Atypical chest pain
- Hyperventilation
- Irritable bladder
- Fibromyalgia
- Repetitive strain injury
- Chronic back pain
- Chronic pelvic pain
- Multiple chemical sensitivity syndrome
- Atypical facial pain

in admitting patients to a medical bed. Such patients who are referred to liaison services usually have severe symptoms or lengthy histories of multiple symptoms, or severe chronic pain, possibly complicated by opiate dependence. In medical out-patient clinics, patients with MUS are much more common – approximately 40% of all new referrals to medical out-patient clinics in the UK have MUS.[53] Liaison services which offer out-patient assessment and treatment will receive many referrals of patients with moderate to severe MUS. The availability of treatment varies but usually involves a combination of antidepressant and psychological treatment. Many patients describe symptom clusters and they may be given a diagnosis that reflects their particular constellation of symptoms (Box 28.5).

A systematic review of the course and prognosis of MUS concluded that 50–75% of patients improve, whereas 10–30% deteriorate over time. The severity and number of symptoms at baseline influence the prognosis and more serious conditions are associated with a poorer outcome.[54]

Fabricated or feigned physical symptoms

Some people intentionally produce or feign symptoms of illness or disability in a persistent and maladaptive fashion. This can include self-inflicted wounds, false reports of cancer or serious illness, and abuse of medication (e.g. warfarin) to produce a physical disorder. There are many individual case reports that describe the ingenious ways people can fabricate illness and sometimes fool doctors into unnecessary surgery or treatment. In some cases the outcome can be fatal.

The term *factitious disorder* is used to describe such states if there is no obvious external motivating reason. This allows cases of fraud, where people feign illness in order to extort money, to be excluded from psychiatric nosology. Doctors usually begin to suspect factitious disorder when there is a discrepancy between the physical presentation of symptoms and the results of detailed investigations. A patient may complain of haemoptysis and even produce fresh blood (the patient may produce the blood only after visiting the bathroom alone), but all investigations will be normal.

Relatively little is known about factitious disorders, as individuals are often very reluctant to engage in any kind of treatment or help. Childhood neglect and abuse are common and it is assumed that people with factitious disorder are in some way trying to obtain care and support for themselves, albeit in a maladaptive and potentially dangerous manner. Little is known about the long-term outcomes, as few individuals offered follow-up remain in contact with services.

> Suspect factitious disorder if there is a discrepancy between the physical presentation of symptoms and the results of detailed investigations.

There is no clear agreement among liaison psychiatrists as to the best way to manage such patients, who constitute a small proportion of total referrals per year to liaison services but whose assessments and management on medical and surgical wards are usually complex, time-consuming and difficult.

Some psychiatrists advocate gentle confrontation, provided there is clear evidence of symptom feigning or fabrication. Other psychiatrists prefer to manage such patients by encouraging staff to reward non-illness-seeking behaviour and to provide the patients with a face-saving way of improving without confrontation. There is no empirical evidence as to which method is best.

Mental health problems in pregnancy

Liaison services receive many referrals from antenatal clinics and wards if the general hospital to which they provide a service also has a maternity unit.[55] Less than half of the mental health trusts in the UK provide specialised perinatal psychiatric liaison, although such provision has been recommended by the National Institute for Health and Clinical Excellence (NICE).[55]

Generic liaison services are unable to provide a comprehensive service, which should be the remit of specialised perinatal services; however, in the absence of such services, generic liaison services usually provide ward consultation liaison advice and out-patient assessment and support while women are in contact with hospital maternity services.

Women with a history of severe affective disorder, particularly bipolar disorder, are at high risk, estimated to be at least 50%, of becoming ill in the days and weeks following delivery. As the average length of stay for delivery is now 1 day, most women have been discharged home with their baby before signs of severe mental illness develop. It is therefore essential, and recommended by NICE,[55] that all women are asked in pregnancy about their previous and current mental health and that proactive plans are put in place for the management of their risk in the peripartum period.

Women with a history of severe mental illness may relapse during pregnancy and the most common reason for this is that they have discontinued medication, for fear of its effects on the unborn child.

Other common perinatal problems referred to liaison services include:

- development of depression in pregnancy, which may warrant treatment with antidepressants and specialist advice
- depression and multiple social problems where there may be risk issues related to the woman or the unborn baby
- a repeated history of self-harm, where there may be issues involving assessment of risk (staff on maternity units find in-patients who harm themselves extremely difficult to manage)
- a history of childhood adversity and sexual abuse
- asylum seekers with a history of severe trauma and rape in the country from which they have fled
- severe alcohol and drug problems (11% of maternal deaths overall and 57% of the psychiatric causes of maternal death involve substance misuse)
- multiple unexplained physical symptoms during pregnancy
- feigning physical symptoms related to pregnancy, such as vaginal bleeding.

For issues related to managing mental health in pregnancy, see also Chapter 20.

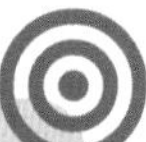

Postpartum women with a history of severe affective disorder, particularly bipolar disorder, have a high risk of becoming mentally ill in the days and weeks after delivery. Many will have been discharged home before the signs of severe mental illness appear.

Interface between liaison psychiatry and primary care

Problems with anxiety and depression in those who present with symptoms due to a physical illness are commonly missed in primary care, resulting in unnecessary suffering and disability.[56–58] General practitioners (GPs) have a key role in helping people to cope with physical illness and in facilitating a natural psychological adjustment. In addition, GPs need to recognise when patients with physical illness are becoming depressed and treat them accordingly. They also need to feel confident in managing patients whose physical symptoms remain unexplained.

Primary care is charged with providing care for common mental health problems and contributing to health promotion, but there is a lack of clarity about who should lead the care of those with chronic, complex and disabling non-psychotic problems.

A joint report from the Royal College of Psychiatrists and Royal College of General Practitioners[1] highlighted the need for closer working between liaison psychiatry services and primary care for patients with complex physical and psychological needs. It stated:

> Multidisciplinary liaison psychiatry services, which have been traditionally hospital-based, can provide valuable community support and training for staff, including GPs, active case managers and other primary care professionals. Treatment can also be offered for patients with severe and complex needs (if appropriate resources are available).

In recent years, 'tier 2' services have been developed which sit between primary and secondary care and are run by specialist GPs. They are intended to provide more rapid access for patients with particular problems, for example eye problems or musculoskeletal symptoms, and avoid unnecessary, costly referral to secondary care. Liaison psychiatry has already been successfully incorporated into some integrated clinical assessment and treatment services (ICATs), which means that patients with certain physical health problems such as musculoskeletal symptoms can rapidly access appropriate physical and mental healthcare within the same tier 2 service.

Liaison outreach to primary care services can help GPs by offering supervision to help manage patients with complex needs and accept GP referrals. These liaison services are far from universal and there is a wide gap between hospital-based and community-based liaison services for patients with complex physical and mental health needs.

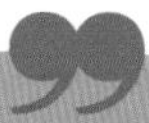

Summary

Liaison services are involved in the assessment and treatment of patients with complex physical and mental health problems in the general hospital setting. The prevalence of psychological problems and psychiatric illness in the general hospital is high, yet rates of detection and treatment are low. Failure to detect and treat mental health problems in patients with physical illness results in a variety of negative outcomes, including: increased mortality, increased length of stay in hospital, increased disability, poorer quality of life and increased health costs.

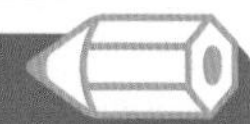

Learning points

- Liaison psychiatry is the specialty of psychiatry that focuses upon the diagnosis, treatment and management of patients with concurrent physical and mental health problems.
- Meta-analyses and randomised controlled trials have shown that collaborative care models are effective in improving outcome in patients with physical and psychological problems.
- Meta-analyses have reported the value of using both psychological treatment and antidepressants in patients with medically unexplained symptoms.
- The prevalence of significant mental illness in patients admitted to an acute medical setting is approximately 28% and a further 40% have subclinical symptoms of anxiety/depression.
- Mental health problems often go unrecognised in patients in the general hospital setting.
- Adverse effects of comorbid mental health problems in people with physical illness result in poorer quality of life, increased health costs, increased length of stay, poorer outcome, greater morbidity and increased mortality.
- Liaison services see a range of mental health problems including: psychological reaction to physical illness; delirium; dementia; acute disturbance; self-harm; alcohol-related problems; medically unexplained symptoms; feigned or fabricated illness; mental health problems in pregnancy; and severe mental illness.
- Leventhal's self-regulation model of health and illness is a useful framework for understanding people's response to illness.
- Delirium occurs in about 15–20% of all general admissions to hospital and in up to 60% of admissions of elderly patients. The detection and management of delirium in the general hospital setting are often very poor.
- Approximately 35% of elderly people admitted to an acute general ward will have dementia and a further 20% will have mild cognitive impairment.
- Self-harm is one of the top five reasons for emergency department attendance in the UK.
- Risk assessment for self-harm should be used to focus interventions where necessary, leading to a risk management programme incorporating multi-agency working, such as social and psychiatric services working together with the acute hospital departments.
- Approximately 20% of all male patients admitted to acute medical wards will have alcohol-related problems; the prevalence is much lower for women.
- There is good evidence that detection followed by a brief alcohol intervention results in significant reductions in alcohol consumption after discharge.
- In medical out-patient clinics, patients with MUS are very common and approximately 40% of all new referrals to medical out-patient clinics in the UK have MUS.

References

1 Royal College of Psychiatrists, Royal College of General Practitioners. *The Management of Patients with Physical and Psychological Problems in Primary Care: A Practical Guide.* College Report CR152. Royal College of Psychiatrists, 2009.

2 Academy of Medical Royal Colleges. *Managing Urgent Mental Health Needs in the Acute Trust.* Academy of Medical Royal Colleges, 2008.

3 Leentjens AFG, Boenink AD, Sno HN, *et al.* The guideline 'consultation psychiatry' of the Netherlands Psychiatric Association. *J Psychosomatic Res* 2009; **66**: 531–5.

4 Gilbody S, Bower P, Whitty P. Costs and consequences of enhanced primary care for depression: systematic review or randomised economic evaluations. *Br J Psychiatry* 2006; **189**: 297–308.

5 Katon W, Von Korff M, Bush T, *et al.* A randomized trial of psychiatric consultation with distressed high utilizers. *Gen Hosp Psychiatry* 1992; **14**: 86–98.

6 Smith GR, Monson AC, Ray DC. Psychiatric consultation in somatisation disorder. *New Engl J Med* 1986; **314**: 1407–13.

7 Smith GR, Rost K, Kashner TM. A trial of the effect of a standardized psychiatric consultation on health outcomes and costs in somatising patients. *Arch Gen Psychiatry* 1995; **52**: 238–43.

8 Bower P, Gilbody S, Richards D, *et al.* Collaborative care for depression in primary care: making sense of a complex intervention – review and meta-regression. *Br J Psychiatry* 2006; **189**: 484–93.

9 Unützer J, Katon W, Callahan CM, *et al.* Collaborative care management of late-life depression in the primary care setting: a randomized controlled trial. *JAMA* 2002; **288**: 2836–45.

10 National Institute for Health and Clinical Excellence. *Depression in Adults with a Chronic Physical Health Problem: Treatment and Management.* Clinical Guidance CG91. NICE, 2009.

11 O'Malley PG, Jackson JL, Santoro J, *et al.* Antidepressant therapy for unexplained symptoms and symptom syndromes. *J Fam Pract* 1999; **48**: 980–90.

12 Jailwala J, Kroenke K. Pharmacological treatment of the irritable bowel syndrome: a systematic review of randomized controlled trials. *Ann Intern Med* 2000; **133**: 136–47.

13 O'Malley PG, Balden E, Tomkins G, *et al.* Treatment of fibromyalgia with antidepressants: a meta-analysis. *J Gen Intern Med* 2000; **15**: 659–66.

14 Herzog T, Stein B, Soellner W, *et al* (eds). *Konsiliar- und Liaisonpsychosomatik und Psychiatrie.* Schattauer, 2003.

15 Saravay SM. Psychiatric interventions in the medically ill: outcome and effectiveness research. *Psychiatr Clin N Am* 1996; **19**: 467–80.

16 Levenson JL, Hamer RM, Rossiter LF. A randomized controlled study of psychiatric consultation guided by screening in general medical inpatients. *Am J Psychiatry* 1992; **149**: 631–7.

17 Gater RA, Goldberg DP, Evanson JM, *et al.* Detection and treatment of psychiatric illness in a general medical ward: a modified cost–benefit analysis. *J Psychosom Res* 1998; **45**: 437–48.

18 Levitan SJ, Kornfeld DS. Clinical and cost benefits of liaison psychiatry. *Am J Psychiatry* 1981; **138**: 790–3.

19 Strain JJ, Lyons JS, Hammer JS, *et al.* Cost offset from a psychiatric consultation–liaison intervention with elderly hip fracture patients. *Am J Psychiatry* 1991; **148**: 1044–9.

20 Schubert DSP, Billowitz A, Gabinet L, *et al.* Effect of liaison psychiatry on attitudes toward psychiatry, rate of consultation, and psychosocial documentation. *Gen Hosp Psychiatry* 1989; **11**: 77–87.

21 Scot J, Fairbairn A, Woodhouse K. Referrals to a geriatric consultation–liaison service: description and evaluation. *Int J Geriatr Psychiatry* 1988; **7**: 347–50.

22 de Leo D, Baiocchi A, Cippolone B, *et al.* Psychogeriatric consultation within a general hospital. *Int J Geriatr Psychiatry* 1989; **4**: 135–41.

23 Swansick GRJ, Lee H, Clare AW, *et al.* Consultation–liaison psychiatry: a comparison between two service models for geriatric patients. *Int J Geriatr Psychiatry* 1994; **9**: 495–9.

24 Creed F, Morgan R, Fiddler M, *et al.* Depression and anxiety impair health-related quality of life and are associated with increased costs in general medical inpatients. *Psychosomatics* 2002; **43**: 302–9.

25 Cepoiu M, McCusker J, Cole MG, *et al.* Recognition of depression by non-psychiatric physicians – a systematic literature review and meta-analysis. *J Gen Intern Med* 2008; **23**: 25–36.

26 Ng TP, Niti M, Tan WC, *et al.* Depressive symptoms and chronic obstructive pulmonary disease: effect on mortality, hospital, readmission, symptom burden, functional status and quality of life. *Arch Intern Med* 2007; **167**: 60–7.

27 Holmes JD, House AO. Psychiatric illness in hip fracture. *Age Ageing* 2000; **29**: 537–46.

28 Egede LE, Zheng D, Simpson K, *et al.* Comorbid depression is associated with increased health care use and expenditures in individuals with diabetes. *Diabetes Care* 2002; **25**: 464–70.

29 Barth J, Schumacher M, Herrmann-Lingen C. Depression as a risk factor for mortality in patients with coronary heart disease: a meta-analysis. *Psychosom Med* 2004; **66**: 802–13.

30 van Melle J, de Jonge P, Spijkerman T, *et al.* Prognostic association of depression following myocardial infarction with mortality and cardiovascular events: a meta-analysis. *Psychosom Med* 2004; **66**: 814–22.

31 Fan VS, Ramsey SD, Giardino ND, *et al.* Sex, depression, and risk of hospitalization and mortality in chronic obstructive pulmonary disease. *Arch Intern Med* 2007; **167**: 2345–53.

32 Bronnum-Hansen H, Stenager E, Stenager EN, *et al.* Suicide among Danes with multiple sclerosis. *J Neurol Neurosurg Psychiatry* 2005; **76**: 1457–9.

33 Himelhoch S, Weller WE, Wu AW, *et al.* Chronic medical illness, depression, and use of acute medical services among medicare beneficiaries. *Med Care* 2004; **42**: 512–21.

34 Guthrie E, Jackson J, Shaffer J, *et al.* Psychological disorder and severity of inflammatory bowel disease predict health-related quality of life in ulcerative colitis and Crohn's disease. *Am J Gastroenterol* 2002; **97**: 1994–9.

35 Lauzon C, Beck CA, Thao H, *et al.* Depression and prognosis following hospital admission because of acute myocardial infarction. *Can Med Assoc J* 2003; **168**: 570–1.

36 Leventhal H, Benyamini Y, Brownlee S, *et al.* Illness representations: theoretical foundations. In *Perceptions of Health and Illness: Current Research and Applications* (eds KJ Petrie, J Weinman): 19–45. Harwood Academic, 1997.

37 Meagher D. Delirium: optimising management. *BMJ* 2001; **322**: 144–9.

38 Leentjens AF, Diefenbacher A. A survey of delirium guidelines in Europe. *J Psychosom Res* 2006; **61**: 123–8.

39 Bourne RS, Tahir TA, Borthwick M, *et al.* Drug treatment of delirium: past, present and future. *J Psychosom Res* 2008; **65**: 273–82.

40 Royal College of Psychiatrists. *Who Cares Wins: Improving the Outcome of Older People Admitted to General Hospitals – Guidelines for the Development of Liaison Mental Health Services for Older People.* Faculty Report. Royal College of Psychiatrists, 2005.

41 Kannabiran M, Deshpande S, Walling A. Cross-sectional survey of disturbed behaviour in patients in general hospitals in Leeds. *Postgrad Med J* 2008; **84**: 428–31.

42 Dennis MS. Suicide and self-harm in older people. *Qual Ageing Older Adults* 2009; **10**: 16–23.

43 Hawton K, Harriss L. Deliberate self-harm in people aged 60 years and over: characteristics and outcome of a 20 year cohort. *Int J Geriatr Psychiatry* 2006; **21**: 572–81.

44 Kapur N, Cooper J, Rodway P, *et al.* Predicting the risk of repetition after self harm: cohort study. *BMJ* 2005; **330**: 394–5.

45 Powell J, Geddes J, Hawton K, *et al.* Suicide in psychiatric hospital in-patients: risk factors and their predictive power. *Br J Psychiatry* 2000; **176**: 266–72.

46 Suyemoto KL. The functions of self-mutilation. *Clin Psychol Rev* 1998; **18**: 531–54.

47 National Confidential Inquiry into Suicide and Homicide by People with Mental Illness. *Annual Report: England and Wales.* University of Manchester, 2009.

48 Chick J, Lloyd G, Crombie E. Counselling problem drinkers in medical wards: a controlled study. *BMJ* 1985; **290**: 965–7.

49 McManus S, Hipkins J, Haddad P, *et al.* Implementing an effective intervention for problem drinkers on medical wards. *Gen Hosp Psychiatry* 2003; **25**: 332–7.

50 Crawford M, Patton R, Touquet R, *et al.* Screening and referral for brief intervention of alcohol-misusing patients in an emergency department: a pragmatic randomised controlled trial. *Lancet* 2004; **364**: 1334–9.

51 Hillemacher T, Bayerlein K, Wilhelm J, *et al.* Recurrent detoxifications are associated with craving in patients classified as type 1 according to Lesch's typology. *Alcohol* 2006; **41**: 66–9.

52 Booth BM, Blow C. The kindling hypothesis: further evidence from a US national study of alcoholic men. *Alcohol* 1993; **28**: 593–8.

53 Nimnuan C, Hotopf M, Wessely S, *et al.* Medically unexplained symptoms – an epidemiological study in seven specialities. *J Psychosom Res* 2001; **51**: 361–7.

54 Hartman TC, Borghuis MS, Lucassen PLBJ, *et al.* Medically unexplained symptoms, somatisation disorder and hypochondriasis: course and prognosis. A systematic review. *J Psychosom Res* 2009; **66**: 363–77.

55 National Institute for Health and Clinical Excellence. *Antenatal and Postnatal Mental Health: Clinical Management and Service Guideline.* Clinical Guideline 45. NICE, 2007.

56 Goldberg D, Huxley P. *Common Mental Disorders: A Bio-social Model.* Routledge, 1992.

57 Chew-Graham CA, Hogg T. Patients with chronic physical illness and co-existing psychological morbidity: GPs' views on their role in detection and management. *Primary Care Psychiatry* 2002; **8**: 35–9.

58 Burroughs H, Morley M, Lovell K, *et al.* 'Justifiable depression': how health professionals and patients view late-life depression; a qualitative study. *Fam Pract* 2006; **23**: 369–77.

29

Old age psychiatry

David Anderson

A range of health problems become more frequent as people get older and comorbidity increases. This chapter describes the diagnosis, investigation and management of these frequently interrelated problems, with emphasis on the effect of medication on ageing physiology and physical and mental pathology. Liaison with primary and secondary care is important, as are risk assessment and general health measures.

Introduction

The separation of physical and mental health in older people is usually a false distinction, as a 'psychiatric' syndrome is often a physical disorder. For example, dementia results from degenerative brain disease or systemic medical conditions, and delirium, predominantly a condition of later life, is always due to physical causes and is a common presentation of acute physical illness in later life. Late-onset psychosis affects up to 20% of non-demented older people by age 85[1] and is more likely to have physical causes than psychosis in younger age groups.[2]

Comorbidity characterises later life.[3] A study of Canadian family practices found that 98% of people aged over 65 years had an average of 6.4 chronic conditions.[4] Knowledge of the physical causes and consequences of mental disorder and its treatment is therefore fundamental to the diagnosis and management of all older people. Balancing physical and mental health gains is fundamental to good treatment and with older people they are inextricably linked.

> Physical illness increases the incidence of mental disorder and *vice versa*. Up to 15% of the over 65s have depression, with rates substantially higher if there is physical illness.

Physical illness increases the incidence of mental disorder and *vice versa*. For example, the community prevalence of depression among people aged over 65 years is 10–15%, but in the presence of physical illness or disability it is substantially higher (Table 29.1). Conversely, untreated depression in later life increases natural mortality rates two- or threefold, most such deaths being from cardiovascular disease or cancer, while treated depression may not.[5] Depression is as significant a risk factor for coronary heart disease as smoking or diabetes.[6]

The most common comorbidities are cardiovascular disease, chronic obstructive pulmonary disease, arthritis, osteoporosis, diabetes, Parkinson's disease, stroke, sensory impairment, prostatism and malignancy. Impaired renal function, malnutrition and polypharmacy complicate treatment. Infection, constipation, dizziness, falls, pain and limited mobility occur frequently. Older people are frequently under the care of other secondary health services.

Somatoform disorders are far less common with older people and medically unexplained symptoms are usually associated with physical conditions or depression.[7]

Physical illnesses

Organic brain syndromes

Dementia

Dementia is the most strikingly age-related medical condition, with 97.8% of cases having onset after age 65; the prevalence rate rises from 1.3% among those aged 65–69 years to 20.3% among those aged 85–89.[8]

Dementia is an organic brain syndrome with a physical cause (Box 29.1). Medical investigation of dementia is required in every case, including neuroimaging.[9] The underlying pathology is recognised by the pattern of disease progression, risk factors and results of investigation. Differentiating these pathologies is important for management and medical treatment.

Vascular risk predisposes to vascular dementia and Alzheimer's disease.[10] Controlling vascular risk in middle age may be the most promising means of reducing the incidence of dementia on the basis of current evidence. Smoking cessation and controlling diabetes, hypertension, cholesterol, heart conditions and alcohol consumption are part of treatment. Around 30% of people with diabetes, particularly type 2, develop cognitive impairment and are 1.6 times more likely to develop dementia, probably due to small-vessel vascular brain disease.[11]

Vascular risk predisposes to vascular dementia and Alzheimer's disease. Controlling vascular risk in middle age may be the most promising means of reducing the incidence of dementia.

Table 29.1 Prevalence of depression in different contexts and conditions

Context/condition	Prevalence (%)
Care homes	16–44
General hospital	29
Primary care attenders	30
Dementia	25
Neurological disorders	24
Parkinson's disease	50
Huntington's disease	40
Stroke	
acute	25
at 12 months	16
at 36 months	30
Myocardial infarction	
acute and at 12 months	15–30
Coronary heart disease	
major depression	20
minor depression	27
Cancer	20
Chronic obstructive pulmonary disease clinic	42

Box 29.1 Causes of dementia

Degenerative

- Alzheimer's disease
- Vascular brain disease
- Mixed Alzheimer's and vascular disease
- Dementia with Lewy bodies
- Frontotemporal
- Parkinson's disease
- Huntington's disease
- Creutzfeld–Jakob disease
- Progressive supranuclear palsy
- Gerstmann–Straussler syndrome

Potentially reversible

- Normal-pressure hydrocephalus
- Cerebral tumour
- Subdural haematoma
- Anaemia
- System failure – cardiac, respiratory, hepatic, renal
- Hypothyroidism
- Hypercalcaemia
- Alcohol related
- Neurosyphilis

Box 29.2 Common causes of delirium

- Infection
- Dehydration
- Electrolyte imbalance
- System failure – cardiac, respiratory, hepatic, renal
- Cardiac arrhythmia
- Stroke
- Seizure
- Cerebral trauma
- Hypo- and hyperglycaemia
- Hypercalcaemia
- Acute blood loss
- Acute abdomen
- Alcohol – intoxication, withdrawal
- Prescribed drugs – anticholinergics, psychotropics, opiates, anticonvulsants, any excessive use
- Illicit substances

A small proportion of cases are due to reversible conditions that examination and investigation must identify (Box 29.1).

Delirium

Delirium is a common non-specific presentation of acute physical illness in older people that doctors must recognise and try to prevent.[12] Urgent medical investigation is needed as treatment is that of the underlying condition (Box 29.2). Mortality is high and the condition is often complicated by falls, incontinence and pressure sores.

Depression and comorbidity

Late-onset depression is more likely to be associated with physical illness than is depression at younger ages. Physical illness may present like depression (pseudodepression), making it more difficult to interpret biological symptoms; management of the physical illness is therefore likely to be essential to treatment. The comorbidity will affect the treatment approach and how and where treatment is delivered.

Antidepressant drugs may benefit physical health, even in the absence of antidepressant effects, but can also have detrimental physical effects.

Parkinson's disease and dementia with Lewy bodies

Parkinson's disease is the second most common neurodegenerative condition affecting older people and incidence increases with age. The prevalence of depression, cognitive impairment, dementia and psychosis is unusually high among those with the disease. They are a powerful predictor of quality of life and outcome. The treatment of psychiatric conditions that arise in those with Parkinson's disease is complex, as they tend to respond little to L-dopa.[13,14]

Cognitive impairment, typically impaired frontal executive function (the dysexecutive syndrome), occurs in uncomplicated Parkinson's disease. Up to 80% of people with the disease develop dementia over 8 years, 50% have depression at some point, which does not seem to be a reaction to motor disability, and 50% experience psychotic symptoms, typically visual hallucinations and sometimes delusions.[13] Apathy and anxiety are common and the dopamine dysregulation syndrome (which involves impulse control disorders) is a complication of the drugs taken for motor symptoms.[15] All people with suspected Parkinson's disease should be seen by a specialist as there are other parkinsonian syndromes.[13] Current thinking is that neurotransmitter abnormalities are the cause of these problems.

Dementia with Lewy bodies is a related condition with the same molecular biochemistry (synucleinopathy), although there is uncertainty whether they are part of a spectrum or distinct.[16] Dementia with Lewy bodies is the fourth most common cause of dementia. It is characterised by a triad of fluctuating cognitive impairment, visual hallucination and Parkinsonism.[17] Perfusion single-photon emission tomography (SPECT) and dopamine transporter (DAT) imaging are valuable diagnostic aids (see below).

Treating Parkinson's disease or dementia with Lewy bodies is complicated, as drugs that improve motor symptoms may induce psychiatric symptoms and drugs for psychiatric symptoms (antipsychotics and antidepressants) may increase motor symptoms. People

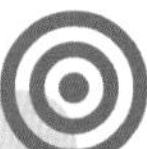

Cognitive impairment, psychosis and depression are common in Parkinson's disease, arising directly from neurotransmitter and neuropathalogical consequences of the condition. It is still important to consider other contributing factors and alternative explanations.

with dementia with Lewy bodies are particularly prone to develop the neuroleptic sensitivity syndrome, causing lethargy, confusion, tremor, rigidity, falls and even death. Parkinsonism occurring within dementia with Lewy bodies is less responsive to L-dopa (about 25% benefit) than that within Parkinson's disease, where response is a diagnostic criterion.

The evidence base for antidepressant treatment is poor; what evidence there is may be best for nortriptyline.[18] Uniquely, it seems, pramipexole, a dopamine agonist, has antidepressant properties superior to sertraline[19] and it may be worth discussing, with the patient's Parkinson's disease specialist, the suitability of using this for motor symptoms in a patient who is depressed. Antidepressants have to be considered cautiously if monoamine oxidase inhibitor B (MAOI-B) drugs are taken for motor symptoms.

Parkinson's disease is a good example of the need for medical and psychiatric knowledge in diagnosis and treatment. Management requires skill to balance the treatment of motor and psychiatric symptoms.

Cardiovascular disease

Vascular risk is relevant to dementia and depression, and uncompensated heart failure or cardiac dysrhythmia are potential causes of delirium. Carotid artery occlusion and microemboli may cause vascular brain disease and are associated with Alzheimer's disease.[20]

Cardiovascular disease in general is a risk factor for depression and, conversely, depression is a risk factor for ischaemic heart disease. Selective serotonin reuptake inhibitors (SSRIs) have been shown to be safe and effective for severe or recurrent depression after myocardial infarction and with unstable angina.[21,22] They may reduce the risk of subsequent fatal and non-fatal cardiac ischaemia.[23] This protective effect is not dependent on their antidepressant effect and is probably due to a reduction in platelet coagulability not apparent with tricyclic antidepressants.[24]

Stroke

Stroke is a cause of vascular dementia and depression. There is lack of evidence for benefit from psychological treatment for depression, but post-stroke depression responds to antidepressants (OR=2.58 compared with placebo). However, it is not possible to recommend a particular antidepressant drug.[25] An SSRI may improve frontal executive function after stroke even in the absence of an antidepressant effect.[26] Patients with new stroke or transient ischaemic attack should be referred to a stroke service. Older people are less likely to receive optimal secondary prevention with drugs.[27]

> **Stroke is a cause of dementia and depression. Post -stroke depression responds to antidepressants but there is no evidence for benefit from psychological treatment.**

Vascular depression

This concept developed from studies of older people with depression who were shown to have cerebral ischaemia on magnetic resonance imaging (MRI)[28] and ischaemia seems to be the underlying cause.[29] Severe deep white-matter lesions in frontal and basal ganglia areas are characteristic. It is quite refractory to conventional treatment and there is interest in the treatment potential of drugs that improve cerebral blood flow.[30] The pathogenetic complexity of this condition is discussed by Teper & O'Brien.[31]

Chronic obstructive pulmonary disease

This population can be particularly difficult to engage, as they tend to present psychological barriers to treatment, but findings from a behavioural and problem-solving approach to overcome these barriers with attention given specifically to the disability arising from the chronic obstructive pulmonary disease is promising.[32] Acute exacerbation may cause delirium. Steroids affect mood state.

Physical examination

All psychiatrists have been trained to perform a basic physical examination and maintaining that skill is a necessary competency for working with older people. Delirium requires very thorough examination and the services of other medical specialists.

A lot can be gleaned from observation and simple examination of appearance, sensory impairment, motor

Box 29.3 Investigations often required with older patients presenting with mental health problems

Routine

- Haematology
- Biochemistry – electrolytes; renal function; hepatic function; calcium metabolism; glucose; B12 and folate
- Thyroid function

Selective

- Electrocardiography
- X-ray
- Syphilis serology
- Structural neuroimaging – magnetic resonance (MR) or computerised tomography if no MR
- Functional neuroimaging – single-photon emission computerised tomography (SPECT) – HMPAO SPECT and FP-CIT SPECT (DAT)

See text for indications for other imaging techniques.

abnormalities, gait, pulse, respiration and peripheral neurological signs. This is so important with older people that it should be seen as an extension of a routine mental state examination. Because most older people in the community are seen by mental health services in their own home, where there is no access to medical equipment, these observational skills must be well developed.

Diagnosis and investigation

In addition to a good physical examination, older people will almost always require medical investigation. Physical symptoms due to known comorbidity, as well as unexplained symptoms, are common. Older people more often present illness in atypical forms. Simple laboratory investigation will be sufficient in most cases where the medical history is known (Box 29.3).

Hypothyroidism presents with a range of mental disturbances and older people frequently have none of the classical signs or symptoms.[33] Syphilis serology should be performed if indicated from personal history. HIV infection is becoming an issue, with reports of increasing rates of new infection in older people and an estimate that by 2015, 50% of people living with HIV will be over the age of 50.[34]

Problems of glucose metabolism, hypercalcaemia, electrolyte disturbance or anaemia may have no physical manifestations. Cardiac or respiratory problems may need further specialist investigation. Unexplained dizziness, collapse or falls should have assessment by a physician or falls service.

Neuroimaging is beginning to have real diagnostic significance, particularly with dementia. Routine structural imaging is recommended, preferably MRI, for all suspected cases of dementia.[9] This gives information on neurodegenerative pathology and is needed to exclude space-occupying lesions. Magnetic resonance imaging gives more information about cerebral ischaemia, including subcortical vascular changes, than does computerised tomography (CT).

Perfusion single-photon emission computerised tomography (SPECT) is valuable for distinguishing frontotemporal from other cortical dementias and Lewy body diseases (synucleinopathies). Dopamine transporter (DAT) scans image presynaptic dopamine integrity with high sensitivity and specificity in the diagnosis of Parkinson's disease, as well as possible and probable dementia with Lewy bodies.[9,35,36]

Monitoring

Monitoring of physical health applies to all patients but specific things will apply to some, for example: renal and thyroid function with lithium salts, blood sugar and $HbA1_c$ in diabetes, weight gain, blood glucose and lipids for those on antipsychotics, and sodium levels with SSRIs (see below).

Prescribed medications

Many drugs for physical illnesses can cause psychiatric disturbance and psychotropic drugs can affect the physical health of older people. The vast majority of older people will be taking drugs for their physical health and the psychiatrist will need to be familiar with their purpose and effects. If an older person develops any new symptom following a new drug, always consider its withdrawal before anything else.

Older people are more susceptible than younger people to adverse drug effects. Altered physiology in those with physical illness, polypharmacy, changes in pharmacokinetics and pharmacodynamics make drug prescribing a more subtle and thoughtful process.

Moreover, simple, even mild, side-effects may have more serious consequences, such as dry mouth causing ulceration and infection that prevent eating, mild postural hypotension causing falls and fractures, and sedation, constipation or tremor impairing independent function. The rate of admission to hospital due to adverse drug reactions is four times higher in older people, although repeat admission is predicted by comorbidity and not advancing age in the older age group.[37]

Ageing brings physiological change that alters the distribution, clearance and metabolism of drugs. Reduction in renal clearance and elimination, liver size, lean body mass, hepatic enzyme activity and serum albumin may occur with chronic disease; malnutrition and ageing are important to appreciate.

Polypharmacy is common: 20% of patients aged over 70 take five or more prescribed drugs.[38] This increases risk of drug interactions, adverse effects, falls, hospital admission, length of hospital admission, readmission and mortality.[39]

The potential for drug interactions must be considered carefully and drugs prescribed at the lowest possible dose. Drugs that will interact to induce hypotension and sedation (which include many psychotropic drugs) are a prominent concern in clinical practice. Dose titration is more gradual than with younger people, as prolonged half-life causes accumulation. Risks must be discussed with the patient and/or carer, depending on the person's capacity to consent to treatment.

Whenever writing a new prescription for an older patient, consider whether any drugs can be discontinued, after discussion with the patient's physician. Stopping or changing a drug to another class may reduce the risk of drug interaction. Examples are: replacing a diuretic when considering lithium or an SSRI; stopping a beta-blocker if prescribing an antidepressant (remembering that venlafaxine increases blood pressure in 10% of patients); using pramipexole or changing an MAOI-B in Parkinson's disease; using an alternative to a non-steroidal anti-inflammatory (NSAID) with lithium or an SSRI to reduce the risk of toxicity or gastrointestinal bleeding, respectively,

> Polypharmacy is common in older people: 20% of patients aged over 70 take five or more prescribed drugs, increasing the risk of drug interactions and adverse effects.

> Remember, especially in older people, that medication for physical illness may cause psychiatric disturbance and psychotropic drugs can affect physical health.

Adherence is improved by simplifying drug regimens. Can administration be reduced to once daily? Could all medicines be given at the same time of day, when a carer can supervise? Would a liquid, orodispersible or patch form be better?

Prescribed drugs are among the most common causes of delirium and any drug in a predisposed person can be responsible (Box 29.2).

Particular considerations

Anticholinergics

Anticholinergic drugs are the most likely to cause delirium.

Antipsychotics

These should be prescribed with considerable caution as they increase the risk of falls, confusion, sedation, infection, hospital admission and mortality. There is good evidence that they are overprescribed to people with dementia.[40]

Olanzapine and risperidone increase the risk of cerebral ischaemia two- to threefold. It is therefore recommended that they are not prescribed to people with dementia, those over 80 or those with high vascular risk.[41] It is likely these risks are a class effect of antipsychotic drugs in general, both atypical and typical,[42] and the risk of sudden cardiac death is the same for typicals and atypicals and is dose related.[43]

The risk of diabetes, weight gain and dyslipidaemia with antipsychotics is much less than it is in younger people and many studies find no significant increase and little difference between typical and atypical antipsychotics, but checking blood glucose and lipid profile is still recommended before treatment, after 3–4 months and then annually.[44]

Antidepressants

Newer antidepressants are probably safer overall than older drugs, particularly in relation to cardiac risk. The SSRIs seem particularly prone to cause hyponatraemia,

The risk of hyponatraemia with SSRIs increases with age and with concomitant use of diuretics. Hyponatraemia can resemble depression with lethargy, slowness and anorexia. Very low sodium levels may cause delirium and seizures.

usually within 4 weeks,[45] and this risk increases with age and with the use of diuretics. Hyponatraemia can resemble depression, with lethargy, slowness and anorexia; very low sodium levels cause delirium or seizures.

Drugs that inhibit serotonin reuptake increase the risk of bleeding, especially upper gastrointestinal bleeding, and in at-risk patients may require co-prescribing of a gastroprotective agent.[46]

Lithium salts

The elimination of lithium is totally dependent on renal function, which declines with age. The typically quoted therapeutic range is based on younger adult populations and older people may become lithium toxic within this range. Estimated glomerular filtration rate (eGFR) should be measured before treatment and to monitor renal function. It is preferable and usually clinically sufficient to maintain levels at the low end of the therapeutic range.

Early toxicity is indicated by increasing hand tremor, incoordination, slowed thought processes or nausea. Where this is suspected or merely in doubt, or while awaiting plasma lithium estimation, withdraw treatment. Older males with prostatism are prone to gradual lithium accumulation secondary to even mild obstructive uropathy.

Older people are more likely to be taking diuretics or NSAIDs, which increase plasma lithium levels. In hot weather, even in temperate climates, fluid depletion occurs with older people and lithium levels rise.

Primary care

Most psychiatry with older people is a collaboration with primary care teams. Local agreements for shared care with, for example, the GP performing screening investigations and providing medical history have advantages and save time. Mental disorders in later life in primary care have been described in detail in a text covering all healthcare for older people.[7]

Community pharmacists can often advise on better medicine management and compliance. Delivering medicines to people's homes and blister packs are services of particular value to older people, many of whom have difficulty collecting drugs or organising complicated medicine regimens. People with dementia forget to take medicines and so often need clear arrangements for supervision.

Many community services are essential for the physical well-being of older people. For example, foot care from chiropodists may be vital for an older person with a physical disability or foot care may be neglected by a person with dementia. The consequences of loss of mobility can be devastating (neglect, pressure sores, infection, incontinence, isolation) and loss of independent function can be the main reason for a move into a care home.[47]

Sensory impairment increases with age and may be relevant to the aetiology of mental disorder.[2] The impairment should be corrected; opticians, ophthalmology and audiology services may be required.

Dental care is often neglected by people who are mentally ill. Older people are more likely to be edentulous or to wear dentures, which may become ill fitting as gums shrink with ageing; poor dentition in turn may affect diet.

Many people seen by older people's mental health teams will have long-term conditions and may be attended by district nurses for diabetes, ulcers, incontinence or stoma care. Close working will improve overall care. Community mental health teams need a good relationship with their physical health counterparts.

Hospitals

Two hospital environments need to be considered.

Mental health

Admitting older people requires as much attention to their physical health as mental health. Uncertainty about medical history or medication should be clarified immediately with the GP.

Germane to any management plan are thorough physical examination and investigation and proper recording of physical impairments, disabilities and handicaps, including vision, hearing, nutrition and dentition. Physiotherapists and occupational therapists

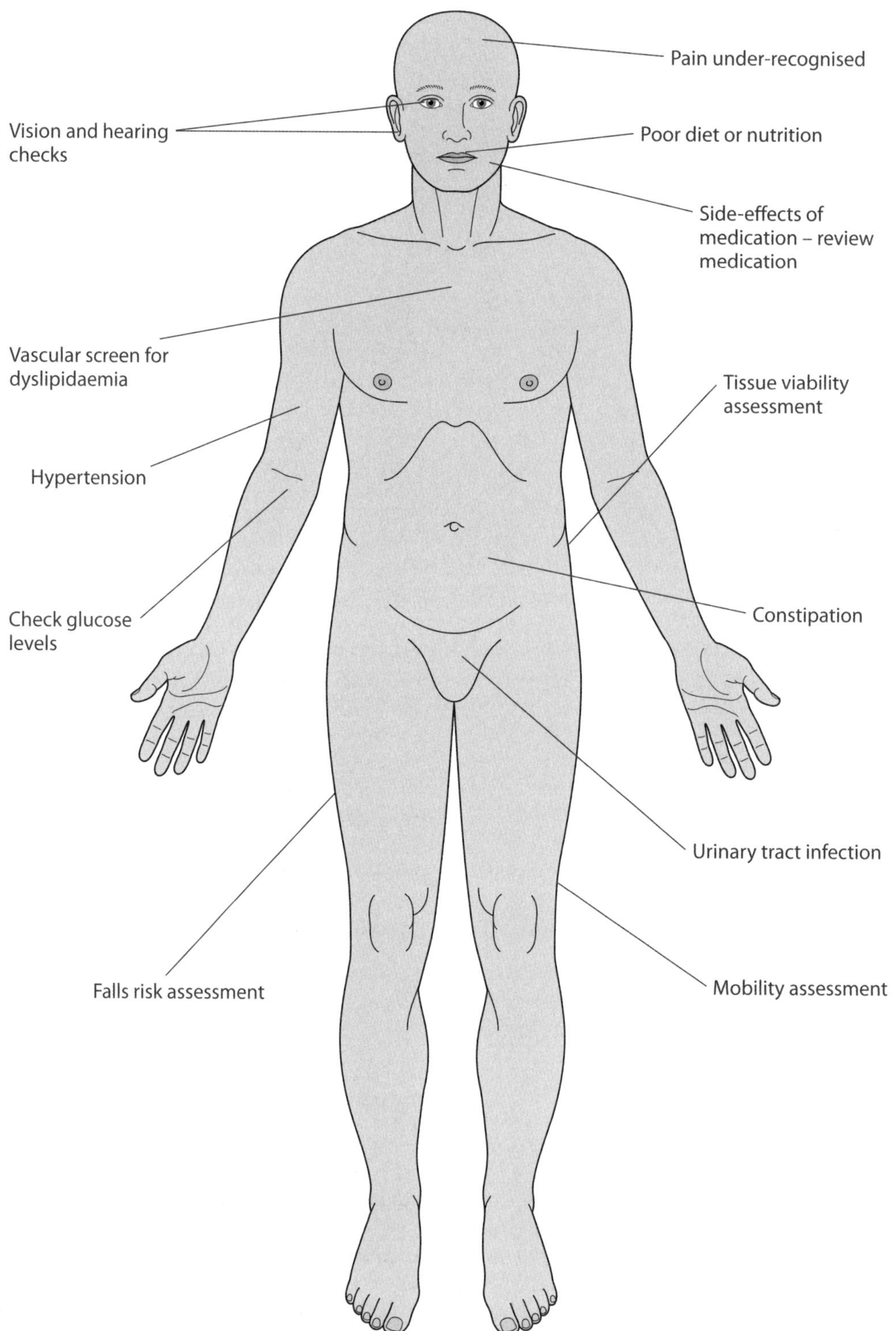

Fig. 29.1 Health risks in the elderly that need to be checked.

are valuable in assessment and management. Screening for vascular risk includes glucose and lipid levels, although in people aged 85 or more with no history of cardiovascular disease classical vascular risk factors, including the Framingham risk score (see Chapter 12), may not be a good predictor of cardiovascular mortality.[48]

Risk assessment includes mobility, falls, pressure sores and continence, particularly for people with dementia. Admitting a person with dementia to an unfamiliar environment like hospital may increase risk. A thorough review and rationalisation of medicines should give consideration to compliance, drug interactions and risk.

Hospitals are dangerous places for older people, as they expose them to an unfamiliar environment and risk of infection and accident. Infections, falls and constipation are particularly common. Poor diet (see below), dentition, lack of exercise and drugs contribute to constipation, which becomes more common with increasing age.[49] It is a cause of pain, behaviour disorder and faecal smearing in people with more severe dementia. Knowing the evidence base for rational investigation and treatment of infection and constipation is important.

Pain is underrecognised and undertreated in people with dementia and may manifest as behaviour disturbance.[50] People with dementia admitted to hospital with hip fracture are half as likely to receive pain relief as people without dementia undergoing the same procedure.[51]

Developing simple protocols for common physical illness with a physician colleague and close liaison with a geriatrician can improve physical healthcare and outcome.

General hospitals

Two-thirds of National Health Service beds are occupied by people over the age of 65. Up to 60% of this age group admitted to general hospital will have or will acquire a mental disorder during an acute hospital admission. In turn, mental disorder is an independent predictor of poor outcome in terms of mortality, length of stay, loss of independent function and institutionalisation.[52]

Liaison psychiatry services for older people are increasingly common and improve outcome, partly because general care teams have very limited mental health expertise.[53,54] Psychiatrists working with older people in the general hospital will encounter serious comorbidity and will need considerable knowledge and skill in both physical and mental health; they should liaise closely with medical and surgical colleagues.[55]

When older people with mental health problems are discharged to the community there needs to be careful planning and coordination of services. Mental illness is a predictor of readmission and further use of healthcare services.[56,57]

Liaison services are a good way of forming strong relationships with medical and surgical colleagues. They also improve the quality of care in general hospitals.[58]

Care homes

Of those in care homes, 50–80% suffer dementia and up to 40% depression.

Care home workers receive very little training yet care for people with complex comorbidity and disability.[59] People with dementia are often prescribed antipsychotic drugs inappropriately and without review, for example in place of good, stimulating, person-centred care. Antipsychotic drugs increase mortality and can lead to serious decline in physical health. The indications for prescribing them are clear in national guidelines, which should be followed.[9] Continuation should be reviewed after 3 months and drug withdrawal considered.[60]

Community matrons focus on long-term conditions to prevent admission to hospital. They review people in care homes routinely but generally have little knowledge of mental health. Developing a parallel mental health process of care-home liaison teams to work alongside them would provide high-quality coordinated physical and mental healthcare. Care-home liaison has been shown to improve quality of life and reduce antipsychotic drug prescribing, GP time and days spent in hospital.[61,62]

General health

Advice on healthy living applies as much to older as younger adults. In a large study of people originally enrolled in the Cardiovascular Health Study, five lifestyle factors (exercise, diet, smoking, alcohol intake and body mass index) accounted for 89% of new cases of diabetes mellitus developing after age 65.[63] Preventing, improving and optimally treating physical illness contribute to the prevention and treatment of mental illness and *vice versa*.

A healthy diet is a basic requirement but difficult for some older people, particularly those who are mentally ill, isolated or disabled. Access to, preparation and cost of healthy food can be a problem with low income, disability or being unable to shop. Limited exposure to sunlight makes the housebound or those in care vulnerable to vitamin D deficiency. Food and vitamin supplements are needed by some. Studies show that at least 10% of people over the age of 65 in the UK are at medium or high risk of malnutrition; single-nutrient deficiencies are much more common, with 29% of independent older people and 35% of those in institutions being folate deficient, and 14% and 40% vitamin C deficient, respectively; 10–60% of older people in hospitals and care homes are malnourished and 70–80% of those with malnutrition leave hospital without that diagnosis having been made.[64] The number of undernourished older people leaving National Health Service hospitals increased 85% in the 10 years up to 2005.[65]

Exercise is important for health and can be more difficult for older people. Maintaining mobility is also critical for independence and quality of life. There is evidence that exercise helps prevent and treat depression in later life.

Alcohol use disorders are common but underrecognised. They may lead to cognitive impairment and depression; patients tend to present with deteriorating physical health. Alcohol withdrawal is more severe and prolonged in older people. Treatment is equally important in later life but approaches to detection, defining safe drinking limits and intervention may be different.[66]

Palliative care is often needed and people with dementia who develop other terminal illnesses receive less palliative care, including pain relief, than people without dementia.[67] It is valuable to involve palliative care teams early and agree approaches to treatment and where care should be provided.

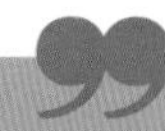

Summary

Multimorbidity of physical and mental illness characterises later life. The diagnosis of late-onset mental disorder will always require appreciation of physical health, and medical investigation and treatment plans will incorporate physical and mental health needs. The prevention and treatment of physical illness will reduce the risk of mental illness and improve recovery and *vice versa.* With comorbidity it is vital to consider the effects of both conditions and ensure treatment of one does not make the other worse.

The interplay between physical and mental healthcare is more obvious on a day-to-day basis in the psychiatry of later life than in other psychiatry specialties. Those working with older people will need to have developed knowledge and skills in both areas of healthcare, and the diagnosis, assessment and management of older people will require a more sophisticated appreciation of their interaction.

The complexity of treatment, the prescribing of drugs and their effect on physical health require careful thought, a broad knowledge and close collaboration with primary and secondary care and with other specialists, both in the community and in hospitals. With an ageing population there will be need of more care professionals with this range of skills.

References

1 Ostling S, Palsson SP, Skoog I. The incidence of first onset psychotic symptoms and paranoid ideation in a representative population sample followed from age 70–90 years: relation to mortality and later development of dementia. *Int J Geriatr Psychiatry* 2007; **22**: 520–8.

2 Anderson D. Clinical assessment and differential diagnosis. In *Principles and Practice of Geriatric Psychiatry* (eds M Abou-Saleh, C Katona, A Kumar): 599–603. John Wiley, 2010.

3 Fortin M, Soubhi H, Hudon C, *et al.* Multimorbidity's many challenges: time to focus on the needs of this vulnerable and growing population. *BMJ* 2007; **334**: 1016–17.

4 Fortin M, Bravo G, Hudon C, *et al.* Prevalence of multimorbidity among adults seen in family practice. *Ann Fam Med* 2005; **3**: 223–8.

5 Ryan J, Carriere I, Ritchie K, *et al.* Late-life depression and mortality: influence of gender and antidepressant use. *Br J Psychiatry* 2008; **192**: 12–8.

6 Van der Kooy K, Van Hout H, Marwijk H, *et al.* Depression and the risk for cardiovascular disease: a systematic review and meta-analysis. *Int J Geriatr Psychiatry* 2007; **22**: 613–26.

7 Anderson D, George J. Psychiatry. In *Practical Geriatric Problems in Primary Care* (eds M Gosney, T Harris): 271–300. Oxford University Press, 2010.

8 Knapp M, Prince M, Albanese E, *et al. Dementia UK: The Full Report.* Alzheimer's Society, 2007.

9 National Institute for Health and Clinical Excellence. *Dementia: Supporting People with Dementia and Their Carers in Health and Social Care.* Clinical Guideline CG42. NICE, 2006.

Learning points

- If older people say they are ill, they usually are – they tend not to feign illness.
- Any change in an older person's behaviour or function usually signifies a new morbid process.
- Beware of short psychiatric histories; the patient is usually physically ill.
- Prescribing is an opportunity to stop and review medications.
- Psychotropic drugs must be introduced carefully and gently.
- Always try to simplify medication regimens.
- If new symptoms follow a newly prescribed drug, stop it.
- Always check thyroid function.
- Prostatism and hot weather can lead to lithium toxicity.
- Do not forget the importance of eyes, ears, teeth, feet and bowels.
- Very demented people communicate pain and distress by behaviour disturbance.
- Do not miss delirium.
- Develop a general hospital liaison psychiatry team to improve relationships with medical and surgical colleagues.

10 Kivipelto M, Helkala EL, Laakso MP, *et al.* Midlife vascular risk factors and Alzheimer's disease in later life: longitudinal, population based study. *BMJ* 2001; **322**: 1447–51.

11 Strachan MWJ, Price JF, Frier BM. Diabetes, cognitive impairment and dementia. *BMJ* 2008; **336**: 6.

12 Anderson D. Preventing delirium in older people. *Br Med Bull* 2005; **73**: 1–10.

13 National Institute for Health and Clinical Excellence. *Parkinson's Disease: National Clinical Guidelines for Diagnosis and Management in Primary and Secondary Care.* NICE, 2006.

14 Miyasaki JM, Shannon K, Voon V, *et al.* Practice parameter: evaluation and treatment of depression, psychosis and dementia in Parkinson's disease (an evidence based review) – report of the Quality Standards Subcommittee of the American Academy of Neurology. *Neurology* 2006; **66**: 996–1002.

15 Giovannoni G, O'Sullivan JD, Turner K, *et al.* Hedonistic homeostatic dysregulation in patients with Parkinson's disease on dopamine replacement therapies. *J Neurol Neurosurg Psychiatry* 2000; **68**: 423–8.

16 McKeith I. Dementia with Lewy bodies and Parkinson's disease with dementia: where two worlds collide. *Pract Neurol* 2007; **7**: 374–82.

17 McKeith IG, Dickson DW, Lowe J, *et al.* Diagnosis and management of dementia with Lewy bodies: third report of the DLB consortium. *Neurology* 2005; **65**: 1863–72.

18 Menza M, Dobkin RD, Marin H, *et al.* A controlled trial of antidepressants in patients with Parkinson's disease and depression. *Neurology* 2009; **72**: 886–92.

19 Barone P, Scarzella L, Marconi R, *et al.* Pramipexole versus sertraline in the treatment of depression in Parkinson's disease. *J Neurol* 2006; **253**: 601–7.

20 Purandare N, Burns A, Daly KJ, *et al.* Cerebral emboli as a potential cause of Alzheimer's disease and vascular dementia: case-controlled study. *BMJ* 2006; **332**: 1119–22.

21 Glassman AH, O'Connor CM, Califf RM, *et al.* Sertraline treatment of major depression in patients with acute MI or unstable angina. *JAMA* 2002; **288**: 701–9.

22 Lesperance F, Frasure-Smith N, Koszycki D, *et al.* Effects of citalopram and interpersonal psychotherapy on depression in patients with coronary artery disease: the Canadian Cardiac Randomised Evaluation of Antidepressant and Psychotherapy Efficacy (CREATE) trial. *JAMA* 2007; **297**: 367–79.

23 Berkman LF, Blumenthal J, Burg M, *et al.* Effects of treating depression and low perceived social support on clinical events after myocardial infarction: the Enhancing Recovery in Coronary Heart Disease Patients (ENRICHD) Randomised Trial. *JAMA* 2003; **289**: 3106–16.

24 Serebruany VL, Suckow RF, Cooper TB, *et al.* Sertraline Antidepressant Heart Attack Randomised Trial: Relationship between release of platelet/endothelial biomarkers and plasma levels of sertraline and N-desmethylsertraline in acute coronary syndrome patients receiving SSRI treatment for depression. *Am J Psychiatry* 2005; **162**: 1165–70.

25 Price A, Rayner L, Okon-Rocha E, *et al.* Antidepressants for the treatment of depression in neurological disorders: a systematic review and meta-analysis of randomised controlled trials. *J Neurol Neurosurg Psychiatry* 2011; **82**: 914–23.

26 Narushima K, Paradiso S, Moser DJ, *et al.* Effect of antidepressant therapy on executive function after stroke. *Br J Psychiatry* 2007; **190**: 260–5.

27 Raine R, Wong W, Ambler G, *et al.* Sociodemographic variations in the contribution of secondary drug prevention to stroke survival at middle and older ages: cohort study. *BMJ* 2009; **338**: b1279.

28 Alexopoulos GS, Meyers BS, Young RC, *et al.* 'Vascular depression' hypothesis. *Arch Gen Psychiatry* 1997; **54**: 915–22.

29 Toedorczuk A, O'Brien JT, Firbank MJ, *et al.* White matter changes and late-life depressive symptoms: longitudinal study. *Br J Psychiatry* 2007; **191**: 212–7.

30 Taragano FE, Allegri R, Vicario A, *et al.* A double-blind randomized clinical trial assessing the efficacy and safety of augmenting standard antidepressant therapy with nimodipine in the treatment of 'vascular depression'. *Int J Geriatr Psychiatry* 2001; **16**: 254–60.

31 Teper E, O'Brien JT. Vascular factors and depression. *Int J Geriatr Psychiatry* 2008; **23**: 993–1000.

32 Sirey JA, Raue PJ, Alexopoulos GS. An intervention to improve depression care in older adults with COPD. *Int J Geriatr Psychiatry* 2007; **22**: 154–9.

33 Heinrich TW, Grahm G. Hypothyroidism presenting as psychosis: myxoedema madness revisited. *Prim Care Companion J Clin Psychiatry* 2003; **5**: 260–6.

34 Gebo KA. HIV infection in older people. *BMJ* 2009; **338**: b1460.

35 Walker Z, Jaros E, Walker RWH, *et al.* Dementia with Lewy bodies: a comparison of clinical diagnosis, FP-CIT single photon emission tomography imaging and autopsy. *J Neurol Neurosurg Psychiatry* 2007; **78**: 1176–81.

36 O'Brien JT, McKeith IG, Walker Z, *et al.* Diagnostic accuracy of ^{123}I-FP-CIT SPECT in possible dementia with Lewy bodies. *Br J Psychiatry* 2009; **194**: 34–9.

37 Zhang M, Holman C, D'Arcy J, *et al.* Comorbidity and repeat admission to hospital for adverse drug reactions in older adults: retrospective cohort study. *BMJ* 2009; **338**: a2752.

38 Rollason V, Vogt N. Reduction of polypharmacy in the elderly: a systematic review. *Drugs Ageing* 2003; **20**: 817–32.

39 Milton JC, Hill-Smith I, Jackson SHD. Prescribing for older people. *BMJ* 2008; **336**: 606–9.

40 Banerjee S. *The Use of Antipsychotic Medication for People with Dementia: Time for Action.* Department of Health, 2009.

41 Committee on Safety of Medicines. *Atypical Antipsychotic Drugs and Stroke.* Department of Health, 2004.

42 Schneider LS, Dagerman KS, Insel P. Risk of death with atypical antipsychotic drug treatment for dementia: meta-analysis of randomized placebo controlled trials. *JAMA* 2005; **294**: 1934–43.

43 Ray WA, Chung CP, Murray KT, *et al.* Atypical antipsychotic drugs and the risk of sudden cardiac death. *New Engl J Med* 2009; **360**: 225–35.

44 Holt R. The metabolic side-effects of antipsychotics in elderly patients. *Geriatr Med* 2008; **July**: 399–402.

45 Kirby D, Ames D. Hyponatraemia and selective serotonin reuptake inhibitors in elderly patients. *Int J Geriatr Psychiatry* 2001; **16**: 484–93.

46 Abajo F, Garcia-Rodriguez L. Risk of upper gastrointestinal tract bleeding associated with selective serotonin reuptake inhibitors and venlafaxine. *Arch Gen Psychiatry* 2008; **65**: 795–803.

47 Wanless D, Forder J, Fernandez J-L, *et al. Securing Good Care for Older People: Taking a Long Term View.* King's Fund, 2006.

48 De Ruijter W, Westendorp RJG, Assendelft WJJ, *et al.* Risk of Framingham risk score and new biomarkers to predict cardiovascular mortality in older people: population based observational cohort study. *BMJ* 2009; **338**: a3083.

49 McCallum IJD, Ong S, Mercer-Jones M. Chronic constipation in adults. *BMJ* 2009; **338**: b831.

50 Department of Health. *Living Well with Dementia: A National Dementia Strategy.* TSO (The Sationery Office), 2009.

51 Morrison RS, Siu AL. A comparison of pain and its treatment in advanced dementia and cognitively intact patients with hip fracture. *J Pain Symptom Manage* 2000; **19**: 240–8.

52 Royal College of Psychiatrists. *Who Cares Wins: Improving the Outcome for Older People Admitted to the General Hospital – Guidelines for the Development of Liaison Mental Health Services for Older People.* Faculty Report. Royal College of Psychiatrists, 2005.

53 Anderson D. Liaison psychiatry and mental disorder in older general hospital patients. *CME Geriatr Med* 2005; **7**: 65–69.

54 Royal College of Psychiatrists Centre for Quality Improvement. *Report of the National Audit of Dementia Care in General Hospitals 2011.* Healthcare Quality Improvement Partnership, 2011.'

54 Anderson D, Ooman S. Liaison psychiatry and older people. In *Seminars in Liaison Psychiatry,* 2nd edn (eds E Guthrie, S Rao, M Temple): 265–87. RCPsych Publications, 2012.

55 Kominski G, Andersen R, Bastani R, *et al.* UPBEAT: the impact of psychogeriatric intervention in VA medical centers. *Med Care* 2001; **39**: 500–12.

56 Wilson K, Mottram P, Hussein M. Survival in the community of the very old discharged from medical inpatient care. *Int J Geriatr Psychiatry* 2007; **22**: 974–9.

57 Anderson D. Liaison with medical and surgical teams. In *Principles and Practice of Geriatric Psychiatry* (eds M Abou-Saleh, C Katona, A Kumar): 803–9. John Wiley, 2010.

58 Alzheimer's Society. *Home from Home.* Alzheimer's Society, 2008.

59 Banerjee S. *The Use of Antipsychotic Medication for People with Dementia: Time for Action.* Department of Health, 2009.

60 Ballard C, Powell I, James I, *et al.* Can psychiatric liaison reduce neuroleptic use and reduce health service utilization for dementia patients residing in care facilities? *Int J Geriatr Psychiatry* 2002; **17**: 140–5.

61 Fossey J, Ballard C, Juszczak E, *et al.* Effect of enhanced psychosocial care on antipsychotic use in nursing home residents with severe dementia: cluster randomized trial. *BMJ* 2006; **332**: 756–8.

62 Mozaffarian D, Kamineni A, Carnethon M, *et al.* Lifestyle risk factors and new onset diabetes mellitus in older adults. *Arch Intern Med* 2009; **169**: 798–807.

63 Anderson D, Abou Saleh MT. Nutrition state. In *Principles and Practice of Geriatric Psychiatry* (eds M Abou-Saleh, C Katona, A Kumar): 824–8. John Wiley, 2010.

64 Age Concern. *Hungry to be Heard: The Scandal of Malnourished Older People in Hospital.* Age Concern England, 2006.

65 O'Connell H, Chin A-V, Cunningham C, *et al.* Alcohol use disorders in elderly people – redefining an age old problem. *BMJ* 2003; **327**: 664–7.

66 Sampson EL, Gould V, Blanchard MR, *et al.* Differences in care received by patients with and without dementia who died during acute hospital admission: a retrospective case note study. *Age Ageing* 2006; **35**: 187–9.

30

Physical effects of eating disorders

Sabine Woerwag-Mehta, Iain C. Campbell and Janet Treasure

Eating disorders can affect the physical health of individuals. This chapter describes: how to evaluate the impact of eating disorders on physical health, including the extent of nutritional compromise; how eating disorders may affect the body; the key findings on physical examination; and how to manage refeeding when this is indicated.

Introduction

This chapter provides guidance on the assessment and evaluation of the physical status of patients with eating disorders and the physical complications encountered. Physical symptoms may play a key role in motivation to change and engagement in therapy.

Eating disorders include *anorexia nervosa*, *bulimia nervosa* and the most common presentation in all age groups, *eating disorder not otherwise specified* (EDNOS), that is, eating disorders which do not strictly fulfil diagnostic criteria (ICD-10 or DSM-IV) for either anorexia nervosa or bulimia nervosa. In contrast to those with anorexia nervosa, adolescents with bulimia nervosa or EDNOS often appear physically healthy, with few symptoms and signs of physical illness.

When do eating disorders appear?

The onset of anorexia nervosa is commonly in adolescence, with a peak age between 15 and 18 years of age, but it can occur as early as 8 years of age; the peak presentation for bulimia nervosa is slightly later, in early adulthood. Anorexia nervosa has a lifetime prevalence of 0.9–2.2% in women and 0.2–0.3% in men; bulimia nervosa is more common and has a lifetime prevalence of 1.5–2% in females and 0.5% in males.[1] The incidence of bulimia nervosa is almost 2.5 times higher in urbanised than in rural areas and 5 times higher in large cities.[2]

The consequences of eating disorders

All eating disorders have major consequences for the individual. Anorexia nervosa:

- is potentially life-threatening
- often runs a chronic relapsing course
- frequently has residual symptoms,[3] despite 66% recovery in the long term[4]
- is associated with a high rate of suicide, with the highest mortality ratio of any psychiatric illness[5,6]
- has a median duration of 6 years
- among all the psychiatric disorders, is second only to schizophrenia in terms of time spent in in-patient settings[7]

Adolescents with bulimia nervosa and eating disorders not otherwise specified often appear physically healthy, with few symptoms and signs of physical illness.

- is associated with high levels of comorbidity
- can pose a substantial burden to carers, relatives, health services and financial resources.

Only a minority of those with the condition seek treatment.[8]

Physical effects of eating disorders

The calorie–protein malnutrition caused by eating disorders affects all organs. Physical symptoms are common in the acute and chronic state and short and long-term physical complications (Table 30.1) can occur. It is important to spot dangerous and life-threatening physical symptoms early and try to prevent long-term chronic complications and physical disabilities. An organic cause should always be considered for unexplained weight loss and a thorough medical investigation carried out before the diagnosis of an eating disorder is made.

Table 30.1 Physical complications in eating disorders in binge-purging anorexia nervosa, anorexia nervosa, bulimia and eating disorder not otherwise specified

System	Acute physical complications	Chronic complications
Metabolic	Hypoglycaemia; hypophosphataemia; osteopenia	Amenorrhoea; polycystic ovaries; hypothyroidism; ⇧ cortisol; inappropriate antidiuretic hormone (ADH) secretion
Metabolic	⇩ Sodium, potassium, phosphate, calcium, chloride, magnesium and zinc	⇧ Free fatty acids; hyper- or hypocholesterolaemia; osteoporosis
Cardiovascular	Hypotension; arrhythmias; electrocardiographic changes	⇩ Cardiac index, blood pressure and heart rate; ⇩ left ventricular mass; ⇩ left ventricular end systolic and diastolic diameter; ⇔ ejection fraction; ⇧ peripheral resistance; congestive heart failure; mitral valve prolapse; pericardial effusion; refeeding oedema
Pulmonary	Pneumothorax; pneumomediastinum	
Gastrointestinal	Haematemesis; gastroduodenal ulcer; ⇩ motility	Mallory–Weiss syndrome; pancreatitis; steatohepatitis; superior mesenteric artery syndrome; enlarged parotid glands
Renal	⇧ Urea and creatinine; oliguria, anuria	Pre-renal and renal failure
Neurological	Metabolic seizures; metabolic encephalopathy	Anomalies on computerised tomography, magnetic resonance imaging, positron emission tomography; cognitive impairment
Immunological		⇩ Cellular immunity; ⇩ complement factors
Dermatological		Russell's sign; dry skin; brittle and lanugo hair, hair loss; brittle nails; yellowish skin (hypercarotenaemia); dental erosions; petechiae; acrocyanosis; pitting oedema; erythema ab igne; acrodermatitis; pellagra; scurvy

Key: ⇩ Decreased ; ⇧ increased; ⇔ unchanged.
Source: Woerwag-Mehta *et al*, 2010.[9] Reproduced with permission.

Table 30.2 Physical findings that can be used to evaluate medical severity or nutritional compromise in people with eating disorders

	Examination	Moderate risk	High risk
Nutrition	Body mass index (BMI) (kg/m^2)	< 15	< 13.5
	BMI centile	< 3	< 2
	Weight loss per week (kg)	> 0.5	> 1.0
	Purpuric rash		+
Circulation	Systolic blood pressure (mmHg)	< 90	< 80
	Diastolic blood pressure (mmHg)	< 60	< 50
	Postural drop (mmHg)	> 10	> 20
	Pulse rate (beats per min)	< 55	< 50
	Oxygen saturation		< 90%
	Extremities		Oedematous
Core temperature		< 35.5 °C	< 34.5 °C
Investigations	Full blood count, urea, electrolytes (including PO_4), liver functions tests, albumin, creatinine kinase, glucose	Concern if outside normal limits	K < 3.0 mmol/l; Na < 135 mmol/l; PO_4 < 0.8 mmol/l
	Electrocardiography	Rate < 60	Rate < 50

Source: Woerwag-Mehta *et al*, 2010.[9] Reproduced with permission.

There are several physical parameters that can be used to evaluate medical severity or nutritional compromise in people with eating disorders (Table 30.2).

Physical examination

The physical examination is an important part of an eating disorder assessment. It should be performed when the patient first presents and repeated if there are new or changing physical symptoms or any rapid decrease or increase in weight. Be aware that symptoms may not always be reported due to malnutrition, embarrassment, stoicism, denial, lack of energy and depression. Patients may consider the physical examination as unimportant or invasive and may be concerned about the resulting treatment or outcome and feel criticised.

Before the physical examination is begun, explain its purpose to the patient and reach an agreement about its extent. It is advisable to conduct it in the presence of someone trusted by the patient. The examination room should provide privacy and allow the patient to feel comfortable. An evaluation of the degree of emaciation and other physical signs while the patient remains fully dressed is difficult. An eating disorder examination does not include a rectal, pelvic or breast examination.

Observe the patient's general appearance, strength, steadiness, movement and gait and their affect and behaviour with those who have accompanied them.

The physical examination should include:

- weight, height and calculation of body mass index (BMI – see below)
- muscle strength
- the cardiovascular, respiratory, abdominal and central nervous systems
- skin, oropharynx and teeth.

Anthropometry (discussed below) is an accurate and reliable method to estimate body fat but requires expertise and training. The most commonly used parameter to determine a patient's risk in terms of weight loss and response to treatment is therefore BMI,

Symptoms in eating disorders may not always be reported due to malnutrition, embarrassment, stoicism, denial, lack of energy and depression.

which is calculated, using the same equipment and at the same time of day each time, as follows.

Height measurement

Read and apply the instructions given for the equipment and ensure the scale is installed correctly, or ask a colleague familiar with the scale to show how to use it. The general rules are:

- ask the patient to remove shoes and stand with heels, buttock and shoulders in line, facing the measurement tool
- the patient's back and head should be straight and the arms hanging loosely at the sides with palms facing the thighs
- the patient should take a deep breath to help straighten the spine
- take the reading in metres at the highest point of the skull.

Weight measurement

The scale should be placed on a hard, flat surface. It should be calibrated accurately at zero before use. Measure the weight before a meal and ask the patient to empty the bladder before the measurement. Shoes should be removed, as should clothing (except underwear and shirt). The patient should stand unassisted, as still as possible, in the middle of the platform. Read the weight and record in kilograms.

Body mass index

A BMI chart is available at http://nhlbisupport.com/bmi/bmi-m.htm (imperial measure equivalent at www.caloriecounting.co.uk/resources/charts/bmi.htm). It is calculated by dividing the patient's weight (in kilograms) by the square of the height (in metres) and so is clinically easy to establish. Body mass index has become the standard measure to assess obesity and underweight states even though it gives no indication of body composition, making simplistic assumptions about the distribution of muscle, bone and fat mass; this may lead to false health evaluations of both under- and overweight states. For example, athletes who have a high lean body mass have a high BMI but are not obese and elderly people (who generally have low muscle bulk and bone density) may have a low BMI but still be obese (see p. 17). Body mass index is difficult to interpret in young children who are growing or whose height is stunted by illness.

Weight measurement may be very stressful for a patient with an eating disorder and some will try artificially to raise their weight by drinking a lot of water, binge-eating or wearing hidden heavy items.

BMI percentiles

The growth of children is usually documented against a BMI growth chart, which allows comparison with typical values for other children of the same age. A BMI below the 5th percentile is considered underweight and above the 95th percentile obese. To determine whether children, young adolescents and short people are growing normally, the BMI percentile rather than BMI should be followed over time; a change in a patient's percentile is a more accurate indicator of weight loss or gain than BMI (see p. 338).

Anthropometry

Estimates of total body fat by anthropometry can be accurate, reliable and inexpensive, but without training and experience such anthropometric measurements are not reliable. The most important skill to learn is how to determine the measurement site and how much tissue to 'pinch'. The callipers should measure the thickness of the skin *and* subcutaneous tissue, not just skin, and must not include muscle.

The cardiovascular system

Cardiovascular impairment as a consequence of eating disorders is based on:

- loss of cardiac muscle through starvation
- an imbalance between cardiac sympathetic and parasympathetic nervous system activity
- acute and chronic depletion of intravascular volume, due to hypovolaemia, with increased peripheral resistance
- electrolyte disturbances.

Cardiac complications pose an acute and life-threatening risk in eating disorders, causing one-third of adult deaths. In adolescents, functional and structural cardiac anomalies are already present in the early stages of illness,[10] but appear to resolve when treated early.[11]

Owing to the adaptive mechanisms of starvation, most malnourished patients present with a slow heart rate (60–80 beats per minute) and low systolic blood pressure.

Common clinical cardiovascular findings in anorexia nervosa include the following.

- *Low blood pressure due to reduced stroke volume.* This requires close monitoring. A clinical picture of tachycardia in combination with low systolic pressure suggests acute fluid loss or heart failure and should be investigated urgently. Sinus bradycardia (i.e. a cardiac rate below 60 beats/min) is due to an increase in vagal tone[12,13] and electrocardiographic (ECG) monitoring should be considered. With *extreme* sinus bradycardia (a heart rate less than 50 beats/min during the day or less than 45 beats/min at night), admission to hospital for cardiac monitoring and gradual weight gain is recommended.[14]
- *Potentially fatal arrhythmias*, mainly due to electrolyte disturbances (most commonly hypokalaemia and hypophosphataemia), require instant assessment by a medical team.
- *Pericardial effusion.* This is often a silent finding, which resolves spontaneously and does not compromise cardiac function. Inflammatory markers and protein status should be checked to rule out infection and hypoalbuminaemia.
- *Loss of cardiac muscle and decreased thickness of the left ventricular wall.* These occur due to starvation. Reduced cardiac output has been documented in anorexia nervosa before treatment.[15] These findings resolve with gradual weight restoration.[16]
- *Changes in orthostatic heart rate and blood pressure.* These may occur due to decreased venous return as a result of atrophic peripheral muscles and volume depletion, and present as syncope. They may resolve with weight gain and can be used as an objective measure of medical stability in anorexia nervosa.[17]
- *Mitral valve prolapse (MVP).* This is thought to develop as a result of reduced left ventricular mass and weight loss.[18] It has been found in up to 37% of patients with a history of anorexia nervosa and is strongly associated with cardiac arrhythmias, adding to risk.[19]

In addition, ECG abnormalities have been reported in 35–95% of patients.[20] Decreased voltage in all ECG leads requires clinical assessment for hydration status and cardiac output. A prolonged QTc (see Chapter 12) should be discussed with a cardiologist. Controversy surrounds the role and impact of prolonged QTc interval in eating disorders, which may be exacerbated by medications (e.g. antipsychotics).

In summary, cardiac complications can occur acutely and they can lead to death. The treatment approach should focus on gradual weight restoration with careful cardiac monitoring from the time of diagnosis to ensure safe restoration of cardiac function.[16] Cardiac complications should be discussed with a medical team.

Fluid and electrolytes

In patients with eating disorders, the main clinical features associated with fluid and electrolyte disturbances are hypo- and hypervolaemia:

- Hypovolaemia presents with dry skin, dry mucous membranes, cold and acrocyanotic extremities and delayed capillary refill time. Serum sodium tends to be in the upper normal range and urea and creatinine concentrations are normal or elevated.
- Hypervolaemia can present with electrolyte disturbances such as low to normal serum sodium levels. Hydration should be established gradually, since rapid rehydration can lead to dangerous volume overload, followed by cardiovascular collapse and heart failure, along with dangerous electrolyte disturbances.

Patients with binge-purging anorexia nervosa and bulimia nervosa may present with unpredictable metabolic changes, including hypokalaemia, hypochloraemia, metabolic alkalosis and hyperaldosteronism due to self-induced and often concealed vomiting. Serial measurements to evaluate fluid and electrolyte status are necessary. Laxative misuse and less commonly diuretic misuse may also contribute to electrolyte disturbances (e.g. laxative misuse may especially affect magnesium levels). Serum phosphate levels may rapidly fall in some patients with anorexia nervosa during refeeding and this can result in serious and dangerous complications, such as arrhythmias. This occurs usually in the first 2 weeks of treatment, so phosphate levels should regularly be checked when feeding is initiated.

The skeletal system

Common complications of eating disorders include the following:

- *Osteopenia.* This defined as a bone mineral density (BMD) 1–2.5 standard deviations (s.d.) below the

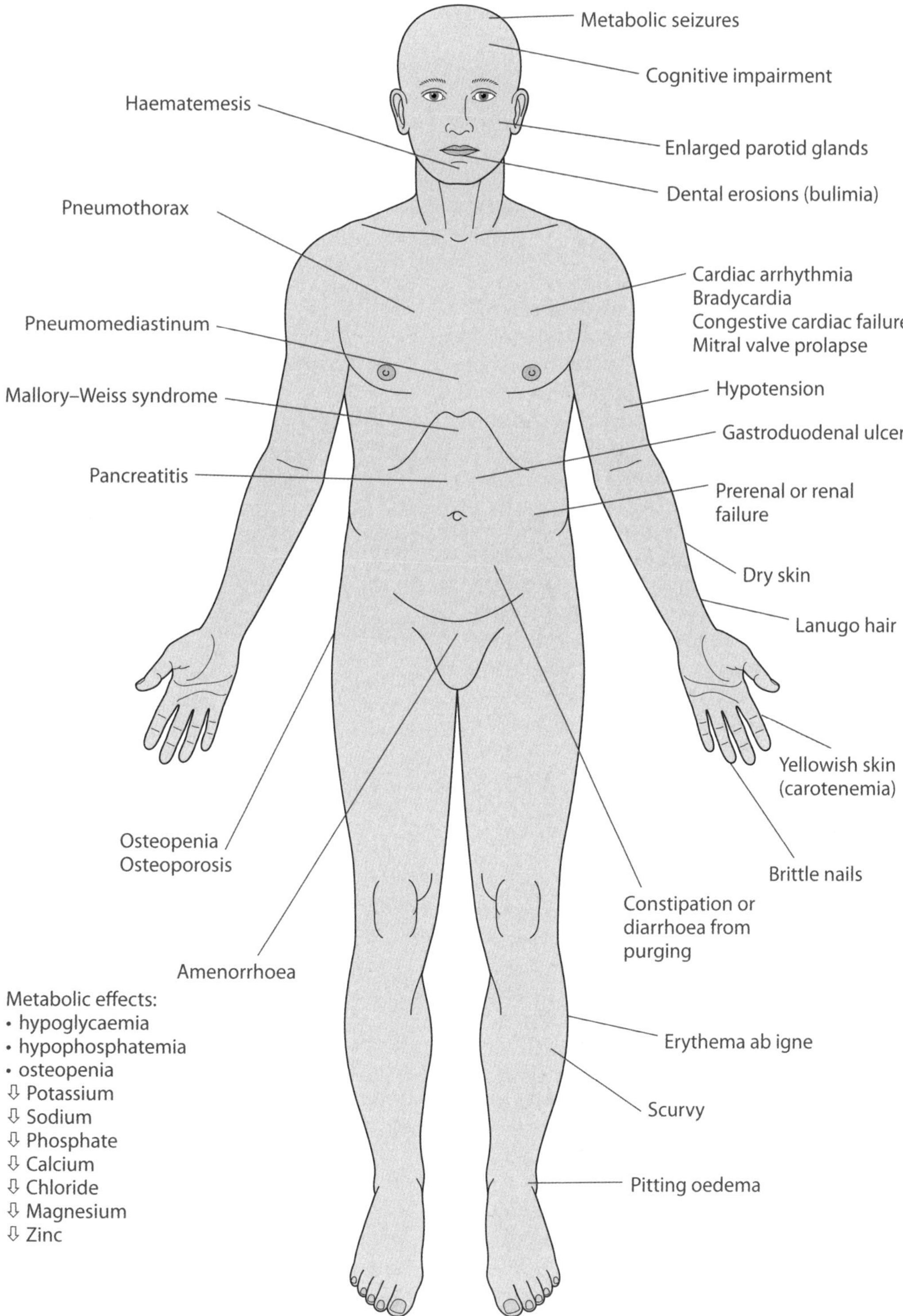

Fig. 30.1 Physical complications of anorexia nervosa, binge-purging anorexia nervosa, bulimia and eating disorders not otherwise specified.

Fracture risk doubles with each decrease of 1 s.d. in bone mass density. More than 50% of women with anorexia nervosa have a bone mass density below fracture threshold and 92% reach a bone density 1 s.d. below the norm.

mean peak bone density for age and gender, as measured by the gold standard dual-emission X-ray absorptiometry (DEXA) scanning.

- *Osteoporosis.* Osteoporosis often follows osteopenia. It is defined as 2.5 s.d. or more below the mean value of BMD for age and gender. It leads to long-term complications and disability,[16,21–26] with an increased rate of immobilising fractures, kyphoscoliosis and chronic pain.

Low BMD occurs early and bone loss is seen within 1 year in some patients. Cortical as well as trabecular bone is affected and there is a long-term risk of permanent bone loss. Lumbar spine, radius and proximal femur are the most commonly affected sites.[27,28] Fracture risk doubles with each decrease of 1 s.d. in BMD.[29] More than 50% of women with anorexia nervosa have a BMD below fracture threshold and 92% reach a bone density 1 s.d. below the norm.[30,31] The risk of fractures has been reported in several studies. Compared with healthy controls, the fracture rate is increased up to seven-fold in patients with a mean duration of anorexia nervosa of 5.8 years.[23]

The pathophysiological mechanisms leading to osteoporosis in anorexia nervosa are multifactorial and not fully understood.[32] Around 60–80% of the peak bone density is determined by genetic predisposition, while nutritional and hormonal factors account for the other 20–40%. Bone mineral density increases gradually during childhood and early adolescence, with peak bone density being achieved in healthy individuals at puberty.

Anorexia nervosa developing in early adolescence is associated with failure to achieve peak bone density, complete puberty and establish mature sexual function both in girls and boys. There is a much higher bone loss compared with those who develop anorexia nervosa in adulthood. At any age, eating disorders lead to an uncoupling of bone metabolism with suppression of bone formation as well as enhanced bone absorption, with a net decrease in bone turnover.[33,34]

Factors that predict development of osteoporosis are:

- low BMI
- low lean body mass and weight[30]
- onset at menarche
- onset, severity and type of eating disorder, with anorexia nervosa bearing the highest risk and worst outcomes.[35]

Until clinical trial results are available, three therapeutic strategies seem promising: first, enhancement and supplementation of nutrition, calcium supplementation and establishment of healthy weight; second, stimulation of bone formation; and third, suppression of bone absorption.

In summary, optimising bone growth and mineralisation is best achieved with weight restoration, the basis for the resumption of normal menstrual physiology. In addition, where diet does not provide adequate calcium and vitamin D, supplementation of the recommended daily allowance to a total daily intake of 1200–1500 mg calcium and 400 IU vitamin D should be considered optimal. Moderate weight-bearing exercise should be encouraged and resistance exercise should be promoted.

Gastrointestinal system

Gastrointestinal complaints and complications are common in eating disorders. Patients experience:

- post-prandial bloating
- oesophageal reflux
- constipation, with increased intestinal gas, faecal impaction, paradoxical diarrhoea and early satiety.

These symptoms occur due to reduced gastrointestinal motility with delayed gastric emptying. A range of symptoms are due to vomiting and purging; others are due to laxative misuse or the combination of both.

The effect of repeated vomiting

Repeated vomiting can cause the following:

- *Abnormal oesophageal peristalsis, decreased lower oesophageal sphincter tone, oesophageal reflux and oesophagitis.* The replacement of the normal epithelium of the oesophagus with squamous, pre-cancerous epithelium (Barrett's syndrome) requires

Repeated vomiting can cause acute gastro-oesophageal bleeding, oesophageal stricture and teeth staining, decalcification, erosion and loss.

endoscopic follow-up. Bisphosphonate treatment increases the risk of oesophagitis and oesophageal stricture.
- *Oesophageal tear* (Mallory–Weiss syndrome). This occurs at the junction of the stomach and the oesophagus and is caused by the physical trauma of vomiting; it can lead to significant gastrointestinal bleeding.
- *Gastric rupture* (Boerhaave syndrome). This may present with severe pain, sepsis and shock, and requires urgent surgical intervention.

Patients with binge-purging anorexia nervosa and bulimia nervosa may present with unpredictable metabolic changes, including hypokalaemia, hypochloraemia and metabolic alkalosis.

Chronic laxative use

This has a variety of effects, including:
- compromise of normal peristaltic function, leading to alternating episodes of diarrhoea and constipation
- gastrointestinal bleeding, with occult or frank blood loss
- weakness of the muscles of the pelvic floor, leading to rectal prolapse, faecal impaction and faecal incontinence.

Effects of eating disorders on the gastrointestinal system

Eating disorders can have a range of effects on the gastrointestinal system itself:
- *Enlarged parotid and submandibular glands.* This classical clinical finding can be caused by protein–calorie malnutrition. It resolves when the eating disorder is treated successfully.
- *Unilateral tender swelling of a parotid gland.* This, though, is rare. It is caused by infection (acute suppurative parotitis), for example with *Staphylococcus*. It can be prevented with adequate hydration and good mouth hygiene.
- *Fatty liver changes and gallstones.* These also occur rarely. They are due to hyperlipidaemia in the context of malnutrition and recurrent weight loss.
- *Acute or chronic pancreatitis.* Patients can present with recurrent and acute abdominal pain, nausea or vomiting. Measurements of serum amylase and lipase, in conjunction with ultrasound and computerised tomography scans establish the diagnosis. Excessive alcohol consumption or biliary tract disease should be explored as the underlying cause.

In addition, a foreign body or bezoar can cause acute and chronic gastrointestinal symptoms, ranging from feelings of discomfort and feeling bloated and nauseous to acute intestinal obstruction.

Perfusion of the superior mesenteric artery may be compromised in very low-weight patients (superior mesentery artery syndrome). Subsequent ischaemia of the upper intestinal tract may cause bloating and epigastric abdominal pain after eating. The diagnosis is confirmed on imaging by demonstrating a narrowed third part of the duodenum with proximal dilation of the bowel. Parenteral feeding may be required.

Type 1 diabetes mellitus and inflammatory bowel disease along with other organic illnesses may mimic or coexist with eating disorders. It is therefore important to initiate a thorough medical work-up as part of a psychiatric assessment.

Dental health

Decalcification, erosion and staining of the teeth, increased temperature sensitivity and caries, gum recession, gum friability and bleeding, tooth loss, and decalcification of the lingual, palatal and posterior occlusal teeth are caused by gastric acid during vomiting and poor nutrition. Amalgams are resistant to acid and become more obvious as enamel erosion progresses. Scurvy (vitamin C deficiency) causes swollen and bleeding gums.

Nervous system

Brain function and structure, spinal cord and muscles are affected by eating disorders:
- Muscle weakness is common, is usually due to malnutrition and improves with refeeding. Myopathy can occur due to deficiency of magnesium, calcium, potassium, phosphorus, vitamin C or protein–calorie malnutrition, and to major tranquillisers and ipecac. Smooth-muscle wasting (e.g. diaphragm, heart) is due to protein–calorie malnutrition.
- Cerebrovascular events are rare. Most central nervous system symptoms are reversible with weight gain

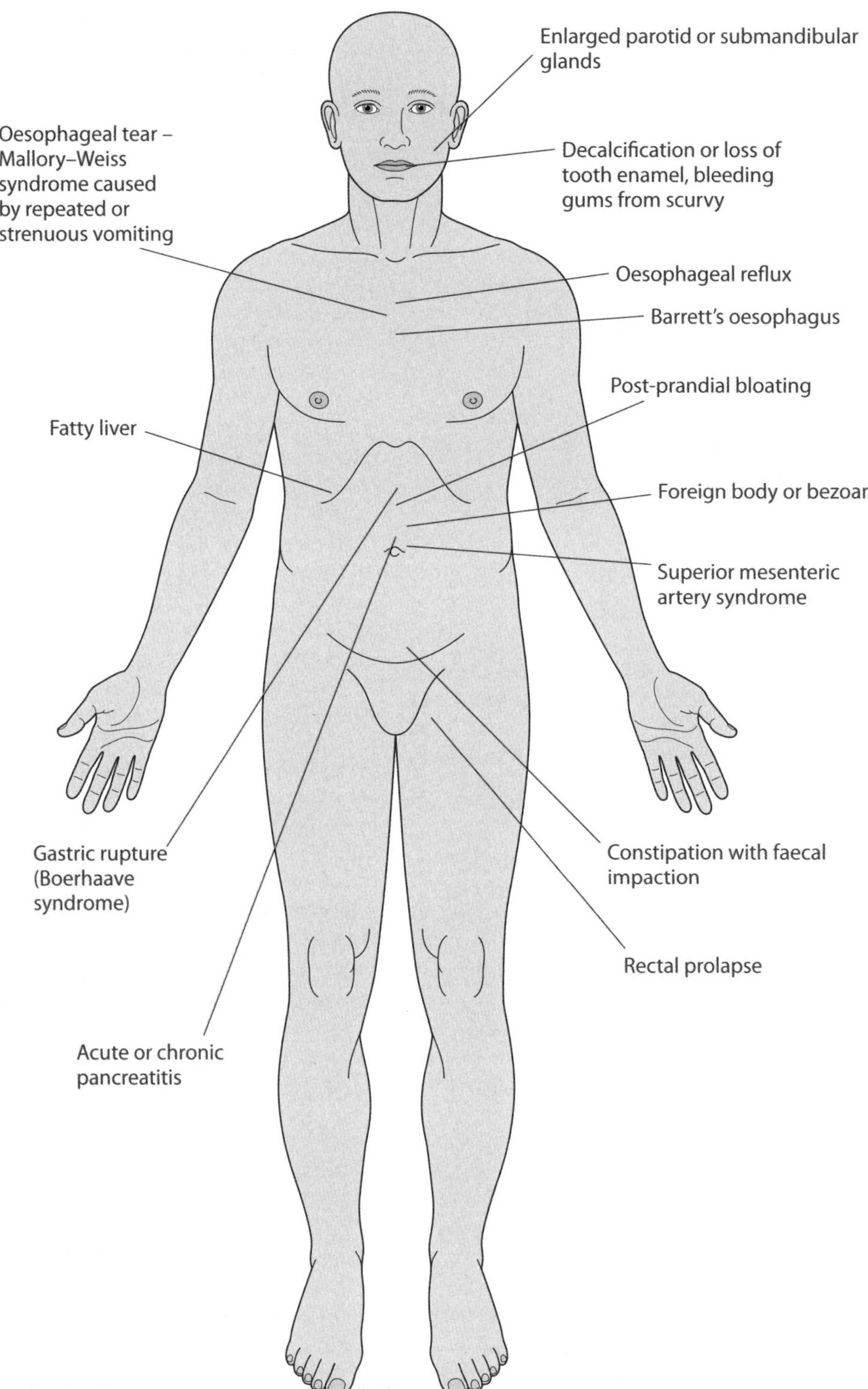

Fig. 30.2 Gastrointestinal complications of eating disorders.

Brain functions are affected by weight loss and are likely to recover with weight gain. Cognitive deficits due to vitamin deficiencies require early vitamin replacement therapy to achieve a good outcome. Patients at low weight may not be able to engage effectively in psychological interventions.

and respond to prompt recognition and treatment of protein–calorie malnutrition and deficiencies of magnesium, calcium, phosphorus, thiamine and vitamins C, B6 and B12.

- Organic brain syndrome caused by malnutrition is common and patients may be unable to understand complex concepts. Psychotherapy may therefore not be possible until the patient's cognition has improved. Structural changes of the brain occur predominantly on the right and involve prefrontal, temporal and mesiotemporal regions and the hypothalamus.[36] Volume reduction in the amygdala and hypocampal formation, changes to the pituitary gland,[37] enlarged ventricular volume, dilated sulci and reduction in both white and grey matter have been described. Despite good reversibility of white matter deficits with weight gain and normalisation of eating behaviours, significant grey-matter reduction can persist beyond recovery.[38–40]

Subacute combined degeneration of the cord can occur involving the dorsal column and pyramidal tract. It presents with impaired joint position and vibration sense and upper motor neuron weakness. When patients are most malnourished and particularly when they are sedated, attention must be given to preventing pressure sores and pressure neuropathies. Pressure neuropathies are most likely to occur over the ulnar nerve at the elbow, the radial nerve behind the upper arm, and the lateral peroneal nerve at the neck of the fibula. Neuropathy due to vitamin B12, pyridoxine and protein–calorie malnutrition and B vitamin excess can occur.

The endocrine system

Hypothalamus–pituitary axis dysfunction due to acute and chronic stress is thought to be the key aspect of endocrine dysfunction in eating disorders and may be mediated by dysregulation of corticotrophin-releasing hormone.[41] Delayed puberty is one of the cardinal complications in adolescents with anorexia nervosa and is defined as a delay of more than 2 s.d. beyond the mean for age and gender, with an absence of progression through expected sexual maturity rating stages. Evaluating delayed puberty involves obtaining a detailed history of all organ systems and conducting a thorough physical examination in the context of an assessment of growth pattern and a review of records of previous height and weight. A family history of growth pattern, including parental height measurements, is invaluable. Reports of pubertal development of both parents as well as maternal age of onset of menarche are important. A paediatric opinion is best sought for sexual maturity ratings and further endocrinology investigations. Some criteria for the assessment of delayed pubertal maturation in females and males are shown in Table 30.3.

Amenorrhoea is one of the ICD-10 and DSM-IV diagnostic criteria for anorexia nervosa. Both primary amenorrhoea (absence of menarche at the age of 16, or absent normal pubertal milestones at the age of 14) and secondary amenorrhoea (menstruation has ceased for 3 months in a female with a history of regular cyclical bleeding, or 6 months in a female with a history of irregular menstruation) can occur in eating

Table 30.3 Criteria for delayed puberty in females and males

Females	Males
Absence of breast development beyond age 13.5	Absence of testicular growth (> 2.5 ml) by age 14
Absence of pubic hair development beyond age 14	Absence of pubic hair development beyond age 15
Absence of menarche by age 16	
More than 5 years elapsed between breast development and menarche	More than 5 years elapsed from initiation and completion of testicular growth

disorders. With primary amenorrhoea, a careful medical assessment is necessary to rule out an organic cause.

Body mass index, calorie intake and exercise are strongly associated with menstrual dysfunction.[42] The weight required for menstruation to return is highly individual but can be predicted by the weight at which menstruation ceased.[43] Fat mass is important for preservation of normal menstrual function and this is in part mediated through leptin secretion.[44] Pregnancy, even though a rare event in young females with eating disorders, can occur. Amenorrhoea may be reported and pregnancy should be excluded by obtaining a pregnancy test and a detailed clinical history, including sexual activities.

Haematology

Most adolescents with eating disorders present with haematological results within the normal range, although mild to severe lymphocytopenia, neutropenia and thrombocytopenia can occur; pancytopenia and bone marrow hypoplasia have been reported.[45] Patients with anorexia nervosa who have leukopenia do not appear to be at a higher risk of infection compared with healthy controls.[46]

Anaemia, usually microcytic, hypochromic iron deficiency, is common in eating disorders, especially in growing adolescents, with a peak prevalence of up to 14% between the ages of 11 and 19 years. It is less common in adolescent females with anorexia nervosa, possibly due to increased iron storage secondary to the contraction of the circulating blood volume, as well as amenorrhoea being a protective factor.[47,48]

When present in anorexia nervosa, other causes of chronic blood loss such as inflammatory bowel disease, malabsorption syndromes and parasitic infections (among other chronic illnesses) should be considered. In bulimia nervosa, iron-deficiency anaemia may occur due to mucosal damage and secondary blood loss through the gastrointestinal tract.

The erythrocyte sedimentation rate (ESR) is useful to differentiate between anorexia nervosa and other organic causes of malnutrition such as chronic inflammatory and infectious processes and other systemic illnesses, and fibrinogen is commonly low in patients with anorexia nervosa. Weight and weight change predict the biochemical measurements to only a small degree.

Refeeding

Weight gain should be the first treatment priority in patients with anorexia nervosa, because of the acute physical risk and the adverse effects of starvation on emotions and mind, which can compromise the effective use of psychological interventions. Target weight gains are:

- for out-patients, an average weekly weight gain of 0.5 kg
- for in-patients, a weight gain of 0.5–1 kg.

Weight gain at a rate of 0.5–1 kg/week requires an additional intake of 3500–7000 calories per week. Careful physical monitoring during this process is important since life-threatening electrolyte disturbances and mineral and vitamin deficiencies may occur, especially during the early stages of refeeding in patients:

- at high risk, defined as a very low weight (e.g. below 12 kg/m^2)
- with a history of severe dietary restraint
- who vomit frequently, misuse laxatives or binge
- with concurrent medical conditions such as diabetes, infection or major organ failure.

People with anorexia nervosa and their carers should be informed if the risk to physical health is high. Refeeding of very low weight patients should be carried out in an in-patient setting under the supervision of an experienced team. Pregnant women with either current or remitted anorexia nervosa should be considered for more intensive prenatal care to ensure adequate nutrition and fetal development. In out-patient settings, carers and families can be effectively involved in helping to achieve weight gain (the Maudsley approach).[49,50]

Untoward consequences of refeeding can be minimised by starting the patient on relatively small amounts of food and increasing the quantities progressively. A sudden increase in metabolic load may precipitate biochemical decompensation, and an excessive protein intake can be hazardous in patients with underlying renal or hepatic impairment.

A range of complex electrolyte disturbances can occur during refeeding due to complex shifts of electrolytes between intracellular and extracellular compartments – the *refeeding syndrome*. The use of intravenous fluids may compound this problem. Hypokalaemia, hypophosphataemia, hypomagnesaemia and hypocalcaemia may occur.[12,51,52] Electrolyte deficiencies may require oral or intravenous replacement, depending on their severity. Electrocardiographic monitoring is strongly recommended in all cases of electrolyte disturbance and during intravenous replacement.

Feeding against the will of the patient should be an intervention of last resort in the care and management of anorexia nervosa. It is a highly specialised procedure, requiring expertise in the care and management of those with severe eating disorders and the associated physical complications. It should be done only in the context of the Mental Health Act 1983 or Children Act 1989 and the legal basis for any such action must be clear.[53,54]

The outcome

Several medical predictors for poor outcome and course of disease have been reported alongside psychological predictors. Medical factors include:

- low body weight at initial presentation
- high creatinine levels
- low albumin levels
- premorbid obesity in bulimia nervosa.

However, given the wide rage of uncertainty, Steinhausen *et al* propose that clinicians should refrain from prognostic statements regarding individual patients.[55,56]

Summary

Anorexia nervosa is associated with severe physical complications which can occur during the acute and chronic states and during recovery, with potentially irreversible long-term implications for health and a significant risk of death. Patients with bulimia nervosa and EDNOS often appear physically healthy, with fewer symptoms and signs of physical illness than those with anorexia nervosa. Careful on-going monitoring of medical parameters from the onset of treatment is essential to ensure the safe recovery of all patients with eating disorders. Close liaison with the medical professions and specialists in the field of eating disorders may be required to manage physical complications safely.

References

1 Keski-Rahkonen A, Raevuori A, Hoek H. Epidemiology of eating disorders: an update. In *Annual Review of Eating Disorders. Part 2* (eds S Wonderlich, JE Mitchell, M De Zwaan, *et al*): 58–68. Radcliffe Publishing, 2008.

2 van Son GE, van Hoeken D, Bartelds AIM, *et al.* Urbanisation and the incidence of eating disorders. *Br J Psychiatry* 2006; **189**: 562–3.

3 Wade TD, Bergin JL, Tiggermann M, *et al.* Prevalence and long-term course of lifetime eating disorders in an adult Australian twin cohort. *Aust N Z J Psychiatry* 2006; **40**: 121–8.

4 Keski-Rahkonen A, Hoek HW, Susser ES, *et al.* Epidemiology and course of anorexia nervosa in the community. *Am J Psychiatry* 2007; **164**: 1259–65.

5 Berkman ND, Lohr KN, Bulik CM. Outcomes of eating disorders: a systematic review of the literature. *Int J Eat Disord* 2007; **40**: 293–309.

6 Birmingham CL, Su J, Hlynsky JA, *et al.* The mortality rate from anorexia nervosa. *Int J Eat Disord* 2005; **38**: 143–6.

7 McKenzie JM, Joyce PR. Hospitalization for anorexia nervosa. *Int J Eat Disord* 1992; **11**: 235–41.

8 Hudson JL, Hiripi E, Pope HG Jr, *et al.* The prevalence and correlates of eating disorders in the national comorbidity survey replication. *Biol Psychiatry* 2007; **61**: 348–58.

9 Woerwag-Mehta S, Treasure J, Birmingham J. Children and adolescents. In *Medical Management of Eating Disorders,* 2nd edn (eds C Laird Birmingham, J Treasure): 161–8. Cambridge University Press, 2010.

10 Panagiotopoulos C, McGridle BW, Hick K, *et al.* Electrocardiographic findings in adolescents with eating disorders. *Pediatrics* 2000; **105**: 1100–5.

11 Mont L, Castro J, Herreros B. Reversibility of cardiac abnormalities in adolescents with anorexia nervosa after weight recovery. *J Am Acad Child Adolesc Psychiatry* 2003; **42**: 808.

12 Palla B, Litt IF. Medical complications of eating disorders in adolescents. *Pediatrics* 1988; **81**: 613–23.

13 Dec GW, Biederman J, Hougen TJ. Cardiovascular findings in adolescent inpatients with eating disorders. *Psychosom Med* 1987; **49**: 285–90.

14 Golden NH, Katzman DK, Kreipe RE, *et al.* Eating disorders in adolescents: position paper of the Society for Adolescent Medicine. *J Adolesc Health* 2003; **33**: 496–503.

15 Goldberg SJ, Comerci GD, Feldman L. Cardiac output and regional myocardial contraction in anorexia nervosa. *J Adolesc Health Care* 1988; **9**: 15–21.

16 Turner J, Bulsara M, McDermott B, *et al.* Predictors of bone density in young adolescent females with anorexia nervosa and other dieting disorders. *Int J Eat Disord* 2001; **30**: 245–51.

17 Shamin T, Golden NH, Arden M, *et al.* Resolution of vital sign instability: an objective measure of medical stability in anorexia nervosa. *J Adolesc Health* 2003; **32**: 73–7.

18 Galetta F, Franzoni F, Prattichizzo F, *et al.* Heart rate variability and left ventricular diastolic function in anorexia nervosa. *J Adolesc Health* 2003; **32**: 416–21.

19 Johnson GL, Humphries LL, Shirley PB, *et al.* Mitral valve prolapse in patents with anorexia nervosa and bulimia nervosa. *Arch Intern Med* 1986; **146**: 1525–9.

20 Casiero D, Frishman W. Cardiovascular complications of eating disorders. *Cardiol Rev* 2006; **14**: 227–31.

21 Bachrach L, Guido D, Katzman D, *et al.* Decreased bone density in adolescent girls with anorexia nervosa. *Pediatrics* 1990; **86**: 440–7.

22 Lenkh C, De Zwaan M, Bailer U, *et al.* Osteopenia in anorexia nervosa: specific mechanisms of bone loss. *J Psychiatr Res* 1999; **33**: 349–56.

23 Soyka L, Grinspoon S, Levitsky L, *et al.* The effect of anorexia nervosa on bone metabolism in female adolescents. *J Clin Endocrinol Metab* 1999; **84**: 4489–96.

24 Soyka L, Misra M, Frenchman A, *et al.* Abnormal bone mineral accrual in adolescent girls with anorexia nervosa. *J Clin Endocrinol Metab* 2002; **87**: 4177–85.

25 Jagielska G, Wolanczyk T, Komender J, *et al.* Bone mineral density in adolescent girls with anorexia nervosa – a cross-sectional study. *Eur Child Adolesc Psychiatry* 2002; **11**: 57–62.

26 Castro J, Toro J, Lazaro L, *et al.* Bone mineral density in male adolescents with anorexia nervosa. *J Am Acad Child Adolesc Psychiatry* 2002; **41**: 613–8.

27 Grinspoon S, Thomas E, Pitts S, *et al.* Prevalence and predictive factors for regional osteopenia in women with anorexia nervosa. *Ann Intern Med* 2000; **133**: 790–4.

28 Mishra M, Aggaral A, Miller K, *et al.* Effects of anorexia nervosa on clinical, haematological, biochemical and bone density parameters in community-dwelling adolescent girls. *Pediatrics* 2004; **114**: 1574–83.

29 Cummings S, Black D, Nevit M, *et al.* Bone density at various sites for prediction of hip fractures. *Lancet* 1993; **341**: 72–5.

30 Herzog W, Minne H, Deter C, *et al.* Outcome of bone mineral density in anorexia nervosa patients 11.7 years after first admission. *J Bone Miner Res* 1993; **8**: 597–605.

31 Zipfel S, Beaumont P, Russel J, *et al.* Osteoporosis in eating disorders. *Eur Eat Disord Rev* 2000; **8**: 108–16.

32 Grinspoon S, Miller K, Coyle C, *et al.* Severity of osteopenia in oestrogen-deficient women with anorexia nervosa and hypothalamic amenorrhea. *J Clin Endocrinol Metab* 1999; **84**: 2049–55.

33 Stephanis N, Mackintosh C, Abraha H, *et al.* Dissociation of bone turnover in anorexia nervosa. *Ann Clin Biochem* 1998; **35**: 709–16.

34 Bolton J, Patel S. Osteoporosis in anorexia nervosa. *J Psychosom Res* 2001; **50**: 177–8.

35 Zipfel S, Sebel M, Lowe B, *et al.* Osteoporosis in eating disorders: a follow-up study of patients with anorexia and bulimia nervosa. *J Clin Endocinol Metab* 2001; **86**: 5227–33.

36 Uher R, Treasure J. Brain lesions and eating disorders. *J Neurol Neurosurg Psychiatry* 2005; **6**: 852–7.

37 Giordiano GD, Renzetti P, Parodi RC, *et al.* Volume measurement with magnetic resonance imaging of hippocampus–amygdala formation in patients with anorexia nervosa. *J Endocrinol Invest* 2001; **24**: 510–14.

38 Neumarker KJ, Bzufka WM, Dudeck U, *et al.* Are there specific disabilities of number processing in adolescent patients with anorexia nervosa? Evidence from clinical and neuropsychological data when compared to morphometric measures from magnetic resonance imaging. *Eur Child Adolesc Psychiatry* 2000; **9** (suppl 2): 111–21.

39 Golden NH, Ashtari M, Kohn MR, *et al.* Reversibility of cerebral ventricular enlargement in anorexia nervosa, demonstrated by quantitative magnetic resonance imaging. *J Pediatr* 1996; **128**: 159–65.

40 Katzman DK, Lambe EK, Mikulis DJ, *et al.* Cerebral grey matter and white matter volume deficits in adolescent girls with anorexia nervosa. *J Pediatr* 1996; **129**: 794–803.

41 Connan F, Lightman AS, Treasure J. Biochemical and endocrine complications. *Eur Eat Disord Rev* 2000; **8**: 144–57.

42 Poyastro PA, Thornton LM, Plotonicov KH, *et al.* Patterns of menstrual disturbance in eating disorders. *Int J Eat Disord* 2007; **40**: 424–34.

43 Swenne I. Weight requirements for return of menstruation in teenage girls with eating disorders, weight loss and secondary amenorrhoea. *Acta Paediatr* 2004; **93**: 1449–55.

44 Miller KK, Grinspoon S, Gleysteen S, *et al.* Preservation of neuroendocrine control of reproductive function despite severe undernutrition. *J Clin Endocrinol Metab* 2004; **89**: 4434–8.

45 Swenne I. The significance of routine laboratory analyses in the assessment of teenage girls with eating disorders and weight loss. *Eat Weight Disord* 2004; **9**: 269–78.

46 Bowers TK, Eckert E. Leukopenia in anorexia nervosa: lack of increased risk of infection. *Arch Intern Med* 1978; **138**: 1520–3.

47 Swenne I. Haematological changes and iron status in teenage girls with eating disorders and weight loss – the importance of menstrual status. *Acta Paediatr* 2007; **96**: 530–3.

48 Kennedy A, Kohn M, Lammi A, *et al.* Iron status and haematological changes in adolescent female inpatients with anorexia nervosa. *J Paediatr Child Health* 2004; **40**: 430–2.

49 Lock J, Le Grange D. *Treatment Manual for Anorexia Nervosa: A Family Based Approach,* 2nd edn. Guilford Press, 2012.

50 Le Grange D, Lock J. *Treating Bulimia in Adolescents: A Family Based Appraoch.* Guilford Press, 2009.

51 Connan F, Lightman-Stafford I, Landau S, *et al.* An investigation of hypothalamic-pituitary-adrenal axis hyperactivity in anorexia nervosa: the role of CRH and AVP. *J Psychiatr Res* 2007; **41**: 131–43.

52 Greenfield D, Mickley D, Quinlan DM, *et al.* Hypokalemia in out-patients with eating disorders. *Am J Psychiatry* 1995; **152**: 60–3.

53 Royal College of Psychiatrists. *Guidelines for the Nutritional Management of Anorexia Nervosa.* Council Report CR130. Royal College of Psychiatrists, 2005.

54 National Institute of Health and Clinical Excellence. *Nutritional Support in Adults.* Clinical Guideline 32. NICE, 2006.

55 Steinhausen HC, Boyadjieva S, Grgoroiu-Serbanescu M, *et al.* A transcultural outcome study of adolescent eating disorders. *Acta Psychiatr Scand* 2000; **101**: 60–6.

56 Steinhausen HC, Seidel R, Winkler Metzke C. Evaluation of treatment and intermediate and long-term outcome of adolescent eating disorders. *Psychol Med* 2000; **30**: 1089–98.

Learning points

- Physical examination is an important part of any assessment of an eating disorder; it should involve all organ systems and the calculation of the patient's BMI. Physical symptoms may be concealed by patients, so observation and evaluation of the physical state is crucial to ensure safe and effective treatment.
- Cardiac complications can pose an acute life-threatening risk. They cause a third of adult deaths in this population. During treatment, careful monitoring is required to avoid disrupting cardiac function.
- Electrolyte disturbances can lead to severe complications during the illness, especially during the early stages of refeeding. Electrolyte levels should be carefully monitored during treatment.
- Patients with anorexia nervosa are at high risk of developing osteopenia and osteoporosis. Loss of bone density occurs early in the course of the illness and may not be fully reversible with weight restoration. Bone fractures due to osteoporosis may lead to significant physical disability at a young age in these patients.
- In children and adolescents, bone maturation and growth may be affected by anorexia nervosa. Bone development should be regularly evaluated and recorded using growth charts.
- Gastrointestinal complaints are common in patients with eating disorders. These are due to reduced gastrointestinal motility, gastric emptying and behaviour related to the eating disorder, such as vomiting, purging and laxative use.
- Severe life-threatening gastrointestinal complications, although rare, require instant medical attention.
- Brain structure and brain, spinal cord and muscle function are affected by eating disorders. Cognitive functions are likely to improve with weight gain.
- Patients at low weight may not be able to understand complex concepts and so may not engage in psychological interventions.
- Impaired cognitive function may be due to vitamin deficiencies. Early replacement therapy is crucial to optimise recovery.
- Endocrine abnormalities are primarily associated with disturbances of the hypothalamus–pituitary axis. For example, disturbances of the menstrual cycle are common in eating disorders and usually resolve with weight gain.
- Young patients with anorexia nervosa may experience a delay in pubertal maturation and primary amenorrhoea. These usually resolve once the eating disorder is treated successfully.

Section IV

Medical emergencies and injuries

31

Emergency medicine

Josephine Tuthill and Christy Lowe

The outcome of medical emergencies can be improved by optimal management. This chapter provides information about the recognition of acute illness, the assessment of a collapsed patient, anaphylaxis and various physical consequences of self-harm. It describes how to manage fits, the unconscious patient, chest pain and sepsis, as well as other topics. The chapter aims to provide the information that is needed to manage the initial stages of a range of medical emergencies.

Introduction

In an emergency, patient outcomes can be significantly improved by rapidly identifying and treating life-threatening problems, providing first aid and beginning initial treatment while awaiting specialised assistance. This chapter covers the principles behind rapid assessment of an acutely unwell patient and the medical emergencies that may commonly be faced in any psychiatric setting. We have included diagnosis-specific management plans, differential diagnoses to consider and, although clinical discretion should be applied, we have recommended when and where to seek help if faced with a medical emergency. Note that *all* doses given in this chapter are *adult* doses.

Recognising acute illness

Acute illness is usually preceded by abnormalities of physiological parameters. *Early warning* scores, or *patient at risk* (PAR) scores (Table 31.1), have been devised to identify patients who may need urgent medical intervention or escalation to an area with a higher level of medical care. Scores are based upon abnormalities of vital signs and parameters and should include the type and speed of escalation required, and the frequency of required monitoring. Very occasionally acutely unwell patients may have a low score, so clinical discretion must be applied.

Some units have a specialised team or an intensive-care outreach team which regularly reviews patients who have a high score. Utilise these teams as appropriate.

The analgesic ladder

Analgesia should be considered early and given rapidly. The prescription of analgesic agents should be guided by pain severity and pain score, as well as current medications and any allergies. Pain scoring is the patient's evaluation of their pain severity with a score from 0 to 10, with 10 being the worst pain imaginable:

- Mild pain, score 1–4: prescribe paracetamol (oral or intravenous), ibuprofen or aspirin.
- Moderate pain, score 5–6: prescribe codeine phosphate, dihydrocodeine, diclofenac, tramadol.

Table 31.1 Modified 'patient at risk' (PAR) scoring system

Score	3	2	1	0	1	2	3
Central nervous system response				Alert	Drowsy	Responds to pain	
Respiratory rate (breaths/min)		<8		9–14	15–20	21–30	>30
Pulse rate (beats/min)		<40	40–50	51–100	100–110	111–130	>130
Systolic blood pressure (mmHg)	<70	71–80	81–100	101–199		>200	

Score of 4 or above. Immediate review by doctor; or call 999 for an emergency ambulance to transfer the patient; or call the local accident and emergency department (A&E) to advise of the patient's immediate transfer.
Score of 3. Call for doctor review within 1 hour; or if no doctor is available, then appropriate treatment options must be considered, including transfer of patient to A&E.
Score of 2. Increase frequency of observations and inform nurse in charge/senior nurse on duty (minimum frequency of observations is hourly for scores of 2 and above).
Score of 0 or 1. Continue observations at current frequency.

Reported in Rees & Mann, 2004.[1]

- Severe pain, score ≥7: prescribe morphine (oral, intravenous or intramuscular), and Entonox® may be useful.

Before prescribing aspirin or non-steroidal anti-inflammatory drugs (NSAIDs) enquire about relative contraindications such as asthma, indigestion, peptic ulceration.

Rapid assessment: the ABCDE approach

A systematic assessment, based on recognised guidelines,[2] should be performed to ensure life-threatening problems are treated rapidly, in an appropriate order, and nothing is overlooked. This should be instituted while waiting for assistance from the hospital 'crash team' or external emergency services. Life-threatening problems should be treated as they are identified, before progressing to the next stage of the assessment, with regular reassessment of the patient. A useful systematic rapid assessment is the ABCDE approach, described below.

Personal safety

Ensure your own personal safety – assess your surroundings and observe the patient and whether they look unwell. 'Shake and shout': ask conscious patients how they are, shake unconscious patients while doing so.

A. Airway and cervical spine

Stabilise the cervical spine if there is any suspicion of injury to it. The head should be held still and in line with the rest of the spine by placing hands on each side of the head. If possible, ask an assistant to immobilise the cervical spine with a collar and sandbags.

Assess airway patency. Noisy breathing occurs in partial airway obstruction. Silent breathing with strenuous respiratory movements signifies complete airway obstruction. In anyone with a decreased level of consciousness (score ≤8 on the Glasgow Coma Scale – see below) assume impending airway obstruction.

Maintain the airway using a head tilt and chin lift or jaw thrust. Airway adjuncts may be required, such as a Guedel airway, nasopharyngeal airway, tracheal intubation, or tracheostomy.

Start high-flow oxygen 15 litres/minute via a non-rebreather mask. Use suction for secretions. Place the patient on their side or in a head-up tilt if there is no contraindication.

B. Breathing

Assess oxygen saturations, respiratory rate, pattern of breathing, tracheal positioning, bilateral chest expansion (is it equal?) and resonance, and auscultate the chest. Treat any pathology (e.g. tension pneumothorax – Table 31.2) when it is found.

If the patient is apnoeic or hypoventilating, start bag-mask ventilation and immediately obtain assistance from someone trained to intubate.

Table 31.2 Clinical features of pneumothorax and pulmonary oedema

Pneumothorax	Pulmonary oedema
Reduced expansion, hyperresonance, diminished breath sounds on affected side. In tension pneumothorax the trachea is deviated away from the affected side	Tachypnoeic, raised jugular venous pressure, fine lung crackles bilaterally, wheeze (cardiac asthma)

Aim to maintain the patient's oxygen saturations as close to normal as possible (> 97%). Oxygen should still be given to those with chronic obstructive pulmonary disease (COPD), to minimise end-organ damage. However, close observation for respiratory depression is required. Aim for saturations of at least 90–92%. Obtain an ABG (arterial blood gas) to ensure optimal management if facilities are available.

C. Circulation

Assess hand colour and temperature, capillary refill time (normal < 2 s), heart rate, blood pressure and jugular venous pressure (JVP), and apply pressure to any area of haemorrhage. Obtain a 12-lead electrocardiogram (ECG).

Insert two large-bore (14- or 16-gauge) cannulae into accessible veins and send blood samples for urgent full blood count (FBC), renal profile, clotting and cross-match.

If normotensive, a 500 ml bolus of crystalloid should be administered over 5–10 minutes. If hypotensive or if there are signs of circulatory compromise, 1 litre of crystalloid should be rapidly administered. For those with known cardiac failure, close monitoring of fluid status is required. Aim to resuscitate to the patient's normal blood pressure if known. Urethral catheterisation will enable urine output and thus fluid balance to be accurately evaluated.

D. Disability

Assess the patient's level of consciousness using either the Glasgow Coma Scale (GCS) (Table 31.3; for an extended version of the GCS see Chapter 4, Box 4.4) or the AVPU scoring system (Box 31.1, full version is in Chapter 4, Box 4.3).

Table 31.3 Glasgow Coma Scale (GCS)

		Score
Eye response	Open spontaneously	4
	Open to verbal stimuli	3
	Open to pain	2
	No response	1
Verbal response	Talking and orientated	5
	Confused or disorientated	4
	Inappropriate words	3
	Incomprehensible sounds	2
	No response	1
Motor response	Obeys commands	6
	Localises pain	5
	Flexion/withdrawal to pain	4
	Abnormal flexion to pain	3
	Extension to pain	2
	No response	1

The GCS score is the sum of the scores achieved in each section. For example, GCS 11/15 (E3, V3, M5). The minimum score is 3.

Check the drug chart for other causes of a decreased conscious level (e.g. opioids, benzodiazepines).

Box 31.1 AVPU scoring system

Alert
Responsive to **V**oice
Responsive to **P**ain
Unresponsive

A GCS score of ≤ 8 or an AVPU rating of P or U means that patients are unlikely to be able to protect their own airway. The airway should be assessed and protected if necessary. Anaesthetic support may be urgently required. Check pupil size, equality and reactivity by shining light from a pen-torch into each eye. Look for direct and consensual pupillary responses. Check blood glucose. If < 3 mmol/l give 50 ml of 10% glucose intravenously. Repeat every minute until the patient regains consciousness, or until a total of 250 ml has been administered.

Box 31.2 AMPLE history

- **A**llergies
- **M**edications (e.g. anticoagulants, insulin, beta-blockers)
- **P**ast medical history
- **L**ast meal
- **E**vents surrounding the current episode

E. Exposure

Fully expose the patient and perform a head-to-toe examination. Maintain dignity and aim to prevent unnecessary heat loss. If not already gained, an AMPLE history (Box 31.2) should be obtained at this point.

Further information

The UK Resuscitation Council has produced some useful materials, including the book *Advanced Life Support*,[2] as well as a basic (Fig. 31.1) and an advanced life support algorithm (Fig. 31.2).

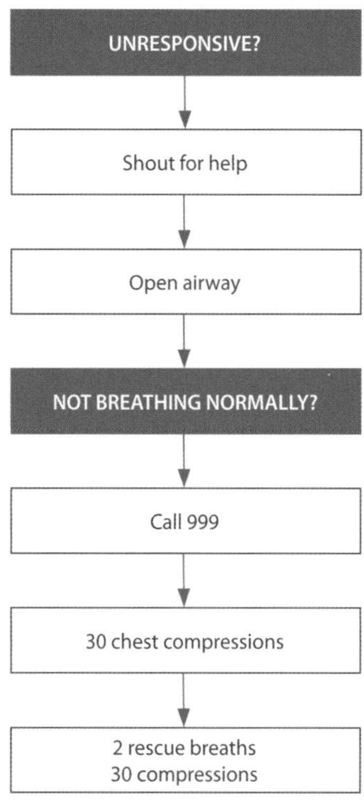

Fig. 31.1 Basic life support algorithm. Reproduced with permission of the UK Resuscitation Council.[2]

Anaphylaxis

Anaphylaxis is a life-threatening and severe systemic allergic reaction which occurs rapidly after contact with an allergen.[3] The common causes are listed in Box 31.3 (for more detail see Doshi *et al*[4]). Onset depends on the nature and extent of exposure and occurs within minutes, but can be delayed by several hours.

Patients with a higher risk of developing anaphylaxis include those with severe asthma, cardiovascular or pulmonary disease, mastocytosis, or predisposing concurrent medication, for example beta-blockers and angiotensin converting enzyme (ACE) inhibitors.

Recognising anaphylaxis

Diagnosis is based on a history of exposure to a triggering agent or event and rapid evolution of symptoms over minutes or hours. A triad of features is likely:[5]

- sudden onset and rapid progression of symptoms
- life-threatening problems with airway, breathing or circulation
- skin and/or mucosal changes, such as flushing, urticaria and angioedema.

The common symptoms are listed in Table 31.4. Note that cutaneous changes *alone* do not support a diagnosis of anaphylaxis.

Differential diagnosis

The differential diagnoses include:[6]

- acute asthma
- acute generalised hives
- syncope
- inhaled foreign body
- non-allergic angioedema (e.g. hereditory angioedema or angioedema caused by ACE inhibitors)
- other causes of shock – septic, cardiogenic, hypovolaemic
- psychological – panic attack, Munchausen's syndrome.

Box 31.3 Common causes of anaphylaxis

- Food: nuts, fish, shellfish, milk, eggs, soy and wheat
- Medications: antibiotics, non-steroidal anti-inflammatory drugs (NSAIDs), including aspirin, X-ray contrast medium
- Latex
- Stings or venoms
- Allergen immunotherapy injections

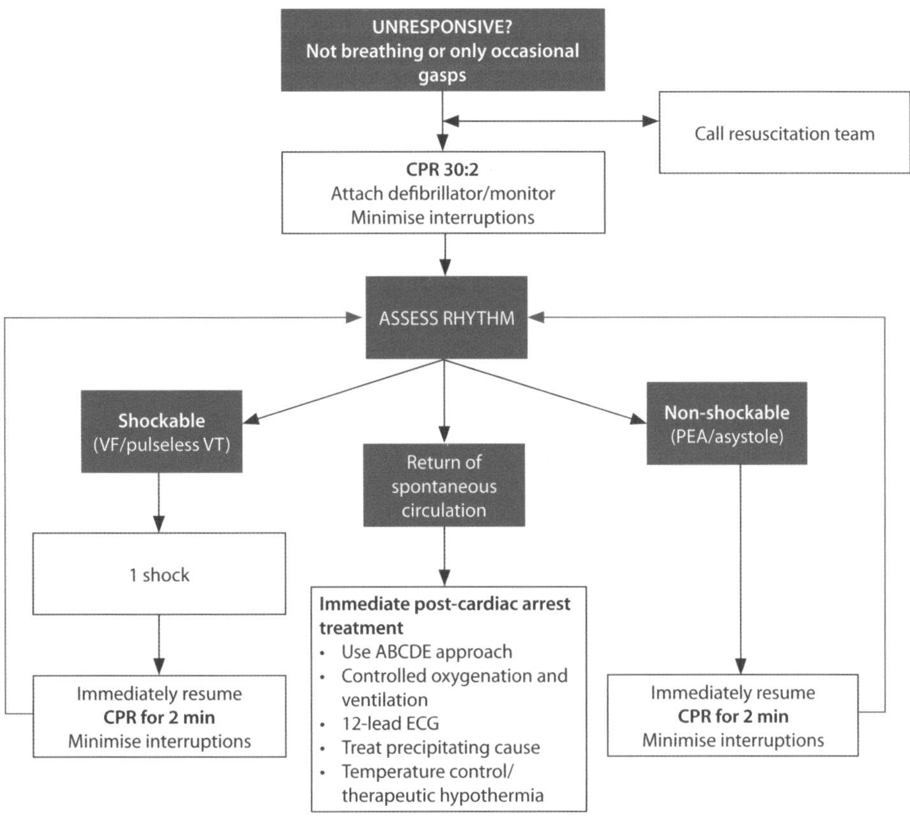

During CPR
- Ensure high-quality CPR: rate, depth, recoil
- Plan actions before interrupting CPR
- Give oxygen
- Consider advanced airway and capnography
- Continuous chest compressions when advanced airway in place
- Vascular access (intravenous, intraosseous)
- Give adrenaline every 3–5 min
- Correct reversible causes

Reversibe causes
- Hypoxia
- Hypovolaemia
- Hypo-/hyperkalaemia/metabolic
- Hypothermia

- Thrombosis – coronary or pulmonary
- Tamponade – cardiac
- Toxins
- Tension pneumothorax

Fig. 31.2 Advanced life support algorithm. Reproduced with permission of the UK Resuscitation Council.[2] CPR, cardiopulmonary resuscitation; ECG, electrocardiogram; PEA, pulseless electrical activity; VF, ventricular fibrillation; VT, ventricular tachycardia.

Table 31.4 Common symptoms in anaphylaxis

System	Examples	Percentage of patients affected
Cutaneous	Urticaria, angioedema, flushing, itching	90%
Respiratory	Dyspnoea, wheeze, stridor, hypoxia	70%
Gastrointestinal	Abdominal pain, vomiting	40%
Cardiovascular	Hypotension	10–30%

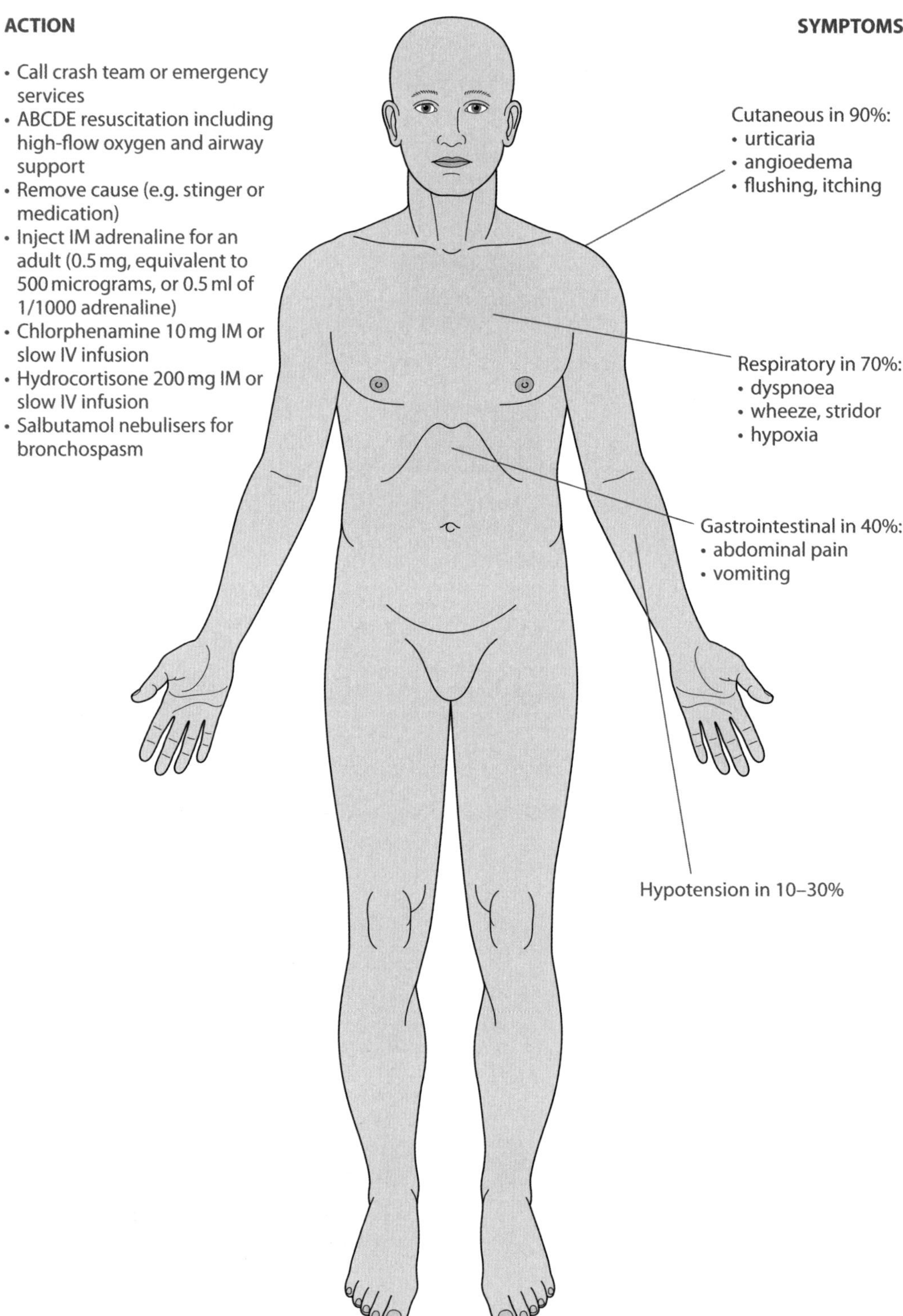
ACTION
• Call crash team or emergency services
• ABCDE resuscitation including high-flow oxygen and airway support
• Remove cause (e.g. stinger or medication)
• Inject IM adrenaline for an adult (0.5 mg, equivalent to 500 micrograms, or 0.5 ml of 1/1000 adrenaline)
• Chlorphenamine 10 mg IM or slow IV infusion
• Hydrocortisone 200 mg IM or slow IV infusion
• Salbutamol nebulisers for bronchospasm
SYMPTOMS
Cutaneous in 90%:
• urticaria
• angioedema
• flushing, itching
Respiratory in 70%:
• dyspnoea
• wheeze, stridor
• hypoxia
Gastrointestinal in 40%:
• abdominal pain
• vomiting
Hypotension in 10–30%

Fig. 31.3 Anaphylaxis, action and symptoms. IM, intramuscular, IV, intravenous

Initial management

The Working Group of the Resuscitation Council makes the following recommendations:[5]

- contact emergency services or 'crash team' immediately
- make an ABCDE assessment and implement high-flow oxygen and airway support
- lie patient flat and raise legs (unless precluded by vomiting or breathlessness)
- remove the causative agent (e.g. stop intravenous infusions, remove stinger)
- administer intramuscular adrenaline if the patient is in respiratory difficulty, has airway swelling, or shock:
  - adult dose = 0.5 mg (equivalent to 500 μg or 0.5 ml 1:1000 adrenaline)
  - use the patient's own adrenaline auto-injector (e.g. EpiPen) if more immediately available, although this will give a smaller dose than recommended above
  - inject into anterolateral aspect of middle third of the thigh
  - repeat adrenaline administration after 5 minutes if no improvement
- intravenous fluids: give adult patients a fluid challenge of 500 ml to 1 litre Hartmann's solution or normal saline. May require up to 1–2 litres
- chlorphenamine – 10 mg intramuscular or slow intravenous infusion
- hydrocortisone – 200 mg intramuscular or slow intravenous infusion
- salbutamol nebulisers for bronchospasm
- continue to monitor vital signs and reassess regularly.

Less severe cases – wheeze or mild difficulty breathing only – may be managed with salbutamol nebulisers.

Secondary cardiorespiratory arrest

Start cardiopulmonary resuscitation (CPR) immediately and use the doses of adrenaline indicated in the ALS guidelines.[2]

Continuing management

Admission and observation are required for a minimum of 6 hours to an area where there are facilities for managing airway and circulatory problems. Biphasic reactions are infrequent but an early recurrence of symptoms may occur 1–72 hours after the initial episode.

Patients should be referred to an allergy clinic for allergy testing and risk assessment.

Individuals at high risk should carry an adrenaline auto-injector (EpiPen) and be trained in its use. Triggers should be avoided and risk factors should be optimised.[4]

Written, personalised, anaphylaxis emergency action plans for patients at risk may be beneficial.[4]

Further information

As well as the works cited above,[5,6] the website of the Anaphylaxis Campaign is a useful source of further information (www.anaphylaxis.org.uk).

Self-harm

Hanging

Hanging is the most common method of suicide in the UK, with around 2000 cases each year. Ten per cent of cases occur in a controlled environment, such as hospital or police custody. Hanging comprises three-quarters of psychiatric in-patient suicides.[7]

The pre-hospital mortality rate is approximately 80%,[7] but incomplete hanging has a survival rate of 80–90%. Survival is proportional to hanging time and good outcome is associated with a hanging time of less than 5 minutes.[8]

Commonly associated injuries include: cerebral anoxia, laryngotracheal fractures, carotid injuries, cervical spine fractures and hyoid bone fractures.[9]

Initial management

Gunnell *et al* make the following recommendations:[7]

- Stabilise the cervical spine.
- Lift the patient to remove pressure on the neck.
- Cut or remove the ligature (avoid cutting the knot as it may be required for medico-legal investigation).
- Make an assessment using the ABCDE approach.
- Commence CPR if there is no pulse.
- Transfer the patient to an area with emergency facilities.

If possible, obtain a history regarding patient positioning, knot placement, drop and type of ligature used.

Prevention

Prevention is crucial and it should be noted that complete suspension is not essential for successful hanging. Partial suspension (sitting or standing) is adequate to obtain the required neck pressure. Ligature points (e.g. hooks or door handles) and materials which may be used for suspension (e.g. shoe laces or dressing gown cord) should be removed or minimised for high-risk patients. If they cannot be removed, the area and patient must be closely controlled and monitored.

Overdose

Assess with the ABCDE approach.

History (from patient and those close to patient)

Enquire about timing, substance taken, concurrent medications, allergies and whether alcohol was consumed. Check bottles and packets for names and quantities.

Examination

Assess pupils and record GCS. Perform a full systemic examination.

Investigations

These should include:

- basic observations
- ECG
- ABG
- blood tests, including FBC, urea and electrolytes (U&E), liver function tests (LFTs), clotting screen, glucose, paracetamol and salicylate levels.

Management

If the substance ingested and precise amount are known, consult TOXBASE (www.toxbase.org) for up-to-date advice on medications, household products, plants, fungi and chemicals. The site details toxicity, likely symptoms and complications, and provides information regarding the level of medical care that will be required. The UK National Poisons Information Service is also contactable on 0844 892 0111.

If the drug has been taken within the past hour, activated charcoal can bind to the drug and reduce absorption. The dose is 50 g taken orally. Like other oral medications it should not be given if the patient has a reduced conscious level, as there is risk of aspiration in these patients. A few drugs and substances are not bound by charcoal: iron, lithium, ethanol, ethylene glycol, methanol, and strong acids and alkalis. There is no advantage to using charcoal in these situations.

Common poisons and their antidotes are listed in Table 31.5.

Patients who are suspected to have taken an overdose should be referred to the emergency department or medical on-call team immediately to ensure adequate monitoring and timely assessment.

Overdose is also discussed in Chapter 28.

Ingestion of foreign bodies

Foreign bodies may be ingested by adults with psychiatric disorders but rarely cause problems unless they become lodged in the oesophagus or are of a harmful nature. Potentially harmful foreign bodies include:

- sharp objects e.g. open safety pins, needles, broken glass, razor blades
- more than one magnet (magnets attract and the resultant pressure may cause ulceration, bowel wall necrosis, perforation, or fistula formation)
- toxic substances, often in the form of button/disc batteries (used for watches and cameras) and items containing lead
- very long or bulky objects.

Table 31.5 Common poisons and their antidotes

Poison	Antidotes
Beta-blockers	Glucagon, atropine
Benzodiazepines	Flumazenil
Digoxin	Digibind (digoxin antibodies)
Iron salts	Desferrioxamine
Methanol	Ethanol, fomepizole
Opiods	Naloxone
Organophosphates	Atropine, pralidoxime
Paracetamol	N-acetylcysteine, methinonine
Warfarin	Vitamin K, clotting factors, FFP (fresh frozen plasma)

Adapted from *Oxford Handbook of Emergency Medicine*.[10]

History

Note the type of object, and the presence of dysphagia, vomiting, abdominal pain or chest pain.

Examination

Look for signs of complications: oesophageal rupture (subcutaneous emphysema of the neck) or peritonitis.

Investigations

Plain chest X-ray can be performed for radio-opaque foreign bodies to confirm passage through the narrowest point, the gastro-oesophageal junction. If the object is benign and has passed the gastro-oesophageal junction, then there are unlikely to be any further complications and no intervention is required. However, if a potentially harmful foreign object has been ingested an urgent referral to the surgical team should be made, as endoscopic removal may be necessary.

Management

Monitor patients for signs of bowel obstruction or perforation. There is no need to examine stools for the foreign body unless it is of value, as objects may take up to 6 weeks to pass through the digestive tract.[10]

If the patient is choking, the algorithm shown in Fig. 31.4 should be followed.

Deliberate cutaneous insertion of foreign bodies

Deliberate insertion of foreign bodies is a relatively unusual form of self-harm. A full history should be obtained and the underlying psychiatric issues addressed. Assess neurovascular status and limb function, and examine for signs of infection.

The range of possible objects and injuries means that management varies considerably. Surgical intervention is likely to be required if there is evidence of functional deficit or infection, or if the object is not easily removable. In the presence of multiple objects, management plans should be tailored to functional status, infection, underlying psychiatric dysfunction and whether the patient is likely to persist with the behaviour.[11]

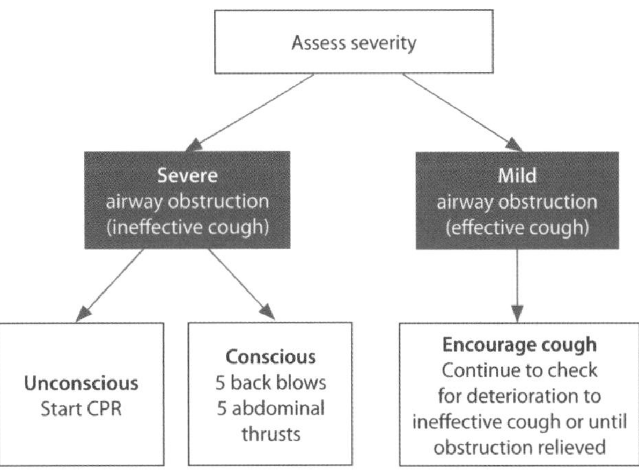

Fig. 31.4 Algorithm for the management of an adult who is choking. Reproduced with permission of the UK Resuscitation Council.[2] CPR, cardiopulmonary resuscitation.

Carbon monoxide poisoning

Carbon monoxide is produced by incomplete combustion and poisoning often results from breathing fumes from a car exhaust or partly burnt fuel. Carbon monoxide reduces blood oxygen-carrying capacity by binding more strongly to haemoglobin than does oxygen, leading to tissue hypoxia.[12]

Early symptoms of carbon monoxide poisoning include nausea, vomiting, headache and general malaise. Hyperventilation, as well as respiratory failure, cardiac arrhythmias, myocardial infarction and cerebral oedema may occur.[12] Neurological and psychiatric features may manifest after exposure, and may improve over time.[12]

High-flow oxygen (100%) should be continued until the blood carboxyhaemoglobin levels fall to less than 10%.[12] Patients should be assessed in a general hospital with facilities for measurement of carboxyhaemoglobin levels and pH[12]. Oxygen saturations via pulse oximetry

> Oxygen saturations using pulse oximetry are misleading in carbon monoxide poisoning.

are misleading in carbon monoxide poisoning. The patient should be deemed to be medically fit before psychiatric assessment or admission to a psychiatric unit

Further information

As well as the TOXBASE website of the National Poisons Information Service (www.toxbase.org; tel. 0844 892 0111), see a chapter in the *Oxford Textbook of Medicine* on poisoning by drugs and chemicals by Vale *et al.*[12] More generally, see Wyatt *et al*'s *Oxford Handbook of Emergency Medicine.*[13]

Wounds and lacerations

Undertake an ABCDE assessment. Apply pressure to any areas of haemorrhage.

The history should cover:

- mechanism of injury
- time of injury
- hand dominance
- comorbidities
- tetanus status.

The examination should reveal the wound size, shape and depth. Determine whether foreign bodies are present. Assess neurovascular status and integrity of deep structures, e.g. tendons.

Wound care

1. Clean

Use 0.9% saline or sterile water and sterile gauze. Pressure irrigation using a syringe and broken-off green needle may be required (take care to avoid eye splashes).

2. X-ray

Obtain at least two views of all wounds where there is injury with metal, china or glass fragments to ensure any foreign body has been removed before wound closure.

3. Closure

The type of closure should be tailored to the wound:

- *Superficial, simple, straight wounds less than 2 cm long, with well opposed edges.* Use skin glue. Apply glue to dry wounds and hold edges in place for 60 seconds until glue has set. Do not use near eyes or joints.
- *Superficial wounds and skin flap lacerations in areas of skin not under tension.* Use steri-strips. Leave 3–5 mm gaps between steri-strips and do not use over joints. Steri-strips can be used in conjunction with skin glue.
- *Wounds overlying joints and wounds greater than 2 cm.* These need sutures. The size of thread to use and the time to suture removal depends on the site of the wound.

Do not close wounds which:

- are over 12 hours old
- require tension to close
- are associated with joint, tendon or neurovascular involvement
- are bite or puncture wounds
- have a foreign body *in situ*
- are heavily contaminated or infected.

4. Tetanus vaccination?

The need for administration depends on whether the patient is up to date with vaccinations and boosters and whether or not the wound is tetanus prone. Tetanus-prone wounds include:

- heavily contaminated wounds (especially those contaminated with soil or faeces)
- wounds requiring surgical intervention but where this is delayed by over 6 hours
- puncture-type injuries
- a significant degree of devitalised tissue
- wounds containing a foreign body
- concomitant sepsis.

Treat immunosupressed patients the same as those who have had incomplete immunisation. Wounds over 12 hours old may require a higher dose of immunoglobulin.

See the relevant section in an up-to-date *British National Formulary* (BNF) for current and more detailed guidelines, including drug doses.

5. Antibiotics?

Prescribe antibiotics if the wound:

- is visibly dirty
- is infected
- is a puncture or bite wound
- involves bone.

Also prescribe antibiotics if the patient has valvular heart disease or has had a splenectomy. Be guided by local National Health Service trust guidelines.

Head injury

Any injury to the head, with the exclusion of superficial lacerations, comprises a head injury. The most common causes are falls, assault and road traffic accidents. In psychiatric patients, self-inflicted injuries from head-banging, for example, may occur.

The vast majority of head injuries, 90%, are classified as minor or mild and will simply require 24 hours of observation, which can often be managed at home. However, signs of intracranial haemorrhage and skull fracture must be recognised early.

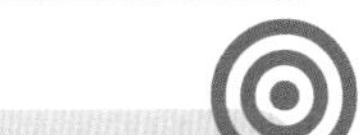

Clinically important brain injury should be excluded before signs or symptoms are attributed to alcohol or medications.

Initial first aid and assessment

Assess using the ABCDE approach. Consider whether the mechanism of injury is sufficient that the patient will need stabilisation of the cervical spine. Significant mechanisms of injury in which the cervical spine must be protected are:[14,15]

- fall from elevation (over 1 m or 5 stairs)
- axial load to the head
- motor vehicle collision at high speed (> 100 km/h, rollover, ejection)
- score on the GCS ≤14 on initial assessment by the healthcare professional
- neck pain or tenderness
- focal neurological deficits
- paraesthesia in the extremities
- other clinical suspicion of cervical spine injury.

Cervical spine immobilisation should remain in place until full assessment by the emergency department has been completed.

History

Try to ascertain:

- time of injury
- mechanism of injury
- anticoagulant medications
- alcohol or recreational drug consumption
- symptoms, including headache, visual disturbance, loss of consciousness, amnesia, drowsiness, vomiting, fitting, focal neurology.

Examination

Perform a full neurological examination, including GCS, pupil size and reactivity. Look for haemotympanum (blood behind tympanic membrane), bruising behind the ears or around the eyes, cerebrospinal fluid or blood leaking from ears or nose, scalp lacerations, bruising, or evidence of a skull fracture.

If there is any of the following, the patient should be referred for emergency assessment:[15]

- decreased conscious level (GCS ≤14)
- focal neurology (e.g. dysphasia, abnormal gait, weakness)
- sign of skull fracture or penetrating injury
- any seizure since the injury
- high-energy head injury (e.g. fall from >1 m or 5 stairs)
- any loss of consciousness since the injury
- persistent headache not relieved by simple analgesia
- vomiting since the injury
- previous cranial neurosurgical interventions, bleeding or clotting disorder
- current anticoagulant therapies
- drug or alcohol intoxication
- age over 65
- suspicion of non-accidental injury
- concern by the injured patient regarding the diagnosis.

See also Chapter 32, pp. 447–8.

Management

If admission or referral for emergency assessment is not required, patients should be observed for 24 hours by a sensible adult. Mild symptoms of headache, nausea and impaired concentration may last up to 2 weeks following injury. Patients should avoid alcohol, sedative medications, contact sports, driving and operating machinery until fully recovered.

Patients should be reassessed by their general practitioner or emergency department if their headache is not resolved by simple analgesia.

Further information

The National Institute for Health and Clinical Excellence (NICE) has provided guidance on head injuries.[15]

Fractures and joint injuries

Initial assessment

Make an assessment following the ABCDE approach. The history should cover the mechanism of injury, site, severity and nature of pain. Also enquire about sensory or motor deficits. Examine the injured area (Box 31.4), the joints above and below, and assess neurovascular status.

Signs suggestive of a fracture include deformity, bony tenderness and the patient's unwillingness to move the affected joint or bear weight. People with these features will need an X-ray.

Also see Chapter 32.

Management

If a fracture is suspected, the patient should be referred to the emergency department. Analgesia should be provided and the affected area should be splinted.

Fractured neck of femur

The patient is typically elderly and osteoporotic. Common mechanisms of injury include tripping or collapse. The affected limb will be shortened and externally rotated and pain may occur in the hip or groin, or radiate down towards the knee. Patients will be unable to raise the leg straight. Suspect a fractured neck of femur in the elderly if they are unable to weight-bear or are 'off legs'. Strong analgesia (preferably intravenous) and intravenous fluids should be administered. Operative management is required.

Ankle fracture

Ankle fractures commonly involve the medial or lateral malleoli, and occur as a result of forced twisting or angulation of the ankle joint. Management will depend on the type of fracture and success of reduction.

Box 31.4 Examining a fracture or joint injury: look, feel, move

- *Look*: Deformity? Bruising? Open wounds? Swelling?
- *Feel*: Localise areas of tenderness, assess peripheral pulses and sensation
- *Move*: Range of movement (active and passive). Assess tendons and ligaments

Open fracture

These are fractures where a wound leads to communication between the fracture haematoma and the outside environment. First aid is required to reduce the subsequent risk of infection:

- provide strong analgesia
- splint the affected limb
- remove gross contamination from the wound
- lavage with large quantities of normal saline or Hartmann's solution
- cover open areas with a sterile dressing
- antibiotics should be administered within the first 3 hours, to decrease risk of infection; a first-generation cephalosporin is recommended, although this should be tailored to the contaminant and local environment.[16]

Rapid referral to orthopaedics is required for assessment.

Tetanus vaccination should be administered if required (see above).

Soft-tissue injuries without fracture

Apply ice, elevate to reduce inflammation and provide good analgesia to ensure the patient is able to mobilise. Encourage exercise to promote healing and prevent stiffness. Utilise physiotherapy services if available.

Collapse

The commonest cause of collapse is a simple faint or vasovagal event. A good history from the patient and a collateral history from any witnesses will help to determine the cause.

Differential diagnoses include:

- epilepsy (see Fig. 31.5)
- arrhythmias (e.g supraventricular tachycardia)
- hyperventilation or panic attack
- vertebro-basilar insufficiency or carotid sinus syncope – both precipitated by different head movements
- hypotension, possibly precipitated by medication (e.g. glyceryl trinitrate, beta-blockers, antihypertensives)
- sepsis or infection

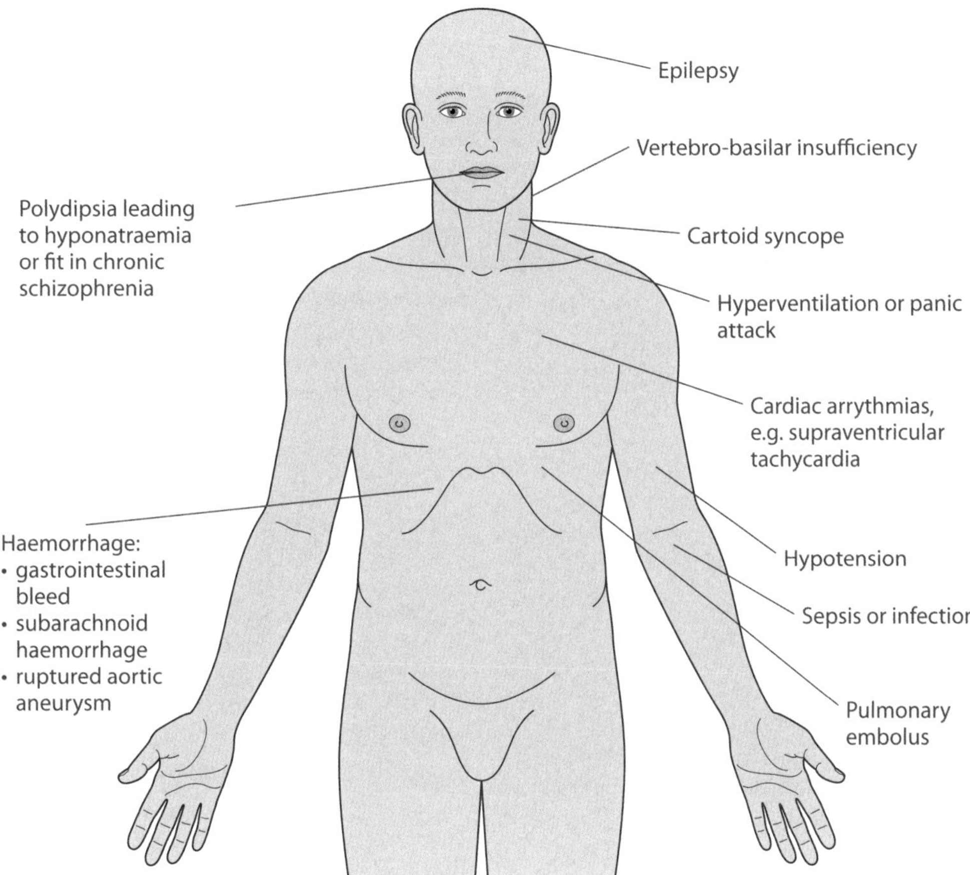

Fig. 31.5 Differential diagnosis of collapse.

- haemorrhage – ectopic pregnancy, ruptured aortic aneurysm, gastrointestinal bleed, subarachnoid haemorrhage
- pulmonary embolus
- polydipsia leading to hyponatraemia (e.g. in chronic schizophrenia).

Simple faint

A simple faint is often precipitated by warm settings, prolonged standing, stress, large meals, starvation, or alcohol. Light-headedness, sweatiness, nausea and visual disturbance are common preceding symptoms. Twitching movements may occur if the patient is kept upright and they may be mistaken for a seizure.

Cardiac cause

Pallor and sweating may be present and recovery is often rapid with no post-ictal phase. Ascertain whether there is any history of chest pain, palpitations or similar episodes. Collapse on exertion is of concern.

Seizures

Usually no warning signs occur, but there can be a cry or shout, followed by tonic–clonic movements. Tongue-biting, incontinence and frothing at the mouth suggest a generalised seizure. Patients tend to have post-ictal confusion and drowsiness. (Differentiation between faints and seizures, see Box 14.1, p. 176.)

Initial management of the collapsed patient

Assess using the ABCDE approach. Initiate oxygen if the patient has collapsed in a hospital department.

History

Determine what the patient was doing at the time of collapse and whether there was a loss of consciousness. Gather information about previous similar episodes, medical history and medications, and enquire about preceding symptoms such as chest pain, palpitations, dizziness or breathlessness.

Examination

Perform a full systemic examination. In particular, look for tongue-biting, evidence of incontinence, focal neurology, and injuries sustained at the time of collapse (e.g. to hip, spine or head).

Investigations

Investigations should include basic observations (including postural blood pressures), ECG, blood glucose, FBC, U&E and other tests if specifically indicated. If infection is suspected as a precipitant, search for a focus and perform urinalysis and a chest X-ray. Perform a pregnancy test in women of child-bearing age (i.e. 11–60 years).

Decide who needs referral or follow-up

If the patient has had a full recovery with a normal examination and investigations, then admission and referral are unlikely to be required.

If there are persisting symptoms, abnormal examination or investigations, or worrying features (e.g. heart failure, structural heart disease, coronary heart disease or family history of sudden death), then patients should be referred for admission under the medical team.

The unconscious patient

Any unconscious patient needs immediate referral to the emergency department or medical on-call team.

While awaiting assistance, a rapid assessment should be performed and treatment may need to be initiated before the diagnosis is known.

Common causes of unconsciousness include:

- hypoglycaemia
- drug overdose
- head injury
- stroke
- subarachnoid haemorrhage
- convulsions
- alcohol intoxication

Other causes to consider are respiratory, cardiac, renal or hepatic failure, arrhythmias, haemorrhage, anaphylaxis, sepsis, hypo- or hyperthermia, diabetic ketoacidosis/hyperosmolar hyperglycaemic non-ketotic coma (DKA/HONK) and psychogenic coma (Box 31.5).

Initial management

Assess the patient following the ABCDE approach.

Ensure that the airway is protected, the blood glucose level is checked, and give intravenous thiamine (Pabrinex®) if you suspect the patient is an alcoholic or is malnourished (although note that Pabrinex® occasionally may cause anaphylaxis) (see Chapter 22).

Collateral history

Establish how and where the patient was found, preceding complaints, the possibility of self-harm or trauma, medical history (including overdose and self-harm), medications and recreational drug use. Obtain medical or general practitioner's notes.

Examination

A full systemic examination is warranted. Look for illness, localising signs, injury or deliberate self-harm. Check wallet, clothes and medic alerts for additional information about identity and medical history.

Look for clues as to cause of the unconsciousness (Table 31.6).

Box 31.5 Psychogenic coma

The patient pretends to be unconscious. Suspect psychogenic coma if observations are within the normal range, eyelashes flicker when touched, or if the patient's hand avoids impact when dropped above their face. Note that all other causes must be actively excluded before this diagnosis is made.

Investigations

Investigations should include: blood glucose, FBC, U&E, clotting, paracetamol and salicylate levels if suspected overdose, ECG, ABG, chest X-ray (infection, aspiration, trauma, tumour, oedema?) and a CT scan of the head (infarct, bleed, infection, tumour?).

Table 31.6 Clues to cause of unconsciousness episode

Difficulty	Possible causes
Tachypnoea	Poisoning, pneumonia/sepsis, diabetic ketoacidosis, obstructed airway
Bradypnoea	Poisoning, raised intracranial pressure
Bradycardia	Hypoxia, beta-blocker/digoxin poisoning, complete heart block
Tachycardia	Hypoxia, supraventricular/ventricular tachycardia, sepsis
Atrial fibrillation	Can cause cerebral infarct
Small pupils and bradypnoea	Opioid overdose
Dilated pupils	Tricyclic overdose
Hypothermia	Can cause coma

The fitting patient

Common causes of fits are:

- epilepsy
- head injury
- hypoglycaemia
- alcohol withdrawal
- brain tumour
- infection
- cerebral infarction
- haemorrhage
- hypoxia
- toxins.

Seizure management

If the patient is actively fitting and unconscious, seizures need to be terminated as soon as possible (Table 31.7) to reduce the risk of cerebral damage.

Table 31.7 Algorithm for the fitting patient

Time frame	What to do
0–5 minutes	ABCDE approach. Give high-flow oxygen, protect the airway (e.g nasopharyngeal airway) and monitor oxygen saturations, heart rate and blood pressure
	Establish intravenous access
	Check blood glucose: administer 50 ml of 50% dextrose if hypoglycaemic
	If ≥ 20 weeks pregnant, give magnesium sulphate 4 mg intravenously over 10 min
	Give slow intravenous thiamine (Pabrinex®) if you suspect alcoholism or malnourishment
5–20 minutes	Call for help – 999, 'crash team' (2222), or medical on-call team
	Give lorazepam 4 mg intravenously (diazepam 5 mg intravenously, if lorazepam is unavailable)
	Repeat lorazepam 4 mg intravenously (or diazepam) if still fitting after 5–10 min
	Obtain ABG and save blood for FBC, U&E, glucose, calcium, liver function tests, cultures, and drug levels if overdose is suspected
20–40 minutes	Commence phenytoin infusion (15 mg/kg in 0.9% saline intravenously at 50 mg/min) with ECG monitoring, or phenobarbital sodium* (10 mg/kg at not more than 100 mg/min, maximum dose 1 g)
	Call anaesthetist
40–60 minutes	General anaesthetic and transfer to intensive-care unit

ABG, arterial blood gas; FBC, full blood count; U&E, urea and electrolytes.
*Avoid in hepatic impairment. If IV access is unavailable, can give rectal diazepam or buccal midazolam (see p. 179).

Post-seizure management

Examine for injuries relating to the seizure (e.g. head injury). For patients who are known to have fits, if the seizure is short, self-limiting and like their usual seizures, there is no need for admission if the patient has fully recovered. They can be looked after by a responsible adult and followed up by their general practitioner.

When to refer

Patients with a 'first fit' should be seen by the medical on-call team, even if they have fully recovered, so that a full assessment and blood tests can be done. In those who are known to fit, if the seizure is prolonged the patient will need transfer to an emergency department, or referral to the medical on-call team for a full assessment of aetiology.

Patients who have seizures should not drive (or do other activities which could result in their or others' death or disability if they have a seizure while doing those activities). It is their responsibility to inform the Driver and Vehicle Licensing Agency (DVLA); if they do not, seek advice from the DVLA website (www.dvla.gov.uk).

Suspected stroke

A stroke, or cerebrovascular accident (CVA), or similar neurological symptoms lasting less than 24 hours (transient ischaemic attack, TIA) is characterised by the acute onset of a focal neurological abnormality. The cause is either cerebral infarction (80%) or cerebral haemorrhage (20%).

Management was well publicised in the media through a campaign on the need to act 'FAST' (www.nhs.uk/Actfast/Pages/stroke.aspx). The 'FAST' approach helps to speed recognition of stroke (Table 31.8).

Patients who have had a stroke are now considered for thrombolytic treatment, by the stroke thrombolysis team, if they arrive at the emergency department within 3 hours of the symptom onset and meet the criteria – obviously the quicker they arrive, the better their outcome is likely to be.

Differential diagnoses for stroke include:

- hypoglycaemia
- Todd's paresis

Table 31.8 The 'FAST' approach to recognition of stroke

Assess	Points to note
Face	Has the patient's face fallen on one side? Can they smile?
Arms	Can they raise both arms and keep them there?
Speech	Is their speech slurred?
Time	Time to call 999 if you see any single one of these signs

Any patient with a focal neurological deficit will need immediate transfer to the emergency department or referral to the medical on-call team. If you have facilities to hand, give oxygen while waiting for the ambulance crew.

- hemiplegic migraine
- meningitis or encephalitis
- Bell's palsy
- brain abscess
- head injury
- tumour.

See Table 31A for the ABCD2 scoring system for the assessment of the short-term risk of stroke following a transient ischaemic attack (TIA).

Emergency complications of psychiatric medications

All medications have side-effects and risks, and psychiatric medications are no different. Some common reactions and their acute management are outlined below. For information on the diagnosis and treatment of cardiac arrhythmias secondary to antipsychotic medication, see Chapter 12.

Antipsychotics

Extrapyramidal symptoms (or acute dystonic reactions) – for example facial spasm, torticollis and limb stiffness – are common with a number of antipsychotics, such as haloperidol and phenothiazines, although other medications can also cause these reactions. Symptoms can be delayed by up to a week.

Treat with 5 mg intravenous or intramuscular procyclidine, repeated after 10 minutes if no relief is apparent. Patients may need 5 mg tablets three times a day for a number of days if symptoms recur. Prescriptions should be reviewed and, if possible, alterations made to limit future reactions.

Neuroleptic malignant syndrome may occur in patients taking antipsychotics. Clinical features include: fever, muscular rigidity, tachycardia, variations in blood pressure and altered consciousness. As this is a potentially fatal condition, it is advisable to discontinue antipsychotic medication immediately. Test for a raised white-cell count and raised creatinine phosphokinase (CPK) levels. Assess whether to call for medical assistance to treat circulatory, respiratory and renal disorders. Treatment is with intravenous dantrolene.

Clozapine

Three per cent of patients taking clozapine develop agranulocytosis and are at risk of developing life-threatening sepsis. Regular blood tests should be performed as part of routine monitoring.

If a patient on clozapine develops a fever, sore throat or any other sign of infection, a full blood count must be done to assess neutrophil count. If neutropenic, the patient should be referred to the medical on-call team for consideration of intravenous antibiotics.

Monoamine oxidase inhibitors (MAOIs)

These drugs inhibit the metabolism of serotonin, noradrenaline, tyramine and other amines. Their effects can last for 2 weeks after being stopped.

There is a risk of sudden hypertensive reactions with amine-rich foods (e.g. red wine, cheese, Marmite) or other medications (e.g. L-dopa, amphetamine). Hypertension and tachycardia are triggered by the release of noradrenaline and can cause intracerebral haemorrhage.

Measure heart rate and blood pressure if you suspect this and refer to the medical on-call team.

Lithium

Nausea, vomiting, confusion and cerebellar signs should make you suspect lithium toxicity. Other medications can trigger lithium toxicity, notably diuretics, anticonvulsants, selective serotonin reuptake inhibitors (SSRIs) and calcium channel blockers.

Examine for tremor, twitching, slurred speech, drowsiness and coma. Take blood for Lithium levels (check you use the correct tube for your local laboratory), and U&E. Refer to the medical on-call team.

Selective serotonin reuptake inhibitors

Serotonin syndrome mostly occurs when a patient starts or increases the dose of SSRIs and may occur when two medications that increase serotonin levels are taken, such as tryptans and SSRIs. Clinical features include agitation, fever, sweating, vomiting, diarrhoea, altered consciousness, poor coordination, tremor, myoclonus, hyper-reflexia, tachycardia and labile blood pressure. Hallucinations can also occur.

As serotonin syndrome is potentially fatal, the SSRI should be immediately discontinued. Exclude infection, neuroleptic malignant syndrome and drug toxicity from illicit drugs (e.g. cocaine). Take blood for blood cultures, FBC, U&E, thyroid function, CPK and drug toxicology. Treat symptoms and physiological changes, for example with benzodiazepines, ventilation, intravenous fluids and muscle relaxants. Refer to the medical on-call team as necessary.

When SSRIs are discontinued, monitor for relapse of depression and increase in suicide risk.

Further information

The *British National Formulary* and the associated website are useful sources of information (http://bnf.org/bnf), as are the Toxbase drug database (www.toxbase.org) and the *Maudsley Prescribing Guidelines.*[17] In addition, you should know the number of your dispensing pharmacist.

Acute red eye

Patients can develop an acute red eye with no history of trauma. Common causes are conjunctivitis, acute iritis and anterior uveitis, acute closed-angle glaucoma and subconjunctival haemorrhage.

Assessment must include visual acuity (ideally using a Snellen chart), and pupil size and reactivity. Patients must be urgently referred to an ophthalmologist if there is:

- any suspicion of reduced visual acuity
- any pupillary abnormality
- a corneal abnormality.

Differential diagnoses for the acutely red eye are discussed further below, along with presenting features and management.

Conjunctivitis

Conjunctivitis can be allergic, viral, bacterial or chemical in origin. Patients often complain of a sensation of foreign body in one or both eyes. The conjunctiva is red and lid swelling may be present. Pupils and visual acuity are normal. Viral and allergic conjunctivitis have a watery discharge. A sticky discharge suggests a bacterial cause.

Management

Use antibiotic drops or ointment (e.g. chloramphenicol or fusidic acid) for 5 days. Careful hygiene is required to prevent spread to others or to the unaffected eye. Symptoms should improve in 4 days.

Acute iritis (acute uveitis)

This recurrent, relapsing condition affects the young and middle-aged. Patients present with pain, reduced vision, watery discharge and 'floaters'. It is associated with sarcoidosis, ulcerative colitis, AIDs and ankylosing spondylitis. Examination findings include: reduced acuity, small pupil (may be irregularly shaped), photophobia and a tender eye (when palpated through the eyelid).

Management

Refer to an ophthalmologist urgently. Steroid eye drops, investigation and follow-up will be required.

Acute closed-angle glaucoma

This occurs in long-sighted middle-aged and elderly patients and may be precipitated by pupil dilation at night (or in the dark) or by anticholinergic drugs. The patient presents with severe pain, headache, nausea or vomiting and reduced visual acuity. Examination reveals a semi-dilated oval shaped pupil with a hazy swollen cornea. The eye feels tender and firm when palpated.

Management

Refer to an ophthalmologist urgently and provide analgesia.

Other causes of red eye

Subconjunctival haemorrhage is a painless haemorrhage over the sclera. If otherwise well, with no history of recent head injury or bleeding disorder and normal blood pressure, then the patient can have general practitioner follow-up. The haemorrhage may take several weeks to resolve.

External hordeolum (stye) is a bacterial infection of the base of the eyelash. Advise hot compresses, antibiotic ointment or drops. No referral is required.

Orbital cellulitis is swelling and erythema of the skin around the eye, associated with fever. Patients should be urgently referred to an ophthalmologist.

Chest pain

A thorough history, examination and ECG will frequently enable an accurate diagnosis of chest pain to be made.

The differential diagnoses are:

- cardiac – myocardial infarction, angina, aortic dissection, pericarditis
- gastrointestinal – gastro-oesophageal reflux, peptic ulcer, oesophageal spasm, pancreatitis
- pulmonary – pulmonary embolism, pneumonia, pneumothorax
- musculoskeletal – rib fracture, muscle spasm, costochondritis
- diabetic ketoacidosis
- psychological.

Initial management

Assess the patient using the ABCDE approach, and aim to exclude any immediately life-threatening causes such as tension pneumothorax.

The history should cover:

- character of pain (site, radiation, nature, severity, onset, duration, alleviating or exacerbating factors)
- associated symptoms (cough, haemoptysis, breathlessness, nausea, vomiting, palpitations)
- trauma to chest
- recent exertion
- previous similar episodes
- cardiac risk factors (hypertension, diabetes, smoking, hypercholesterolaemia, family history of heart disease).

The patient will need a full systemic examination, looking for:

- murmurs
- heart failure
- crackles
- bronchial breathing
- tenderness over the chest wall
- evidence of deep venous thrombosis.

> Musculoskeletal and psychogenic chest pain should be viewed as diagnoses of exclusion until more sinister causes have been excluded.

Investigations should include: basic observations; ECG; chest X-ray; ABG, FBC, U&E, D-dimer, and baseline and 12-hour troponin.

Myocardial infarction

This may be confirmed by ischaemic ECG changes: new-onset left bundle branch block (LBBB), ST elevation/depression, T-wave inversion.

If chest pain is cardiac-sounding in nature, worse or lasting longer than the patient's usual angina, or if ECG changes are present, contact the emergency services or the on-call medical team. Administer:

- high-flow oxygen
- glyceryl trinitrate spray (if systolic blood pressure is >90 mmHg)
- 300 mg chewable/crushed/soluble aspirin
- analgesia as required (e.g. morphine).

Patients with myocardial infarction may be suitable for thrombolysis or primary coronary angioplasty.

Pulmonary embolism

Suspect pulmonary embolism if the patient has pleuritic chest pain, haemoptysis and significant dyspnoea (often of sudden onset). Arterial blood gas will show hypoxia but chest X-ray may be normal. Changes on ECG include: sinus tachycardia, S1Q3T3, RBBB (right bundle branch block), AF (atrial fibrillation). D-dimer can be used to exclude pulmonary embolism in those thought to be at low risk of pulmonary embolism, but cannot be used to exclude pulmonary embolism in those who are at moderate to high risk.

If pulmonary embolism is suspected, refer the patient to the medical on-call team as definitive diagnosis requires further imaging with CT, pulmonary angiography or V/Q (ventillation perfusion) scan. If the patient is unstable, or massive pulmonary embolism is suspected, contact the emergency services or hospital 'crash team'. Massive pulmonary embolism may precede cardiac arrest.

Initiate treatment with high-flow oxygen to maintain saturations and administer a therapeutic dose of low-molecular-weight heparin (use with caution for patients with severe renal failure). In massive pulmonary embolism, aggressive fluid resuscitation may be required to maintain adequate right ventricular filling pressure.

Further investigations should include consideration of risk factors: immobility, malignancy and coagulation disorders. Chest pain is also discussed in Chapter 12.

Sepsis

Sepsis is a reaction to infection and ranges from minor signs and symptoms through to multiple organ dysfunction. Mortality is high, rising from 25–30% in severe sepsis to 40–70% in septic shock[18] and is directly correlated with the number of failed organs and time to treatment.

Sepsis is also discussed in Chapters 23 and 28.

Diagnosis

A high clinical index of suspicion, rapid diagnosis, and early, aggressive treatment are vital for improving outcome. Signs include: fevers and rigors, tachycardia, tachypnoea, flushing and warm, vasodilated peripheries.

Sepsis progression is indicated in Fig. 31.6.

Systemic inflammatory response syndrome

Suspect sepsis in anyone who meets the criteria for systemic inflammatory response syndrome (SIRS):

- body temperature ≥38°C or ≤36°C
- heart rate ≥90 beats/min
- respiratory rate ≥20/min or $PaCO_2$ < 4.3 kPa
- white blood count ≥12 000/ml or ≤4000 cells/ml, or ≤10% bands (immature neutrophils).

Sepsis

Sepsis is defined as suspected or known infection with at least two of the criteria for systemic inflammatory response (SIRS) met.

Severe sepsis

Sepsis is 'severe' when there are signs of organ dysfunction:

- hypotension with systolic blood pressure <90 mmHg
- altered mental state
- hyperglycaemia in the absence of diabetes
- hypoxaemia (SpO_2 < 93% or PaO_2 < 9 kPa)
- oliguria (urine output < 0.5 ml/kg/h)
- coagulopathy (international normalised ratio > 1.5 or platelets < 100)
- raised serum lactate (> 2 mmol/l).

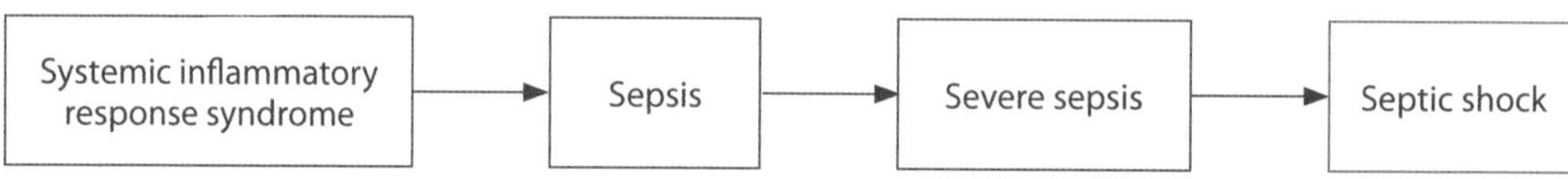

Fig. 31.6 Sepsis progression.

Septic shock

This is sepsis with hypotension unresponsive to a rapid fluid challenge of between 500 ml and 2 litres.

Initial management

Use the ABCDE approach to assessment.

Check the patient's history for clues as to the source of infection: respiratory, gastrointestinal, urinary tract, skin, bone or neurological symptoms.

A full systemic examination should be performed – respiratory, cardiovascular, abdominal, neurological, ears, throat and skin.

Investigations should include FBC, U&E, liver function tests, C-reactive protein, blood cultures (three sets if the patient's temperature is > 38°C) and urinalysis (ideally from mid-stream urine) for microscopy and culture. Also consider chest X-ray and stool cultures.

If sepsis is suspected, the patient should be referred to the medical on-call team or emergency department for assessment and management.

However, the following should be done as early as possible (and certainly within the first 6 hours) to improve outcome.

- Obtain cultures (blood, urine, etc.) before administering antibiotic therapy.
- Give broad-spectrum antibiotics as soon as possible after cultures are obtained (time to antibiotics should ideally be less than an hour). Choose the antibiotic agent according to the NHS trust protocol and suspected source.
- Measure serum lactate if the facilities (e.g. ABG machine) are available.
- Administer intravenous fluids if the patient is hypotensive, or if lactate levels are > 4 mmol/L. Give a fluid challenge of 20 ml/kg crystalloid.
- Maintain central venous saturations. Utilise high-flow oxygen if appropriate.

Common causes of in-patient sepsis include urinary and respiratory infections.

Further information

The website of the Surviving Sepsis Campaign is useful (www.survivingsepsis.org).

Acute urinary retention

Acute urinary retention presents with inability to pass urine associated with suprapubic pain. Pain is often spasmodic in nature and progressively worsens.

Common causes include:

- prostatic hyperplasia
- urethral stricture
- prolapsed intervertebral disc
- medication (tricyclics, antihistamines, anticholinergics, antihypertensives, alcohol, opioids)
- urethral stones or blood clots
- urinary tract infection, overfilling or severe constipation ('acute on chronic')
- pregnancy, particularly if associated with a retroverted uterus
- pelvic tumour
- genital herpes
- urethral rupture secondary to trauma
- multiple sclerosis.

Diagnosis

History

Enquire about symptoms of urinary infection, prostatic hypertrophy, spinal cord compression, previous urological complaints and medications.

Examination

The physical examination should have the following components:

- abdominal (uncomfortable, palpable bladder which is dull to percussion?)
- neurological (lower limb weakness or sensory loss?)
- rectal (reduced anal tone, loss of peri-anal sensation, or prostate hypertrophy?) (see Fig. 31.7).

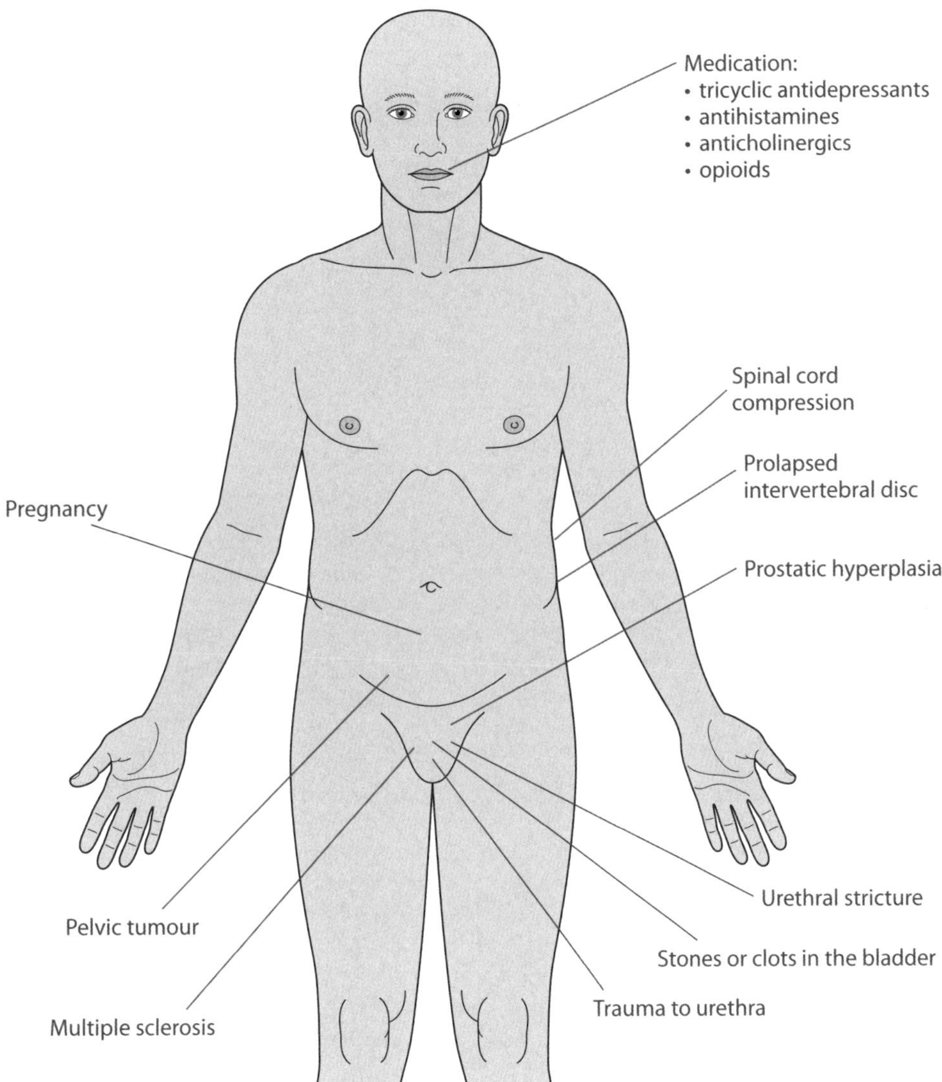

Fig. 31.7 Causes of acute urinary retention.

Investigations

A handheld bladder ultrasound scanner can be used to confirm retention. A large volume of urine in the bladder (over 400–500 ml) which cannot be voided is indicative of retention. Normal bladder capacity is 400–600 ml.

Initial management

If there is a high suspicion or evidence of cord compression (decreased anal tone or abnormal lower-limb neurology) (see pp. 295, 296), emergency services should be contacted immediately, or an urgent referral to neurosurgery or orthopaedics should be made if the patient is an in-patient.

- Provide analgesia.
- Attempt conservative measures to aid urination, such as privacy, running water or standing the patient up.
- If conservative treatment fails, insert a urethral Foley catheter to decompress the bladder.
- Measure the volume of urine retained.
- Perform a urine dip and send for culture if appropriate.
- Assess for the underlying cause.

- Refer to urology. Out-patient follow-up and investigation are likely to be required.

Contraindications to urethral catheterisation are evidence or suspicion of trauma (i.e. blood at the urethral meatus) and urethral stenosis.

Diarrhoea and vomiting

The most common cause of diarrhoea and vomiting is gastroenteritis. However, the differential diagnoses are wide and include: appendicitis, ulcerative colitis, constipation (overflow diarrhoea), rectal tumour, overdose and medication (antibiotics, laxative misuse).

History

Enquire about frequency, duration, consistency of stools and vomit, food ingested, contacts, foreign travel, systemic symptoms (abdominal pain, fever), weight loss, and medications.

Examination

Examine the patient's abdomen and assess their fluid status.

Investigations

Basic observations are required and blood tests if clinically indicated. Stool cultures should be obtained if the patient is in an institution, has a history of foreign travel, or if a bacterial or parasitic cause is suspected.

Treatment

If gastroenteritis is suspected, oral rehydration is the mainstay of treatment. Oral rehydration therapy (e.g. Dioralyte) is effective and well tolerated by most patients. Intravenous rehydration may be required if severe dehydration is present or if the patient is unable to tolerate oral fluids. Antibiotics may be required for some infectious causes. Consult local infectious disease guidelines.

In-patients with diarrhoea should be isolated until symptoms settle and hospital infection control should be informed.

Emergency equipment recommended for a psychiatry department

Psychiatrists would expect to have access within 3 minutes to adequate resuscitation equipment as this is the standard set by NICE guidance on the management of medical emergencies. Box 31.6 lists the emergency equipment that should be made available on various wards.

Box 31.6 Emergency equipment

Observation/monitoring equipment

- Blood pressure monitor, pulse oximeter, thermometer
- Blood glucose (BM) machine

Examination equipment

- Stethoscope, tongue depressor, pen torch, tendon hammer, auroscope, ophthalmoscope

Basic ward equipment

- ECG machine, large-bore cannulae, intravenous fluids, giving sets, needles, syringes, gauze, blood bottles, oxygen, oxygen masks, airway adjuncts, Foley catheter, steri-strips, wound glue, suture pack, wound dressings, cervical collar, sandbags and tape

Crash trolley (tailor contents to local National Health Service trust policy)

- Automated electronic defibrillator
- Emergency medications – adrenaline, atropine, adenosine, amiodarone, lidocaine, magnesium sulphate
- Airway equipment – oropharyngeal (Guedel) airway, nasopharyngeal airway, laryngeal mask airway, laryngoscope, endotracheal tube, oxygen masks and, if required, oxygen supply
- Intravenous access – cannulation equipment, intravenous fluids (crystalloid), sharps bin, syringes, blood bottles, needles, arterial blood gas (ABG) syringes (if access to an ABG analyser is available)

Summary

Medical emergencies occur at any time and anywhere. Having the confidence to deal with all emergencies is the realm of the expert, but members of the team should be able to manage those described here, even if this is restricted to recognising acute illness, carrying out an ABCDE rapid assessment and providing initial management pending the arrival of the emergency services, or alerting someone who can. All members of staff in contact with patients should have the ability and confidence to commence cardiopulmonary resuscitation and have the basic knowledge to start supportive treatment when a patient becomes acutely unwell.

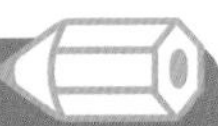

Learning points

- In a medical emergency, patient outcomes are significantly improved by rapid identification of life-threatening problems, first aid and initial treatment
- Analgesia should be considered early and given rapidly
- A Glasgow Coma Score ≤8 or an AVPU rating of P or U indicates that the patient may not be able to protect their airway
- The website TOXBASE contains useful advice on the toxicity of ingested substances (www.toxbase.org)
- Clinically important brain injury must be excluded before signs or symptoms are attributed to drugs or alcohol
- Refer a collapsed patient to the medical on-call team when there are persistent symptoms, abnormalities on physical examination or investigations, or other worrying features
- Patients with a 'first fit' should be referred to the medical 'on-call' team, even if they have recovered
- In suspected stroke, use the FAST system to speed recognition
- After TIA, use the $ABCD^2$ system to identify patients with an early risk of stroke
- Following myocardial infarction, arrange immediate transfer to hospital for consideration for coronary angioplasty to restore coronary artery flow
- Common causes of in-patient sepsis include urinary tract and respiratory infections
- In-patients with diarrhoea should be isolated until symptoms settle and infection should be reported to the infection control team

References

1 Rees JE, Mann C. Use of the patient at risk scores in the emergency department: a preliminary study. *Emerg Med J* 2004; **21**: 698–9.

2 Resuscitation Council (UK). *Advanced Life Support,* 6th edn. Resuscitation Council (UK), 2011.

3 Sampson HA, Muñoz-Furlong A, Campbell RL, *et al.* Second Symposium on the Definition and Management of Anaphylaxis: Summary Report. *Ann Emerg Med* 2006; **47**: 373–80.

4 Estelle F, Simons R. Anaphylaxis: recent advances in assessment and treatment. *J Allergy Clin Immunol* 2009; **124**: 625–36.

5 Doshi D, Foex B, Body R, *et al. Guideline for the Management of Acute Allergic Reaction: Guidelines for Emergency Medicine Network.* College of Emergency Medicine, 2009.

6 Working Group of the Resuscitation Council (UK). *Emergency Treatment of Anaphylactic Reactions.* Guidelines for Healthcare Providers. Resuscitation Council (UK), 2008 (http://www.resus.org.uk/pages/reaction.pdf).

7 Gunnell D, Bennewith O, Hawton K, *et al.* The epidemiology and prevention of suicide by hanging: a systematic review. *Int J Epidemiol* 2005; **34**: 433–42.

8 Vander KL, Wolfe R. The emergency department management of near-hanging victims. *J Emerg Med* 1994; **12**: 285–92.

9 Salim A, Martin M, Sangthong B, *et al.* Near-hanging injuries: a 10-year experience. *Injury* 2006; **37**: 435–9.

10 Wyatt J, Illingworth R, Graham C, et al. *Oxford Handbook of Emergency Medicine*, 3rd edn. Oxford University Press, 2006.

11 Wraight WM, Belcher HJCR, Critchley HD. Deliberate self-harm by insertion of foreign bodies into the forearm. *J Plast Reconstr Aesthet Surg* 2008; **61**: 700–3.

12 Vale JA, Bradberry SM, Bateman DN. Poisoning by drugs and chemicals. In *Oxford Textbook of Medicine*, 5th edn (eds DA Warrell, TM Cox, JD Firth): 1271–323. Oxford University Press, 2010.

13 Wyatt JP, Illingworth RN, Graham CA, *et al. Oxford Handbook of Emergency Medicine*, 4th edn, revised. Oxford University Press, 2012.

14 Stiell IG, Wells GA, Vandemheen KL, *et al.* The Canadian C-spine rule for radiography in alert and stable trauma patients. *JAMA* 2001; **286**: 1841–8.

15 National Institute for Health and Clinical Excellence. *Head Injury: Triage, Assessment, Investigation and Early Management of Head Injury in Infants, Children and Adults.* Clinical Guideline CG56. NICE, 2007.

16 Cross WW, Swiontkowski MF. Treatment principles in the management of open fractures. *Indian J Orthop* 2008; **42**: 377–86.

17 Taylor D, Paton C, Kapur S. *Maudsley Prescribing Guidelines*, 10th edn. Taylor and Francis, 2010.

18 Lever A, Mackenzie I. Sepsis: definition, epidemiology, and diagnosis. *BMJ* 2007; **355**: 879–83.

19 Johnston SC, Rothwell PM, Nguyen-Huynh MN, *et al.* Validation and refinement of scores to predict very early stroke risk after transient ischaemic attack. *Lancet* 2007; **369**: 283–92.

20 National Institute for Health and Clinical Excellence. *Stroke: Diagnosis and Initial Management of Acute Stroke and Transient Ischaemic Attack (TIA).* NICE, 2008.

Appendix

Table 31A Transient ischaemic attack (TIA) – ABCD^2 scoring system to evaluate the risk of stroke 2 days later

Each item scores 1 point	Score	Each item scores 2 points	Score
A Patient aged ≥60 years	1		
B Blood pressure ≥140/90 mmHg	1		
C Speech disturbance and no weakness	1	Unilateral weakness	2
D1 Duration of symptoms 10–59 minutes	1	Duration >60 minutes	2
Duration of symptoms <10 minutes	0		
D2 Diagnosed with diabetes	1		
Sum scores from both columns to give total:			

The risk of having a stroke 2 days after a TIA varies with the total number of ABCD^2 points: 0–3 low risk (1%), 4–5 moderate risk (4%), 6–7 high risk (8%).[19] **Patients with an ABCD^2 score ≥4 or a score of ≤3 but who have had two TIAs in one week are 'high risk' and should be started on aspirin 300 mg and referred for immediate specialist assessment and consideration of cerebral imaging.**[20] Patients with an ABCD^2 score of ≤3 should receive specialist assessment within 1 week. If vascular territory or pathology is uncertain, urgent brain imaging should be arranged independent of the ABCD^2 score.[20]

Partly adapted from: National Institute for Health and Clinical Excellence, 2008.[20]

32

Minor injuries

Murad El-Salamani

This chapter describes minor injuries to the head, face, chest, upper limb (including the hand) and lower limb. Illustrations are used to highlight key features of the injuries and their management. The author recommends that an expert opinion be sought if there is any doubt about whether an injury is minor or if treatment by a specialist is needed.

Introduction

This chapter is not intended to be a comprehensive account of minor trauma. The aim is rather to help a healthcare provider to deal with the commonest types of minor injuries. If, after assessment, you have any concerns that an apparently minor injury may be more serious, you should refer the patient immediately to the nearest emergency department for more comprehensive and expert assessment.

Minor head injury

Trauma to the head causing no or brief loss of consciousness with or without a short period of amnesia and no more than one episode of vomiting is usually followed by full recovery. Examination should include as a minimum:

- the Glasgow Coma Scale (GCS) (see Chapter 4, Box 4.4, p. 36)
- neck examination
- pupils reaction to light and accommodation (note that although pupil dilatation with sluggish reaction is a sign of severe head injury, it can occur unilaterally in the absence of serious head injury, due to direct trauma occurring in close proximity of the eye)
- cranial nerve examination
- motor tone, power and reflexes compared on both sides.

Note that an X-ray of the skull is rarely required. Start the examination with a review of eye opening, verbal responses to questions and motor function, and document the outcome using the GCS. Document the score according to the response demonstrated. For example, E3 V3 M5. Keep a record of the score, so that any deterioration (or improvement) can be easily identified.

A more serious head injury warrants a computerised tomography (CT) brain scan to determine whether there has been internal compromise to brain function. If so, the patient should be immediately transferred to the nearest emergency department.

The patient may need a CT brain scan when:[1]

- the GCS score is less than 13 on initial assessment in the emergency department
- the GCS score is less than 15 at 2 hours after injury on assessment in the emergency department

- there is a suspected open or depressed skull fracture
- there is any sign of basal skull fracture (haemotympanum, 'panda' eyes, and cerebrospinal fluid leakage from the ear or nose, or bruising over the mastoid – Battle's sign).
- the patient has a post-traumatic seizure
- the patient has a focal neurological deficit
- there is more than one episode of vomiting
- the patient has amnesia for events more than 30 minutes before the injury.

There are specific circumstances when an urgent CT scan is warranted:

- loss of consciousness or amnesia at any time after the injury (adults)
- when the patient is over 65 years of age
- where there is coagulopathy (history of bleeding, clotting disorder, current treatment with warfarin)
- there was a dangerous mechanism of injury (e.g. a pedestrian or cyclist struck by a motor vehicle, an occupant ejected from a motor vehicle, or a fall from a height of greater than 1 m or five stairs).

Facial injuries

Injuries to the face occur for a variety of reasons, but more frequent causes are road traffic accidents, assaults and accidental falls. Injuries include wounds and fractures of the nasal bone, mandible, orbital bones and cheek bone (zygoma). Associated neck injuries are not uncommon.

Wounds on the face

The following wounds should be referred to an appropriate specialist.

- Wound in the medial corner in the lower lid (Fig. 32.1a) may involve the lachrymal drainage system, resulting in overflow of tears (epiphora) (Fig. 32.1b). Refer to an ophthalmic surgeon.
- When the wound crosses the margin of the lid (Fig. 32.1a) the edges should be closed with sutures and perfectly approximated, otherwise a gap is created in the margin when the eye lids are shut, causing epiphora.

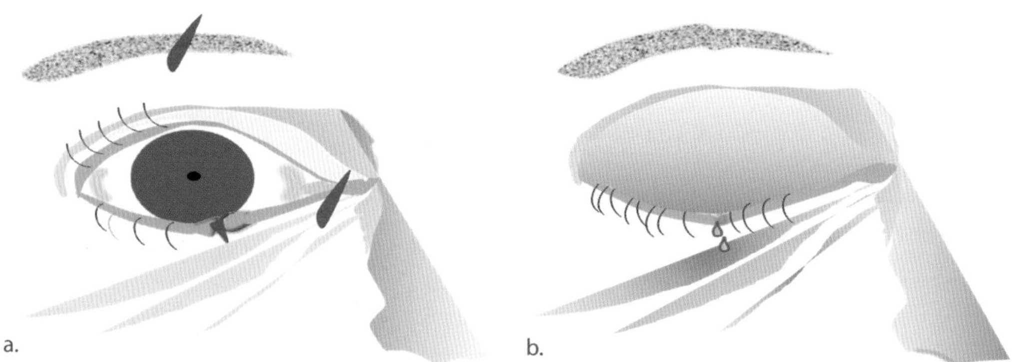

Fig 32.1 Eye wounds. a. Eye wounds involving the medial angle of the eye, wounds crossing the margin of the lids and eyebrow. b. Complications of inappropriate closure of wounds.

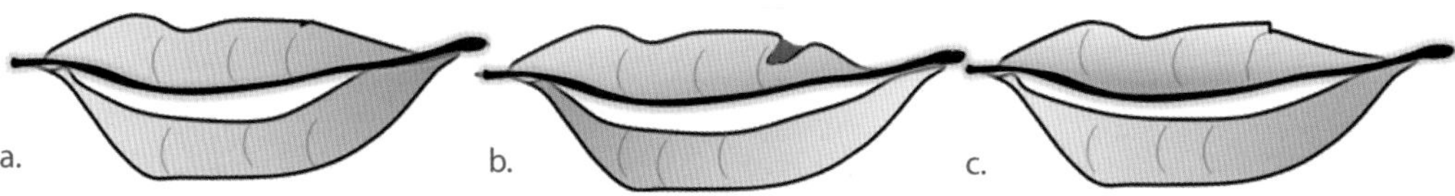

Fig. 32.2 Mouth wound. a. Before injury, b. After injury, c. Improper repair.

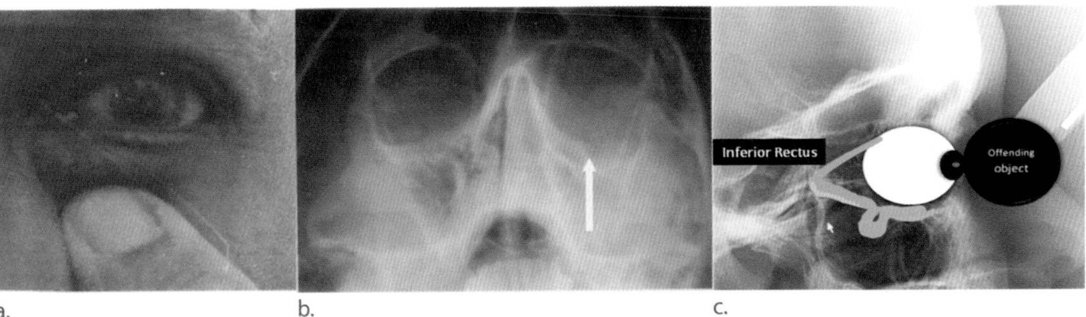

a. b. c.

Fig. 32.3 Eye wound. a. Palpation of the lower orbital margin. b. X-ray showing a step in the lower orbital margin. c. Blow-out fracture.

- Wounds crossing the eyebrow (Fig. 32.1a) or the lip margin (Fig. 32.2b,c) will heal with a disfiguring scar if not accurately approximated. Refer to a plastic surgeon.

Nasal bone injury

Nose bleeds (epistaxis) are common after nasal bone injury; they usually stop spontaneously and rarely need packing. Look for the following:

- *Deformity*. This is usually obvious in the first few hours before the swelling and is easy to correct by simple manipulation. No anaesthesia required. It helps if the patient is given a mirror to see the deformity. The patient usually asks for the manipulation and is grateful to see the result.
- *Late presentation*. Swelling will be well established, so refer to an ear, nose and throat (ENT) surgeon.
- *Septal haematoma* appears as a bulge on both sides of the septum, causing obstruction of the passages; this requires *immediate* referral to the ENT surgeon.

An X-ray of the nasal bone is not required.

Orbital, peri-orbital and mid-face injuries

These may include orbital floor fracture. Look for:

- *Double vision (diplopia)*. This may be due simply to the peri-orbital swelling. In the absence of a fracture no treatment is needed.
- *Facial paraesthesia on the upper lip and upper teeth and gum*. This may be due to transient nerve damage to the infra-orbital nerve (neuropraxia). In the absence of a displaced fracture, the initial treatment is conservative.
- *A 'step' on the lower orbital margin on palpation*. Comparison with the other orbit is helpful to diagnose the fracture.
- *Restricted eye movements, in particular upward gaze compared with the movements of the other eye*. This indicates a blow-out fracture of the floor of the orbit with entrapment of the inferior rectus muscle. This occurs owing to the offending object causing increased intra-ocular pressure. In this case, X-ray of the facial bones may show a 'teardrop' in the maxillary sinus (Fig. 32.3a,b,c). If so, urgent referral to the maxillo-facial surgeon is needed.

Injury to the cheek bone (zygoma)

This presents with tenderness of the zygomatic arch. Look for deformity (which may be obvious) and restricted mandibular movements.

X-rays of the zygoma *and* facial bones are required to confirm or exclude a fracture of the zygoma (Fig. 32.4).

Injuries to the mandible

You should assume that bleeding from the gum indicates a fracture in the mandible until proven otherwise. Look for:

- *dislocation of the temporomandibular joint (TMJ)* – this is associated with malocclusion and dribbling of saliva
- *loss of tongue control* – this indicates instability of the fracture and requires urgent referral to a maxillo-facial unit; note that most mandibular fractures are stable.

Manipulation of the TMJ will require sedation of the patient.

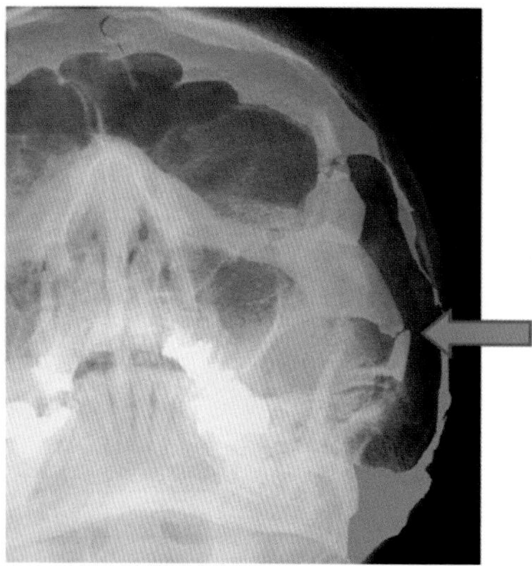

Fig. 32.4 Fracture of the left zygoma.

Antibiotic cover is required for fractures associated with wounds of the gum.

Chest injury

This may present as a minor injury but is usually very painful. Look for the following.

- *Restricted breathing.* This can lead to serious complications, including pneumonia and pulmonary embolism. It requires immediate transfer to the emergency department.
- *Any disturbance of cardiac rhythm.* This suggests cardiac contusion. Monitor cardiac rhythm and arrange immediate transfer to the emergency department.
- *Signs of respiratory distress.* These include:
  - increased breathing rate or respiratory effort, such as using an accessory muscle of respiration, neck muscles, flared nostrils, abdominal muscles
  - surgical emphysema, indicated by crepitus (a 'crinkling sensation') when palpating neck and chest
  - decreased breath sounds
  - severe pain not controlled by simple analgesia, which can lead to respiratory distress and failure.

Any sign of respiratory distress warrants immediate transfer to the emergency department.

Injury to the circumflex branch of the axillary nerve may occur in shoulder dislocation and with a fractured neck of the humerus. It causes deltoid muscle weakness, detected by loss of sensation on the tip of the shoulder.

The treatment for simple chest contusion is analgesia, such as co-codamol and non-steroidal anti-inflammatory drugs (NSAIDs), prescribed as regular doses until the breathing effort returns to normal.

Injuries to the upper limb

Shoulder injuries

Look for evidence of dislocation:

- Compare the contours of the shoulders on the normal and injured sides – an anterior dislocation may have a depression in the affected shoulder but a posterior dislocation may look normal.
- On the dislocated side, the hand cannot be placed on the uninjured shoulder.

Reducing a shoulder dislocation needs analgesia and adequate muscle relaxation (such as intravenous midazolam).

Fractured humerus

This usually occurs at the surgical neck of the bone.

Apply a 'collar and cuff' to allow the weight of the arm to reduce the fracture.

Rotator cuff sprain

Supraspinatus muscle injury restricts the first 20–30 degrees of abduction. Infraspinatus muscle injury restricts external rotation of the shoulder. Subscapularis muscle restricts adduction of the arm.

Fractured clavicle and dislocation of the acromio-clavicular joint

Treatment is conservative. Apply a broad arm sling, not a collar and cuff.

Fracture dislocation at the acromio-clavicular joint may require internal fixation. Refer to an orthopaedic surgeon.

In adults, a fracture of the head of the radius and in children a supracondylar fracture may not be seen on the initial X-ray. A joint effusion may be the only tell-tale sign. You should repeat the radiograph after 10 days, when a fracture may be more apparent.

Elbow injuries

Injuries to the elbow can occur by direct trauma or by falling on the outstretched hand. The most common injuries are sprains, fracture of the head of the radius and fracture of the olecranon process; in children, supracondylar fracture and avulsion fracture of the medial epicondyle are common.

In a normal elbow you can palpate a symmetrical triangle formed by the olecranon and the medial and lateral epicondyles (Fig. 32.5). The forearm moves in extension, flexion, pronation and supination. In the injured elbow, extension is the first movement to become restricted and is the last to recover. An inability to extend the elbow against resistance may occur with an olecranon fracture. Restricted supination indicates injury to the head of the radius.

Swelling, deformity and bruising are the usual signs of a fracture. Tenderness over the head of the radius commonly results from falling on an outstretched hand.

A painful lateral epicondyle (tennis elbow) can result from minor trauma.

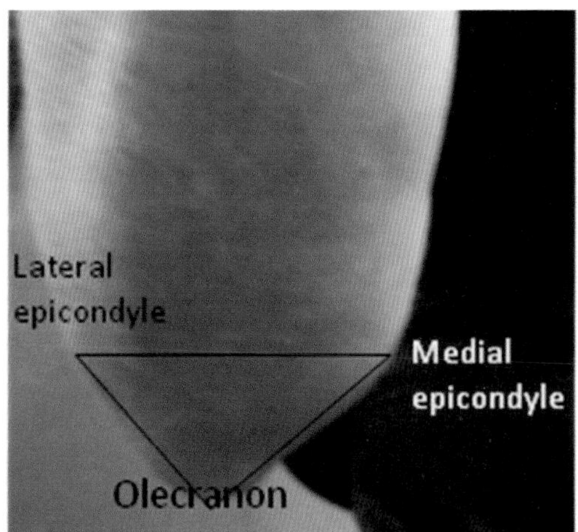

Fig. 32.5 Symmetrical triangle formed by the olecranon and the medial and lateral epicondyles.

Wrist injuries

Sprained wrist

Although very common, a sprained wrist is always difficult to diagnose without an X-ray, as there will always be bony tenderness. Even when only soft tissues are injured, differentiation between soft tissue and bone tenderness is hard.

Simple support is usually sufficient, but if the pain is severe, a splint or even a cast may be required.

Colles fracture

These injuries are common in people aged over 50; most are due to a slip and fall, usually backwards, on the dorsi-flexed hand with radial deviation in supination of the forearm. Look for a 'dinner fork deformity', which is usually the result of dorsal displacement of the radius (Fig. 32.6). Deformity over the ulnar styloid suggests a fracture. Manipulation may be required, depending on the degree of displacement and the age/general condition of the patient.

Smith fracture

This is mostly seen in a younger age group and is often incurred by a fall forwards onto the outstretched hand while running. The hand becomes static on the ground while the momentum carries the forearm dorsally. Look for anterior displacement of the hand on the radius. On an X-ray, a Smith fracture is a mirror image of a Colles fracture.

Hand injuries

Hand injuries lead to a disproportionate number of negligence cases. Early referral to the hand surgeon is recommended whenever nerve or tendon injury is suspected.

If the wound is on the dorsum of the hand, ensure there has been no nerve or tendon injury. Then treat as you would any skin wound.

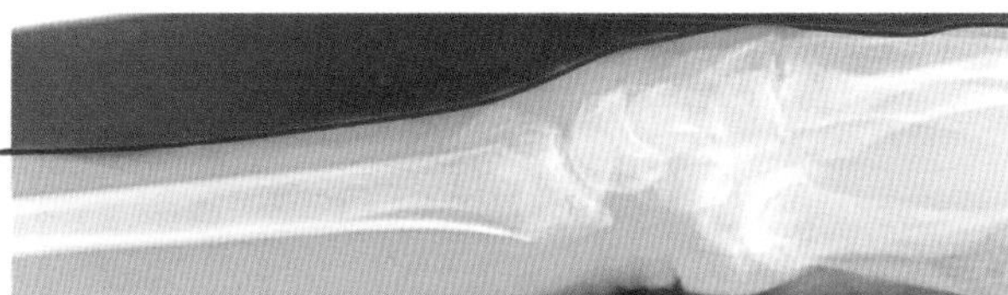

Fig. 32.6 Colles fracture.

If the wound is on the palm of the hand, nerve and tendon injuries must similarly be excluded.

Wounds caused by blunt trauma are usually followed by marked swelling and should not be closed. Dressing only should be applied.

Scaphoid injury

There is usually a history of falling on the outstretched hand. Look for:

- tenderness in the anatomical snuffbox
- tenderness on the scaphoid tubercle
- pain on axial thumb compression
- pain on pronation with ulnar deviation of the wrist.

If more than one of the above is present, request an X-ray for scaphoid fracture (Fig. 32.7). Apply firm support to the wrist and hand. If the fracture is confirmed, a scaphoid cast must be applied until the patient is seen by an orthopaedic surgeon.

Triquetral injury (a common hand bone injury)

This typically occurs following hyperextension or hyperflexion of the wrist. Look for tenderness on the dorsum of the hand over the triquetral bone. On an X-ray (Fig. 32.8), a small chipped fracture may be seen dorsally on the lateral projection only.

Metacarpal fractures

These injuries are usually obvious on simple inspection.

In fractures involving the metacarpal neck, look for the following:

- *Displacement or angulation of the neck of the index and middle metacarpals.* If either is present, refer the patient for manipulation.
- *Angulation of the ring and little metacarpals.* Up to 70 degrees of angulation is acceptable, as the metacarpals' mobility will compensate for the deformity. Treatment is aimed at making the patient comfortable. Support the metacarpal in a wool and crêpe bandage or plaster of Paris.
- *Fracture shaft of the metacarpal.* This requires immobilisation in a cast in an acceptable position as the fracture is usually unstable. Refer the patient to orthopaedics.

Injury to the thumb

Sprain of the metacarpo-phalangeal joint

Sprain of the metacarpo-phalangeal joint (MCPJ) is extremely painful and recovers very slowly. X-rays are always needed to exclude a fracture. Support in a bandage or splint is usually required.

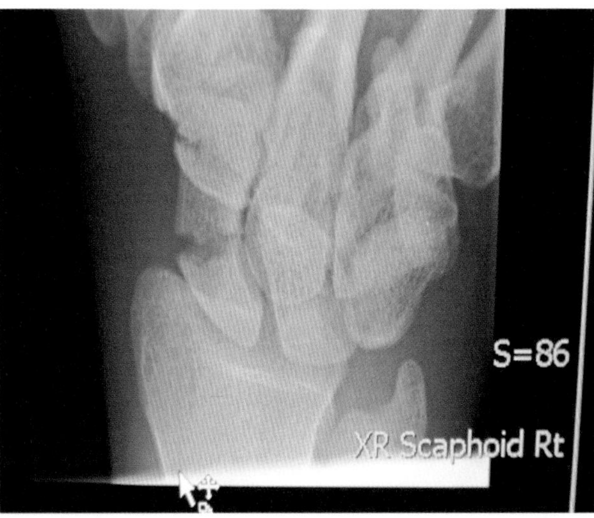

Fig. 32.7 Scaphoid fracture.

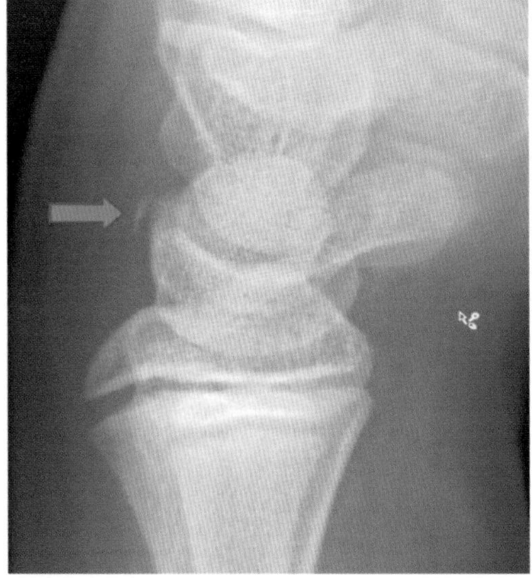

Fig. 32.8 Triquetral fracture

Games keeper's thumb

This is a rupture of the ulnar collateral ligament at the MCPJ. Look for abnormal thumb abduction – with the joint flexed, the injured thumb abducts to a wider angle than the uninjured thumb. This may follow hyperabduction injury or ligamentous rupture. Refer the patient to an orthopaedic surgeon for support in a cast or repair.

Bennett fracture

This is a fracture of the base of the metacarpal (Fig. 32.9) due to either striking a solid object (such as a skull or wall) or a fall onto the thumb. It is nearly always accompanied by subluxation or dislocation of the thumb. Look for:

- instability of the carpo-metacarpal joint of the thumb
- pain and weakness of the pinch grasp
- pain, swelling and bruising around the base of the thumb and over the carpo-metacarpal joint of the thumb.

Treatment is manipulation with immobilisation in a cast or internal fixation. Referral to an orthopaedic surgeon is essential as the thumb is important for many hand functions.

Injury to the fingers

Look for rotational deformity. Ask the patient to make a fist; the fingers should all point to the scaphoid and the nails should all be facing dorsally. If not, there may be a fracture (Fig. 32.10).

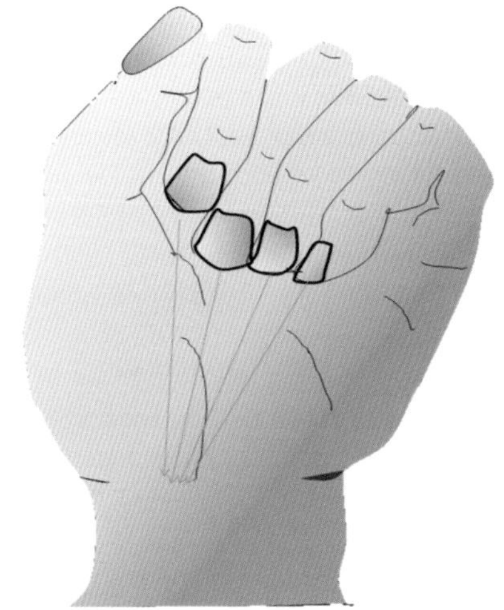

Fig. 32.10 Fingers' direction on making a fist.

An undisplaced fracture can be treated by strapping the injured finger to the neighbouring finger. A displaced fracture can be manipulated under digital block and treated in neighbour strapping.

If the finger is painful and appears crooked, swollen, or is bent at a strange angle and cannot be bent or straightened, the injury is most likely a dislocation. Ensure there is no nerve injury before giving anaesthesia and reduction by manipulation. Always assess the

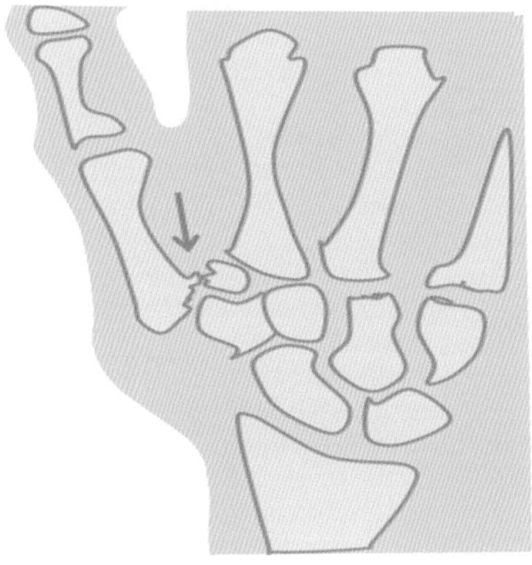

Fig. 32.9 Bennett fracture.

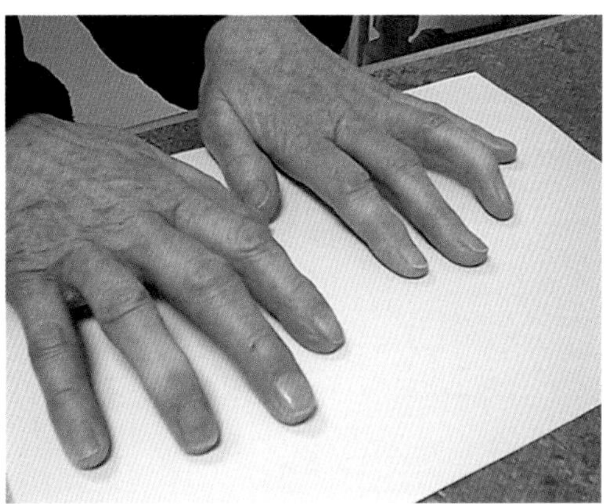

Fig. 32.11 Bilateral mallet deformity of the ring fingers.

integrity of the tendons and the collateral ligaments afterwards.

A mallet deformity is due to a hyperflexion injury to the distal interphalangeal joint of a finger leading to rupture of the extensor tendon (Fig. 32.11). This may be accompanied by an avulsion fracture at the base of the distal phalanx. In this case it is a painful injury. Whether or not a fracture exists the treatment is by a mallet splint.

Wounds to the distal phalanx

Linear wounds are painful and bleed profusely. They are treated by steri-strips and simple dressings.

Partial amputation of the tip of distal phalanx

If bone is exposed, refer the patient to the orthopaedic team for bone trimming to allow closure without tension.

If bone is not exposed, options are simple dressing until healing or by 'V–Y' advancement flap (Fig. 32.12).

If the amputated part of the finger is found it should not be discarded but wrapped in gauze, put in a plastic bag, and the bag put in ice, and sent with the patient, as it can be used as a graft (Fig. 32.13).

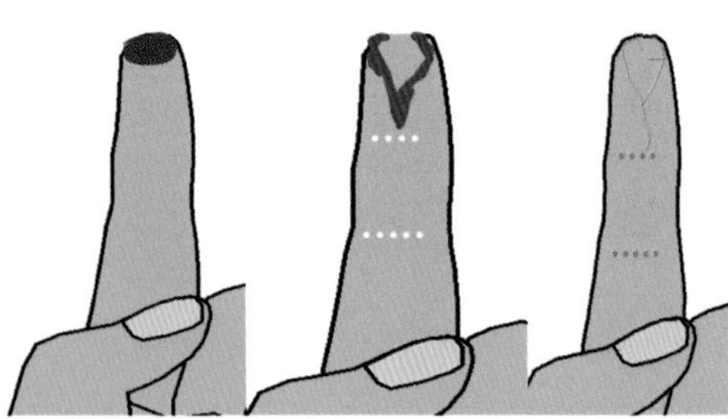

Fig 32.12 V–Y plasty.

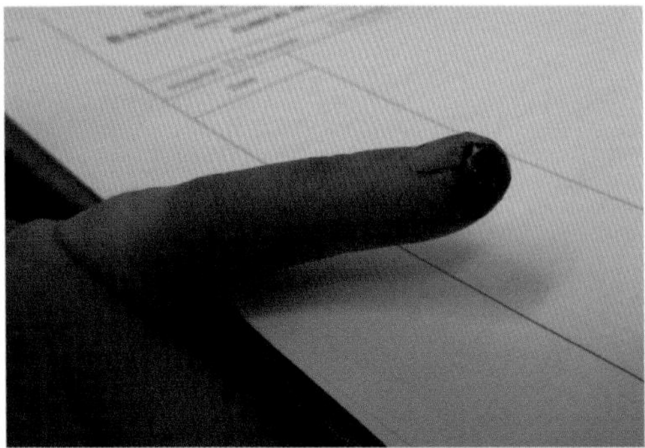

Fig. 32.13 Appearance of skin 2 weeks after it was grafted. Patient had normal tip after 6 weeks..

Pulp fat loss from the terminal phalanx

On a finger (not necessarily on a thumb), this will require amputation of the phalanx.

Wounds to the dorsal surface of the proximal phalanx

These need exploration for tendon injury. Examination alone cannot exclude middle slip rupture of the extensor expansion, which may present later with Buttonnière deformity.

Examination for flexor tendon injury

- *Flexor digitorum superficialis (FDST).* This inserts into the base of the distal phalanx. Immobilise the proximal interphalangeal joint and ask the patient to flex the distal phalanx.
- *Flexor digitorum profundus (FDPT).* This is inserted more distally. Immobilise all uninjured fingers in full extension of the distal interphalangeal joint and ask the patient to flex the finger.

In 75% of patients the FDST is immobilised and the patient can only use the FDPT.

Injuries to the lower limb

Knee injuries

In the acute stage a firm diagnosis can be very difficult to reach. The intention at this stage is to exclude serious injury that requires immediate referral to an orthopaedic surgeon.

If the patient is able to raise the leg straight, this will exclude rupture of the patellar tendon and more serious internal injuries.

If effusion occurs within the first 4–6 hours, the injury is likely to be a haemarthrosis, which is associated with a more serious injury, such as fracture or rupture of the cruciate ligaments.

According to the Ottawa rules,[2] an X-ray is required for knee injury only with any of these findings:

- patient is aged 55 or more
- isolated tenderness of the patella
- tenderness at the head of the fibula
- inability to flex to 90 degrees
- inability to bear weight, both immediately and in the emergency department (patients are asked to take four steps to test whether they are able to transfer weight twice onto each lower limb regardless of limping).

Ankle sprain

The most common injury encountered is the inversion type, when the sole of the foot is facing towards the opposite ankle at the time of injury. It can cause sprain of the lateral ligament, especially the weakest part (the anterior talofibular ligament) and a traction fracture of the base of the fifth metatarsal.

Eversion injury may cause a fracture of the medial malleolus (because the medial ligament is stronger) and may be associated with fracture of the fibula proximally.

Always examine the foot, leg, knee and the Achilles tendon. Achilles tendon injury is diagnosed by the classical history of a sensation of a thumb in the back of the ankle and examination by palpation for a gap in the tendon and Simmonds' test (squeezing the calf should produce passive plantar flexion of the foot in an intact tendon).

An ankle X-ray is required only if there is any pain and bruising in the malleolar zone and either of these findings (Fig. 32.14):

- bone tenderness on the malleolus when it is palpated on its posterior surface (Fig. 32.15)
- inability to bear weight both immediately and in the emergency room.

A foot X-ray is required if there is any pain in the mid-foot zone and any of these findings:

- bony tenderness on the navicular (Fig. 32.16)
- bony tenderness on the base of fifth metatarsal (Fig. 32.17)
- inability to bear weight both immediately and in the emergency department.

Treatment of the sprained ankle consists of support bandage, elevation and cold compression. Exercise should be encouraged.

Fracture of the tip of the lateral malleolus

Fracture of the tip of the lateral malleolus below the syndosmosis can be treated as a sprain, depending on the severity of symptoms.

Toe injuries

Big toe

Fracture with involvement of the first metatarsal-phalangeal joint requires referral to the orthopaedic team as this fracture can later be complicated with hallux rigidus.

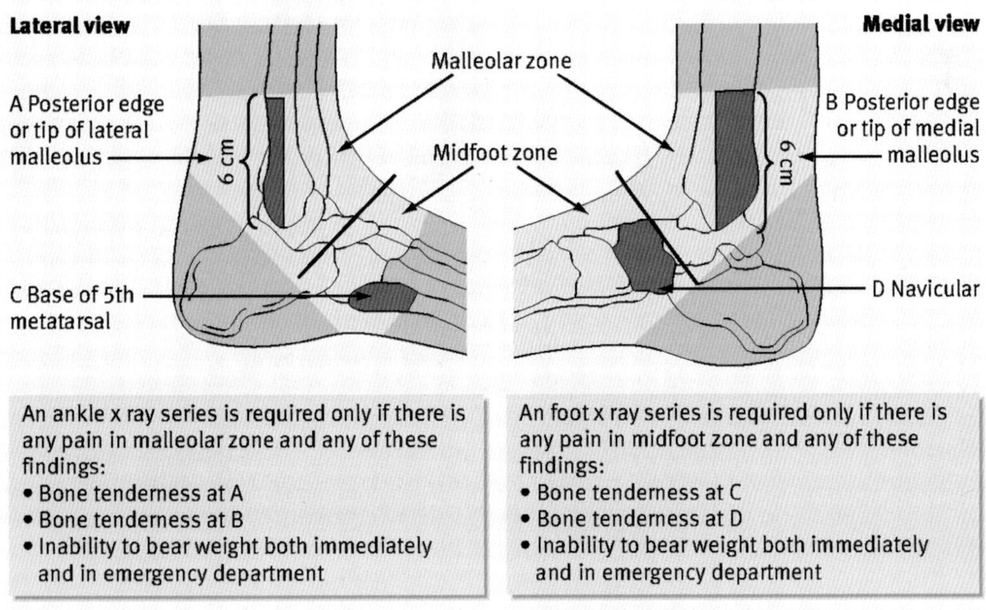

Fig. 32.14 Ottawa ankle rules. Source: Bachmann *et al*, 2009.[3] Reproduced with permission.

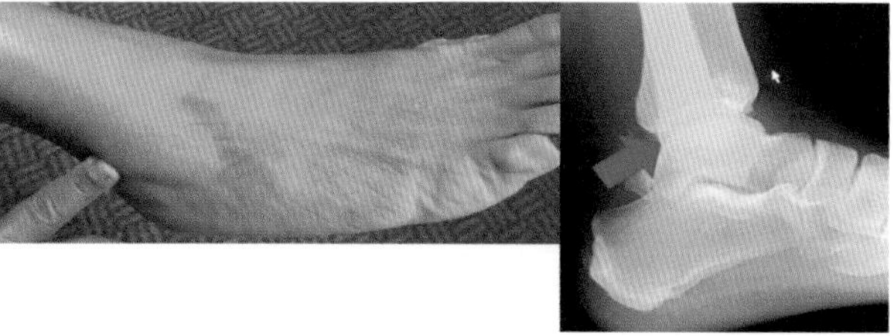

Fig 32.15 Palpation of lateral malleolus.

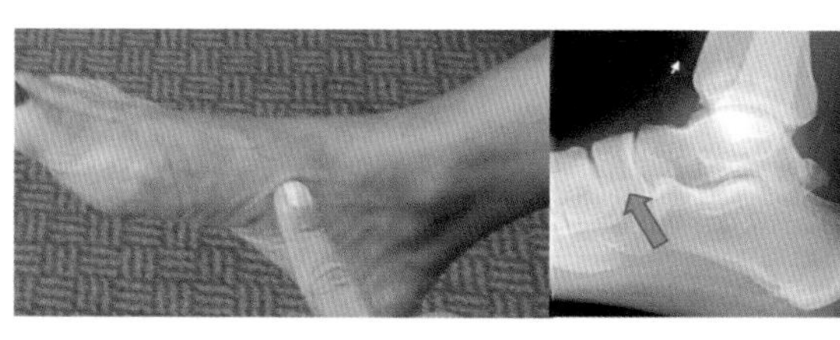

Fig. 32.16 Palpation of the navicular.

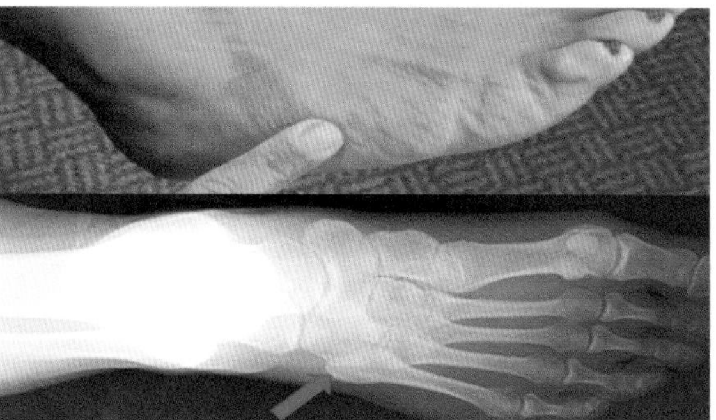

Fig. 32.17 Palpation of the base of 5th metatarsal.

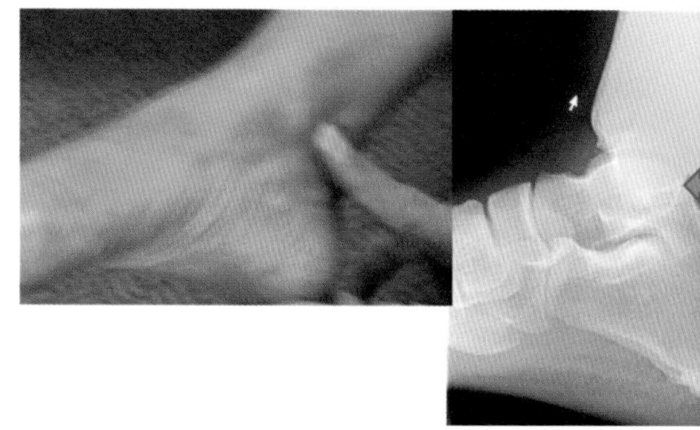

Fig 32.18 Palpation of the medial malleolus.

Other toes (fracture or dislocation)

Unless associated with a deformity interfering with the ability of the patient to wear a shoe (Fig. 32.19) the treatment involves strapping the toe to its healthy neighbour until pain settles. X-rays are not usually required. When there is such deformity (Fig. 32.19) X-ray, manipulation and reduction will be needed.

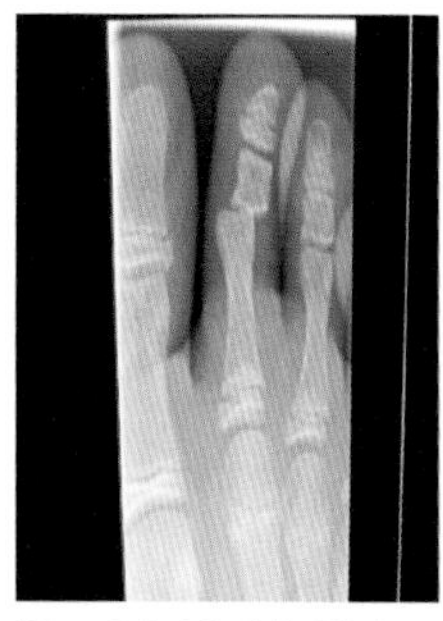

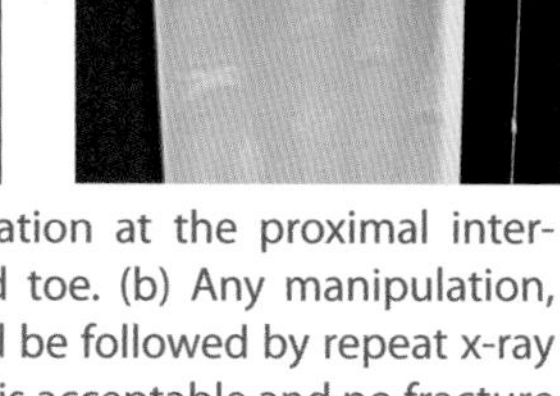

Fig. 32.19 (a) Dislocation at the proximal interphalangeal joint, 2nd toe. (b) Any manipulation, even if simple, should be followed by repeat x-ray to check the position is acceptable and no fracture occurred during manipulation.

Summary

Minor injuries can worry both patients and staff, especially injuries that arise 'out of hours'. The information in this chapter should help staff to know how to assess and treat such injuries.

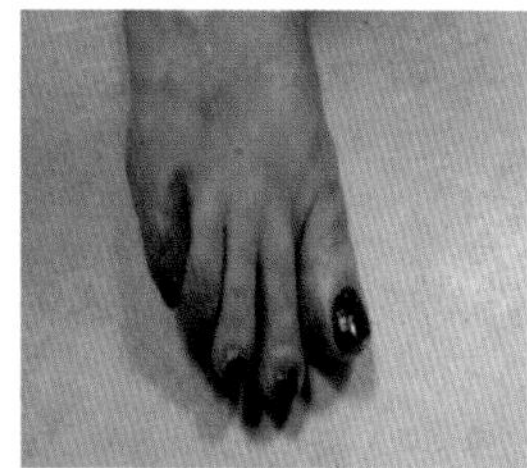

Fig. 32.20 Little toe fracture with no deformity.

References

1 National Institute for Health and Clinical Excellence. *Triage, Assessment, Investigation and Early Management of Head Injury in Infants, Children and Adults.* Clinical guideline CG56. NICE, 2007.

2 Stiell IG, Greenberg GH, Wells GA, *et al.* Prospective validation of a decision rule for the use of radiography in acute knee injuries. *JAMA* 1996; **275**: 611–5.

3 Bachmann LM, Kolb E, Koller MT, *et al.* Accuracy of Ottawa ankle rules to exclude fractures of the ankle and mid-foot; systematic review. *BMJ* 2009; **339**: b2901.

Recommended reading

Adams B, Depiesse F. Specific injuries by anatomic site: Ankle and foot injuries. In *IAAF Medical Manual* (http://www.iaaf.org/medical/manual/index.html).

Allonby-Neve CL, Okereke CD. Current management of facial wounds in UK accident and emergency departments. *Ann R Coll Surg Engl* 2006; **88**: 144–50.

Dincer D. *Injuries of the Hand and Wrist.* International Boxing Association, 2007 (www.aiba.org/documents/site1/Commissions/Medical/Hand%20and%20Wrist%20Injuries.pdf).

Fingertip injuries and amputations. OrthoInfo, 2011 (http://orthoinfo.aaos.org/topic.cfm?*topic*=A00014).

Gomersall C, Calcroft R. Chest injuries. ICU web, 1993 (www.aic.cuhk.edu.hk/web8/chest_injuries.htm).

Khan K, Bruker P. Ankle acute injuries. In *Encyclopaedia of Sports Medicine and Science* (ed TD Fahey), 1998 (www.sportsci.org/encyc/ankacuinj/ankacuinj.html).

Levy DB. Soft tissue knee injury. Medscape (http://emedicine.medscape.com/article/826792-overview).

Mancini MC. Blunt chest trauma. Medscape (http://emedicine.medscape.com/article/428723-overview).

Oussedik S, Jenabzadeh R. Chest wall injuries. Sports Injury Bulletin (www.sportsinjurybulletin.com/archive/chest-wall-injuries.htm).

Scottish Intercollegiate Guidelines Network. *Early Management of Patients with a Head Injury (A National Clinical Guideline 110).* SIGN, 2009.

Semer ND. Facial lacerations. In *Practical Plastic Surgery for Nonsurgeons*: 145–159. Hanley & Belfus, 2001.

Thoracic trauma. TRAUMA.ORG (www.trauma.org/archive/thoracic/CHESTintro.html).

Yates DW. The NICE head injury guidelines. *Emerg Med J* 2003; **20**: 117.

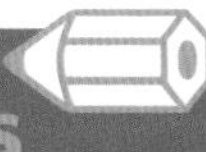

Learning points

- Minor injuries can occur at any time to anyone
- Be prepared to deal with minor injuries
- In head injury, assess using the Glasgow Coma Scale and don't forget to document the score
- Signs of potential major head injury include: more than momentary loss of consciousness, repeat vomiting, suspected skull fracture, seizure, declining Glasgow Coma Scale, more than 30 minutes of pre-trauma amnesia or focal neurological deficit.
- With facial injury, refer for assessment and accurate repair any wound that involves the inner corner of the lower eyelid, or crosses the eyebrow, lip margin or the margin of the lid.
- Refer any wound to the nose that causes a bulge to the septum which obstructs the nasal passages
- Refer to a specialist when eye movements are restricted following a blow to the orbit or mid-face.
- Following chest trauma, signs of serious injury include difficulty breathing or respiratory distress, or cardiac rhythm abnormalities – immediate referral to hospital is necessary.
- Signs of a limb fracture may be subtle – look for swelling, deformity and bruising.
- Be aware that, to avoid potential litigation, early referral is to be recommended in suspected nerve or tendon damage.
- Follow the Ottawa rules after an ankle injury – this will avoid unnecessary X-ray.

Index

Compiled by Linda English

Page numbers in *italics* refer to figures, tables and boxes